Infectious Causes of Cancer

Infectious Disease

SERIES EDITOR: *Vassil St. Georgiev*

Infectious Causes of Cancer

Targets for Intervention

Edited by

James J. Goedert, MD

Viral Epidemiology Branch, National Cancer Institute
Rockville, MD

Humana Press ❄ Totowa, New Jersey

This publication is printed on acid-free paper. ∞
ANSI Z39.48-1984 (American Standards Institute) Permanence of Paper for Printed Library Materials.

Cover design by Patricia F. Cleary.

Cover photos from: Figs. 3 and 8 of Chapter 10, *Kaposi's Sarcoma and Other HHV-8-Associated Tumors*, by Chris Boshoff.

Printed in the United States of America. 10 9 8 7 6 5 4 3 2 1

Library of Congress Cataloging in Publication Data

Infectious causes of cancer : targets for intervention / edited by James J. Goedert.
    p. ; cm. -- (Infectious disease)
  Includes bibliographical references and index.
  ISBN 0-89603-772-X (alk. paper)
    1. Microbial carcinogenesis. I. Goedert, James J. II.Infectious disease (Totowa, N.J.)
  [DNLM: 1. Neoplasms--etiology. 2. Helicobacter pylori--pathogenicity. 3. Oncogenic
  Viruses--pathogenicity. QZ 200 I4343 2000]
  RC268.57 .I5727 2000
  616.99'4071--dc21

                                                    99-057865

Preface

During his 1996 reelection campaign, Bill Clinton's slogan of "Building a Bridge to the 21st Century" was lampooned widely and became hackneyed. The need for more and better communication links among medical subspecialties, however, is undeniable as we enter the era of molecular medicine. Prior to the acquired immunodeficiency syndrome (AIDS) epidemic, professional communication between oncologists and infectious disease specialists was limited almost exclusively to consultations for neutropenic fever during cancer chemotherapy. AIDS patients required the broader expertise of oncologists, dermatologists, pathologists, pulmonologists, and infectious disease physicians, with the latter becoming primary caregivers during the decade between the discovery of human immunodeficiency virus (HIV) in 1984 and the development of combination antiviral chemotherapy in the 1990s. The spectacular efficacy of highly active antiretroviral therapy (HAART) against HIV and AIDS is a model likely to be repeated, as drugs are discovered not so much by their efficacy against an overt disease, but rather by their design to block specific molecules in critical pathways underlying the disease. *Infectious Causes of Cancer: Targets for Intervention* reviews neoplasms in which certain viruses, bacteria, and parasites play critical roles, anticipating that they will be likely targets for drugs or vaccines.

Cancers are the most thoroughly studied of a growing list of chronic diseases previously thought to be noninfectious. As such, they provide lessons that are likely to apply more broadly.

Lesson one is that the infection must be persistent or chronically active to play a role in a complex disease such as cancer. Putative "hit-and-run" mechanisms are likely an artifact of insensitive methods for detecting the infection. A corollary is that many infectious agents, such as Epstein–Barr virus (EBV), human papillomaviruses (HPVs), and *Helicobacter pylori* (*H. pylori*), much like neoplastic cells, have evolved ways to evade immune recognition. For some infections, the activity of the infection and the risk of the cancer is markedly increased by acquired or, rarely, congenital immune deficiency.

Lesson two is that the relationship between infection and cancer, like that between any single host gene and cancer, is never a simple cause-and-effect. Through interactions with the human host, most of the implicated infections are cofactors that indirectly increase the probability of critical genetic mutations. Age at infection and host immunogenetics often have a major influence on susceptibility to EBV-related Burkitt's lymphoma and nasopharyngeal carcinoma and to *H. pylori*-related gastric cancer (Chapters 5, 6, and 21, respectively). Because the odds of the critical genetic mutations are low, the corollary of this lesson is that most infected people do not develop cancer.

Lesson three is that the infection may not be necessary for the cancer phenotype. As classical examples, Burkitt's lymphoma and hepatocellular carcinoma do occur without EBV infection and hepatitis B or C virus (HBV, HCV) infections, respectively. This implies that pathways that affect the occurrence of genetic mutations and the resulting cancer are accessible by noninfectious mechanisms. These include spontaneous c-*myc*/immuno-globulin gene rearrangement of a pre-Burkitt's B lymphocyte; alcoholic hepatitis, cirrhosis, and precancerous clonal regeneration of the liver; and others. The exceptions are noteworthy, since squamous cell carcinoma of the cervix probably does not occur without a "high-risk" HPV infection, nor Kaposi's sarcoma without human herpesvirus type 8 (HHV-8) infection.

Lesson four is that a substantial part of the disease process and of the tumor tissue itself results from responses such as inflammation, lymphedema, sclerosis, and neovascularization that are ancillary to the cancer cell. Hodgkin's disease (Chapter 7) is a prototype, in which the cancerous, EBV-infected Reed–Sternberg cells are few and far between.

Lesson five is that cancer often can be prevented by preventing the infection or the immune deficiency that allows it to persist or reactivate. Likewise, remissions of the cancer often can be induced by successful early treatment of the infection or the underlying immune deficiency.

Lesson six is that "cancer" or "malignancy" can be difficult to define. Two examples resulting from uncontrolled EBV infection, fulminant X-linked lymphoproliferative disease and post-transplant lymphoproliferative disease, present and often must be treated as highly aggressive non-Hodgkin's lymphomas, irrespective of oligo-, poly-, or monoclonality. As nicely reviewed in Chapter 1, difficulties with basic definitions such as "cancer," "infection," "dissemination," and "spread" are not new to infectious disease oncology. The practicing physician already is familiar with "remission" and "cure," which are so difficult to define as to depend more upon consensus than certainty.

Infectious Causes of Cancer: Targets for Intervention is intended to serve as an introduction to infectious disease oncology for practitioners. It has only five overview chapters on the major human carcinogenic infections (herpesviruses, retroviruses, papillomaviruses, hepatitis viruses, and *H. pylori*). Most of the other chapters focus on specific neoplasms, often adding perspectives to the six aforementioned lessons. Each of the chapters—including the overviews, the specific neoplasms, and those that are more oriented to research frontiers—reviews the history and current status of its topic and provides a vision of the future in terms of prevention and treatment of the disease, the underlying infection, or both. The goal is to bridge the disciplines and not to present detailed recapitulations of virology, bacteriology, parasitology, and oncology, all of which are available elsewhere.

Mechanisms of Neoplasia: *Targets of Opportunity*

Oncogenic infections increase the risk of cancer through expression of their genes in the infected cells. Occasionally, these gene products have paracrine effects, leading to neoplasia in neighboring cells. More typically, it is the infected cells that become neoplastic. These viral, bacterial, and parasitic genes and their products are obvious candidates for pharmacologic interruption or immunologic mimicry, promising approaches for drugs or possibly vaccines.

Herpesviruses, especially EBV and, since its discovery in 1994, human herpesvirus 8 (HHV-8, also known as Kaposi's sarcoma-associated herpesvirus), are the most extensively studied and best characterized infections that cause cancer in humans (Chapters 2–10). They are relatively large DNA viruses with an approximately 140,000 basepair genome that codes for more than 80 genes, including those for building daughter virions during the "lytic" portion of their life cycle, as well as regulatory genes that enable the infection to persist in "latency" for prolonged periods. Several of the regulatory genes have human homologs that apparently were pirated by the virus during mammalian evolution and that probably contribute to its evolutionary survival and to human disease. As a rule, the DNA of EBV and HHV-8 does not integrate into the human genome. Rather, during "latency" the extrachromosomal ("episomal") herpes DNA is copied during mitosis, yielding progeny cells that are likewise latently infected with episomal herpes DNA. Uncontrolled proliferation of these latently infected progeny cells characterizes EBV- and HHV-8-associated neoplasms. Proliferation of both the EBV-associated lymphoproliferative diseases and of HHV-8-associated Kaposi's sarcoma seems to be highly sensitive to the severity of the cell-mediated immune deficiency that occurs with AIDS, with pharmacologic suppression of allograft rejection, and with the congenital X-linked lymphoproliferative disease originally described by Purtilo *(1) (see also,* Chapter 3*)*. In other neoplasms, such as endemic (African) Burkitt's lymphoma and nasopharyngeal carcinoma, EBV is able to evade immune recognition by masking or downregulating critical antigens.

Retroviruses and their lentivirus cousins are RNA viruses with a pathognomonic enzyme, reverse transcriptase, that enables them to make a DNA "provirus" copy of their genome and to integrate it permanently into the genome of the infected host cell. Rare cases of Non-Hodgkin's lymphoma (NHL) among persons with AIDS appear to result from activation of a protooncogene owing to upstream integration of HIV in macrophages (Chapter 13). However, the overwhelming way that HIV causes cancer is by destroying cellular immunity, thus dysregulating HHV-8 and leading to Kaposi's sarcoma (Chapter 10), dysregulating EBV, leading to some AIDS NHLs (Chapter 8), and perhaps other indirect and paracrine effects of dysregulated cytokines and growth factors. The effects of HIV on cellular immunity are not a major focus of this book. It should be noted, however, that there is clear, if incomplete, recovery of cellular immunity and reduction in risk of some cancers that occurs with interruption of the replication of HIV through drugs that interfere with reverse transcriptase and especially those specifically designed to interfere with the viral protease enzyme *(2)*. The prototype human retrovirus, human T-lymphotropic virus type I (HTLV-I), causes transformation of T lymphocytes and highly aggressive adult T-cell leukemia/lymphoma (ATL) through poorly characterized mechanisms that probably include transactivation of cellular genes controlling growth by HTLV-I's *tat* gene and possibly alteration of cellular immunity (Chapters 11 and 12). Anti-HIV drugs have little or no activity against HTLV-I, illustrating the specificity of each virus's reverse transcriptase and protease.

HPVs encompass more than 100 genotypes of small, related DNA viruses that have a strong tropism for epithelial cells. The major oncogenic agents for humans are HPV-16, HPV-18, and several others that are sexually transmitted and cause cancer of the cervix, penis, and anus (Chapters 14 and 15). HPV-16 and -18 appear to transform infected cells when their episomal circular genome is broken open and integrated into the host genome, allowing marked upregulation and expression of their E6 and E7 proteins. Unlike the E6 and E7 proteins of nononcogenic HPVs (such as type 1, which causes common warts), those of HPV-16 and -18 have strong affinity for the p53 and Rb pathways, respectively. Interference with both the p53 and the Rb pathways allows unregulated cell cycling and failure to undergo apoptosis (normal cellular senescence), increasing the likelihood of additional mutations. A possible role for HPVs in other squamous cell carcinomas, such as those of the skin and oropharynx, is uncertain, although the mechanisms appear to be the same (Chapter 16). HPV-16 virus-like particle and E6 recombinant protein vaccines are currently in clinical trials in hopes of reducing the major HPV diseases, cervical and anal cancers.

The two oncogenic hepatitis viruses, HBV and HCV, are phylogenetically unrelated but do share the ability to establish chronic active infection, inflammation (hepatitis), cell death, scarring (cirrhosis), and clonal, nodular regeneration of the liver (Chapters 17 and 18). Because this sequence appears to underlie virtually all cases of hepatocellular carcinoma, there should be several opportunities for intervention. Unfortunately, the mechanisms for this sequence of events are largely unknown. HBV, however, has been well studied and has the advantage of two natural animal models, the woodchuck and ground squirrel hepatitis viruses, both of which cause hepatocellular carcinoma in their respective species. HBV is a partially double-stranded DNA virus; it uses an RNA intermediate and a reverse transcriptase for its replication; and it can integrate into the host genome. The integration appears to drive the liver tumor in the animal models and may contribute directly to human hepatocellular carcinoma. HCV, an RNA virus that cannot integrate into the host genome, increases the risk of hepatocellular carcinoma indirectly. These primarily include the sequence of inflammation, cell death, scarring, and nodular regeneration with increased chance of a proneoplastic genetic mutation. The cancer risk increases with all insults to the liver, including HBV, HCV, alcoholism, and other hepatotoxins. Aflatoxin B1, a fungal contaminant of peanuts and other food staples in parts of Africa and China, is associated with a highly specific mutation of the *p53* cancer suppressor gene and greatly increases the risk of hepatocellular carcinoma among people with chronic HBV infection.

A similar sequence of inflammation, scarring, and regeneration, probably contributes to the development of squamous cell bladder cancer. This neoplasm, which is unusual in industrialized societies, is closely tied to heavy, chronic bladder infestation by *Schistosoma haematobium*, a helminthic parasite that infects some 200 million people in endemic regions of Africa (Chapter 24). The same may also be true for the reported association of cholangiocarcinoma with chronic infection by the liver flukes, *Opisthorchis viverrini* and *Clonorchis sinensis*, which are summarized in depth elsewhere *(3)*. Risk of cancer with these chronic parasitic infections may be increased or actually depend on vitamin deficiencies, polymorphisms in detoxification or activation enzymes of the human host, superinfection by bacteria, or several of these.

Chronic bacterial infections (and perhaps also chronic helminth and fluke infections) generate reactive oxygen species that, like aflatoxin B1, can be genotoxic and may contribute to the odds of mutation in a gene that increases neoplasia *(4)*. Such a mechanism is postulated specifically for the clear associations between *Salmonella typhi* and gallbladder cancer and between *H. pylori* and gastric cancer (Chapters 23 and 21, respectively). It should be noted that these infections generate relatively little inflammation and scarring and that, instead, they are associated with mucosal atrophy and a high risk of adenocarcinomas rather than squamous cell carcinomas. Identification of the mechanisms for these associations may not be immediately important, since these bacteria can be eradicated by antibiotics and, for *Salmonella typhi*, by cholecys-tectomy. However, these mechanisms could have broader implications for understand-ing and preventing or treating noninfectious adenocarcinomas.

Inability of the immune system to eradicate a chronic infection appears to underlie the association between *H. pylori* and B-cell non-Hodgkin's lymphoma of the mucosa-associated lymphoid tissue (MALT) of the stomach (Chapter 22). It seems that bacte-rial antigens are passaged and presented by the M cells (specialized epithelial cells) of the gut to Peyer's patches where B lymphocytes are recruited, activated, and circulated back to the mucosa where they are maintained by T-cell signaling. Regression can occur with either eradication of the *H. pylori* or with blockade of the T-cell signaling. A similar continuous feedback-loop mechanism has been postulated for the association of chronic HCV infection with type 2 mixed cryoglobulinemia and other B-cell disor-ders that may include NHL (Chapter 19).

The Infectious Disease Universe

The polymerase chain reaction (PCR) revolution led to a rapid discovery of novel viruses, bacteria, and parasites and to a recognition of our ignorance of how these organisms relate to human beings. At least two recently discovered viruses, the DNA transfusion-transmissible virus (TTV) and the RNA GB-virus C (also known as hepa-titis G virus), establish chronic, active infections in peripheral blood lymphocytes, but as yet have no known chronic disease *(5,6)*. Perhaps they are symbionts and cause no disease in humans. The discoveries of HCV, HHV-8, *Tropheryma whippelii* (the Whipple's disease bacterium), and *Bartonella henselae* (the agent of cat scratch dis-ease) parallel a growing body of literature supporting the association of chronic viral or bacterial infections with atherosclerosis, Alzheimer's disease, rheumatoid arthritis, type 1 diabetes mellitus, and other nonmalignant chronic diseases.

On the frontiers of this universe are cancers of high incidence, viruses of high preva-lence, and novel associations. Investigators are searching for homologs of mouse mam-mary tumor virus (MMTV) or interactions with endogenous retroviruses in human breast cancer (Chapter 27). One model posits that breast cancer is an MMTV zoonosis acquired from domestic mice *(7)*. Others are investigating simian virus 40 (SV40), which causes mesothelioma, osteosarcoma, and brain tumors when injected into new-born hamsters and which contaminated poliovirus vaccines administered to tens of millions of people from the mid-1950s to the early 1960s (Chapter 26). The human polyomaviruses, BK virus and JC virus, are related to SV40 and cause cystitis and progressive multifocal leukoencephalopathy, respectively, in immune-deficient patients. Discoveries are certain to come from these frontiers. As with explorations of the New World, however, they may not bring back the anticipated gold of definitive disease associations, but instead may provide fundamental insights to be exploited with unforeseen technologies.

James J. Goedert

REFERENCES

1. Purtilo DT, Yang JPS, Cassel CK, Harper R, Stephenson SR, Landing BH, Vawter GF. X-linked recessive progressive combined variable immunodeficiency (Duncan's disease). Lancet 1975; 1:935–941.
2. Centers for Disease Control Surveillance for AIDS-defining opportunistic illnesses, 1992-1997. Morbid Mortal Weekly Rep 1999; 48 (No. SS-2): 1–22.
3. Thamavit W, Shirai T, Ito N. Liver flukes and biliary cancer. In: Parsonnet J (ed.) Microbes and Malignancy: Infection as a Cause of Human Cancers. New York: Oxford University Press,1999, pp. 346–371.
4. Christen S, Hagan TM, Shigenaga MK, Ames BN. Chronic inflammation, mutation, and cancer. In: Parsonnet J (ed.) Microbes and Malignancy: Infection as a Cause of Human Cancers. New York: Oxford University Press,1999, pp. 35–88.
5. Nishizawa T, Okamoto H, Konishi K, et al. A novel DNA virus (TTV) associated with elevated transaminase levels in posttransfusion hepatitis of unknown etiology. Biochem Biophys Res Commun 1997; 241:92–97.
6. Linnen J, Wages J, Zhang-Keck ZY, Fry KE, et al. Molecular cloning and disease association of hepatitis G virus: a transfusion-transmissible agent. Science 1996; 271:505–508.
7. Stewart THM, Sage RD, Stewart AFR, Cameron DW. Breast cancer incidence highest in the range of one species of house mouse, *Mus domesticus*. Brit J Cancer 2000; 82:446–451.

Contents

Glossary of Abbreviations

3-Hydroxyanthranilic acid (3-OHAA)

Amino acid (aa)
α-Fetoprotein (α-FP or AFP)
AIDS Clinical Trials Group (ACTG)
Adult T-cell leukemia (ATL)
Antibody-dependent cellular cytotoxicity (ADCC)
Acute lymphoblastic leukemia (ALL)
Acquired Immunodeficiency Syndrome (AIDS)
Avian leukosis virus (ALV)
Anal squamous intraepithelial lesion (ASIL)

Baboon endogenous virus (BaEV)
N-Butyl-N-(4 hydroxybutyl) nitrosamine (BBN)
Basal cell carcinoma (BCC)
Basic fibroblast growth factor (bFGF)
Burkitt's lymphoma (BL)
Bovine leukemia virus (BLV)
BK virus (BKV)

Chemokine receptors (CCRs)
Cytotoxin-associated gene A (Cag)
Common B-cell acute lymphoblastic leukemia (cALL)
Computed axial tomography (CAT)
Covalently closed circular DNA (cccDNA)
Centrocyte-like cell (CCL)
Centers for Disease Control and Prevention (CDC)
Chronic lymphocytic leukemia (CLL)
Coding DNA (cDNA)
Colony forming units (cfu)
Cytomegalic inclusion disease (CID)
Cellular interference factor (CIF, including CIF-I and CIF-II)
Cervical intraepithelial neoplasia (CIN)
Carcinoma *in situ* (CIS)
Cell-mediated immunity (CMI)
Cytomegalovirus (CMV)
Central nervous system (CNS)
Complement C3d receptor (CD21)
Cyclooxygenase 2 (COX-2)

Complete remission (CR)
Core viral genes (C)
Cottontail rabbit papillomavirus (CRPV)
Cyclin-dependent kinases (CDKs)
Cyclin-dependent kinase inhibitors (CKI)
Cyclosporin A (CsA)
Cervical squamous intraepithelial lesion (CSIL)
CXC chemokine receptors (CXCRs)
Cytotoxic T lymphocytes (CTLs)

Duck hepatitis B virus (DhBV)
Diffuse large B-cell lymphoma (DLBCL)
Drosophila melanogaster Tenascin gene (TNM)

Early viral genes (E)
Early antigen (EA)
Early antigen-diffuse (EA-D)
Early antigen-restricted (EA-R)
Epstein–Barr nuclear antigen (EBNA, including EBNA1,2,3A,3B, and 3C)
Epstein–Barr encoded RNAs (EBERs)
Epstein–Barr virus receptor (CD21)
Epstein–Barr virus (EBV, including subtypes EBV1 and 2)
Epidermal growth factor receptor (EGFR)
Equine infectious anemia virus (EIAV)
Enzyme-linked immunosorbent assays (ELISAs)
Epidermodysplasia verruciformis (EV)
Etoposide (VP-16)

FLICE inhibitory protein (FLIP)
Fibrosing cholestatic hepatitis (FCH)
Fine needle aspiration (FNA)

Gastroesophageal junction (GE)
Gastric *Helicobacter*-like organisms (GHLO)
G-protein-coupled receptor (GPCR)
Geometric mean titer (GMT)
Granulocyte macrophage colony stimulating factor (GM-CSF)
Granulocyte colony stimulating factor (G-CSF)
Glycoprotein (gp)
Group antigen (gag)
Growth regulated oncogene alpha (Gro-α)
General Register Office for Scotland (GROS)
Ground squirrel hepatitis virus (GSHV)
Glutathione-S-transferase-μ (GSTM1)

Highly active antiretroviral therapy (HAART)
HTLV-associated myelopathy/ Tropical spastic paraparesis (HAM/TSP)
Hematopoietic stem cell transplantation (HSCT)
Hepatitis A virus (HAV)

Hepatitis B core antigen (HBcAg)
Hepatitis B e antigen (HBeAg)
Hepatitis B surface antigen (HBsAg)
Hepatitis B virus (HBV)
Hepatitis C virus (HCV)
Hepatocellular carcinoma (HCC)
Helicobacter pylori (*H. pylori*)
Hodgkin's Disease (HD)
Hodgkin Reed–Sternberg Cell (H-RS)
Human endogenous retrovirus (HERV)
Human endogenous retrovirus type K (HERV-K)
Human foamy virus (HFV)
Hepatitis G virus (HGV, also known as GB virus-C)
Human herpesvirus 6 (HHV-6)
Human herpesvirus 7 (HHV-7)
Human herpesvirus 8 (HHV-8)
Human immunodeficiency virus (HIV)
Human immunodeficiency virus type 1 (HIV-1)
Human leukocyte antigen (HLA)
Human papillomavirus (HPV)
Human retrovirus 5 (HRV-5)
High-grade squamous intraepithelial lesion (HSIL)
Herpes simplex virus 1 (HSV-1)
Herpes simplex virus 2 (HSV-2)
Human T-cell lymphotropic virus type I (HTLV-I)
Human T-cell lymphotropic virus type II (HTLV-II)
Hypervariable region (HVR)
Herpesvirus saimiri (HVS)
Humorally mediated hypercalcemia of malignancy (HHM)

Immediate early (IE)
Interferon (IFN)
Immunoglobulin (Ig)
Immunocytoma/ lymphoplasmacytic lymphoma (Ic)
Interleukin 2 (IL-2)
Interleukin 6 (IL-6)
Infectious mononucleosis (IM)
Immunoglobulin heavy chain variable region genes (V_H)
Inducible nitric oxide synthase (iNOS)
Interleukin (IL)
Inverse polymerase chain reaction (IPCR)
Interferon regulated factor (IRF)
Information and Statistics Division (ISD)
Intravenous drug use, intravenous drug user (IVDU)

JC virus (JCV)

Kaposi's sarcoma-associated herpesvirus (KSHV)

Late viral genes (L)
Leukocyte activated killer cells (LAK)
Latency associated transcript (LAT)
Live attenuated varicella vaccine (LAVV)
Lactate dehydrogenase (LDH)
Loop electrosurgical excision procedure (LEEP)
Latent membrane protein (LMP, including LMP1 and 2)
Leader protein (LP)
Lewis b histo-blood group antigen (Leb)
Lewis b-binding adhesin (BabA)
Lymphoepithelial lesion (LEL)
Leukocyte inhibitory factor (LIF)
Lymphocyte depleted Hodgkin's disease (LDHD)
Large loop excision of the T zone (LLETZ)
Lymphoctye predominant Hodgkin's disease (LPHD)
Lymphoma study group (LSG)
Low-grade squamous epithelial lesion (LSIL)
Long-terminal repeat (LTR)
Long unique coding region (LUR)

Macrophage colony stimulating factor (M-CSF)
Macrophage inhibitory proteins (MIPs)
Mycobacterium avium complex (MAC)
Multicenter AIDS Cohort Study (MACS)
Mucosa associated lymphoid tissue (MALT)
Mixed cryoglobulinemia (MC)
Multicentric Castleman's disease (MCD)
Mixed Cellularity Hodgkin's Disease (MCHD)
Monoclonal gammopathy of undetermined significance (MGUS)
Monotypic lymphoproliferative disorders of undetermined significance (MLDUS)
Multiple myeloma (MM)
Mouse mammary tumor virus (MMTV)
MMTV-like viruses (HML)
N-Methyl-*N*-nitro-*N'*-nitrosoguanidine (MNNG)
N-Nitrosomethylurea (MNU)
Multiple sclerosis (MS)
Men who have sex with men (MSM)
Murine leukemia virus (MuLV)

Non-A non-B hepatitis (NANBH)
Natural killer cells (NK)
National Cancer Institute (NCI)
Nuclear factor-κB (NF-κB)
Non-Hodgkin's Lymphoma (NHL)
Nonisotopic *in situ* hybridization (NISH)

Nodular lymphocyte predominant Hodgkin's disesase (NLPHD)
N-Nitrosomethyl-dodecyclamine (NMDCA)
Non-melanoma skin cancer (NMSC)
N-Nitroso compounds (NNC)
Nasopharyngeal carcinoma (NPC)
Nonstructural viral genes (NS)
Nodular sclerosis Hodgkin's disease (NSHD)

Oral squamous cell carcinoma (OSCC)
Open reading frames (ORFs)

Polycyclic aromatic hydrocarbons (PAH)
Positron emission tomography (PET)
Pneumocystis carinii pneumonia (PCP)
Platelet derived growth factor (PDGF)
Primary effusion lymphoma (PEL)
Peripheral blood mononuclear cells (PMBC)
Polymerase chain reaction (PCR)
Porcine endogenous retrovirus (PERV)
Peripheral blood (PB)
Protein induced by vitamin K absence or antagonism (PIVKA-II, also known as
     Des-Γ-carboxy prothrombin)
Parathyroid hormone releasing protein (PTHrP)
Posttransplant lymphoproliferative disorder (PTLD)
Protein phosphatase 2A (PP2A)

Revised European-American-Lymphoma classification (REAL)
Rat embryo fibroblast (REF)
Rheumatoid factor (RF)
Restriction fragment length polymorphism (RFLP)
Representational difference analysis (RDA)
Radioimmunoassay (RIA)
Reactive nitrogen oxide species (RNOS)
Reactive oxygen species (ROS)
Retinblasoma gene (Rb) and protein (pRb)
Reed–Sternberg cell (RS)
Reverse transcriptase (RT)
Reverse transcriptase polymerase chain reaction (RT-PCR)

Salmonella typhi and *paratyphi* (*S. typhi* and *S. paratyphi*)
SLAM-associated protein (SAP)
Simian immunodeficiency virus (SIV)
Simian virus 40 (SV40)
Squamous cell carcinomas (SCCs)
Severe combined immune deficiency (SCID)
Surveillance, Epidemiology, and End Results (SEER)
Socioeconomic status (SES)
San Francisco General Hospital (SFGH)
Simian foamy virus (SFV)

Squamous intraepithelial lesion (SIL)
Signaling lymphocyte-activation molecule (SLAM)
SLAM-associated protein (SAP)
Spasmolytic polypeptide (SP)
Single-stranded conformational polymorphism (SSCP)
Single-stranded DNA (SSDNA)
Sexually transmitted disease (STD)
Simian T-lymphotrophic virus (STLV)
Surface glycoproteins (SU)

Tandem repeats of tandemly repeated sequences (TR)
Drosophila melanogaster Tenascin gene (TNM)
Transporter protein associated with antigen presentation (TAP)
Transitional cell carcinoma (TCC)
Transforming growth factor β (TGF-β)
T helper cell type 1 (Th-1)
T helper cell type 2 (Th-2)
T-cell receptor (TCR)
Transmembrane glycoproteins (TM)
Tumor necrosis factor (TNF)
Tumor necrosis factor-α (TNF-α)
Transforming growth factor-β (TGF-β)
Tropical spastic paraparesis (also known as HTLV-associated myelopathy,
       HAM/TSP)
Tumor necrosis factor receptor (TNFR)
TRAF adaptor protein (TRADD)
Tumor necrosis factor receptor-associated (TRAF)
Transfusion-transmitted virus (TTV)
Transformation zone (TZ)

Untranslated region (UTR)
Ultraviolet (UV)

Vacuolating cytotoxin (VacA)
Virus-associated hemophagocytic syndrome (VAHS)
Viral capsid antigen (VCA)
Vascular epithelial growth factor-A (VEGF-A)
Vascular epithelial growth factor receptor 3 (VEGFR-3)
Virus-like particle (VLP)
Varicella-zoster virus (VZV)

World Health Organization (WHO)
Woodchuck hepatitis virus (WHV)
Women's Interagency Health Study (WIHS)

X-linked lymphoproliferative disease (XLP)

Z EBV replication activator protein (ZEBRA)

Contributors

CHRIS BOSHOFF, MRCP, PhD • *Glaxo Wellcome Research Fellow, Departments of Oncology and Molecular Pathology, University College, London, UK;* **Chapter 10** *corresponding author: The Cancer Research Campaign Viral Oncology Group, Departments of Oncology and Molecular Pathology, University College London, 91 Riding House Street, London W1P 8BT, United Kingdom, Facsimile: +44-(0)20-7679-9555 E-mail: c.boshoff@ucl.ac.uk*

JUDY A. BREUER, PhD • *Department of Virology, St Bartholomew's and Royal London School of Medicine and Dentistry, Queen Mary and Westfield College, London, UK*

JOHN A. G. BUCHANAN • *Department of Oral Medicine, St Bartholomew's and Royal London School of Medicine and Dentistry, Queen Mary and Westfield College, London, UK*

GERTRUDE CASE BUEHRING, PhD • *Program in Infectious Diseases, School of Public Health, University of California Berkeley, Berkeley, CA*

CHRISTINE P. J. CAYGILL, PhD• *Barrett's Oesphagus Registry, Barrett's Oesophagus Foundation, Department of Surgery, Royal Free Hospital, London, UK;* **Chapter 23** *corresponding author: UK National Barrett's Oesophagus Registry, Lady Sobell Gastrointestinal Unit, Wexham Park Hospital, Slough, Berkshire SL2 4HL, United Kingdom, Telephone: +44-1753-633-655 Facsimile: +44-1753-512-859*

DING-SHINN CHEN, MD • *Professor of Medicine and Director of Hepatitis Research Center, National Taiwan University College of Medicine and National Taiwan University Hospital, Taipei, Taiwan;* **Chapter 17** *corresponding author: Graduate Institute of Clinical Medicine, Department of Internal Medicine, National Taiwan University College of Medicine, National Taiwan University Hospital, 7 Chung-Shan South Road, Taipei 100, Taiwan, Telephone: +886-2-23970800 ext. 7307 Facsimile: +886-2-23317624 E-mail: kjh@ha.mc.ntu.edu.tw*

KUM COOPER, MB, BCH, FCPATH, FRCPATH, DPHIL • *Department of Pathology, University of Vermont, Burlington, VT*

JACK R. DAVIS, MT(ASCP) • *Department of Pathology/Microbiology, University of Nebraska Medical Center, Omaha, NE*

GUY DE THÉ, MD • *Retrovirus Department, Institut Pasteur, Paris, France;* **Chapter 5** *corresponding author: Institut Pasteur, Retrovirus Department, 28, rue du Dr Roux, 75015 Paris, France, Facsimile: +33-1-45-68-89-31 E-mail: dethe@pasteur.fr*

CLODOVEO FERRI, MD • *Dipartimento Medicina Interna, Rheumatology Unit, University of Pisa, Pisa, Italy;* **Chapter 19** *corresponding author: Dipartimento Medicina Interna, Rheumatology Unit, University of Pisa, Via Roma 67, 56126 Pisa, Italy, Telephone: +39-50-558601 or 550582 Facsimile: +39-50-558601 or 550582 E-mail: c.ferri@int.med.unipi.it*

JAMES G. FOX, DVM • *Division of Comparative Medicine and Bioengineering and Environmental Health, Massachusetts Institute of Technology, Cambridge, MA;* **Chapter 20** *corresponding author: Division of Comparative Medicine and Bioengineering and Environmental Health, Massachusetts Institute of Technology, 77 Massachusetts Ave., Bldg. 16, Rm. 825, Cambridge, MA 02139, Telephone: +1-617-253-1757 Facsimile: +1-617- 258-5708*

JAMES J. GOEDERT, MD • *Chief, Viral Epidemiology Branch, National Cancer Institute, Rockville, MD;* **Editor**: *Viral Epidemiology Branch, National Cancer Institute, 6120 Executive Blvd., Room 8012, MSC 7248, Rockville, MD 20852 Telephone: 301-435-4724 Facsimile: 301-402-0817 E-mail: goedertj@mail.nih.gov*

JOHN L. GRANER, MD • *Division of International Medicine, Department of Internal Medicince, Mayo Clinic, Rochester, MN;* **Chapter 1** *corresponding author: Department of General Internal Medicine, Mayo Clinic, Division of Internal Medicine, Mayo Building, W12B, 200 First Street SW, Rochester, MN 55905 USA, Telephone: +1-507-284-9739, Facsimile: +1-507-538-0298, E-mail: ganer.john@mayo.edu*

MEL F. GREAVES, PhD, MRCPath, HonMRCP • *Chester Beatty Laboratories, Leukaemia Research Fund Centre, Institute of Cancer Research, London, UK;* **Chapter 25** *corresponding author: Leukaemia Research Fund Centre, Institute of Cancer Research, Chester Beatty Laboratories, 237 Fulham Road, London SW3 6JB, United Kingdom, Telephone: +44-171-352-8133 ext 5160 Facsimile: +44-171-352-3299 E-mail: m.greaves@icr.ac.uk*

TIMOTHY G. GREINER, MD • *Department of Pathology/Microbiology, University of Nebraska Medical Center, Omaha, NE*

THOMAS G. GROSS, MD, PhD • *Division of Hematology/Oncology, Children's Hospital Medical Center, Cincinnati, OH*

CATHERINE A. HARWOOD • *Center for Cutaneous Research, St Bartholomew's and Royal London School of Medicine and Dentistry, Queen Mary and Westfield College, London, UK*

BRIAN G. HERNDIER, PhD, MD • *Departments of Pathology and Laboratory Medicine, University of California, San Francisco, CA*

MICHAEL J. HILL, PhD, DSc, FRCPath, ECP • *Headquarters, Moat Cottage, Church End, Sherfield-on-Loddon, Hook, UK*

LINDA J. HOFFMAN • *Departments of Pathology and Infectious Diseases and Microbiology, University of Pittsburgh Cancer Institute, University of Pittsburgh, Pittsburgh, PA*

SARAH JACKSON, PhD • *Centre for Cutaneous Research, St Bartholomew's and Royal London School of Medicine and Dentistry, Queen Mary and Westfield College, London, UK*

FRANK J. JENKINS, PhD • *Departments of Pathology and Infectious Diseases and Microbiology, University of Pittsburgh Cancer Institute, University of Pittsburgh, Pittsburgh, PA;* **Chapter 2** *corresponding author: Division of Behavioral Medicine and Oncology, University of Pittsburgh Cancer Institute, 3600 Forbes Avenue, Suite 405, Pittsburgh, PA 15213 USA, Telephone: +1-412-624-4630 Facsimile: +1-412-647-1936 E-mail: fjenkins@pop.pitt.edu*

HAL B. JENSON, MD • *Chief of Pediatric Infectious Diseases, Departments of Pediatrics and Microbiology, University of Texas Health Science Center, San Antonio, TX;* **Chapter 9** *corresponding author: Division of Pediatric Infectious Diseases, Departments of Pediatrics and Microbiology, University of Texas Health Science Center, 7703 Floyd Curl Dr., San Antonio, TX 78284-7811 USA, Telephone: +1-210-567-5301 Facsimile: +1-210-567-6921 E-mail: jenson@uthscsa.edu*

JIA-HORNG KAO, MD, PhD • *Graduate Institute of Clinical Medicine and Department of Internal Medicine, National Taiwan University College of Medicine and National Taiwan University Hospital, Taipei, Taiwan*

MICHAEL C. KEW, MD, PhD, DSc, FRCP • *Department of Medicine, MRC/CANSA/University Molecular Hepatology Research Unit, Medical School, Johannesburg, South Africa;* **Chapter 18** *corresponding author: MRC/CANSA/University Molecular Hepatology Research Unit, Department of Medicine, Medical School, 7 York Road, Parktown 2193, Johannesburg, South Africa, Telephone: +27-11-488-3626 Facsimile: +27-11-643-4318 E-mail: 014anna@chiron.wits.ac.za*

ARPAD LANYI, PhD • *Department of Pathology/Microbiology, University of Nebraska Medical Center, Omaha, NE*

IRENE M. LEIGH, DSc • *Centre for Cutaneous Research, St Bartholomew's and Royal London School of Medicine and Dentistry, Queen Mary and Westfield College, London, UK;* **Chapter 16** *corresponding author: Centre for Cutaneous Research, St Bartholomew's and Royal London School of Medicine and Dentistry, Queen Mary and Westfield College, 2 Newark Street, London E1 2AT, United Kingdom, Telephone: +44-171-295-7170 Facsimile: +44-171-295-7171 E-mail: i.leigh@icrf.icnet.uk*

ALEXANDRA M. LEVINE, MD • *USC/Norris Comprehensive Cancer Center, University of Southern California School of Medicine, Los Angeles, CA;* **Chapter 8** *corresponding author: USC/Norris Comprehensive Cancer Center, 1441 Eastlake Ave., MS 34, Rm. 3468, University of Southern California School of Medicine, Los Angeles, CA 90033 USA, Telephone: +1-323-865-3913 Facsimile: +1-323-865-0060 E-mail: hornor@hsc.usc.edu*

CATHERINE LEY, PhD • *Division of Epidemiology, Department of Health Research and Policy, Stanford University, Stanford, CA;* **Chapter 21** *corresponding author: Division of Epidemiology, Department of Health Research and Policy, Redwood Bldg. T221, Stanford University, Stanford, CA 94305-5405 USA, Telephone: +1-650-723-7274 Facsimile: +1-650-725-6951 E-mail: cley@leland.stanford.edu*

MASAO MATSUOKA, MD, PHD • *Laborotory of Virus Immunology, Research Center for AIDS, Institute for Virus Research, Kyoto University, Kyoto, Japan;* **Chapter 12** *corresponding author: Laboratory of Viral Immunology, Institute for Virus Research, Kyoto University, 53-1 Shogoin Kawahara-cho, Sakyo-ku, Kyoto 606-8507, Japan, Telephone: +81-75-751-4048, Facsimile: +81-75-751-4049, E-mail: mmatsuok@virus1.virus.kyoto-u.ac.jp*

MICHAEL S. McGRATH, MD, PHD • *Departments of Laboratory Medicine, Pathology and Medicine, University of California, San Francisco, CA;* **Chapter 13** *corresponding author: San Francisco General Hospital, 1001 Potrero St., Building 80, Ward 84, San Francisco, San Francisco, CA 94110 USA, Telephone: +1-415-206-3858 Facsimile: +1- 206-3765 E-mail: mmcgrath@sfaids.ucsf.edu*

JANE M. McGREGOR • *Centre for Cutaneous Research, St Bartholomew's and Royal London School of Medicine and Dentistry, Queen Mary and Westfield College, London, UK*

PAULA G. O'CONNOR, MD • *Hematology–Oncology Fellow, AIDS Research Center, Dana Farber/ Partners Cancer Care, Massachusetts General Hospital, Harvard Medical School, Boston, MA*

JOEL M. PALEFSKY, MD • *Departments of Laboratory Medicine, Medicine and Stomatology, University of California, San Francisco, San Francisco, CA;* **Chapter 15** *corresponding author: Departments of Laboratory Medicine, Medicine and Stomatology, 505 Parnassus Avenue, Room M1203, Box 0126, University of California, San Francisco, San Francisco, CA 94143 USA, Telephone: +1-415-476-1574 Facsimile: +1-415-476-0986 E-mail: joelp@labmed.ucsf.edu*

JULIE PARSONNET, MD • *Departments of Medicine and of Health Research and Policy, Stanford University, Stanford, CA*

STEFANO PILERI, MD • *Unità di Anatomia Patologica ed Emolinfopatologia, Dipartimento di Oncologia ed Ematologia, Università di Bologna, Bologna, Italy*

CHARLOTTE M. PROBY • *Centre for Cutaneous Research, St Bartholomew's and Royal London School of Medicine and Dentistry, Queen Mary and Westfield College, London, UK*

NANCY RAAB-TRAUB, PHD • *Department of Microbiology and Immunology, Lineberger Comprehensive Cancer Center, The University of North Carolina at Chapel Hill, Chapel Hill, NC;* **Chapter 6** *corresponding author: Lineberger Comprehensive Cancer Center, Campus Box 7295, School of Medicine, The University of North Carolina at Chapel Hill, Chapel Hill, NC 27599-7295 USA; Telephone: +1-919-966-1701 Facsimile: +1-919-966-9673 E-mail: nrt@med.unc.edu*

MARJORIE ROBERT-GUROFF, PHD • *Basic Research Laboratory, National Cancer Institute, National Institutes of Health, Bethesda, MD;* **Chapter 27** *corresponding author: National Institute of Health, National Cancer Institute, Basic Research Laboratory, 41 Library Drive, Building 41, Room D804, Bethesda, MD 29892-5055 USA, Telephone: +1-301-496-2114 Facsimile: +1-301-496-8394 E-mail: guroffm@exchange.nih.gov*

DAVID T. SCADDEN, MD • *Massachesetts General Hospital, Dana Farber/ Partners Cancer Care, Harvard Medical School, Boston, MA; Chapter 7 corresponding author: AIDS Research Center and Massachusetts General Hospital Cancer Center, Massachusetts General Hospital, Harvard Medical School, 149 13th Street, room 5212, Boston, MA 02129 USA, Telephone: +1-617-726-5615 Facsimile: +1-617-726-4691 E-mail: scadden.david@mgh.harvard.edu*

THOMAS A. SEEMAYER, MD • *Department of Pathology/Microbiology, University of Nebraska Medical Center, Omaha, NE; Chapter 3 corresponding author: Department of Pathology/Microbiology, University of Nebraska Medical Center, 983135 Nebraska Medical Center, Omaha, NE 68198-3135 USA, Telephone: +1-402-559-4244 Facsimile: +1-402-559-6018 E-mail: taseemay@unmc.edu*

KEERTI V. SHAH, MD, PHD • *Department of Molecular Microbiology and Immunology, School of Public Health, Johns Hopkins University, Baltimore, MD; Chapter 26 corresponding author: Department of Molecular Microbiology and Immunology, Johns Hopkins School of Public Health, 615 N. Wolfe Street, Baltimore, MD 21205, Telephone: +1-410-955-3189 Facsimile: +1-410-955-0105 E-mail: kvshah@jhsph.edu*

BRUCE SHIRAMIZU, MD • *Department of Pediatrics and Medicine, John A. Burns School of Medicine, University of Hawaii, Honolulu, HI*

ALAN STOREY • *Centre for Cutaneous Research, St Bartholomew's and Royal London School of Medicine and Dentistry, Queen Mary and Westfield College, London, UK*

JANOS SUMEGI, MD, PHD • *Department of Pathology/Microbiology, University of Nebraska Medical Center, Omaha, NE*

MONALISA SUR, MB, BS, DCPATH, FCPATH, MMED, DIPRCPATH • *Department of Anatomical Pathology, Medical School, University of the Witwatersrand, South African Institute for Medical Research, Johannesburg, South Africa; Chapter 24 corresponding author: Department of Anatomical Pathology, University of Witwatersrand, Johannesburg, P. O. Box 4280, Cresta 2118, South Africa, Telephone: +27-83-309-4474 Facsimile: +27-11-642-9185 E-mail: mlsur@hotmail.com*

LODE J. SWINNEN, MD • *Division of Hematology/Oncolgy, Cardinal Bernardin Cancer Center, Department of Medicine, Loyola University, Chicago, Maywood, IL; Chapter 4 corresponding author: Department of Medicine, Division of Hematology/Oncology, Cardinal Bernadin Cancer Center, Loyola University Medical Center, Building 112, Room 245, 2160 South First Avenue, Maywood, IL 60153 USA, Telephone: +1-708-327-3142 Facsimile: +1-708-327-3219 E-mail: lswinne@luc.edu*

TIMOTHY C. WANG, MD • *Gastrointestinal Unit, Department of Medicine, Massachusetts General Hospital, Boston, MA*

ROBIN A. WEISS, PHD • *Windeyer Institute of Medical Sciences, University College London, London, UK; Chapter 11 corresponding author: Windeyer Institute of Medical Sciences, University College London, 46 Cleveland Street, London W1P 6DB, UK, Telephone: +44-171-504-9554 Facsimile: +44-171-504-9555 E-mail: r.weiss@ucl.ac.uk*

ANDREW C. WOTHERSPOON, MRCPath • *Department of Histopathology, Royal Marsden Hospital, London, UK; **Chapter 22** corresponding author: Department of Histopathology, Royal Marsden Hospital, Fulham Road, London SW3 6JJ, United Kingdom, Telephone: +44-171-352-7348 Facsimile: +44-171-352-7348 E-mail: Andrew.Wotherspoon@rmh.nthames.nhs.uk*

ANNA LINDA ZIGNEGO, MD • *Dipartimento Medicina Interna, University of Florence, Florence, Italy*

HARALD ZUR HAUSEN, MD • *Deutsches Krebsforschungszentrum, Heidelberg, Germany; **Chapter 14** corresponding author: Deutsches Krebsforschungszentrum, Im Neuenheimer Feld 280, 69120 Heidelberg, Germany Telephone: +49-6221-422850 Facsimile: +49-6221-422840 E-mail: zurhausen@dkfz-heidelberg.de*

I
Background

History of Infectious Disease Oncology, from Galen to Rous

John Graner

The possibility that cancer might spread via an infectious mechanism has been considered for centuries. As the concepts of infectious disease and tumor changed, so also did the proposed relationships between the two. To understand the hypotheses raised regarding the transmissibility of malignancy, an understanding of how authorities in each era regarded the concepts of malignancy and infectious diseases is required. The sections that follow have been subdivided accordingly.

We begin our historical review with the 18th century, as relatively little consideration was given to the possibility of a link between infectious diseases and cancer prior to that time. There are several reasons why this was the case. The most important is the simple fact that, despite a few anecdotal remarks to the contrary *(1)*, tumors were not generally observed to spread from one person to another, nor did they demonstrate an epidemic pattern of development within a community. In addition, before the 18th century, the general concept of infection was only poorly understood. We refer the reader interested in theories of tumor causation prior to the 18th century to the monographs by Rather *(2)* and Wolff *(3)*.

THE 18TH AND EARLY 19TH CENTURIES

Introduction

The second half of the 18th century was a period of great theoretical confusion in medicine. For many, the ancient theories of disease causation had lost their traditional authority, but no new and unified system of concepts arose to take their place. Not surprisingly, the terminology of the period reflects this confusion. The old cancer term "scirrhus" came to be used in a variety of different ways. Also, words such as "germ" and "infection" possessed entirely different meanings than they do today. We therefore begin this section with a brief review of the way in which these terms were used by authors of the period. This is followed by subsections discussing period concepts of cancer causation, and the nature and spread of infectious diseases. Finally, we discuss early considerations of the possible infectious transmission of malignancies.

From: *Infectious Causes of Cancer: Targets for Intervention*
Edited by: J. J. Goedert © Humana Press Inc., Totowa, NJ

NOTES ON TERMINOLOGY

"Scirrhus"

No other term was used so consistently by ancient authors in discussions of malignancy as was "scirrhus" (also at times spelled "schirrus"). Depending on the era in which the author was writing, this word was used variously either to denote a malignancy, or a tumor that could potentially become so—what would now be termed a premalignant lesion. Derived from the Latin *scirros* (taken, in turn, from the Greek σκιρρος, meaning a firm swelling), this word originally denoted the extreme hardness of the lesion.

With rare exception, from the time of Galen until the end of the 18th century, the scirrhus was looked upon as a premalignant entity, capable of transforming into a cancer only under certain poorly understood circumstances. Traditionally, the most important predictive elements of malignant transformation were considered to be the quantity and quality of black (melancholic) bile associated with the lesion *(4)*.

By the 18th century, less credence was given to the tenets of traditional Galenic humoralism, and the contributions of black bile to the transformational process were often left unmentioned (although, as noted below, tacit references to the black humor remained). Boerhaave, for example, considered the scirrhus capable of becoming a true cancer under the following conditions:

> If a Schirrus by long standing, increasing, and motion of the adjacent parts is thus moved, that the neighbouring Vessels around its edges begin to inflame, it's become malignant, and from its likeness to a Crab, is now called a Cancer, or Carcinoma. *(5)*

Aitken, writing in 1782, echoes the opinion of Boerhaave. He likewise considers "scirrhosity" a "predisposition to cancerous ulcer," such changes occurring when the lesion is "attacked by inflammation" *(6)*.

Buchan, in his immensely popular textbook of domestic medicine, also agreed with traditional doctrine insofar as he considers cancer an extreme case of scirrhus: "If the tumour becomes large, unequal, of a livid blackish, or leaden colour, and is attended with violent pain, it gets the name of an occult cancer" *(7)*.

At the turn of the century, the term "scirrhus" gradually came to be used in another sense, as representing not a precancerous lesion, but a true cancer. For example, Thomas, writing in 1815, defined the scirrhus by its malignant nature, considering it the "occult or primary stage" of a cancer *(8)*. Similarly, Pearson, writing in 1793, used the word to denote a hard malignant growth *(9)*.

In contrast to most other authorities, however, Pearson did not consider "tumor," or swelling, to be a necessary component of the scirrhus, and so broadens the concept considerably *(10)*. Rather, to him, true scirrhus was defined primarily by its malignant behavior and not its firmness, true cancers being "dangerous in their nature, (and) difficult in their cure" *(11)*. Pearson also challenged the widely held notion that the "induration and defective sensibility" of a lesion in and of itself could be taken as proof that the lesion is cancerous *(12)*. Nor did he believe that the firmness of a lesion necessarily predicts its predisposition to malignant behavior.

By the second half of the 19th century, "scirrhus" had undergone yet another transformation in meaning, now being used to define only one particular form of cancer, based upon its microscopic appearance. Another term also used for this form of tumor was the "carcinomatous sarcoma" of Abernethy *(13).* The term again made reference to the stony hard nature of the lesion *(14).*

Cancer "Germs" and Cancer "Infection"

Particularly confusing in the context of the present topic is the use of the word "germ" by 19th century medical authors in their descriptions of tumor spread. While we now understand the term to denote a disease-causing microorganism, it was then used in its more original meaning, as that principle "from which any thing springs" *(15).*

Thus, when Wood, in his 1858 *Practice of Medicine,* referred to "the conveyance of (cancer) germs" from one part of the body to another *(16),* he is not advocating a true infectious etiology of cancer, as this would imply an infectious mode of spread to the affected individual. Rather he is referring only to a vague sort of seminal property possessed by some entity associated with malignancy, perhaps, as proposed by Virchow, the "liquid exuded in cancerous tissues," allowing it to arise in areas of the body separate from its primary location. He even used the term "infection" to describe this spreading process within the body in a clearly analogous sense, thereby comparing it to the process by which an infectious disease spreads within a community, or from person to person.

Many other writers of the period referred to the "germs" of cancer in a similar manner. For example, Joseph Bell, in a lecture given in 1857, after stating that "no object similar to the cancer cell has been found in the minute organisms either of the animal or vegetable worlds," then went on to say that "cancer cells may be formed in the body, from germs or corpuscles" *(17).* Again, he was here referring only to some sort of generative entity, the true nature of which remains unknown. Likewise, Campbell De Morgan, discussing the unfortunate tendency of cancer to recur after operation, refers to the "continued development of germs which were not included in the extirpation of the tumour" *(18),* without thereby assigning any particular identity to those entities.

Even more confusing in the literature of the period is the occasional use of the word "infection" in reference to the spread of cancer within the human body. Wood's reference, cited earlier, is one example of such usage.

Thus, De Morgan discussed malignant growths that "infect neighbouring and distant parts" without thereby considering cancer an infectious disease in the true sense *(19).* Billroth used the term in a similar manner. As a matter of fact, for him, "malignant" and "infectious" were synonymous terms *(20).*

Even Virchow, in his famous work on cellular pathology, mentioned the "infecting" powers of malignancies in his discussion of metastatic spread *(21).* He also referred to tumor juices as "contagious," and draws an analogy between tumor spread and smallpox *(22).* Again, he was not thereby referring to cancer spread from one individual to another in a truly infectious manner, but rather to different organs within the same individual.

Use of "infection" in this manner may have been confusing even to the author's contemporary readers. After all, a medical dictionary of the period defines it as "a synonim (sic) of contagion" *(23),* and by all accounts this is the way in which the term was generally used.

Waldeyer probably recognized this confusion, and so made the distinction explicit in 1867, when he stated that only in the sense that the epithelial cancer cell is capable of generating its own supporting stroma is the so-called "infectious theory" of cancer valid *(24)*. He also believed that although cancer cells resembled "entozoal germs" in their ability to reproduce themselves, they were of human, rather than animicular, origin.

EARLY CONCEPTS OF CANCER CAUSATION

Because cancer was defined only by its clinical behavior, it was impossible for the clinician of the period seeing a lesion for the first time to recognize it as malignant. He could not even call a hard tumor a "scirrhus" if by that term he meant a definitely cancerous lesion. A suspicious growth could at best be considered only potentially malignant until its subsequent behavior could be ascertained.

Some form of humoral disease theory remained in vogue from the time of Galen until well into the 19th century. Since the 1500s, several powerful attacks on Galenist doctrine had been made, most notably by Paracelsus, "the Luther of medicine" *(25)*, in the 16th century, and van Helmont in the 17th. In his 17th century work on fevers, Willis also explicitly rejected traditional Galenistic theory when he states, "We do not allow of the Opinion of the Ancients, That the Mass of Blood consists of the four Humours, viz Blood, Flegm, Choler, and Melancholy" *(26)*.

"Iatrochemistry," a modified form of humoralism emphasizing hermetic chemical concepts rather than the traditional Galenic humors, increased in popularity over the course of the 17th century, so that by the century's end traditional Galenism was considered antiquated by the more progressive physicians *(27)*.

Nevertheless, popular theory of tumor causation throughout most of the 17th century continued to embrace vital, humoral theory, in the form of the so-called "lymphatic humoralism" of Astruc and Peyrilhe *(28)*. The lymphatic vessels had been discovered in 1628, and scirrhus was now considered to be the product of an abnormal accumulation of lymph, which could later degenerate into cancer *(29)*.

Needless to say, the various humoral systems of disease failed to provide the physician the practical knowledge required to practice medicine effectively. In the words of William Osler, "What disease really was, where it was, how it was caused, had not even begun to be discussed intelligently" *(30)*.

Practicing physicians were very aware of this shortcoming. In the 17th century, Sydenham's concentration on the clinical characteristics of disease *(31)*, and in the 18th, Morgagni's emphasis on anatomical pathology *(32)*, represented attempts at bringing medical theory closer to the bedside.

Unfortunately, however, these efforts had little immediate impact in the field of tumor medicine. As a matter of fact, the clinical antecedents of malignancy were understood little better in the first half of the 19th century than they had been in the 16th, as may be noted from a perusal of some representative writings of the period. For example, Buchan, writing in 1816, provided the following list of the common antecedents to tumor appearance:

> This disease is often owing to suppressed evacuation; hence it proves so frequently fatal to women of a gross habit … It may likewise be occasioned by excessive fear, grief, anger, religious melancholy, or any of the depressing passions … It may also be occasioned by

the long continued use of food that is too hard of digestion, of an acrid nature; by barrenness, celibacy, indolence, colds, blows, friction, pressure or the like ... Sometimes the disease is owing to an hereditary disposition. *(33)*

Buchan's list is very similar to that of Boerhaave's, written a century earlier, elements of which could, in turn, be traced to classical sources:

The cause of a Cancer is ... An alteration in the Circulation of Humors, from the Menstrua, Hemorroids or any other Hemorragy being suppress'd; Barrenness, abstinence from all Venereal Acts; the leaving off of Child-bearing from the Age of 45, to 50; An austere, sharp or hot Diet; the several and even contrary Affections of the Mind, whether Melancholy or Anger, and the like; Any external irritation of the Schirrus by it's Motion, Heat and Acrimony; or Medicines which ... will produce the same Effect, whether outwardly or inwardly applied. *(34)*

The mention of "melancholy" by both Buchan and Boerhaave is rooted in the Galenic concept of the melancholic (black) humors, an excess of which was thought to be the ultimate cause of cancer *(35)*. Such thinking had not progressed noticeably from the attitude of the 16th century surgeon who considered malignancies to be caused by the "humors Melancholicke which come from all the partes of the bodie" *(36)*.

The most important clinical observation of the period was Pott's recognition of the increased incidence of scrotal cancer in chimney sweeps, which he reported in 1775 and again in 1778 *(37)*. Thomas, writing in the early 19th century, included this observation in his section on the subject *(38)*. Otherwise, however, he merely recited the various causes listed by earlier authors. If anything, mid-19th century textbook authors had even less to say regarding the clinical antecedents of cancer than had their predecessors. The old concepts were noted to be fallacious, but nothing new replaced them.

From a pathologist's standpoint, knowledge of cancer likewise remained rudimentary. During the first four decades of the 19th century, one had to rely upon the naked eye, without the aid of significant magnification, to make tissue diagnoses. Little wonder then that there remained great difficulty in diagnosing malignancy by appearance alone. Authorities of the period tended to lump true cancers into the same category as other "tumors," including tubercle (at that time not considered to result from an infectious disease), melanosis, and encephaloid *(39)*.

With the work of Bichat, published in the first years of the 19th century *(40)*, pathologists began thinking more on the tissue level of disease. However, Bichat's studies were carried out without the aid of a microscope, and before the development of these instruments in the 1820s and 1830s, no real advances in tumor histology could be made.

The real breakthrough in pathology came with recognition of the cell as the ultimate structural component of the body. The first description of cancer cells, or "globular bodies," was made by Gluge in 1837 *(41)*. Cell theory had actually begun with the botanists in the first quarter of the 19th century *(42)*. Schwann broadened this concept to include animals in 1838. The same year, Müller recognized the true cellular nature of malignancies *(43)*. With the aid of microscopes of improved accuracy, the new cell theory gradually came to replace the time-honored belief, derived ultimately from the writings of Aristotle, that the fiber constituted the ultimate structural component of life *(44)*.

By the middle of the 19th century, through the pioneering work of Müller and others, a primitive classification system based upon the microscopic appearance of tumor tissue had been devised. Tumors were divided into three main groups: scirrhus, composed predominantly of fibrous tissue, and therefore firm; colloid, made up of loculations containing a gelatinous substance termed "blastema;" and cephaloma or medullary, composed predominantly of recognizable cells *(45,46)*. This last form of malignancy, said to resemble brain tissue, was also at times called "encephaloid" *(47)*, a term probably first used by Bayle and Laennec *(48)*.

One would think that once tumors were found to differ significantly in microscopic appearance, their true diversity would also come to be recognized. Surprisingly, however, such was not the case. All malignancies were still considered variants of a single disease, and different types of cancer, properly speaking, were not thought to exist. Watson offers a defense for this position:

> You may ask upon what principle structures so dissimilar in their physical appearance have been assigned to the same genus? Why, for these reasons. They are all strictly destructive or malignant forms of disease. Although in any shape they are of somewhat rare occurrence, yet when they do occur, two, or all three of the species are often found to coexist in different organs of the same individual ... More than this: if a tumour consisting of one species be amputated, and a fresh growth springs (as too often it does) from the same spot, this secondary growth is frequently of another species ... (T)he facts I have just stated suggest the question, whether instead of being different species of the same genus, they ought not rather to be regarded as mere varieties of the same species. *(49)*

EARLY CONCEPTS OF INFECTIOUS DISEASE: CONTAGION AND MIASMA

While concepts of tumor morphology had changed markedly by the middle of the 19th century, infectious disease theory had not. Such changes were not to occur until several decades later. As a matter of fact, in the United States, owing to the conservatism and scientific backwardness of the American medical profession, theories of infectious disease remained more or less unchanged until the early 1880s *(50)*.

Throughout the 18th and most of the 19th centuries, infectious diseases were considered to be of two major types, contagious and miasmal. The former, represented by such diseases as smallpox, were observed to be transmitted from one individual to another. The latter, the prime example of which was "intermittent fever," were not spread by contact, but rather were observed to affect numerous people in a community in a short period of time *(51)*. Such diseases were therefore thought to be transmitted by a noxious "effluvia" exhaled by areas of rotting vegetation, such as marshes. The term "malaria" came to be used synonymously for this marsh miasm *(52)*.

Regarding this latter form of disease spread, Gregory, in a well-known textbook of the period, stated, "It cannot be disputed that the miasmata of marshes are the most frequent and important exciting causes of intermittent fever" *(53)*. Similarly, Rush considered yellow fever to be "produced by the exhalations from the gutters, and the stagnating ponds of water" *(54)*.

Gallup, in his classic 1815 work on the epidemic diseases of Vermont, defined the two types of diseases in the following manner. Contagion is illness "eliminated from the diseased body in a subtle gas, or by contact, (producing) its likeness in a healthy body," while miasma "is the effect of animal and vegetable decomposition and corruption on the surface of the earth ... eliminating therefrom in the form of a subtle gas or effluvia" *(55)*.

Gallup's description of contagion may have been influenced by the writings of Cullen. Already in the 18th century, the latter had recognized the somewhat arbitrary nature of the distinction between contagion and miasma, and argued that both types of disease spread involved emanations into the atmosphere, one of human (contagion), the other of nonhuman (miasmatal) origin *(56).* He went on to suggest the use of the terms "human" and "marsh" effluvia rather than the general terms "contagion" and "miasma" *(57).* Cullen's suggestion was not generally accepted, however, and this modification, considered somewhat trivial to modern readers, left the underlying traditional theory intact.

Understandably, the decision as to whether a particular disease was miasmal or contagious was sometimes not an easy one to make. Thus, in a footnote to the first page of Armstrong's 1829 work on typhus, his editor stated the following:

> When Dr. Armstrong wrote this article he considered human contagion the primary source of the disease. Since then, however, he has abandoned this opinion, and now believes that marsh effluvium is the cause ... Some very eminent physicians in this country ... still believe in the contagious nature of this disease. *(58)*

Factions were formed, and debate ensued, sometimes heated, as to the mode of transmission of a particular disease. One example of such an exchange was the 1859 argument between contagionist and noncontagionist factions over the origin of yellow fever *(59).*

Still other authors, such as Stokes *(60),* expressed the opinion that no theory could satisfactorily explain all examples of infection. Despite the shortcomings of this dichotomous distinction, no one offered a clear alternative until the advent of the zymogen theory, to be discussed later.

CONSIDERATIONS REGARDING THE INFECTIOUS ETIOLOGY OF TUMORS

When one excludes those "pseudo-references" to cancer as an infectious disease that are the result not of the author's true conviction that cancer represents an infectious process, but rather his analogous use of terms, it may be said with confidence that, prior to the 18th century, very few believed in the infectious etiology of tumors.

Pearson, in his 1793 treatise on cancer, wished to consider all possible etiologies of malignancy, including that of infection. He first investigated the human miasmal possibility (analogous to Cullen's "human effluvia"), by considering the possible "infectious power of the vapour arising from a cancerous sore" *(61).* Stating that "some ... have asserted that the cancerous sore emits a morbiferous effluvium, which can produce the same disease in a sound person," he went on to note that these rare assertions "appear to me very insufficient for the purpose of establishing so important a proposition." He concluded these considerations with the following practical observation:

> Surgeons and their attendants, expose themselves almost every day to the noxious effects of cancerous sores with perfect impunity; from whence it may be safely concluded, that the danger of infection is so small, as not to form an object of serious attention. *(62)*

Pearson next explored the possibility that cancer may be a noneffluvial contagion by assessing "the contagious quality of cancerous matter when applied in a fluid state to an abraded surface." Giving no consideration to a possible animal model of study, he admitted that experimentation would resolve this particular issue, but, "No man ever had, nor ever will have the unwarrantable temerity, to attempt the solution of this pathological doubt, by a method so repugnant to the laws of humanity" *(62).*

He went on to provide a short list of postulated cases of such transmittal, debunking them all. He concluded this section with another practical statement: "Where the disease so frequently occurs, the defect of positive proof, affords a strong presumption against the contagious quality of cancerous matter" *(63).*

As a matter of fact, the experiment that Pearson rejected as immoral was actually conducted by Alibert. Thomas referred to its results as a demonstration of the noncontagiousness of cancer:

> Mons. Alibert inoculated himself and some of his pupils with cancerous matter, and although in some instances inflammation of the part, and of the lymphatics proceeding from it occurred, yet nothing like scirrhus, or cancer succeeded. *(64)*

Joseph Adams, writing in 1795, agreed with Pearson that cases in which fluid from a cancer seems to act like a "morbid poison," producing a similar ulcer in another person, do not represent true examples of malignancy:

> Two cases of this kind … were relieved, one by corrosive sublimate, the other without an operation. It is unnecessary to add that neither could be a true carcinoma. One of them being on the lip of a married lady, proved contagious and fatal to her husband. Here we have an instance of a morbid poison originating from an incurable disease (rather than a cancer), and relieved in the first instance by mercury. The husband was abroad, or might probably have experienced the same relief… *(65)*

Wood, writing in 1858, also addressed the issue of the possible transmissibility of cancer. He stated that "opinion has generally been opposed to this idea." However, he mentioned one experiment that lends support to it. Langenbeck injected cancerous matter into the veins of a dog, which when killed several weeks afterwards, demonstrated cancerous growths in the lungs *(66).* He also mentioned two cases cited by Watson *(67),* of women with cancer of the uterus whose husbands subsequently developed cancer of the penis.

Wood also addressed the possibility that cancer may be a very small "parasitic animal," but continued:

> Strongly in opposition to this notion is the well-established fact, that many of the lower animals are liable to the same disease; whereas parasites are generally peculiar to the species of animal in which they are found. *(68)*

This statement demonstrates well the limited role that living agents were generally thought to play in human disease during this period. Pasteur was not to formulate his germ theory of disease until well into the 1870s *(69),* but parasitic diseases had already been identified. Wood expressed the opinion that because such diseases appeared to infect only a particular species, while many species were found to harbor cancer (which, as noted earlier, was usually still considered a single disease entity, despite its several forms), malignant disease could not fit the parasitic model of causation.

Although most prominent men in the field gave scant consideration to the possibility that cancer may be due to some form of living organism, some notable exceptions to this rule existed. William Gibson, professor of surgery at the University of Pennsylvania, demonstrated a firm belief in the infectious (or, more correctly, "infestuous") nature of cancer. In his 1845 *Practice of Surgery,* he postulated an "animalcular origin" of cancer, "thus giving to cancer an independent vitality." Apparently the parasite (he suggested an insect or worm) was thought to lie dormant in the body, the exciting cause for its activity being some form of trauma sufficient to bring about "such a condition of the part … as to afford a nidus particularly suited to the lodgement and growth of independent beings" *(70).*

Watson, writing in his *Lectures on the Principles and Practice of Physic,* the most popular medical textbook of the period, also expressed the opinion that cancer may be a contagious entity. He stopped one step short of calling it an infectious disease, however. He cited two cases that he himself had witnessed, also cited by Wood, of uterine cancer in a wife and penile cancer in the husband. He also mentioned Langenbeck's experiment, likewise cited by Wood. Based on these observations, Watson stated that "It seems … that the germs of the disease are capable of being transferred from one human being to another; and even to an animal of a different species."
He saw

> plausible grounds for the hypothesis, that the seeds of cancer may be introduced, in some way which eludes observation, from without; that cancerous growths are strictly parasitic, and independent of the body, excepting so far as they derive their pabulum from its juices … But whether this hypothesis be true, or whether the cancer cells and germs are merely morbid elements of the native tissues of the body … remains yet to be determined. *(71)*

Two other lesser known authors of the period who considered cancer a parasitic disease were Carmichael in 1836 and Kuhn in 1861. The former used the term "animal fungus" to describe this proposed entity *(72).* None of these early parasitic theories gained wide acceptance, for the simple fact that the proposed parasites were never discovered.

Although by the mid 1800s a contagious mode of tumor transmission had been repeatedly considered, a miasmal mechanism had not. Perhaps the only well-known author prior to the turn of the century to consider such a possibility was Theodor Billroth. Writing in his mid-century classic *General Surgical Pathology and Therapeutics,* he suggested that goiter (then considered a form of tumor) may be a "chronic endemic-miasmatic" entity. He postulated that infection occurs through the blood, and that the enlargement of the thyroid is "the local expression of a general infection" *(73).* Ironically, a true miasmal theory of cancer was not to arise until the turn of the century, as noted in a subsequent section.

Despite the several suggestions to the contrary, the firm belief in the noninfectious nature of cancer held sway until the very end of the 19th century, not only among most authorities in the field, but also the rank and file of the profession, an independent group who tended to base their opinions primarily on their own clinical experience.

MID- TO LATE 19TH CENTURY

Introduction

By the 1860s the microscope was in wide use. It had come to be recognized by many as a valuable tool in the study of disease, and would ultimately serve to place the study of tumors and infections on the same fundamental basis: the cell. In the field of tumor pathology, we have already made note of the fact that with the advent of microscopic study, a new, albeit rudimentary, histological classification system of cancers was already widely accepted by the 1850s.

The microscopic study of bacterial diseases began in earnest soon after this, but a universally accepted theory of microbial disease, not to mention an understanding of the contribution of microbes to the inflammatory process, were still several decades away. Thus, in the same edition of his textbook in which Watson presents the new microscopic tumor classification system, he continued to refer to the ancient Greek concept of φλεγμονη and the Latin *inflammatio* when discussing the nature of inflammation *(74)*. It is amazing then, that by the turn of the century, thanks to the work of Pasteur, Koch, and others, the germ theory of disease was to be considered dogma by the majority of the scientific medical community.

Tumor Theory in the Mid- to Late 19th Century

Few advances in the knowledge of the clinical antecedents of cancer were made during this period. The next major breakthroughs in this area were not to occur until after the turn of the century.

In the realm of the laboratory, while Schwann and Müller had demonstrated microscopically that tissues were in reality composed of aggregates of cells, they still believed these cells to derive from an amorphous blood-derived cytoblastema, "a kind of repeated spontaneous generation out of a primitive body fluid" *(75)*. Virchow, a one time student of Müller's, also adhered to this concept throughout the 1840s *(76)*. However, by 1854 he began to express some doubts. These misgivings were in part the result of the work of William Addison, who throughout the latter half of the 1840s continued to reject the blastema theory, arguing that cell formation from such a substance had never been convincingly demonstrated *(77)*. In his lectures of 1858, Virchow made the following statement:

> According to Schwann, the intercellular substance was the cytoblastema, destined for the development of new cells. This I do not consider to be correct, but, on the contrary, I have … arrived at the conclusion that the intercellular substance is dependent … upon the cells. *(78)*

As a matter of fact, Virchow had abandoned the blastema theory several years before. Already in 1855 he had made the famous pronouncement, *"Omnis cellula a cellula,"* that is, all cells arise from cells *(79)*.

Virchow went on to substitute the connective tissue for the blastema as the source of cell origin, at least in the case of malignancies. He came to believe that all cancers took their origin from connective tissue elements, and even includes an illustration depicting the development of cancer from connective tissue in his 1858 work (Fig. 1) *(80)*. Parenthetically, in the 1850s tuberculosis was still not considered an infectious disease, and although Virchow clearly recognized the difference between tubercles and other tumors, he believed both types of lesions arose from connective tissue *(81)*.

With powerful authorities such as Virchow to support it, the connective tissue theory of cancer histogenesis was widely accepted from 1855 to 1865. It was finally disproved by Thierch, who demonstrated that epithelial cancer derived from like normal tissue, only later spreading to the connective tissue *(82)*. This view was soon supported by others, including Waldeyer, who in an 1867 article proposed that the only source of epithelial cancer cells is the normal epithelium. He also asserted that metastasis

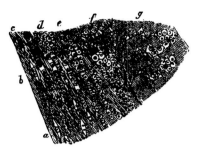

Development of cancer from connective tissue in carcinoma of the breast. *a.* Connective-tissue corpuscles, *b,* division of the nuclei, *c,* division of the cells, *d,* accumulation of the cells in rows, *e,* enlargement of the young cells and formation of the groups of cells[1] (foci—Zellenheerde) which fill the alveoli of cancer, *f,* further enlargement of the cells and the groups. *g.* The same developmental process seen in transverse section. 300 diameters.

Fig. 1. Virchow's depiction of development of carcinoma from connective tissue. (Reprinted from ref. *21,* with permission.)

resulted only from transport of tumor cells about the body. Tumor secretions or "juices" by themselves were not capable of spreading the disease *(83).*

With Waldeyer, tumor theory reached a new level of maturity. His basic tenets, that not only did cells derive only from other cells, but also that tumor cells derived from normal cells of the same type; and that metastatic spread resulted from the spread and multiplication of the primary tumor cells, remain legitimate today.

Infectious Disease Theory: The Bacterial Cause of Disease

To better explain the rise and ultimate triumph of bacterial theory, we must step backward a bit, and return briefly to the early decades of the 19th century. We have said that a controversy existed during this period regarding the contagious nature of specific diseases. This controversy was to reach "epidemic" proportions.

None could deny that such a thing as contagion existed. After all, how else could the transmission of smallpox and rabies by inoculation be explained? However, although some used the term "contagious" to denote only those diseases transmittable in this manner, others used it in its broader, less restricted sense to include all diseases that could be spread from person to person *(84).*

Some anticontagionists used arguments expanding upon the "human miasm" theory to explain the contagious appearance of epidemic diseases. Such arguments were useful at times for social as well as scientific reasons, and played a part in changing official policy on such things as quarantine and public hygiene *(85).*

Before 1860, most 19th century authorities had used chemical rather than microbiological explanations for infectious diseases. In what could be considered the final form of humoralism, chemists, most notably Liebig, had attempted to explain the infectious diseases in terms of fermentation, thought to be a purely chemical process.

At the forefront of this approach to disease explanation was William Farr, who in the 1840s introduced the term "zymogic" to explain the chemical nature of disease causation *(86).* Under this theory, it was thought that infection was spread through chemical particles "thrown from the (diseased) person, or from substances proceeding from the person, ... borne by the air to other persons in full health" *(87)*. One reason for the ultimate acceptance of this theory was that it served to bridge the ever-widening gap between contagionists and noncontagionists, as zymogens could be considered contagions, while at the same time miasmata could be considered capable of creating zymotic materials *de novo (88)*.

However, as the century progressed, it became impossible to ignore the work of microbiological researchers such as Pasteur and Koch. The former's brilliant research during the late 1850s had shown that fermentation, thought by Liebig to be a purely chemical phenomenon, was actually vital, in that it required microorganisms to occur *(89)*.

By the next decade, Pasteur had shown that two diseases of silkworms were due to bacterial infections. To his contemporaries, the most impressive aspect of his theory was its practical value. Utilizing his bacteriological discoveries, he had actually formulated a plan through which the silkworm disease was successfully eliminated *(90)*. When Pasteur came to devise his systematic germ theory in the 1870s, he was already considered an expert in the field, and by this time his opinions carried considerable weight.

Koch was second only to Pasteur in his ability to influence his contemporaries toward a positive reception of the germ theory of disease. His work, especially with tuberculosis, but also with anthrax, diphtheria, and cholera, helped establish these conditions as specific infections. Also, Petri and other students in his laboratory made important improvements in culture technique and other technical innovations. "Koch's postulates," actually devised by his student Löffler, soon became the *sine qua non* for establishing the infectious etiology of a specific disease *(91)*.

Once more, the zymogen theory served to bridge the gap between the old and the new. In light of the breakthroughs in the field of microbiology, the zymogen soon came to be considered a biological, rather than a chemical particle, and eventually zymogens were considered analogous to disease germs *(92)*.

This was another instance in which advancements in technology proved of fundamental importance for the generation and acceptance of new theories. Once the proper techniques for identification and culture of microorganisms were in place, their recognition as etiologic factors in specific diseases proceeded rapidly, and by the turn of the century, when one discussed infectious diseases, it was solely in terms of bacterial theory.

Cancer and Infection

As stated in the previous section, the vast majority of late 19th century researchers did not consider cancer to be an infectious disease. This having been said, it is also true that with the triumph of the germ theory, a number of German and French researchers did attempt to isolate a bacterium from cancer cells. This work is well summarized by Wolff *(93)*. False leads were generated for a time, but were never universally accepted.

Waldeyer was among the majority of researchers who did not believe in any such theory. Writing after the turn of the century, he recognized two authors who considered cancer to be caused by an infectious agent. The first was Rudolf Maier, who suggested that an infectious agent was necessary to transform normal cells into cancer cells. Waldeyer considered this "a completely unsupported hypothesis." The other author cited by Waldeyer is Wilhelm Müller, who thought that epithelioma and carcinoma were infectious diseases, each caused by a different infectious agent. Waldeyer did not support either claim *(94)*.

Samuel Shattock was also interested in attempting "the growth of a specific microphyte from carcinoma." In the Morton Lecture on Cancer, delivered before the Royal College of Surgeons of England in 1894, he reported preliminary observations of "actively moving amoebae" in tissue cultures of cancer cells. He postulated that these organisms could possibly be the transmitters of human malignancy *(95)*.

Shattock was one of those who embraced a protozoal, rather than a bacterial, explanation of cancer. Work was pursued in this field in several laboratories around the turn of the century. A detailed discussion of this research is beyond the scope of this chapter, but is also described in great detail in the monograph by Wolff *(96)*. Suffice it to say that, as was the case with bacteria, all attempts at finding a protozoal cause for cancer were in vain.

At the same time that several laboratories were busily engaged in unfruitful attempts at isolating the illusive cancer "bug," a new population-based miasmal theory of cancer was beginning to gain rather widespread acceptance, not only among members of the medical profession, but the general public as well. This was the so-called "cancer house" theory.

"Cancer Houses"

The "cancer house" theory postulated that certain districts, towns, and even single dwellings possessed a factor subjecting their occupants to an increased risk of cancer. Becoming popular in the last years of the 19th century, it remained so for the next several decades.

In several respects this theory harkened back to those of a hundred years previously. In the first place, its proponents did not rely directly on the new and burgeoning field of microbiology. Rather, they presented what might be considered a modernized version of the old miasmal theory of disease transmission to explain their findings. Second, similar to earlier writers, proponents of this theory considered cancer a unitary disease, with all tumors representing examples of the same underlying disease process *(97)*.

The principal British exponent of this theory was D'arcy Power, who, in an article published in 1899, presented a detailed study of cancer incidence in a single English district *(98)*. In an earlier article he had dismissed the possibility that cancer represented a contagious disease *(99)*, but a miasmal mechanism seemed much more promising. He noted that "much of the country shows the ordinary characters of marsh land," and went on to say that "cancer is the prevailing disease."

Without providing statistics to prove his contention (not to be expected at this early date), Power found the manner in which the disease was distributed "remarkable," noting that it "seems to cling to certain spots and groups of buildings." He found no relationship to the water sources, but did believe that "an unduly large proportion of the cases of cancer occur near the streams which water the district" *(100)*. He saw no evidence of a hereditary influence. He did notice, however, that the inhabitants have "unstable tissues, for ... insanity in its various forms is exceedingly rife, and ... in many of the houses where cancer has occurred there have been one or more cases of insanity."

He also found the distribution of the cancers suggestive:

(O)f the 173 cases of cancer here recorded, 49 occurred in the alimentary canal, 10 in the lip, and 22 in the liver; ... it seems to point to some source of infection gaining access to the body through the digestive system. Yet I do not think that water is the direct infecting agent. There is far more likely to be some intermediate host about which we know nothing at the present time.

In the final analysis he resorted to a miasmal theory to explain his findings:

It is impossible to resist the conclusion that the marshy ground from which the rivers in this district rise, as well as their wooded banks, have some causal connection with the numerous cases of cancer which have been observed. This part of the country must once have been pre-eminently malarious, the inhabitants being constantly "below par." But improved drainage of the land, better sanitation, and a higher standard of living and personal comfort have led to a disappearance of the ague....

Power suggested that another reason malaria may have disappeared from the area, "if we may accept the most interesting inoculation experiments of Professor Bignami," was the elimination of "the particular species of diptera, or gnats, carrying the infective protozoon." He believed he recognized a relationship between malaria and malignancy, in that they seem to "occur in inverse ratio to each other. Where malaria is common, cancer is rare..."

Power postulated that cancer may be

caused by an organism allied to ... the malarial parasite, but differing from it in the fact that it had a much longer incubation period, that it attacked tissues in a more decadent condition, that it no longer confined itself to the blood, but that it was capable of penetrating into the tissues, thereby causing a rapid proliferation of the cells-both epithelial and connective tissue.

He went on to cite several more series of "endemic cancer" taken from the recent literature. He ended his rather lengthy paper by stating:

I cannot help thinking that these cases raise a strong presumption in favour of cancer being an infective disease, to which some are much more susceptible than others ... I do not think that the cause will be found in any given room or house or water supply, notwithstanding the curious instances which have been cited in this paper ... It will almost certainly prove that there is some intermediate host whose chance of detection will increase or diminish with the care which is taken to examine the fauna and flora of the districts where cancer is most prevalent.

I have quoted Power's article at length, as he was perhaps the most influential writer on the subject. Of course, what this and similar reports lacked were the statistical calculations needed to support their assertions.

Power did not hazard a guess as to the nature of the miasmal organism, but Haviland did. After reporting his own series of cancer houses, he suggested that "cancerous neoplasms might possibly belong to a group of maismatic diseases capable of being propagated by spores formed outside the organism" *(101)*.

The subject of cancer houses was still actively discussed in 1914. In an entry in *The Lancet* entitled "Cancer Houses," Gifford Nash reported 10 instances of what he termed "dual cancer," which was malignancy occurring in husband and wife pairs within a relatively short period of time *(102)*. Nash concluded his submission with the statement that in his experience "dual cases of cancer have been far more frequent than dual cases of tuberculosis."

The laboratory equivalent of the cancer house theory was the so-called "cancer cage" theory. This theory, originally propounded by the influential French researcher Amédée Borrel, postulated that tumors in mice and rats were more common to develop in animals housed in certain cages *(103)*.

Borrel derived his theory directly from the cancer house theory. In his words, "There are cancer-ridden cages just as there are homes, streets and countries ridden with cancer." Based on this observation, he also expressed the opinion that cancer is a "miasmatic disease, such as coccidioses or malaria" *(104)*.

The cancer house and cancer cage theories may have been the first and last to invoke a miasmal mechanism of cancer spread. Interest in them appears to have dissipated by the 1920s, and by the 1930s they, along with germ theories of cancer in general, had become objects of derision *(105)*.

EARLY 20TH CENTURY

Concepts of Tumor Etiology

In the early years of the 20th century, the concept of irritation continued to play an important role in the etiologic theories of cancer. The development of cancers at the site of scars had been a long recognized phenomenon. Physical irritation, whether from caustic burns, trauma, or ulcers was also considered a risk factor for acquiring gastric cancer *(106)*. Irritation was likewise thought to be the cause of the malignancies sometimes seen in association with various parasitic infections, such as the hepatic malignancies associated with liver-fluke disease *(107)*, and the bladder cancer associated with schistosomal infection (*see also,* Chapter 24). An interesting sidelight on the latter observation was the awarding of the Nobel Prize in 1926 to Fibiger for his demonstration of the carcinogenic influence of nematodes in rats, a finding that was later disproved *(108)*.

In the realm of chemical carcinogenesis, at the turn of the century little more was known other than Pott's "remarkably prescient" recognition of an increased incidence of scrotal cancer in chimney sweeps *(109)*. However, the years 1900–1915 saw the first evidence of the carcinogenicity of tobacco smoking, betel nut chewing, and biliary calculus *(110)*. Also, by 1920 it had been shown in the animal model that repeated application of tar to the ears of rabbits resulted in skin neoplasms. In 1930, 1,2,5,6-dibenzanthracene was isolated from tar and found to cause cutaneous tumors. These studies led to the recognition, later in the century, of the carcinogenic properties of the polyaromatic hydrocarbons *(111)*.

The carcinogenic property of ultraviolet light was demonstrated in experimental animals in 1928. Soon after X-rays were discovered by Röentgen in 1895 *(112)*, they were also shown to be carcinogenic. Apparently Frieben, in 1902, was the first to report the carcinogenic effect of X-rays in humans *(113)*.

As far as the possible infectivity of tumors is concerned, the following statement by Andrewes, made in 1934, expresses well the opinion that prevailed at the turn of the century:

(T)umours are not infectious. There is no evidence of any value that a tumour either of man or animal is acquired as a result of contact between one individual and another. I say this notwithstanding the vast literature which has accumulated on the subject of so-called cancer houses and, as regards mice, of cancer cages. *(114)*

At the cellular level, it was still not clear in the early decades of the 20th century that chromosomal aberrations were the cause of malignant cellular behavior. Already in 1858 Virchow was describing the division of the nucleoli and nuclei prior to whole cell division *(115)*. By the turn of the century the presence and division of the chromosomes were also established facts, but their function remained unknown *(116)*. And by the mid-1930s, although it was known that "a mutation … depends on some alteration in the genes or chromosomal complex," there was still "no proof that chromosomal or gene alterations are responsible for the various malignant cells" *(117)*.

New Concepts in Microbiology: The Virus

By the turn of the century the knowledge among physicians that bacteria were the cause of numerous infectious diseases was commonplace, the propagation of pathogenic bacteria in the laboratory routine, and manuals of bacteriology ubiquitous. The most important new discovery made during this period was that of the "filterable viruses." Although they could not be seen directly (this would not be accomplished until the advent of the electron microscope many years later) the presence of submicroscopic transmitters of disease was inferred from the fact that certain illnesses could be transmitted via cell-free filtrates.

It had been known for many years that several of the contagious diseases were probably not caused by bacteria, although transmittable by inoculation. Examples included smallpox, hydrophobia, and foot-and-mouth disease of cattle. As a matter of fact, already in 1884 Pasteur had expressed his belief that the cause of hydrophobia was "a microorganism infinitesimally small." *(118)*.

The first disease to be shown to be caused by a cell-free filtrate was tobacco mosaic disease in 1892. Iwanowski used porcelain filters to block the passage of any microscopically visible microbes and demonstrated that the filtrates were nonetheless fully capable of causing the leaf changes associated with the disease.

Recognition of other such diseases soon followed. Foot-and-mouth disease was shown to be transmittable by filtrate in 1898. The same year Iwanowski's findings regarding tobacco mosiac virus were confirmed by Beijerinck. Smallpox, hydrophobia, infantile paralysis, herpes encephalitis, and many others soon followed *(119)*. The term "virus," which had traditionally been used in the general sense of "active or contagious matter" or "poison" *(120)*, now came to denote these postulated submicroscopic entities.

VIRUSES AND MALIGNANCY

Early Research

Perhaps the first researcher to postulate a viral etiology for cancer was Amédée Borrel. He used the term "epitheliosis" for the cellular reaction to the invisible viruses responsible for such diseases as smallpox, cowpox, and sheep-pox, as early as 1903 *(121)*. The term is based on the fact that these entities localize and proliferate in epithelial tissue *(122)*. Considering the viral inclusions to be parasites, he found them analogous to those found in some malignancies, such as the contagious epithelioma of birds *(123)*. He postulated that the viruses causing the tumors were carried to the tissues by nematodes, mites, or other living agents *(124)*. Interestingly, Borrel used the example of cancer cages to support the concept of the viral transmission of cancer *(125)*.

Although the transplantation of a malignant tumor from one animal to another was first carried out successfully in 1876, and several other such studies were reported throughout the remaining decades of the 19th century, no undue attention was given to them *(126)*. The first cell-free transmission of what only in retrospect was recognized to be a malignancy was that of fowl leukemia by Ellermann and Bang in 1908 *(127)*.

Rous and Fowl Sarcoma

After reporting the transmission of fowl sarcoma via tissue in 1910 *(128)*, Peyton Rous went on to report its transmissibility via cell-free filtrate in 1911 *(129)*. In so doing he became the first to describe the cell-free transmission of a solid tumor, and thus the first researcher to provide evidence of a possible viral origin of cancer (*see also*, Chapter 14).

Rous knew of no instance of spontaneous transmission of the tumor in nature *(130)*. He was also careful to report the absence of bacteria or any other "parasitic organism" in filtrate or fresh smears of the tumor surface, and was the first to admit that his findings were "unusual." He concluded his classic report with a word of caution:

> The first tendency will be to regard the self-perpetuating agent active in this sarcoma of the fowl as a minute parasitic organism. Analogy with several infectious diseases of man and the lower animals, caused by ultramicroscopic organisms, gives support to this view of the findings … But an agency of another sort is not out of the question. It is conceivable that a chemical stimulant … might cause the tumor. *(131)*

By 1913 Rous' group had reported two other filterable chicken tumors, a chondrosarcoma *(132)* and a sarcoma with an intracanalicular pattern *(133)*. This third malignancy tended to metastasize to skeletal muscle *(134)*.

Rous also went on, in 1913, to report further work with his first filtrate. He provided evidence that from the tumor, "there can be separated by drying, or filtration, or glycerinization, an agent, presumably living, which, under special conditions, will cause a sarcomatous change in the tissue of a previously normal fowl" *(135)*.

In a 1914 article, Rous and Murphy reported several observations regarding filterable agents. They noted that "association of a foreign body with the filtrate" makes it more likely that tumors will be produced. Diatomaceous earth "elicits … an intense reactive connective tissue proliferation with the formation of giant cells." They noted that secondary growths have themselves yielded a filterable agent that in turn caused tumors. Finally, they reported that the filterable agent not only resists drying, but also gylcerination, freezing, and thawing *(136)*.

Other important articles published by Rous and his group prior to 1932 include a report on the production of antisera to a filterable agent in geese *(137)*, and the report that two types of chicken tumors upon transplantation may give rise to neoplasms of identical character. The postulate is made that tumors of various character may be caused by the same agent *(138)*.

C. H. Andrewes

Another important early researcher in the field of filterable tumor agents was C. H. Andrewes. In 1926 he and Gye reported on the filterability of the Rous fowl sarcoma I virus. They concluded that the virus is indeed filterable, but variably so *(139)*.

Andrewes' next article was a much more important one, in which he reported that six fowls bearing a slowly growing fibrosarcoma, termed "MH1," had been found to possess neutralizing properties in their serum against filtrates of the Rous sarcoma 1 virus. These sera also neutralized filtrates of fowl endothelioma MH2. Andrewes concluded with the following statement:

> There thus appears to be a close immunological relationship between three histologically distinct filterable fowl tumors; presumably they have some antigen in common. Moreover interaction between an antibody and this antigen renders the virus unable to attack the cells and thus give rise to a tumour. One may therefore assume either that the antigen is the virus itself or a part of it or else is an indispensable weapon in its armamentarium. *(140)*

He noted in a follow-up article that "potent antisera were not found in fowls which had borne tumours for less than five months" *(141)*.

In 1932 Andrewes also reported the successful transmission to pheasants of three fowl sarcomata, including the Rous chicken tumor 1, thus demonstrating that the virus could transmit disease from one avian species to another *(142)*. As a matter of fact, the species barrier in tumor virus studies had already been broken by Fujinami and Suzue in 1928, who succeeded in growing a highly malignant strain of chicken myxoma in ducklings, and after 40 generations in ducklings, returning the tumor to chickens *(143)*. Andrewes used this virulent filtrate as one of the three that he subsequently transferred to pheasants.

Richard Shope and Filtrate-Induced Mammalian Tumors

Richard Shope was the first, in 1932, to report a filtrate-induced mammalian tumor *(144,145)*. He concluded the second in a pair of articles on the subject with the following statement:

> The properties of the tumor-producing agent described in this and the preceding paper are all of the group generally considered characteristic of a filtrable virus. The failure to cultivate any organisms from the tumors or to see them in stained sections, together with the tumor-producing agent's resistance to glycerol, its ready filtrability, the type of immunity it induces, its relative host specificity, its production of cytoplasmic inclusions in the epithelial cells of one of its susceptible hosts, and its apparent tropism for one type of tissue, considered collectively, suffice to place it in the general group of filtrable viruses. *(146)*

This discovery was of seminal importance in engendering interest in the field among researchers in the medical profession, most of whom had previously considered the avian tumor inducers of Rous et al. merely interesting curiosities. For those studying mammalian tumors who did not wish to address the issue of an infectious etiology of cancer (still a less than credible topic for many) it must have been reassuring to know that such things as filterable oncogenic agents had been reported only in the field of avian research. Indeed, one commentator on the subject must not have been aware of Shope's work of a year before when he stated, in 1933,

"(T)ransmission of tumours by cell-free extracts … has been observed only in birds and especially in fowls … In discussing the mammalian tumours we have come to the conclusion that (the change in the cell which constitutes malignancy) must be a purely cellular one, not due to an extraneous agent… *(147)*

In 1933 Shope issued another report on the rabbit papilloma *(148)*. This tumor was to become the subject of intense study in the years to follow. The agent responsible was eventually found to be a DNA virus, subsequently labeled "papillomavirus" *(149)*.

The year 1933 was notable also for a report by Furth presenting evidence that the same filterable agent could at different times cause chicken lymphomatosis, myelocytomatosis, or endothelioma *(150)*. Subsequently, other investigators reported similar findings. The underlying reasons for these variations were not to be unraveled until the 1960s, with Rubin's discovery of resistance-inducing factor and Rous-associated virus, and their role as "helpers" of the Rous sarcoma virus *(151)*.

Controversy Surrounding the Nature of the Tumor Agent

Researchers studying filterable tumor transmission used the term "virus" to define what their filtrates did *not* contain: it was not a tumor cell, and it was not a bacteria. What was contained in the filtrate, no one knew. In an important review article on the subject of transmissible fowl tumors, Claude and Murphy discussed the controversy surrounding the nature of the transmissible entity. They started their discussion with the statement:

> (T)he nature of the transmitting agent or agents remains as yet unsettled. The general tendency has been to class them among the filterable viruses. Unfortunately the so-called filterable virus group has been used to a considerable extent for the indiscriminate segregation of disease-producing agents of unknown nature, having in common principally their sub-microscopic size and the fact that they appear to be obligatory parasites of living cells.
> …But it is not easy to expand the theory to explain the variety of types of chicken tumors, each with an agent, not only limited in its action to a definite cell type but after forming its contact with the cell, causing it to grow and differentiate into a specialized type … This has been the principal argument against the virus theory for tumors. *(152)*

The authors further stated that they believe tumor agents to be some sort of "simple substances which belong to the field of biochemistry rather than to that of bacteriology" *(153)*. Until the agents could be further studied biochemically and visualized with the electron microscope, the questions and controversy regarding their ultimate structure and nature would continue.

Notable Viral Research, 1934–1936

Rous' first report of his work with the Shope papilloma was published in 1934. He had given up work on fowl viruses several years before, probably because of the slow acceptance of his research by those who were sure that cancer could not be caused by an infectious agent. Also, he had worked with a "very unfashionable laboratory animal—the chicken" *(154)*. Rous recognized that Shope's discovery not only lended support to his own earlier work, but also provided an animal model much closer phylogenetically to the human species.

In the first of their two initial articles on the Shope virus, Beard and Rous confirmed the malignant potential of the tumor, and noted that the virus is recoverable from the tissue. They also noted that papillomas of the skin are transmittable through virus inoculation, and that these growths "proliferate actively as a rule and frequently cause death" *(155)*.

In their second article on the subject, Beard and Rous reported that injection of a chemical solution of Scharlach R into the skin about a papilloma results in malignant invasion of underlying tissues *(156)*. In a pair of articles the following year, they also reported that the skin papillomas may develop into carcinomas spontaneously *(157,158)*. Shope contributed his own article on the subject the same year, reporting the successful transmission of the virus serially in domestic rabbits *(159)*.

The year 1935 was noteworthy for reports of concentration of avian tumor virus, both the Rous tumor 1 and the Fujinami myxosarcoma, through the use of high-speed centrifuges *(160,161)*. Isolation was confirmed by the disappearance of infectivity of the supernatant and increased infectivity of the centrifuged fraction.

Also in 1935, Rous, McMaster, and Hudack carried out a series of experiments on the interactions between viruses and cells, using vaccinia and the Shope fibroma virus. They used the infectious potential of cell suspensions exposed to virus to determine whether or not the viruses were still present therein. Their conclusion was that "the viruses became fixed on both living and dead cells, and were carried through the washings with them. When now the living cells were exposed to immune serum such virus as they carried was not in the least affected, whereas that associated with killed cells underwent neutralization," Based on these conclusions, the further supposition was made that viruses exposed to living cells "owe their persistence … to an intracellular situation" *(162)*.

In 1936 Rous and colleagues authored a pair of articles on the nature of induced immunity to the papilloma agent. In the first of these articles they reported that whereas the serum of normal domestic rabbits is devoid of viral neutralizing influence, that of animals carrying the papilloma usually exhibits neutralizing power soon after the lesions appear. Although having no influence on established lesions, successful reinoculation is prevented *(163)*.

In the second article Kidd, Beard, and Rous reported that the serum of a rabbit with large lesions resulting from the transplantation of a squamous cell carcinoma that had arisen from a virus-induced papilloma possessed the power to neutralize the virus, whereas the sera of rabbits carrying tar papillomas or the Brown-Pearce carcinoma did not *(164)*. This implied that previous exposure to the tumor virus was necessary to produce neutralizing material in the serum of the tumor host.

In retrospect, one of the most important publications to appear in 1936 was a short one-page article by John Bittner of the Jackson Memorial Laboratory, in which he reports that the incidence of mammary gland tumors in mice is influenced by nursing *(165)*. For the next 20 yr, in a series of more than 40 articles, Bittner and colleagues were to report this phenomenon in great detail, demonstrating the carcinogenic virus of mouse milk *(166)*. (*See also* Chapter 27.)

The next milestone in the history of tumor virology came in 1938 with Balduin Lucké's report of the viral etiology of the frog renal adenocarcinoma *(167)*. Lucké had actually begun work on this malignancy in 1934 *(168)*, but only reported its viral etiology 4 yr later. He found that desiccated and glycerinated tumor tissue injected into the abdomen gave rise to the tumor in a manner similar to inoculation with living tumor. Lucké had initially suspected a viral etiology for this tumor when he discovered that inclusion bodies were present within the tumor cells. His studies on the frog tumor model were to continue well into the 1950s *(169)*.

Poor Reception of Early Efforts in Tumor Virology

A tremendous bias existed at the turn of the century against any notion of an infectious process as a possible cause for cancer. In the words of Gross:

> (I)t is very difficult to suspect the infectious origin of an obscure disease if the contagious nature of the disease is not apparent, if an infectious agent cannot be detected by microscopic … examination of the diseased tissue, and if the disease cannot be transmitted experimentally by inoculation. *(170)*

After the many decades of fruitless efforts to demonstrate an infectious etiology of cancer, researchers were understandably wary, and when positive data finally did surface, in the form of the viral studies outlined previously, it was almost universally ignored. Thus, one textbook author of the period refers to the "wide-spread delusion that contagion is a possible factor in the development of cancer" *(171)*. Another, writing in 1935, seemed blissfully unaware of the work on tumor viruses that had been going on for over 20 yr: "Up to the present time, … no specific microorganismal agent has been discovered (as a cause for cancer), and the greater number of investigators have come to the conclusion that carcinoma is not an infectious disease" *(172)*.

Of course, the investigators themselves acknowledged the fact that cancer was not observed to be an infectious disease. Both Rous and Andrewes mentioned the cancer house concept of the turn of the century, which by now engendered only scorn, as an example of a false lead in this direction *(173,174)*.

Also, the nature of the investigations themselves led to skepticism. During these early years, in the words of a later investigator in the field, "virologists were considered the pariahs of oncological research" *(175)*.

It took many years to prove to the satisfaction of the academic community that filtrate-induced tumors did indeed represent true malignancies. What is more, viruses could not be seen, and remained essentially unidentified. Until they could be better typified there would be disbelief, and such typification was not to occur until later in the century, with improvement of tissue culture techniques and a sufficient maturation of the fields of immunology and molecular biology.

As late as 1950, a large number of pathologists and virologists refused to believe that viruses could cause malignancy *(176)*. Peyton Rous was not awarded the Nobel Prize for his tumor virus research until 1966 (Fig. 2), a full 55 yr after the publication of his most important article on the subject *(177)!*

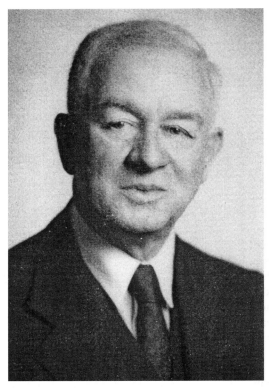

Fig. 2. Peyton Rous. (Reprinted from ref. *118,* with permission.)

REFERENCES

1. Wolff J. The Science of Cancerous Disease from Earliest Times to the Present. New Delhi: Amerind, 1989, p. 433.
2. Rather LJ. The Genesis of Cancer: A Study in the History of Ideas. Baltimore: The Johns Hopkins University Press, 1978.
3. Wolff J. The Science of Cancerous Disease from Earliest Times to the Present. New Delhi: Amerind, 1989.
4. Reedy J. Galen on Cancer and Related Diseases. Clio Medica 1975; 10:227–238.
5. Boerhaave H. Of cancers. In: Delacoste J (ed) Boerhaave's aphorisms: Concerning the Knowledge and Cure of Diseases. Birmingham: The Classics of Medicine Library, 1986, p. 113 (Original publication date 1715).
6. Aitken J. Elements of the Theory and Practice of Physic and Surgery, Vol. II. London: [No publisher given], 1782: 425–426.
7. Buchan W. Domestic Medicine. Leith: A Allardice, 1816, p. 356.
8. Thomas R. The Modern Practice of Physic. New York: Collins, 1815, p. 609.
9. Pearson J. Practical Observations on Cancerous Complaints. London: J Johnson, St. Paul's Church-yard, 1793, p. 6.
10. Ibid, p. 9.
11. Ibid, p. 3 (misnumbered 4 in original text).
12. Ibid, p. 6.
13. Wood G. A Treatise on the Practice of Medicine, Vol. I. Philadelphia: JB Lippincott, 1858, p. 133.

14. Watson T. Lectures on the Principles and Practice of Physic. Philadelphia: Blanchard and Lea, 1851, p. 138.
15. Webster N. An American Dictionary of the English Language. Springfield: George and Charles Merriam, 1848, p. 500.
16. Wood G. A Treatise on the Practice of Medicine, Vol. I. Philadelphia: JB Lippincott, 1858, p. 132.
17. Bell J. On malignant disease. In: Braithwaite W (ed). The Retrospect of Medicine 1857; 35:447–450.
18. De Morgan C. On the use of chloride of zinc in surgical operations and injuries. In: Braithwaite W (ed). The Retrospect of Medicine 1866; 53:147–164.
19. De Morgan C. On cancer. In: Braithwaite W (ed). The Retrospect of Medicine 1874; 64:34–39.
20. Billroth T. General Surgical Pathology and Therapeutics. New York: D Appleton and Company, 1871, p. 553.
21. Virchow R. Cellular Pathology. London: John Churchill, 1860, p. 218.
22. Ibid, p. 219.
23. Hooper R. A Compendious Medical Dictionary. Newburyport: Wm Sawyer, 1809, p. 142.
24. Rather LJ. The Genesis of Cancer: A Study in the History of Ideas. Baltimore: The Johns Hopkins University Press, 1978, p. 151.
25. Osler W. The Evolution of Modern Medicine. New York: Arno Press, 1972, p. 135.
26. Willis T. The London Practice of Physick. New York: The Classics of Medicine Library, 1992, p. 520 (Original publication date 1685).
27. Rather LJ. The Genesis of Cancer: A Study in the History of Ideas. Baltimore: The Johns Hopkins University Press, 1978, p. 30.
28. Ibid, p. 39.
29. Ibid, p. 40.
30. Osler W. The Evolution of Modern Medicine. New York: Arno Press, 1972, p. 183.
31. Swan J (ed). The Entire Works of Dr. Thomas Sydenham. London: E Cave, 1753.
32. Morgagni JB. The Seats and Cause of Diseases. London: A Millar, 1769.
33. Buchan W. Domestic Medicine. Leith: A Allardice, 1816, pp. 356–357.
34. Boerhaave H. Of cancers. In: Delacoste J (ed). Boerhaave's Aphorisms: Concerning the Knowledge and Cure of Diseases. Birmingham: The Classics of Medicine Library, 1986, pp. 113–114 (Original publication date 1715).
35. Reedy J. Galen on cancer and related diseases. Clio Medica 1975; 10:227–238.
36. Lowe P. The Whole Course of Chirurgerie. Birmingham: The Classics of Medicine Library, 1981 [unnumbered page, first page of Chapter 8]. (Original publication date 1597).
37. Pott P. The Chirurgical Works, Vol. II. London: James Williams, 1778, pp. 403–406.
38. Thomas R. The Modern Practice of Physic. New York: Collins, 1815, pp. 609–610.
39. Rather LJ. The Genesis of Cancer: A Study in the History of Ideas. Baltimore: The Johns Hopkins University Press, 1978, p. 62.
40. Bichat X. A Treatise on the Membranes. Boston: Cummings and Hilliard, 1813.
41. Rather LJ. The Genesis of Cancer: A Study in the History of Ideas. Baltimore: The Johns Hopkins University Press, 1978, p. 83.
42. Ibid, p. 84.
43. Müller J. On the finer structure and the forms of morbid tumors. In: Rather LJ, Rather P, Frerichs JB (eds). Johannes Müller and the Nineteenth-Century Origins of Tumor Cell Theory. Canton MA: Science History Publications, 1986, p. 56.
44. Rather LJ, Rather P, Frerichs JB (eds). Johannes Müller and the Nineteenth-Century Origins of Tumor Cell Theory. Canton MA: Science History Publications, 1986, p. 4.
45. Southam G. On the nature and treatment of cancer. In: Braithwaite W (ed). The Retrospect of Medicine 1858; 37:9–15.

46. Flint A. A Treatise on the Principles and Practice of Medicine. Philadelphia: Henry C Lea, 1868, pp. 43–45.
47. Watson T. Lectures on the Principles and Practice of Physic. Philadelphia: Blanchard and Lea, 1851, p. 138.
48. Laennec RTH. A Treatise on the Diseases of the Chest and on Mediate Auscultation. Philadelphia: Desilver, Thomas, 1835, pp. 362–367.
49. Watson T. Lectures on the Principles and Practice of Physic. Philadelphia: Blanchard and Lea, 1851, p. 138.
50. Richmond PA. American attitudes toward the germ theory of disease (1860–1880). Hist Med 1954; 9:428–454.
51. King LS. Transformations in American Medicine from Benjamin Rush to William Osler. Baltimore: The Johns Hopkins University Press, 1991, pp. 70–72.
52. Bartlett E. The History, Diagnosis, and Treatment of the Fevers of the United States. Philadelphia: Lea and Blanchard, 1847, p. 347.
53. Gregory G. Treatise on the Theory and Practice of Physic, Vol. I. Philadelphia: Towar & Hogan, 1826, p. 119.
54. Rush B. Medical Inquiries and Observations, Vols. III and IV. New York: Arno Press, 1972, III: p. 217.
55. Gallup JA. Sketches of Epidemic Diseases in the State of Vermont. Boston: TB Wait & Sons, 1815, p. 86, 87.
56. Cullen W. First Lines of the Practice of Physic. Edinburgh: C Elliot, 1784, p. 78.
57. Ibid, p. 86.
58. Armstrong J., (Leland PW [ed]). Practical illustrations of typhus and other fevers. Boston: Timothy Bedlington, 1829, p. 1.
59. Brieger GH. Editor's Note. In: Brieger GH (ed). Medical America in the Nineteenth Century. Baltimore: The Johns Hopkins Press, 1972, p. 278.
60. Stokes W. Lectures on the Theory and Practice of Physic. Philadelphia: Haswell, Barrington, and Haswell, 1840, pp. 428–429.
61. Pearson J. Practical Observations on Cancerous Complaints. London: J. Johnson, St. Paul's Church-yard, 1793, p. 20.
62. Ibid, p. 22, 23.
63. Ibid, p. 30.
64. Thomas R. The Modern Practice of Physic. New York: Collins, 1815, p. 610.
65. Adams J. Observations on Morbid Poisons, Phagedaena, and Cancer. London: J Johnson, 1795, pp. 173–174.
66. Wood G. A Treatise on the Practice of Medicine, Vol. I. Philadelphia: JB Lippincott, 1858, p. 133.
67. Watson T. Lectures on the Principles and Practice of Physic. Philadelphia: Blanchard and Lea, 1851, p. 140.
68. Wood G. A Treatise on the Practice of Medicine, Vol. I. Philadelphia: JB Lippincott, 1858, p. 133.
69. Bynum WF. Science and Practice of Medicine in the Nineteenth Century. Cambridge University Press, 1996, p. 128.
70. Gibson W. Institutes and Practice of Surgery, Vol. I. Philadelphia: James Kay, Jun and Brother, 1845, p.164.
71. Watson T. Lectures on the Principles and Practice of Physic. Philadelphia: Blanchard and Lea, 1851, p. 140.
72. Wolff J. The Science of Cancerous Disease from Earliest Times to the Present. New Delhi: Amerind, 1989, p. 445.
73. Billroth T. General Surgical Pathology and Therapeutics. New York: D Appleton, 1871, p. 551.
74. Watson T. Lectures on the Principles and Practice of Physic. Philadelphia: Blanchard and Lea, 1851, p. 93.

75. Long ER. A History of Pathology. New York: Dover Publications, 1965, p. 122.
76. Rather LJ. The Genesis of Cancer: A Study in the History of Ideas. Baltimore: The Johns Hopkins University Press, 1978, p. 101.
77. Rather LJ. Addison and the White Corpuscles: An Aspect of Nineteenth-Century Biology. London: Wellcome Institute of the History of Medicine, 1972, p. 125.
78. Virchow R. Cellular Pathology. London: John Churchill, 1860, p. 15.
79. Rather LJ. The Genesis of Cancer: A Study in the History of Ideas. Baltimore: The Johns Hopkins University Press, 1978, p. 124.
80. Virchow R. Cellular Pathology. London: John Churchill, 1860, p. 454.
81. Ibid, p. 478.
82. Rather LJ. The Genesis of Cancer: A Study in the History of Ideas. Baltimore: The Johns Hopkins University Press, 1978, pp. 138–139.
83. Ibid, p. 153.
84. Eyler JM. Victorian Social Medicine: The ideas and methods of William Farr. Baltimore: The Johns Hopkins University Press, 1979, p. 97.
85. Ibid, p. 100.
86. Ibid, p. 103.
87. Barnard FAP. The Germ Theory and Its Relations to Hygiene. In: Brieger GH (ed). Medical America in the Nineteenth Century. Baltimore: The Johns Hopkins Press, 1972, p. 281.
88. Eyler JM. Victorian Social Medicine: The ideas and methods of William Farr. Baltimore: The Johns Hopkins University Press, 1979, p. 104.
89. Bynum WF. Science and Practice of Medicine in the Nineteenth Century. Cambridge University Press, 1996, p. 127.
90. Barnard FAP. The germ Theory and Its Relations to Hygiene. In: Brieger GH (ed). Medical America in the Nineteenth Century. Baltimore: The Johns Hopkins Press, 1972, p. 287.
91. Bynum WF. Science and Practice of Medicine in the Nineteenth Century. Cambridge University Press, 1996, pp. 129–130.
92. Eyler JM. Victorian Social Medicine: The Ideas and Methods of William Farr. Baltimore: The Johns Hopkins University Press, 1979, pp. 105–107.
93. Wolff J. The Science of Cancerous Disease from Earliest Times to the Present. New Delhi: Amerind, 1989, pp. 453–458.
94. Rather LJ. The Genesis of Cancer: A Study in the History of Ideas. Baltimore: The Johns Hopkins University Press, 1978, p. 166.
95. Shattock SG. Abstract of the Morton lecture on cancer. Lancet 1894; 1:1231–1233.
96. Wolff J. The Science of Cancerous Disease from Earliest Times to the Present. New Delhi: Amerind, 1989, pp. 445–562.
97. Haviland A. "Cancer houses." Lancet 1895; 1:1049.
98. Power D. The local distribution of cancer and cancer houses. Practitioner 1899; 62:418–429.
99. Power D. Cancer houses and their victims. Br Med J 1894; 1:1240.
100. Power D. The local distribution of cancer and cancer houses. Practitioner 1899; 62:422.
101. Haviland A. "Cancer houses." Lancet 1895; 1:1050.
102. Nash WG. Cancer houses. Lancet 1914; 1:1149.
103. Borrel A, Gastinel P, Gorescu C. Acariens et cancer. Ann de l'Inst. Pasteur 1909; 23:7–124.
104. Ibid, p. 7.
105. Wood FC. Cancer. In: Herrick WW (ed). Nelson Loose-Leaf Living Medicine, Vol. III. New York: Thomas Nelson & Sons, 1928, p. 165.
106. Strümpell A. A Text-Book of Medicine for Students and Practitioners, Vol. I. New York: D Appleton, 1911, p. 544.
107. Stiles CW. Distomatosis-trematode or fluke infections. In: Osler W, McCrae T (eds). Modern Medicine: Its Theory and Practice, Vol. I. Philadelphia: Lea Brothers, 1907, p. 543.

108. Diamandopoulos GTH. Cancer: an historical perspective. Anticancer Res 1996; 16:1595–1602.

109. Bickers DR. Lowy DR. Carcinogenesis: a fifty-year historical perspective. J Invest Dermatol 1989; 92 (4 Suppl):123S.

110. Garrison FH. An Introduction to the History of Medicine. Philadelphia: WB Saunders, 1929, p. 723.

111. Bickers Dr. Lowy Dr. Carcinogenesis: a fifty-year historical perspective. J Invest Dermatol 1989 (4 Suppl): 1215–1315.

112. Garrison FH. An Introduction to the History of Medicine. Philadelphia: WB Saunders, 1929, p. 721.

113. Diamandopoulos GTH. Cancer: an historical perspective. Anticancer Res 1996; 16:1600.

114. Andrewes CH. Viruses in relation to the aetiology of tumours. Lancet 1934; 2:117–123.

115. Virchow R. Cellular Pathology. London: John Churchill, 1860, p. 306.

116. Bateson W. Mendel's Principles of Heredity. Cambridge University Press, 1909, p. 270.

117. Lewis WH. Normal and malignant cells. Science 1935; 81:545–553.

118. Gross L. Oncogenic Viruses. Oxford: Pergamon Press, 1970, p. 2.

119. Ibid, p. 3.

120. Webster N. An American Dictionary of the English Language. Springfield: George and Charles Merriam, 1848, p. 1238.

121. Borrel A. Épithélioma de la souris. Ann de l'Inst. Pasteur 1903; 17:112–118.

122. Le Guyon R. Borrel et la théorie virusale des cancers. Bull Acad Natl Med 1967; 151:585–593.

123. Ibid, p. 586.

124. Borrel A. Parasitisme et tumeurs. Ann de l'Inst. Pasteur 1910; 24:778–787.

125. Borrel A. Épithélioma de la souris. Ann de l'Inst. Pasteur 1903; 17:112–118.

126. Gross L. Oncogenic Viruses. Oxford: Pergamon Press, 1970, p. 8.

127. Ellermann V, Bang O. Experimentelle Laukämie bei Hühnern. Zent Bakt Parasit 1908; 46:595–609.

128. Rous P. A transmissible avian neoplasm. (Sarcoma of the common fowl.) J Exp Med 1910; 12:696–708.

129. Rous P. A sarcoma of the fowl transmissible by an agent separable from the tumor cells. Exp Med 1911; 13:397–411.

130. Ibid, p. 399.

131. Ibid, p. 409.

132. Tytler WH. A transplantable new growth of the fowl, producing cartilage and bone. J Exp Med 1913; 17:466–480.

133. Rous P, Lange B. The characteristics of a third transplantable chicken tumor due to a filterable cause. A sarcoma of intracanalicular pattern. J Exp Med 1913; 18:651–664.

134. Ibid, p. 660.

135. Rous P. Resistance to a tumor-producing agent as distinct from resistance to the implanted tumor cells. J Exp Med 1913; 18:416–427.

136. Rous P, Murphy JB. On the causation by filterable agents of three distinct chicken tumors. J Exp Med 1914; 19:52–69.

137. Rous P, Robertson OH, Oliver J. Experiments on the production of specific antisera for infections of unknown cause. J Exp Med 1919; 29:305–320.

138. Rous P. On certain spontaneous chicken tumors as manifestations of a single disease. J Exp Med 1914; 19:570–576.

139. Gye WE, Andrewes CH. A study of the Rous fowl sarcoma No. 1: I. Filterability. Br J Exp Pathol 1926; 7:81–87.

140. Andrewes CH. The immunological relationships of fowl tumours with different histological structure. J Pathol Bacteriol 1931; 34:91–107.

141. Andrewes CH. Some properties of immune sera active against fowl-tumour viruses. J Pathol Bacteriol 1932; 35:243–249.

142. Andrewes CH. The transmission of fowl-tumours to pheasants. J Pathol Bacteriol 1932; 35:407–413.

143. Fujinami A, Suzue K. Contribution to the pathology of tumor growth. Experiments in the growth of chicken sarcoma in the case of heterotransplantation. Trans Jpn Pathol Soc 1928; 18:616–622.

144. Shope RE. A transmissible tumor-like condition in rabbits. J Exp Med 1932; 56:793–802.

145. Shope RE. A filtrable virus causing a tumor-like condition in rabbits and its relationship to virus myxomatosum. J Exp Med 1932; 56:803–822.

146. Ibid, p. 817.

147. Cramer W. Discussion on tumours. Proc R Soc Ser B 1933; 113:280.

148. Shope RE. Infectious papillomatosis of rabbits. J Exp Med 1933; 58:607–624.

149. Wold WS, Green M. Historic milestones in cancer virology. Semin Oncol 1979; 6:461–478.

150. Furth J. Lymphomatosis, myelomatosis, and endothelioma of chickens caused by a filterable agent. I. Transmission experiments. J Exp Med 1933; 58:253–275.

151. Burmester BR, Purchase HG. The history of avian medicine in the United States V. Insights into avian tumor virus research. Avian Dis 1979; 23:1–29.

152. Claude A, Murphy JB. Transmissible tumors of the fowl. Physiol Rev 1933; 13:246–275.

153. Ibid, p. 259.

154. Editor. Introduction. Classics in oncology: Peyton Rous (1879–1970). CA Cancer J Clin 1972; 22:21–22.

155. Rous P, Beard JW. A virus-induced mammalian growth with the characters of a tumor (the Shope rabbit papilloma). I. The growth on implantation within favorable hosts. J Exp Med 1934; 60:701–722.

156. Beard JW, Rous P. A virus-induced mammalian growth with the characters of a tumor (the Shope rabbit papilloma). II. Experimental alterations of the growth on the skin: morphological considerations: the phenomena of retrogression. J Exp Med 1934; 80:723–740.

157. Rous P, Beard JW. Carcinomatous changes in virus-induced papillomas of the skin of the rabbit. Proc Soc Exp Biol Med 1935; 32:578–580.

158. Rous P, Beard JW. The progression to carcinoma of virus-induced rabbit papillomas (Shope). J Exp Med 1935; 62:523–548.

159. Shope RE. Serial transmission of virus of infectious papillomatosis in domestic rabbits. Proc Soc Exp Biol Med 1935; 32:830–832.

160. McIntosh J. The sedimentation of the virus of Rous sarcoma and the bacteriophage by a high-speed centrifuge. Proc Pathol Soc Great Br Irel 1935; 41:215–217.

161. Ledingham JCG, Gye WE. On the nature of the filterable tumour-exciting agent in avian sarcomata. Lancet 1935; 1:376–377.

162. Rous P, McMaster PD, Hudack SS. The fixation and protection of viruses by the cells of susceptible animals. J Exp Med 1935; 61:657–688.

163. Kidd JG, Beard JW, Rous P. Serological reactions with a virus causing rabbit papillomas which become cancerous I. Tests of the blood of animals carrying the papilloma. J Exp Med 1936; 64:63–77.

164. Kidd JG, Beard JW, Rous P. Serological reactions with a virus causing rabbit papillomas which become cancerous II. Tests of the blood of animals carrying various epithelial tumors. J Exp Med 1936; 64:79–96.

165. Bittner JJ. Some possible effects of nursing on the mammary gland tumor incidence in mice. Science 1936; 84:162.

166. Gross L. Oncogenic Viruses. Oxford: Pergamon Press, 1970, pp. 238–280.

167. Lucké B. Carcinoma in the leopard frog: its probable causation by a virus. J Exp Med 1938; 68:457–468.

168. Lucké B. A neoplastic disease of the kidney of the frog, *Rana pipiens*. Am J Cancer 1934; 20:352–379.
169. Gross L. Oncogenic Viruses. Oxford: Pergamon Press, 1970, pp. 82–98.
170. Gross L. Viral etiology of cancer and leukemia: a look into the past, present, and future—GHA Clowes memorial lecture. Cancer Res 1978; 38:485–493.
171. Wood FC. Cancer. In: Herrick WW (ed). Nelson Loose-Leaf Living Medicine, Vol. III. New York: Thomas Nelson, 1928, p. 164.
172. McFarland J. Cancer. In: Piersol GM (ed). The Cyclopedia of Medicine, Vol. III. Philadelphia: F. A. Davis, 1935, p. 75.
173. Rous P. The virus tumors and the tumor problem. Harvey Lect 1935; 31:74–115.
174. Andrewes CH. Viruses in relation to the aetiology of tumours. Lancet 1934; 2:117–123.
175. Friend C. The coming of age of tumor virology: Presidential address. Cancer Res 1977; 37:1255–1263.
176. Ibid
177. F. J. C. R. Francis Peyton Rous. Lancet 1970; 1:477.

II
Herpesviruses

2

Overview of Herpesviruses

Frank J. Jenkins and Linda J. Hoffman

INTRODUCTION TO HERPESVIRUSES

What is a Herpesvirus?

Identification of a virus in the family *Herpesviridae* is based on the morphology of the virus particle. Viewed through an electron microscope, the virions of different members of the *Herpesviridae* family are indistinguishable and consist of four distinct components: the core, capsid, tegument, and envelope (Fig. 1) *(1)*. The core contains a double-stranded DNA genome arranged in an unusual torus shape that is located inside an icosadeltahedral capsid that is approx 100 nm in size and contains 162 capsomeres *(2)*. Located between the capsid and the viral envelope is an amorphous structure termed the tegument that contains numerous proteins. The tegument structure is generally asymmetrical, although some virus members (such as human herpesvirus 6 [HHV-6] and human herpesvirus 7 [HHV-7]) have been shown to have well-defined tegument structures *(3,4)*. Presumably, the tegument is responsible for connecting the capsid to the envelope and acting as a reservoir for viral proteins that are required during the initial stages of viral infection *(5,6)*. The outermost structure of the herpes virion is the envelope, which is derived from cell nuclear membranes and contains several viral glycoproteins. The size of mature herpesviruses ranges from 120 to 300 nm owing to differences in the size of the individual viral teguments *(1)*.

The life cycle of all herpesviruses in their natural host can be divided into lytic (resulting in the production of infectious progeny) and latent (dormant) infections. During a lytic infection the virus is replicated and newly synthesized particles are released into the surrounding medium. During a latent infection viral replication is suppressed, resulting in the formation of a quiescent state. The establishment of viral latency is a hallmark of all known herpesviruses. As described below, the sites of lytic and latent infections differ among the various members of the human herpesvirus family.

Herpesvirus Subfamilies

The Herpesvirus Study Group of the International Committee on the Taxonomy of Viruses *(7)* has divided the herpesviruses into three subfamilies, termed alphaherpesvirinae, betaherpesvirinae, and gammaherpesvirinae (Table 1). Membership into a

From: *Infectious Causes of Cancer: Targets for Intervention*
Edited by: J. J. Goedert © Humana Press Inc., Totowa, NJ

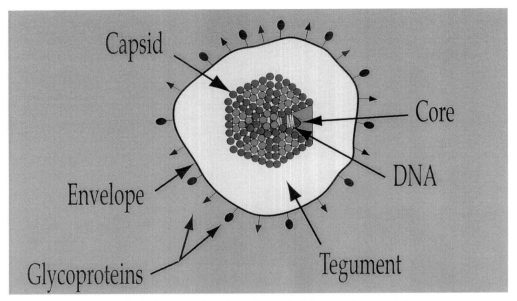

Fig. 1. Schematic drawing of a typical herpesvirus particle.

Table 1
Subfamily Membership of the Human Herpesviruses

Alphaherpesvirinae	Betaherpesvirinae	Gammaherpesvirinae
HSV-1	CMV	EBV
HSV-2	HHV-6	HHV-8
VZV	HHV-7	

particular subfamily is based on biologic and genetic properties (demonstrated in Fig. 2) and has been useful in predicting the properties of newly discovered isolates (such as HHV-6, HHV-7, and human herpesvirus 8 [HHV-8]). The alphaherpesvirinae are characterized by a variable host range, a short replicative cycle in the host, rapid growth and spread in cell culture, and the establishment of latent infections in sensory ganglia *(7)*. Members of this subfamily are often referred to as neurotropic herpesviruses. Among the human herpesviruses, herpes simplex virus 1 (HSV-1), herpes simplex virus 2 (HSV-2), and varicella-zoster virus (VZV) belong to the alphaherpesvirinae. The betaherpesvirinae are characterized by a fairly restricted host range with a long reproductive cycle in cell culture and in the infected host, which often results in the development of a carrier state. Latency is established in lymphocytes, secretory glands, and cells of the kidney as well as other cell types *(8)*. The human herpesviruses cytomegalovirus (CMV), HHV-6, and HHV-7 are members of this subfamily. The gammaherpesvirinae are characterized by a restricted host range with replication and latency occurring in lymphoid tissues, although some members have

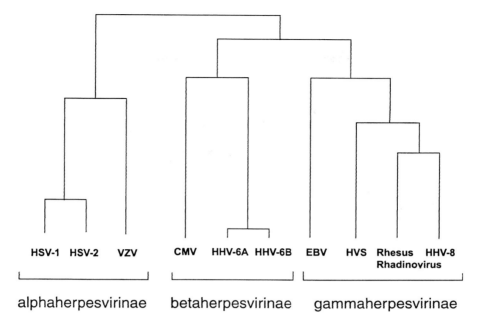

Fig. 2. Genetic relatedness of different herpesviruses. The genetic relationship between different herpesviruses was determined by analysis of the predicted amino acid sequence of the glycoprotein B homolog from each virus. Analysis was performed using the program Pileup from the GCG Sequence Analysis Program.

demonstrated lytic growth in epithelial, endothelial and fibroblastic cells *(7,9)*. Among the lymphoblastic cells, viral replication is generally restricted to either T or B cells. The gammaherpesvirinae subfamily is further divided into two genera, *Lymphocryptovirus* and *Rhadinovirus*. Among the human herpesviruses, Epstein–Barr virus (EBV) is a member of the *Lymphocryptovirus* genus while the newly discovered HHV-8 is a member of the *Rhadinovirus* genus *(10,11)*.

Animal Herpesviruses

Herpesviruses have been found in almost all animal species. Besides the human herpesviruses mentioned previously, herpesviruses have also been identified in nonhuman primates, cattle, horses, pigs, sheep, goats, wildebeests, deer, reindeer, dogs, guinea pigs, hamsters, elephants, cats, mice, harbor seals, shrews, birds, amphibians, reptiles and fish. There are well over 100 different herpesviruses identified to date (reviewed by Roizman and Sears *[1]*). These herpesviruses cause a variety of diseases ranging from inapparent infections to death. In addition, a number of them such as pseudorabies virus in pigs and Marek's disease virus in chickens represent serious threats to agriculture.

Most of the nonhuman herpesviruses can be classified into one of the three subfamilies described earlier. A notable exception is a recently described herpesvirus of elephants *(12)*. Richman and co-workers *(12)* described the detection of a novel herpesvirus of elephants that appears to be responsible for a highly fatal disease among perinatal Asian and African elephants. Separate but highly related strains were isolated from African and Asian elephants that had died from this disease, which was characterized by a sudden onset, edema in the skin of the head and proboscis, cyanosis of the tongue, decreased levels of white blood cells and platelets, and internal hemorrhages. Histologically, basophilic intranuclear inclusion bodies were detected in vascular cells of the heart, liver, and tongue. Death was found to be due to myocardial failure from capillary injury and leakage. Identification of the causative agent as a herpesvirus was based on electron micrographs of viral capsids from infected organs. Sequence analysis of two viral genes and comparison of the DNA sequences of these genes with those of known herpesviruses (representing the three herpesvirus subfamilies), revealed that the two elephant-derived strains may represent a new subfamily. Interestingly, the strain isolated from Asian elephants was present in benign papilloma lesions of African elephants. The authors have suggested that the two strains have crossed species (from African to Asian and from Asian to African elephants). As a result, in their natural host, the viruses cause a benign infection, while in the other elephant species, viral infection results in a fatal disease.

ALPHAHERPESVIRUSES

Human Alphaherpesvirus Members and Associated Diseases

Three human herpesviruses belong to the alphaherpesvirus subfamily: HSV-1, HSV-2, and VZV. HSV-1 and HSV-2 belong to the genus simplexvirus, are very closely related at genetic and nucleic acid levels, and produce similar diseases (reviewed by Whitley and Gnann *(13)*). Clinically, both HSV-1 and HSV-2 cause a variety of syndromes ranging from inapparent infections and self-limiting cutaneous lesions to fatal encephalitis. In addition, both viruses establish and maintain a latent state in nerve cells from which recurrent HSV infections arise.

In a primary infection, HSV enters the body through a mucosal membrane or abraded skin and establishes infection locally in epithelial cells. Viral replication in the epithelial cells results in the amplification of virus, the formation of a virus-filled blister, and the elicitation of both cellular and humoral immune responses. The virus then spreads from the site of primary infection by retrograde transport to the nuclei of sensory neurons that innervate the site of the local infection *(14)*. Studies using animal models have indicated that a limited viral replication occurs within these neurons followed by the establishment of latency. A latent HSV infection is characterized by the presence of viral genomes in the nuclei of sensory ganglia neurons and the absence of viral replication or protein production (reviewed by Hill *[15]*).

A latent HSV infection is maintained for the life of the host, but the virus (in some individuals) can be reactivated periodically to produce infectious virus resulting in asymptomatic shedding or recurrent disease. During reactivation, viral replication occurs within the reactivated neuron, and the virus is transported back down the axon, where it can establish an infection in the epithelia of the skin. Studies using both animal models and human subjects have shown that viral reactivation can be triggered by a variety of stressful or stress-related stimuli including heat, ultraviolet light, fever, hormonal changes, menses and surgical trauma to the neuron *(16–19)*. Although the virus appears to be latent most of the time, HSV infection probably is best characterized as reoccurring reactivations divided by periods of latency.

VZV belongs to the genus varicellavirus and is related genetically at the amino acid sequence level to both HSV-1 and HSV-2 *(20)*. VZV gets its name from the two diseases it causes: the childhood disease varicella (more commonly known as chickenpox) and the adult disease herpes zoster (commonly known as shingles). Varicella is the clinical outcome of a primary VZV infection, while herpes zoster is the result of the reactivation of latent VZV. Although HSV can reactivate frequently, VZV generally reactivates only once during the host's lifetime *(21)*.

VZV is considered to be endemic among most populations *(22)*. The majority of varicella cases occur in children younger than 10 of age and can be epidemic among cloistered children, such as schools, nurseries, etc. A VZV infection begins as a result of direct contact with viral lesions or inhalation of airborne droplets. A primary viremia develops that results in the spread of virus to multiple organs, including the spleen and liver *(23)*. A secondary viremia, mediated by lymphocytes, results in the spread of virus to cutaneous epithelial cells and the development of characteristic "chicken pox" lesions. VZV is communicable at least 1–2 d prior to the onset of a rash and during the presence of the virus-infected lesions.

Epidemiology of Alphaherpesvirus Infections

Epidemiologic studies of HSV-1 and HSV-2 based on clinical symptoms alone are inadequate due to the fact that many primary infections are asymptomatic *(13)*. Primary HSV-1 infections occur most often in young children and present clinically as gingivostomatitis. Primary infection is associated with socioeconomic factors such that individuals in lower socioeconomic classes seroconvert at an earlier age when compared to members of higher socioeconimic classes (reviewed by Whitley and Gnann *[13]*). In the United States, the seroprevalence for HSV-1 increases from 20% to 40% in children under the age of 4 to approx 80% among individuals over the age of 60 *(24)*.

The seroprevalence of HSV-2 is lower than that of HSV-1 primarily because its mode of transmission is most often through sexual encounters. Fleming and colleagues *(25)* recently reported that the age-adjusted seroprevalence of HSV-2 in the United States has risen 30% during the last 13 yr to 20.8% or one in five individuals. These rather disturbing results indicate that sexual transmission of HSV-2 has not abated, but has continued to increase to alarming levels.

Varicella zoster virus is fairly ubiquitous in the general population with the majority of individuals seroconverting during childhood *(26)*. With the advent and use of the live attenuated varicella vaccine (LAVV), which is recommended to be given to pre-school-age children, the incidence of VZV infections should diminish. LAVVhas been shown to be quite effective (85–95%) in preventing development of chickenpox *(27,28)*.

Overview of Replication

Our current understanding of the replication cycle of herpesviruses is due to the extensive amount of research performed on HSV-1 replication. For the purposes of this chapter, we use the replication cycle of HSV-1 as our model for herpesvirus replication. HSV replication begins with the enveloped virus particle binding to the outside of a susceptible cell resulting in a fusion between the viral envelope and cellular membrane (Fig. 3). As a result of membrane fusion, the nucleocapsid enters the cell cytoplasm and migrates to the nuclear membrane. The viral genome is released from the

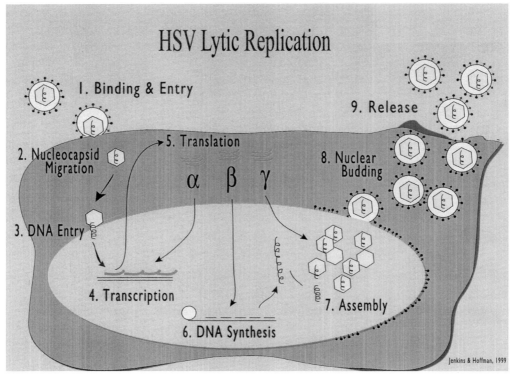

Fig. 3. Schematic of herpes simplex virus replication cycle. **1.** Virus particles bind to specific receptors on cell surface. Fusion occurs between the viral envelope and cell membrane, resulting in the release of the nucleocapsid into the cytoplasm. **2.** Viral nucleocapsid migrates to the nuclear membrane. **3.** Viral DNA is released from the nucleocapsid and enters the nucleus through a nuclear pore. **4.** HSV transcription is initiated in a coordinated, cascade fashion producing the three classes of mRNA, α, β, and γ. Viral mRNA is transported to the cytoplasm where translation occurs. **5.** The different viral proteins are produced and transported to their appropriate cellular location. Alpha (α) proteins are involved in regulation of viral transcription; β proteins are involved primarily in DNA synthesis; γ proteins represent primarily structural proteins. **6.** Synthesis of viral DNA occurs through a rolling circle mechanism in the nucleus producing DNA concatamers. **7.** Empty capsid structures are assembled in the nucleus and unit length viral DNA is packaged into the capsid producing a nucleocapsid. **8.** The nucleocapsid buds through the nuclear membrane and is released from the cell **(9)**.

capsid structure and enters the nucleus through nuclear pores. Once inside the nucleus, viral-specific transcription and translation, and replication of the DNA genome occur.

HSV genes are divided into three major temporal classes (α, β, and γ) that are regulated in a coordinated, cascade fashion (for review see Roizman and Sears [1]). The α or immediate-early (IE) genes contain the major transcriptional regulatory proteins, and their production is required for the transcription of the β and γ gene classes. β proteins are not produced in the absence of α proteins, and their synthesis is required for viral DNA replication. The β proteins consist primarily of proteins involved in viral nucleic acid metabolism. The γ proteins reach peak rates of synthesis after the onset of DNA replication and consist primarily of viral structural proteins.

Once synthesized, the viral DNA is packaged into preformed capsid structures and the resulting nucleocapsid buds through the nuclear membrane, obtaining its envelope. The replication of HSV is fairly rapid, occurring within 15 h after infection, and it is extremely lethal to the cell resulting in cell lysis and death.

Latency

A hallmark of all herpesviruses is the ability to establish and maintain a latent infection. Latency is defined as a state of infection in which the viral genome persists in the infected cell in the absence of any viral replication, although depending on the specific herpesvirus, there may be a limited amount of viral transcription. Latency results in the long-term survival of the virus in its host and is why herpesvirus infections are described as once infected, always infected. Indeed, herpesvirus infections are for life.

Latent herpesvirus infections can be reactivated resulting in the production of a lytic cycle of replication and recrudescent disease. The frequency of reactivation and the type of recrudescent disease varies among the different human herpesviruses.

Members of the alphaherpesvirinae subfamily establish latent infections in sensory ganglia. Evidence from both human and animal models have demonstrated that the site for HSV latency is the neuron *(29–31)*. Identification of the site of VZV latency is less clear with some laboratories advocating the neuron while others point to ganglionic cells surrounding the neuron *(32,33)*.

Neurons latently infected with HSV do not produce virus or detectable virus-specific proteins. While the absence of virus production suggests that viral gene transcription is absent, a small subset of viral transcripts, termed the latency associated transcripts (LATs), are transcribed during active and latent infections *(34–38)*. The function of the LAT transcripts is unclear. Viral deletion mutants indicate that the LATs are not required to establish latent infection *(39,40)*, although a decreased frequency of reactivation in LAT mutants has been reported *(41–44)*.

Reactivation of HSV begins within the latently infected neuron. Following reactivation, the virus is transported down the axon of the neuron and establishes a peripheral infection in the skin. Recurrent HSV infections are generally less severe compared to primary infections both in terms of number of lesions formed and length of appearance *(45)*.

In immunocompetent hosts, active herpes simplex virus infections rapidly stimulate immune responses that function to restrict viral replication and the spread of virus. In addition, the host's immune response is most likely involved in the establishment of latent infections. In fact, the establishment of latency could be viewed as a double-edged sword. It provides the host with a mechanism to limit viral spread and cellular damage while, at the same time, ensuring the persistence and survival of the virus. In HSV-infected neonates and immunocompromised hosts, virus replicates to high titers, often with wide dissemination and generally extensive viral pathology. While the mechanisms involved in controlling HSV replication and establishment of latency are not completely understood, it has become increasingly evident that they involve interactions among nervous, immune and endocrine systems (reviewed in Turner and Jenkins *[46]*).

VZV latency appears to be quite different from HSV. There are no LAT homologs in VZV, and therefore there is no equivalent LAT gene expression during latency. Several laboratories have reported, however, the detection of gene expression from several

VZV genes in latently infected ganglia *(47–49)*. Because these genes also are expressed during a lytic replication, what role, if any, they play in VZV latency is unclear (reviewed by Kinchington *[50]*). Reactivation of latent VZV causes the disease herpes zoster, or shingles. This reactivated disease is quite different from recurrent HSV lesions in that the resulting rash and blisters occur throughout an entire dermatome (an area of the skin that is innervated by a single spinal nerve *[21]*). The appearance of VZV vesicles in a dermatome is evidence that following viral reactivation, the infection spreads throughout the ganglion and is transported to the skin via the numerous axons associated with that ganglion. Fortunately, zoster rarely occurs more than once in a lifetime.

BETAHERPESVIRUSES

Human Betaherpesvirus Members and Associated Diseases

There are three human herpesviruses belonging to the subfamily betaherpesvirinae: CMV, HHV-6, and HHV-7. CMV was originally given the name "salivary gland virus" when it was cultivated in 1956 from several salivary gland tissues *(51–53)*. The more descriptive name of cytomegalovirus was given by Weller in 1960 *(54)*. CMV infects epithelial cells, polymorphonuclear leucocytes, and T cells in the infected host *(55)*.

CMV is a frequent cause of asymptomatic infections in humans. As a result, clinical CMV disease is fairly uncommon except among neonates and immunocompromised individuals *(56)*. Congenital CMV infection is estimated to occur among 1% of all newborns in the United States *(57)*, making it the most common congenital infection. Among the newborns infected with CMV, approx 10% will exhibit clinical symptoms. Congenital CMV infection results in cytomegalic inclusion disease (CID) which presents as a widely disseminated infection with multiorgan involvement. CID is the leading cause of mental retardation, deafness, and other neurologic deficits among neonates *(56)*. In immunocompromised individuals with a cell-mediated deficiency (such as bone marrow and solid organ transplant patients and individuals with AIDS), primary or reactivated CMV infections can result in several life-threatening diseases including interstitial pneumonia, gastroenteritis, hepatitis, and leukopenia *(56)*. In addition, CMV infection can result in graft versus host disease in bone marrow transplant patients and is the leading cause of retinitis among AIDS patients. In apparently healthy adults, a primary CMV infection can result in a heterophile-negative mononucleosis-like disease *(56)*.

CMV is the prototype of the betaherpesvirinae, and until 1986 it was the sole human member of this subfamily. In 1986, a novel virus was isolated from the lymphocytes of individuals with lymphoproliferative disorders *(58)*. This subsequently was found to be a newly discovered herpesvirus and is now termed human herpesvirus 6 (HHV-6). Four years later, in 1990, another novel herpesvirus was isolated from cultured lymphocytes of a healthy adult *(59)*. This virus was found to be highly related, yet distinct from HHV-6 and was given the name human herpesvirus 7 (HHV-7). HHV-6 and HHV-7 are closely related at the genetic level and share homology, to a lesser extent, with CMV. HHV-6 has been shown to have two major variants (A and B) that can be distinguished at the DNA level *(60,61)*. Both HHV-6 and HHV-7 exhibit a T-cell tropism. In addition, HHV-6 has been found to also infect epithelial cells, natural killer (NK) cells, and monocytes *(62)*.

HHV-6 infection is most often asymptomatic, occurring in young children *(8)*. It has been definitively shown to be the causative agent of the childhood disease exanthem subitum (also called roseola infantum), which is characterized by a high fever for 3–5 d followed by a small red rash on the neck and trunk that lasts for 1–2 d *(63)*. HHV-6 variant B is responsible for almost all cases of exanthem subitum, and in a recent study was implicated as the primary cause of emergency room visits, febrile seizures, and hospitalizations among children under the age of 3 yr *(64)*. HHV-6 infections in young children also have been associated with hepatitis, encephalitis, and seizures. Primary infections in healthy adults are rare (due to the high seroprevalence rate among adults) and are associated with heterophile-negative mononucleosis, hepatitis, and lymphadenopathy *(8)*. Among adults, the greatest risk of HHV-6-associated disease is in transplant patients. Solid-organ and bone marrow transplant recipients who reactivate HHV-6 following transplant are at risk for several disorders including a fever and rash, pneumonitis, hepatitis, and neurologic disorders *(8)*. HHV-6 reactivation also has been associated with graft rejection among some renal transplant patients *(65)*. More recently, HHV-6 has been linked to multiple sclerosis (MS) by the detection of viral DNA in MS plaques *(66)* and more than 70% of MS patients have been shown to have evidence of an active HHV-6 infection *(67)*. Definitive proof for a causal role of HHV-6 in MS, however, is still lacking. HHV-7 infection is not associated with any definitive disease although there have been some reports of roseola infantum linked to HHV-7 infection *(68–70)*.

Epidemiology of Betaherpesvirus Infections

Horizontal CMV transmission can occur (1) during birth by direct contact with virus-containing cervical or vaginal secretions, (2) by ingestion of breast milk, (3) by direct contact with saliva, (4) by contact with blood products or upon receiving transplanted tissues, and (5) by sexual transmission *(56)*. Interestingly, the incidence of CMV infections in the United States is not uniform over time, but instead shows peak increases within distinct age groups *(57)*. These increases are seen during the first few months of life (from maternal secretions or breast milk), during the toddler years (from saliva of family members and other children), during the teenage years (from intimate kissing), and during young adulthood (from sexual transmission). Worldwide, CMV infection and seroprevalence is associated with age, geographic location, and socioeconomic status (SES) *(57)*. In developed countries, 40–60% of adults in middle to upper level SES are CMV seropositive compared to more than 80% among those in a lower SES. In contrast, in developing countries more than 80% of all children have seroconverted by the age of 3.

HHV-6 and HHV-7 infections are highly ubiquitous. Seroconversion to HHV-6 occurs predominantly (> 90%) between 1 and 2 yr of age *(71,72)*. HHV-7 infection occurs slightly later, with more than 85% of children seroconverting by age 3 *(73)*.

Betaherpesvirus Latency

The targets for CMV latency in seropositive individuals are peripheral blood and bone marrow derived monocytes *(74)*. Latently infected cells have been shown to express two classes of latency associated transcripts that map to the region of the CMV genome that encodes for the major immediate-early protein. The sites for HHV-6 latency have been reported to include monocytes, macrophages and the salivary glands *(33)*, while the sites for HHV-7 latency have not been clearly defined.

GAMMAHERPESVIRUSES

Human Gammaherpesvirus Members and Associated Diseases

There are currently two human herpesviruses belonging to the gammaherpesvirinae subfamily: EBV and HHV-8. EBV is the prototype for the *Lymphocryptovirus* genus while HHV-8 belongs to the genus *Rhadinovirus*. Members of both genera are characterized by a tropism for lymphoid cells and the ability to induce cell proliferation in vivo resulting in lymphoproliferative disorders.

EBV is well established in the majority of the world's human population. Its prevalence rate stands at > 90%. The majority of primary EBV infections are believed to be asymptomatic *(75)*. While no disease or illness has been associated with a primary EBV infection in healthy infants, in other individuals (particularly in adolescents and young teens), primary EBV can result in infectious mononucleosis. An EBV infection begins with the virus infecting the epithelial layer of the nasopharynx and spreading to nearby B cells. As a result of viral replication, fever, pharyngitis, lymphadenopathy, splenomegaly, hepatocellular dysfunction, and oftentimes skin rashes develop *(76,77)*.

Normally, the immune response to EBV is aggressive, resulting in a rapid elimination of virus-infected cells. The immune response includes the activation of NK cells, antibody-dependent cellular cytotoxicity (ADCC), and EBV-specific cytotoxic T cells (CTL) *(77)*. The immune response controls viral replication, marking the end of the primary infection and forcing the virus into establishing latency in B cells *(78)*.

In 1994, using representational difference analysis Chang and colleagues *(79)*, described the detection of DNA sequences in AIDS-associated Kaposi's sarcoma (KS) lesions belonging to a new human herpesvirus termed Kaposi's sarcoma-associated herpesvirus (KSHV) or HHV-8. The predicted amino acids encoded by these DNA sequences were found to share homology to proteins encoded by herpesvirus saimiri (HVS) and EBV.

HHV-8 DNA has been found in > 95% of all KS tissues *(79–84)*, and in two unusual types of lymphoma termed primary effusion lymphoma (PEL, previously called body-cavity based lymphoma) and multicentric Castleman's disease (MCD) *(85–87)*. The precise role of HHV-8 in the development of these cancers is not known, but is the focus of intensive laboratory efforts (*see* Chapter 10). Currently, there has not been a disease associated with a primary HHV-8 infection.

Epidemiology of Gammaherpesvirus Infections

EBV infection is ubiquitous throughout the world such that by the age of 30, 80–100% of all individuals have seroconverted *(9)*. Seroprevalence among younger individuals varies according to SES, similar to HSV-2 and CMV *(88)*. In developing countries, primary EBV infection occurs during the first few years of life, while in developed countries it occurs more often during adolescence. The primary route of EBV transmission is oral, although limited transmission following transplantation has been reported *(76)*. Approximately 50% of the primary infections occurring during adolescence result in clinical infectious mononucleosis *(88)*.

Seroepidemiology studies of HHV-8, as well as the epidemiology of KS, have indicated that transmission of HHV-8 appears to be primarily through sexual contact. For example, HHV-8 seroprevalence among homosexual men has been significantly linked to multiple sexual partners *(89–91)*. While HHV-8 infection is increased among homosexual men, it is not increased among intravenous drug users, indicating that transmission does not occur significantly through blood inoculation *(92)* (Bernstein, Jacobson, and Jenkins, *unpublished results*). The seroprevalence of HHV-8 among individuals above the age of 15 ranges from 0% to 20% depending on the serologic assay *(93–96)*. HHV-8 infection in children under the age of 15 is rare in the United States and the United Kingdom (Jenkins, *unpublished results) (97)*, but it does occur in KS-endemic regions of Mediterranean and African countries. HHV-8 DNA was been found in saliva, peripheral blood mononuclear cells (PBMCs), and semen of infected individuals *(98–103)*, although not consistently. The exact nature of an HHV-8 infection including location, spread into various tissues, timing of viral shedding, and location of infectious virus remains undetermined at present. Further, the potential for viral transmission by routes other than sexual contact must be investigated, given that there has been some documentation of horizontal transmission from mother to child *(97)*.

Latency

Epithelial cells and B cells are important targets in the life cycle of EBV. Differentiating epithelial cells have been shown to be permissive for lytic replication while B lymphocytes are the primary target for latency and represent a virus reservoir in humans *(77)*. The ability of EBV to establish latent infections in B cells is believed to be directly responsible for the development of several different neoplasms, including endemic Burkitt's lymphoma, undifferentiated nasopharyngeal carcinoma, Hodgkin's disease, and polyclonal B-cell lymphocytosis *(104,105)*. The association of EBV with some of these neoplasms has demonstrated important geographic variations. Both Hodgkin's disease and sporadic Burkitt's lymphoma from Latin America have higher rates of EBV-association than cases from Western countries. Furthermore, the EBV-association in all African Burkitt's lymphoma is unique and exhibits distinctive clinical and pathologic features. A recent investigation of primary intestinal lymphomas of Mexican origin demonstrated the presence of EBV in all examined cases of T-cell non-Hodgkin's lymphomas, Burkitt's lymphoma, and in a proportion of other B-cell non-Hodgkin's lymphomas *(106)*.

In immunologically compromised individuals, EBV can cause a malignant B-lymphocyte proliferation directly linking it to lymphoproliferative disorders, as well as virus-associated hemophagocytic syndrome, certain forms of T-cell lymphoma, and some gastric carcinomas *(107)*. Serologic studies have been largely used to correlate virus presence to the pathogenesis of many these diseases.

Latency of the gammaherpesvirinae is quite unique distinct from that of the alphaherpesvirinae and betaherpesvirinae. EBV infection of B cells triggers the expression of several latent-specific proteins whose functions (among others) are to maintain the EBV genome as an episome in the latently infected B cell and to transform the B cell to ensure long-term survival (reviewed by Kieff and Leibowitz *[9]*.). To accomplish this, EBV latency consists of a complex pattern of viral gene expression. Given that EBV must establish and maintain a latent infection in a relatively short-lived B cell, while

HSV and VZV latency occurs in differentiated and nondividing neuronal cells, perhaps it is not surprising that the pattern of latent viral gene expression is quite different between these virus subfamilies.

The cancers associated with HHV-8 (KS, PEL, MCD) appear to represent a predominantly latent infection, as the majority of the cells express latent proteins and do not produce significant amounts of virus *(108,109)*. Several HHV-8 latent proteins have been identified, but their function is not known. If similar to EBV, these proteins would serve to establish and maintain viral latency. These answers will depend on the development of HHV-8 mutants that can be studied in vitro or in suitable animal models.

SUMMARY

The human herpesviruses induce a variety of illnesses ranging from asymptomatic to life-threatening infections and cancer. The majority of these viruses are acquired during childhood and persist for life. The ability of the herpesviruses to establish and maintain a latent infection adds an additional layer of complexity to the viruses' life cycle and complicates all attempts to eradicate the virus from infected individuals. While much has been learned about the human herpesviruses over the last 30 yr, there is still much more to be learned before they are no longer a serious health threat.

ACKNOWLEDGMENTS

The authors wish to express their appreciation to David Burnikel and Angelica Starkey for their assistance in preparing this manuscript.

REFERENCES

1. Roizman B, Sears AE. Herpes simplex viruses and their replication. In: Roizman B, Whitley RJ, Lopez C (eds). The Human Herpesviruses, 1st edit. New York: Raven Press, 1993, pp. 11–68.
2. Furlong D, Swift H, Roizman B. Arrangement of herpesvirus deoxyribonucleic acid in the core. J Virol 1972; 10:1071–1074.
3. Roffman E, Albert JP, Goff JP, Frenkel N. Putative site for the acquisition of human herpesvirus 6 virion tegument. J Virol 1990; 64:6308–6313.
4. Kramarsky B, Sander C. Electron microscopy of human herpesvirus-6 (HHV-6). In: Ablashi DV, Krueger GR, Salahuddin SZ (eds). Human Herpesvirus 6. Amsterdam: Elsevier, 1992, pp. 59–79.
5. Pellett PE, McKnight JL, Jenkins FJ, Roizman B. Nucleotide sequence and predicted amino acid sequence of a protein encoded in a small herpes simplex virus DNA fragment capable of trans-inducing alpha genes. Proc Natl Acad Sci USA 1985; 82:5870–5874.
6. Batterson W, Roizman B. Characterization of the herpes simplex virion-associated factor responsible for the induction of alpha genes. J Virol 1983; 46:371–377.
7. Roizman B, Carmichael LE, Deinhardt F, de The G, Nahmias AJ, Plowright W, et al. Herpesviridae. Definition, provisional nomenclature and taxonomy. Intervirology 1981; 16:201–217.
8. Kimberlin DW. Human herpesviruses 6 and 7: identification of newly recognized viral pathogens and their association with human disease. Pediatr Infect Dis J 1998; 17:59–68.
9. Kieff E, Liebowitz D. Epstein-Barr virus and its replication. In: Fields BN, Knipe DM, Chanock RM, Hirsch MS, Melnick JL, Monath TP, et al. (eds). Field's Virology, 2nd edit. New York: Raven Press, 1990, pp. 1889–1920.
10. Jones JF, Katz BZ. Epstein-Barr virus infections in normal and immunosuppressed patients. In: Glaser R, Jones JF (eds). Herpesvirus Infections. New York: Marcel Dekker, 1994, pp. 187–226.

11. Boshoff C, Weiss RA. Kaposi's sarcoma-associated herpesvirus. Adv Cancer Res 1998; 75:58–87.
12. Richman LK, Montali RJ, Garber RL, Kennedy MA, Lehnhardt J, Hildebrandt T, et al. Novel endotheliotropic herpesviruses fatal for Asian and African elephants. Science 1999; 283:1171–1176.
13. Whitley RJ, Gnann JWJr. The epidemiology and clinical manifestations of herpes simplex virus infections. In: Roizman B, Whitley RJ, Lopez C (eds). The Human Herpesviruses. New York: Raven Press, 1993, pp. 69–106.
14. Cook ML, Stevens JG. Pathogenesis of herpetic neuritis and ganglionitis in mice: evidence of intra-axonal transport of infection. Infect Immun 1973; 7:272–288.
15. Hill TJ. Herpes simplex virus latency. In: Roizman B (eds). The Herpesviruses. New York: Plenum Press, 1985, p. 175.
16. Carlton CA, Kilbourne ED. Activation of latent herpes simplex virus by trigeminal sensory-root section. N Engl J Med 1952; 246:172.
17. Segal AL, Katcher AH, Bringtman VJ, Miller MF. Recurrent herpes labialis, recurrent apthous ulcers and the menstrual cycles. J Dent Res 1974; 53:797–803.
18. Pazin GJ, Ho M, Jannetta PJ. Herpes simplex reactivation after trigeminal nerve root decompression. J Infect Dis 1978; 138:405.
19. Spruance SL. Pathogenesis of herpes simplex labialis: experimental induction of lesions with UV light. J Clin Microbiol 1985; 22:366–368.
20. Davison AJ, McGeoch DJ. Evolutionary comparisons of the S segments in the genomes of herpes simplex virus type 1 and varicella-zoster virus. J Gen Virol 1986; 67:597–611.
21. Grose C. Varicella zoster virus infections: chickenpox, shingles, and varicella vaccine. In: Glaser R, Jones JF (eds). Herpesvirus Infections. New York: Marcel Dekker, 1994, pp. 117–185.
22. Arvin AM. Varicella-zoster virus. Clin Microbiol Rev 1996; 9:361–381.
23. Gelb LD. Varicella-zoster virus clinical aspects. In: Roizman B, Whitley RJ, Lopez C, (eds). The Human Herpesviruses. New York: Raven Press, 1993, pp. 281–316.
24. Johnson RE, Nahmias AJ, Magder LS, Lee FK, Brooks CA, Snowden CB. A seroepidemiologic survey of the prevalence of herpes simplex virus type 2 infection in the United States. N Engl J Med 1989; 321:7–12.
25. Fleming DT, McQuillan GM, Johnson RE, Nahmias AJ, Aral SO, Lee FK, et al. Herpes simplex virus type 2 in the United States, 1976 to 1994. N Engl J Med 1997; 337:1105–1111.
26. Arvin AM. Varicella-zoster virus: overview and clinical manifestations. Semin Dermatol 1996; 15:4–7.
27. Arvin AM, Gershon A. Live attenuated varicella vaccine. Annu Rev Microbiol 1996; 50:59–100.
28. Krause PR, Klinman DM. Efficacy, immunogenicity, safety, and use of live attenuated chickenpox vaccine. J Pediatr 1995; 127:518–525.
29. Baringer JR, Swoveland P. Recovery of herpes simplex virus from human trigeminal ganglions. N Engl J Med 1973; 228:648.
30. Bastian FO, Rabson AS, Yee CL. Herpesvirus hominis: isolation from human trigeminal ganglion. Science 1972; 178:306.
31. Stevens JG, Cook ML. Latent herpes simplex virus in spinal ganglia of mice. Science 1971; 173:843–845.
32. Gilden DH, Rozenman Y, Murray R, Devlin M, Vafai A. Detection of varicella-zoster virus nucleic acid in neurons of normal tissue thoracic ganglia. Ann Neurol 1987; 22:377–380.
33. Le Cleach L, Fillet A-M, Agut H, Chosidow O. Human herpesviruses 6 and 7. Arch Dermatol 1998; 134:1156–1157.
34. Wechsler SL, Nesburn AB, Watson R, Slanina S, Ghiasi H. Fine mapping of the major latency-related RNA of herpes simplex virus type 1 in humans. J Gen Virol 1988; 69:3101–3106.

35. Wagner EK, Devi-Rao G, Feldman LT, Dobson AT, Zhang YF, Flanagan WM, et al. Physical characterization of the herpes simplex virus latency-associated transcript in neurons. J Virol 1988; 62:1194–1202.

36. Stevens JG, Haarr L, Porter DD, Cook ML, Wagner EK. Prominence of the herpes simplex virus latency-associated transcript in trigeminal ganglia from seropositive humans. J Infect Dis 1988; 158:117–123.

37. Krause PR, Croen KD, Ostrove JM, Straus SE. Structural and kinetic analyses of herpes simplex virus type 1 latency-associated transcripts in human trigeminal ganglia and in cell culture. J Clin Invest 1990; 86:235–241.

38. Rock DL, Nesburn AB, Ghiasi H, Ong J, Lewis TL, Lokensgard JR, et al. Detection of latency-related viral RNAs in trigeminal ganglia of rabbits latently infected with herpes simplex virus type 1. J Virol 1987; 62:3820–3826.

39. Ho DY, Mocarski ES. Herpes simplex virus latent RNA (LAT) is not required for latent infection in the mouse. Proc Natl Acad Sci USA 1989; 86:7596–7600.

40. Steiner I, Spivack JG, Lirrete RP, Brown SM, MacLean AR, Subak-Sharpe J, et al. Herpes simplex virus type 1 latency-associated transcripts are evidently not essential for latent infection. EMBO J 1989; 8:505–511.

41. Natarajan R, Deshmane S, Valyi-Nagy T, Everett R, Fraser NW. A herpes simplex virus type 1 mutant lacking the ICP0 introns reactivates with normal efficiency. J Virol 1991; 65:5569–5573.

42. Block TM, Spivack JG, Steiner I, Deshmane S, McIntosh MT, Lirette RP, et al. A herpes simplex virus type 1 latency-associated transcript mutant reactivates with normal kinetics from latent infection. J Virol 1990; 64:3417–3426.

43. Perng GC, Slanina SM, Ghiasi H, Nesburn AB, Wechsler SL. A 371-nucleotide region between the herpes simplex virus type 1 (HSV-1) LAT promoter and the 2-kilobase LAT is not essential for efficient spontaneous reactivation of latent HSV-1. J Virol 1996; 70:2014–2018.

44. Maggioncalda J, Mehta A, Fraser NW, Block TM. Analysis of a herpes simplex virus type 1 LAT mutant with a deletion between the putative promoter and the 5′ end of the 2.0 kilobase transcript. J Virol 1994; 68:7816–7824.

45. Whitley RJ. Herpes simplex virus infections. In: Glaser R, Jones JF (eds). Herpesvirus Infections. New York: Marcel Dekker, 1994, pp. 1–57.

46. Turner SL, Jenkins FJ. The role of herpes simplex virus in neuroscience. J Neurovirol 1997; 3:110–125.

47. Croen KD, Ostrove JM, Dragovic LJ, Straus SE. Patterns of gene expression and sites of latency in human nerve ganglia are different for varicella-zoster and herpes simplex viruses. Proc Natl Acad Sci USA 1988; 85:9773–9777.

48. Cohrs R, Mahalingam R, Dueland AN, Wolf W, Wellish M, Gilden DH. Restricted transcription of varicella-zoster virus in latently infected human trigeminal and thoracic ganglia. J Infect Dis 1992; 166 (Suppl. 1):S24–S29.

49. Vafai A, Murray RS, Wellish M, Devlin M, Gilden DH. Expression of varicella-zoster virus and herpes simplex virus in normal human trigeminal ganglia. Proc Natl Acad Sci USA 1988; 85:2362–2366.

50. Kinchington PR. Latency of varicella zoster virus; a persistently perplexing state. Front Biosci 1999; 4:d200–211.

51. Rowe WP, Hartley JW, Waterman S, Turner HC, Huebner RJ. Cytopathogenic agent resembling human salivary gland virus recovered from tissue cultures of human adenoids. Proc Soc Exp Biol Med 1956; 92:418–424.

52. Smith MG. Propagation in tissue cultures of a cytopathogenic virus from human salivary gland virus (SVG) disease. Proc Soc Exp Biol Med 1956; 92:424–430.

53. Weller TH, Macauley JC, Craig JM, Wirth P. Isolation of intranuclear inclusion-producing agents from infants with illnesses resembling cytomegalic inclusion disease. Proc Soc Exp Biol Med 1957; 94:4–12.

54. Weller TH, Hanshaw JB. Virological and clinical observation of cytomegalic inclusion disease. N Engl J Med 1962; 266:1233–1344.

55. Mocarski ES. Cytomegalovirus biology and replication. In: Roizman B, Whitley RJ, Lopez C (eds). The Human Herpesviruses. New York: Raven Press, 1993, pp. 173–226.

56. Greenberg MS. Herpesvirus infections. Dent Clin North Am 1996; 40:359–368.

57. Demmler GJ. Congenital cytomegalovirus infection and disease. Adv Pediatr Infect Dis 1996; 11:135–162.

58. Salahuddin SZ, Ablashi DV, Markham PD, Josephs SF, Sturzenegger S, Kaplan M, et al. Isolation of a new virus, HBLV, in patients with lymphoproliferative disorders. Science 1986; 234:596–601.

59. Frenkel N, Schirmer EC, Wyatt LS, et al. Isolation of a new herpesvirus from human CD4[+] T cells. Proc Natl Acad Sci USA 1990; 87:748–752.

60. Ablashi DV, Balachandran N, Josephs SF, Hung CL, Krueger GRF, Kramarsky B, et al. Genomic polymorphism, growth properties, and immunologic variations in human herpesvirus-6 isolates. Virology 1991; 184:545–552.

61. Schirmer EC, Wyatt LS, Yamanishi K, Rodriguez WJ, Frenkel N. Differentiation between two distinct classes of viruses now classified as human herpesvirus 6. Proc Natl Acad Sci USA 1991; 88:5922–5926.

62. Lusso P. Target cells for infection. In: Ablashi DV, Krueger GRF, Salahuddin SZ, (eds). Human Herpesvirus 6. Amsterdam: Elsevier, 1992, pp. 25–36.

63. Yamanishi K, Okuno T, Shiraki K, Takahashi M, Kondo T, Asano Y, et al. Identification of human herpesvirus-6 as a causal agent for exanthem subitum. Lancet 1988; i:1065–1067.

64. Hall CB, Long CE, Schnabel KC, et al. Human herpesvirus-6 infection in children: a prospective study of complications and reactivation. N Engl J Med 1994; 331:432–438.

65. Okuno T, Higashi K, Shiraki K, Yamanishi K, Takahashi M, Kokado Y, et al. Human herpesvirus 6 infection in renal transplantation. Transplantation 1990; 49:519–522.

66. Challoner PB, Smith KT, Parker JD. Plaque-associated expression of human herpesvirus 6 in multiple sclerosis. Proc Natl Acad Sci USA 1995; 92:7440–7444.

67. Soldan SS, Berti R, Salem N, Secchiero P, Flamand L, Calabresi PA, et al. Association of human herpes virus 6 (HHV-6) with multiple sclerosis: increased IgM response. Nat Med 1997; 3:1394–1397.

68. Tanaka K, Kondo T, Torigoe S, Okada S, Mukai T, Yamanishi K. Human herpesvirus 7: another causal agent for roseola (exanthem subitum). J Pediatr 1994; 125:1–5.

69. Hidaka Y, Okada K, Kusuhara K, Miyazaki C, Tokugawa K, Ueda K. Exanthem subitum and human herpesvirus 7 infection. Pediatr Infect Dis J 1994; 13:1010–1011.

70. Ueda K, Kusuhara K, Okada K, et al. Primary human herpesvirus 7 infection and exanthema subitum. Pediatr Infect Dis J 1994; 13:167–168.

71. Briggs M, Fox J, Tedder RS. Age prevalence of antibody to human herpesvirus 6. Lancet 1988; i:1058–1059.

72. Balachandra K, Ayuthaya PI, Auwanit W, Jayavasu C, Okuno T, Yamanishi K, et al. Prevalence of antibody to human herpesvirus 6 in women and children. Microbiol Immunol 1989; 33:515–518.

73. Wyatt LS, Rodriguez WJ, Balachandran N, Frenkel N. Human herpesvirus 7: Antigenic properties and prevalence in children and adults. J Virol 1991; 65:6260–6265.

74. Slobedman B, Mocarski ES. Quantitative analysis of latent human cytomegalovirus. J Virol 1999; 73:4806–4812.

75. Yao QY, Rickinson AB, Epstein MA. A re-examination of the Epstein-Barr virus carrier state in healthy seropositive individuals. Int J Cancer 1985; 35:35–42.

76. Sixbey JW, Nedrud JC, Raab-Traub N, Hanes RA, Pagano JS. Epstein-Barr virus replication in oropharyngeal epithelial cells. N Engl J Med 1984; 310:1225–1230.

77. Schwartzmann F, Jager M, Hornef M, Prang N, Wolf H. Epstein-Barr viral gene expression in B-lymphocytes. Leuk Lymphoma 1998; 30:123–129.

78. Decker LL, Klaman LD, Thorley-Lawson DA. Detection of the latent form of Epstein–Barr virus DNA in peripheral blood of healthy individuals. J Virol 1996; 70:3286–3289.

79. Chang Y, Cesarman E, Pessin MS, Lee F, Culpepper J, Knowles DM, et al. Identification of herpesvirus-like DNA sequences in AIDS-associated Kaposi's sarcoma. Science 1994; 266:1865–1869.

80. Su IJ, Hsu YS, Chang YC, Wang IW. Herpesvirus-like DNA sequence in Kaposi's sarcoma from AIDS and non-AIDS patients in Taiwan. Lancet 1995; 345:722–723.

81. Huang YQ, Li JJ, Kaplan MH, Poiesz B, Katabira E, Zhang WC, et al. Human herpesvirus-like nucleic acid in various forms of Kaposi's sarcoma. Lancet 1995; 345:759–761.

82. Dupin N, Grandadam M, Calvez V, Gorin I, Aubin JT, Havard S, et al. Herpesvirus-like DNA sequences in patients with Mediterranean Kaposi's sarcoma. Lancet 1995; 345:761–762.

83. Collandre H, Ferris S, Grau O, Montagnier L, Blanchard A. Kaposi's sarcoma and a new herpesvirus. Lancet 1995; 345:1043–1044.

84. Boshoff C, Whitby D, Hartziioannou T, Fisher C, van der Walt J, Hatzakis A, et al. Kaposi's sarcoma-associated herpesvirus in HIV-negative Kaposi's sarcoma. Lancet 1995; 345:1043–1044.

85. Cesarman E, Chang Y, Moore PS, Said JW, Knowles DM. Kaposi's sarcoma-associated herpesvirus-like DNA sequences in AIDS-related body-cavity-based lymphomas. N Engl J Med 1995; 332:1186–1191.

86. Nador RG, Cesarman E, Knowles DM, Said JW. Herpes-like DNA sequences in body-cavity-based lymphoma in HIV-negative patient. N Engl J Med 1995; 333:943.

87. Ansari MQ, Dawson DB, Nador R, Rutherford C, Schneider NR, Latimer MJ, et al. Primary body cavity-based AIDS-related lymphomas. Am J Clin Pathol 1996; 105:221–229.

88. Evans AS. Infectious mononucleosis and related syndromes. Am J Med Sci 1978; 276:325–339.

89. Blackbourn DJ, Osmond D, Levy JA, Lennette ET. Increased human herpesvirus 8 seroprevalence in young homosexual men who have multiple sex contacts with different partners. J Infect Dis 1999; 179:237–239.

90. Grulich AE, Olsen SJ, Luo K, Hendry O, Cunningham P, Cooper DA, et al. Kaposi's sarcoma-associated herpesvirus: a sexually transmissible infection? J Acquir Immune Defic Syndr 1999; 20:387–393.

91. Martin JN, Ganem DE, Osmond DH, Page-Shafer KA, Macrae D, Kedes DH. Sexual transmission and the natural history of human herpesvirus 8 infection. N Engl J Med 1998; 338:948–954.

92. Zhang X, Fitzpatrick L, Campbell TB, Badaro R, Schechter M, Melo M, et al. Comparison of the prevalence of antibodies to human herpesvirus 8 (Kaposi's sarcoma-associated herpesvirus) in Brazil and Colorado. J Infect Dis 1998; 178:1488–1491.

93. Chandran B, Smith MS, Koelle DM, Corey L, Horvat R, Goldstein E. Reactivities of human sera with human herpesvirus-8 infected BCBL-1 cells and indentification of HHV-8 specific proteins and glycoproteins and the encoding cDNAs. Virology 1998; 243:208–217.

94. Gao SJ, Kingsley L, Hoover DR, Spira TJ, Rinaldo CR, Saah A, et al. Seroconversion to antibodies against Kaposi's sarcoma-associated herpesvirus-related latent nuclear antigens before the development of Kaposi's sarcoma. N Engl J Med 1996; 335:233–241.

95. Lennette ET, Blackbourn DJ, Levy JA. Antibodies to human herpesvirus type 8 in the general population and in Kaposi's sarcoma patients. Lancet 1996; 348:858–861.

96. Chatlynne LG, Lapps W, Handy M, Huang YQ, Masood R, Hamilton AS, et al. Detection and titration of human herpesvirus-8-specific antibodies in sera from blood donors, acquired immunodeficiency syndrome patients, and Kaposi's sarcoma patients using a whole virus enzyme-linked immunosorbent assay. Blood 1998; 92:53–58.

97. Bourboulia D, Whitby D, Boshoff C, Newton R, Beral V, Carrara H, et al. Serologic evidence for mother-to-child transmission of Kaposi sarcoma-associated herpesvirus infection. JAMA 1999; 280:31–32.

98. Corbellino M, Bestetti G, Galli M, Parravicini C. Absence of HHV-8 in prostate and semen. N Engl J Med 1996; 335:1237–1238.

99. Gupta P, Singh MK, Rinaldo C, Ding M, Farzadegan H, Saah A, et al. Detection of Kaposi's sarcoma herpesvirus DNA in semen of homosexual men with Kaposi's sarcoma. AIDS 1996; 10:1596–1598.

100. Koelle DM, Huang ML, Chandran B, Vieira J, Piepkorn M, Corey L. Frequent detection of Kaposi's sarcoma-associated herpesvirus (human herpesvirus 8) DNA in saliva of human immunodeficiency virus-infected men: clinical and immunologic correlates. J Infect Dis 1997; 176:94–102.

101. Lefrere JJ, Meyohas MC, Mariotti M, Meynard JL, Thauvin M, Frottier J. Detection of human herpesvirus 8 DNA sequences before the appearance of Kaposi's sarcoma in human immunodeficiency virus (HIV)-positive subjects with a known date of HIV seroconversion. J Infect Dis 1996; 174:283–287.

102. Monini P, DeLellis L, Fabris M, Rigolin F, Cassai E. Kaposi's sarcoma-associated herpesvirus DNA sequences in prostate tissue and human semen. N Engl J Med 1996; 334:1168–1172.

103. Smith MS, Bloomer C, Horvat R, Goldstein E, Casparian JM, Chandran B. Detection of human herpesvirus 8 DNA in Kaposi's sarcoma lesions and peripheral blood of human immunodeficiency virus-positive patients and correlation with serologic measurements. J Infect Dis 1997; 176:84–93.

104. Lyons SF, Liebowitz DN. The roles of human viruses in the pathogenesis of lymphoma. Semin Oncol 1998; 25:461–475.

105. Mitterer M, Pescosta N, Fend F, Larcher C, Prang N, Schwartzmann F, et al. Chronic active Epstein-Barr virus disease in a case of persistent polyclonal B-cell lynphocytosis. Br J Haematol 1995; 90:526–531.

106. Quintanilla-Martinez L, Lome-Maldonado C, Ott G, Gschwendtner A, Gredler E, Angeles-Angeles A, et al. Primary intestinal non-Hodgkin's lymphoma and Epstein-Barr virus: high frequency of EBV-infection in T-cell lymphomas of Mexican origin. Leuk Lymphoma 1998; 30:111–121.

107. Okano M, Thiele GM, Davis JR, Grierson HL, Purtilo DT. Epstein-Barr virus and human diseases: recent advances in diagnosis. Clin Microbiol Rev 1988; 1:300–312.

108. Sarid R, Flore O, Bohenzky RA, Chang Y, Moore PS. Transcription mapping of the Kaposi's sarcoma-associated herpesvirus (human herpesvirus 8) genome in a body cavity-based lymphoma cell line (BC-1). J Virol 1998; 72:1005–1012.

109. Zhong W, Wang H, Herndier B, Ganem D. Restricted expression of Kaposi sarcoma-associated herpesvirus (human herpesvirus 8) genes in Kaposi sarcoma. Proc Natl Acad Sci 1997; 93:6641–6646.

3

X-Linked Lymphoproliferative Disease

Thomas A. Seemayer, Timothy G. Greiner, Thomas G. Gross, Jack R. Davis, Arpad Lanyi, and Janos Sumegi

PROLOGUE

The disease discussed in this chapter was discovered 30 yr ago at the autopsy table by a young and very inquisitive pathologist. Within the past year, the mutated gene central to this condition has been cloned and studies are underway to elucidate its normal immunologic function. This review summarizes our present state of knowledge of X-linked lymphoproliferative disease (XLP).

THE DISCOVERY OF XLP

In 1975, Purtilo described three brothers who died (1961, 1969, and 1973) of an acute illness with features of infectious mononucleosis (IM), lymphoblastic leukemia, and hepatic and marrow failure *(1)*. Included in the report were descriptions of three maternally related nephews who had developed agammaglobulinemia after IM, cerebral lymphoma after IM, and ileocecal lymphoma unrelated to IM. These boys, sharing a common ancestor, surname Duncan, defined a new entity, Duncan's disease or X-linked lymphoproliferative disease (XLP), as it later came to be known. In this index publication, he noted that several of the boys had IM during or preceding the terminal event; from this observation, he suggested that the Epstein–Barr virus (EBV) or other viruses were central to the pathogenesis of this condition.

EBV AND THE IMMUNE SYSTEM

EBV, a large (172,000 basepairs) herpesvirus, preferentially infects B lymphocytes in humans and causes lifelong infection. In developing countries, well over 90% of individuals are infected before the age of 2 yr *(2,3)*. In industrialized countries, such as the United States, only 25–40% of children have been infected by the age of 2, but approx 75–90% of individuals will have acquired the infection by the age of 25 *(4)*. Primary infection by EBV results in two main responses, depending on the age of the individual and the maturity of the immune system. If the primary infection occurs in early childhood, the immune response and clinical symptoms are almost always clinically silent, that is, quiescent seroconversion; in contrast, about two-thirds of infected older children and adults will develop overt IM *(2)*.

From: *Infectious Causes of Cancer: Targets for Intervention*
Edited by: J. J. Goedert © Humana Press Inc., Totowa, NJ

Infection occurs following salivary exposure to an individual shedding virus. The virus gains entry to cells through the complement C3d receptor (CD21) *(5)*. Viral replication occurs in the oropharyngeal epithelial cells and released virions then infect B cells in the lymphoid tissues of Waldeyer's ring *(6)*. Once infected by EBV, an individual maintains a lifelong relationship with the virus with about 1 in 10 million B cells in the peripheral blood carrying latent virus *(7)*. The intimate association of mucosal epithelia with oropharyngeal submucosal lymphoid tissues results in the constant release of circulating infected B cells. Viral replication and shedding into salivary excretions are present in at least 15% of seropositive individuals at any given time *(8)*.

The incubation period from infection to development of clinical symptoms of IM generally is 4–6 wk. During this time, increased numbers of B cells are infected and disseminate widely, to proliferate in the germinal centers of lymph nodes and spleen and the sinusoidal and periportal areas of the liver *(2,3)*. In response to this proliferation and dissemination of infected B cells, the immune system responds massively, yet elegantly.

The predominate cellular respondents in IM are large, pleomorphic atypical lymphocytes or "Downey cells" which are CD8$^+$ T lymphocytes, not the infected B cells *(9)*. These cells are highly activated, as evidenced by elevated serum levels of soluble interleukin-2 (IL-2) receptors and soluble CD8, concentrations that correlate with the absolute number of CD8$^+$ cells *(9,10)*. The initial humoral response is nonspecific, resulting in hypergammaglobulinemia and associated autoantibodies production. The latter is illustrated by the production of heterophile antibodies, nonspecific IgM antibodies that agglutinate sheep and horse erythrocytes *(11)*. This immune response is thought to account for the diverse clinical findings that have been observed with primary EBV infection, for example, meningoencephalitis, Guillain-Barré syndrome, Bell's palsy, cerebellar ataxia, oculoglandular syndrome, conjunctivitis, keratitis, uveitis, carditis, arthritis, nephritis, pneumonitis, and hepatitis *(12)*. The manner in which EBV triggers such a response is not known, but the symptoms of IM are attributable to this immune response and the concomitant massive release of inflammatory cytokines, rather than the direct effect of proliferating EBV-infected B cells, as once believed.

In the majority of individuals, this intense nonspecific immune response is subdued through a well-orchestrated immune response consisting of humoral elements, antibody-dependent cellular cytotoxicity, natural killer cell activity, cytokine production, and T-cell immunity; of these, the latter appears to be the most critical *(2,13–18)*. Once the infection is controlled, a delicate balance between host and virus is maintained throughout the lifetime of the infected individual. A fascinating and yet to be explained phenomenon is that younger children usually do not experience the symptoms of IM following primary EBV infection, suggesting that this massive immune response in IM is age related.

If this initial immune response is not controlled, one outcome is fulminant IM, which occurs in approx 1 in 3000 IM cases, about 40–50 cases annually in the United States *(2,3,18–20)*. The explosive lymphoproliferation that occurs in fulminant IM mimics that seen in certain hematologic neoplasms, such as acute lymphoblastic leukemia, and can obscure recognition of fulminant IM as a cause of death. The median age at presentation is 13 yr, with a 1:1 male/female ratio *(9)*. The majority are sporadic and do not represent individuals with XLP.

DIAGNOSIS OF EBV INFECTION

The detection of heterophile antibodies is the most widely utilized test to diagnose IM. However, their presence is not specific for IM; moreover, in young children, especially < 10 yr of age, such antibodies may not be present following EBV infection *(2)*. In this and other settings, EBV serology is necessary to document EBV infection. The first detectable EBV-specific antibody produced following EBV infection is IgM to viral capsid antigen (VCA); this is present during acute IM and occasionally during viral reactivation. Anti-VCA IgG is also detectable early in the course of IM and both IgG and IgM antibodies to VCA may be present by the time an individual seeks medical attention. Anti-VCA IgG titers usually peak 1–2 mo into the clinical illness and gradually decline, yet persist for life. Anti-early-antigen (EA) responses generally appear later than responses to VCA; rises in anti-EA titers are also seen with viral reactivation. IgG titers against EBV nuclear antigen (EBNA) rise slowly over 1–2 yr post-infection and persist for life. The majority of normal individuals have detectable IgG antibodies to EBNA 6 mo following EBV infection *(2)*.

In immunocompromised patients, anti-VCA IgG titers can be greatly elevated, increased EA titers may persist for a long time, yet anti-EBNA antibodies are low or often absent. Caution should be taken when using this latter finding as a diagnostic criterion for XLP, as anti-EBNA antibodies are produced slowly in the normal individual. Thus, although most will have anti-EBNA titers by 6 mo, a delay up to 3 yr has been reported in normal children *(21)*. The diagnosis of EBV-associated atypical lymphoproliferations and of fulminant IM can be difficult because the usual EBV antibody responses may be lacking or unusually high, and the clinical picture may resemble acute leukemia, another malignancy, or overwhelming sepsis *(22)*. An accurate diagnosis may require the immunostaining of lymphoid tissues for EBV latent membrane protein (LMP-1) or molecular analyses including *in situ* (EBV-encoded RNA [EBER]) hybridization, Southern blot hybridization, or polymerase chain reaction studies to demonstrate the viral genome *(22)*.

FEATURES OF XLP

In 1980, Purtilo established the XLP Registry to track the disease, orchestrate research, and provide counseling to clinicians, pathologists, and patients *(23)*.

Unlike some of the other entities in this monograft, XLP is not typified by a standard clinical phenotype. Rather, study of 305 affected males from 88 kindreds in the XLP Registry reveals at least five distinct clinical phenotypes: fulminant IM, generally with virus-associated hemophagocytic syndrome (VAHS), dysgammaglobulinemia, malignant lymphoma, aplastic anemia, and vasculitis. It is not uncommon (22%) that an XLP boy develops several (two or three) different phenotypes over time, for example, fulminant IM years following dysgammaglobulinemia. In addition to boys with diverse phenotypic expressions of XLP, we have diagnosed nine asymptomatic boys (one with chorionic villus sampling) to have inherited the mutated *XLP* gene based upon restriction fragment length polymorphisms (RFLPs) (six cases) or genomic mutational analysis (three cases) (Table 1).

As much of this chapter relates to fulminant IM with VAHS and malignant lymphoma, mention of other XLP phenotypes is in order. Dysgammaglobulinemia, the second most

Table 1
Cumulative Proportion and Survival of Phenotypes of 305 Patients with XLP[a]

Phenotype	No. cases	Cumulative proportion	Mean age at onset/diagnosis	Survival
Fulminant IM	191	63%	5	7%
Dysgammaglobulinemia	92	30%	9	51%
Lymphoproliferative disease/lymphoma	87	28%	6	26%
Aplastic anemia	17	6%	8	18%
Vasculitis	3	1.0%	6.5	0%
Asymptomatic[b]	9	3.0%	N/A	100%

[a] Data from the X-linked lymphoproliferative (XLP) disease registry.

[b] Positive only for genotype by RFLP or mutational analyses.

common expression of XLP, usually is reflected by reduced serum levels of IgG. Lesser numbers of boys manifest increased levels of serum IgM and IgA. Several died subsequently with fulminant IM. Aplastic anemia stems from marrow pancytopenia or pure red cell aplasia; the mechanism(s) responsible for this state is (are) unknown. Similarly, several boys with aplastic anemia subsequently died from fulminant IM. Three boys have developed necrotizing vasculitis, a uniformly lethal condition in this setting.

Overall, 76% of the XLP boys have died, some 70% before 10 yr of age. The most common and virulent form of XLP is fulminant IM with VAHS. Among 191 cases with this phenotype, only 7% have survived (Table 1). Their mean age at onset is 5 yr and the clinical course is explosive, most dying within 1 mo of onset of symptoms. Although other phenotypes fare better, their survival rates also are dismal (Table 1). The oldest survivor is 44 yr old.

Initially, it was believed that the diverse phenotypes of XLP followed exposure to the ubiquitous herpesvirus, EBV. With time, however, we have witnessed boys (approx 10% of the cases) with an XLP phenotype devoid of serologic and/or molecular evidence of EBV infection (24). This issue is discussed later in this chapter.

Prior to the cloning of the *XLP* gene *(see below)*, XLP was diagnosed (with certainty) only when two or more maternally related males manifested an XLP phenotype following EBV infection (25). Although many were thought likely to be "immunodeficient" prior to EBV infection, no definitive laboratory test was available to confirm this diagnosis (24). Many demonstrated a failure to produce IgG antibodies to Epstein–Barr nuclear antigen (EBNA) following EBV infection; as well, some failed to switch Ig isotype (IgM →IgG) after exposure to phage ⌀X174. Yet, as these defects may be seen in other genetically determined immunodeficiencies, they were not deemed specific for XLP. Many families have been studied with RFLP analysis; in some individuals, a presumptive diagnosis was made, albeit with less than absolute certainty; in others, the studies were uninformative.

The definitive treatment for all phenotypes of XLP is allogeneic hematopoietic stem cell transplantation (HSCT) (26). Of the 13 boys thus treated, nine are alive and well; all four who died were over 15 yr at age at time of transplantation. Clinically, fulminant

IM with VAHS is addressed urgently with intense chemotherapy: cyclosporin A to downregulate T cells and etoposide (VP-16) to quell macrophage activation. The survivors should then undergo immune reconstitution with an allogenic HSCT. Hypogammaglobulinemia is treated with monthly IV-IG infusions. This treatment, however, has proved to be less than fully effective as several boys have developed more serious phenotypes of XLP while under this putative "therapeutic umbrella." Lymphoma patients receive chemotherapy, appropriate for the type and stage of disease. Aplastic anemia patients receive conventional treatment for marrow aplasia. The few boys affected with vasculitis received treatment appropriate for vasculitis. Unfortunately, all XLP boys are at subsequent risk for fulminant IM.

EBV INFECTION IN XLP

Unlike the well-orchestrated immune response in normal individuals leading to resolution of symptoms and lifetime control of latently infected B cells, XLP boys who develop fulminant IM with VAHS generate a vigorous but dysregulated and uncontrolled immune response that results in pancytopenia and usually death. Initially, the marrow shows extensive infiltration by lymphoid cells and erythrophagocytosis by histiocytes. Terminally, the marrow shows massive necrosis, cellular depletion, and marked histiocytic hemophagocytosis. Similar tissue reactions occur in the liver, spleen, thymus, and lymph nodes. The lymphocyte infiltration is represented by small numbers of polyclonal populations of EBV (+) B cells admixed with large numbers of activated T cells, both CD8[+] and CD4[+] *(2,19,20,27)*. The T cells, activated by the infected B cells, secrete cytokines that recruit and activate macrophages *(10,20)*. Following infection by EBV, normal individuals develop a T helper cell (Th-1) cytokine response, as witnessed by elevated serum levels of interferon-γ and IL-2. This response is greatly heightened in XLP boys *(10)*, when compared with normal individuals with IM. Quite likely, this dysregulated Th-1 response is central to the chaos and devastation of fulminant IM in XLP and provides the rationale for the employment of potent immunosuppressive agents in such patients. The recent identification of the *XLP* gene will hopefully provide clues to the immune system's response to EBV in XLP, as well as other viral infections.

Since the index description of XLP, many held to the notion that EBV infection was the requisite trigger to unmask clinically the underlying gene defect *(1,28)*. Until 1995, we ascribed to this belief. While usually the case, this is not always true, as illustrated by data from the Registry. Greater than 10% of boys with XLP manifest their immunodeficiency prior to exposure to EBV *(24)*. Interestingly, when fulminant IM, which is always associated with acute EBV infection is excluded, the percentage of boys manifesting the other major XLP phenotypes is similar, regardless of EBV status (Table 2). This suggests that the immune system of these boys may be fundamentally abnormal, independent of its response to EBV. Moreover, this suggests that EBV is of pathogenic relevance in XLP largely because of its ability to catalyze immunologic chaos leading to fulminant IM with VAHS.

Other factors that may contribute to the pathogenesis of XLP are not known. It is reasonable to speculate that other infectious agents may be involved. There are scant but hardly compelling anecdotal data suggesting that the odd XLP boy has an increased complication rate to some viral infections or live virus vaccines. Yet, the vast majority

Table 2
Correlation of Initial XLP Phenotype with EBV Status

Phenotypex	EBV (+) ($n = 50$)	EBV (–) ($n = 33$)
Dysgammaglobulinemia	26	12
Lymphoproliferative disease/lymphoma	20	19
Aplastic anemia	4	2

received routine vaccines without complications, were infected with other viruses without incident, and generated appropriate immune responses to all proteins. The recent identification of the gene defect in XLP should shed much awaited light on the molecular, genetic, biochemical, and immunologic factors central to this disease. Indeed, it has already been shown that the XLP protein interacts with a molecule of T-cell activation and may function normally in suppressing continued T-cell activation and proliferation *(see below)*.

XLP AND MALIGNANT LYMPHOMA

One of the three major phenotypes of XLP is malignant lymphoma, beginning with several patients in the original Duncan pedigree who were so affected. In one, tumor involved the ileum, colon, and pancreas; in a second, lymphoma involved the brain *(1)*. Since these initial cases, 28% of the patients in the Registry have developed malignant lymphoma. The most common types of B-cell lymphoma that occur in XLP are small noncleaved cell (Burkitt's type) and diffuse large cell lymphomas *(29–31)*. In 17 cases reviewed at Nebraska, the tumor distribution has been reported as 45% small noncleaved, 19% large noncleaved, 17.5% large cell immunoblastic, 12.5% mixed cell type, and 6% unclassified. The most common presenting site is the terminal ileum which contains Peyer's patches. Small noncleaved lymphomas are of germinal center origin, a component of the Peyer's lymphoid tissue.

Non-Hodgkin's lymphoma (NHL) in XLP must be differentiated from fulminant IM, as these patients can be misinterpreted as having NHL or acute leukemia. Indeed, in the original description, one XLP boy with fulminant IM was incorrectly diagnosed with acute lymphoblastic leukemia *(1)*. Harrington et al. observed that half of the cases referred to the XLP Registry as malignant lymphoma were fulminant IM on histologic review *(31)*. The histology in NHL is monomorphous with sheets of noncleaved cells or large numerous blastic cells. In fulminant IM, the infiltrate is polymorphous, including lymphocytes, plasma cells, immunoblasts, and microscopic areas of necrosis. This histology is similar to lymphoid expansions witnessed in posttransplant EBV-driven lymphoproliferative disease *(see* Chapter 4.)

EBV has been identified in the DNA of benign lymphoid tissues of XLP patients by hybridization methods *(32)*. However, significant numbers of lymphomas have not been studied beyond anecdotal reports of three EBV-positive cases *(31,33)*.

In 1982, Purtillo reported on the site of origin of 35 cases of lymphoma, of which 26 presented in the terminal ileum. Other sites included the liver, kidney, thymus, tonsils, and, rarely, the psoas muscle *(34)*. In nine cases, IM appeared to evolve into malignant lymphoma. However, most patients with lymphoma had no prior episode of IM, nor were blood or throat washings positive for EBV. One patient was found to have IM following malignant lymphoma. Fifteen patients with a sole presentation of NHL ranged in age from 5 to 15 yr.

Harrington et al. *(31).* described the characteristic presentation and course of XLP patients with NHL and observed that these patients had a median overall survival of 12 mo. Presenting symptoms include fever, nausea, vomiting, and abdominal pain. The majority had "B" symptoms and a normal leukocyte count. Almost all tumors occurred in extranodal sites and all NHL had a diffuse growth pattern. Most patients had localized stage 1 and 2 tumors; a few presented with advanced disease *(30).* The main cause of death has been infection. Several have died of fulminant IM, years after having malignant lymphoma.

Chromosomal translocations have been infrequently described in NHL in XLP, owing primarily to a lack of fresh material and the paucity of such studies. The t(8;14)(q24;q32), commonly seen in pediatric Burkitt's NHL *(see* Chapter 5), has been described *(35,36)* as has a t(8;22) *(37),* both of which include a translocation of the c-*myc* gene.

The XLP registry contains referring pathology reports on 84 cases of lymphoproliferative disorders. In the majority (65%) of cases the type of lymphoma was unspecified and the relevant histologic sections were not available for study. By report, there have been three cases of Hodgkin's disease and eight cases of T-cell lymphoproliferations. The latter group includes three cases of lymphoblastic lymphoma and five cases of lymphomatoid granulomatosis (sometimes referred to as angiocentric immunoproliferative lesions). Unlike the general pediatric population in which lymphoblastic lymphoma constitutes 30–50% of NHL cases, lymphoblastic NHL has been rarely described in XLP *(31).* Now that the *XLP* gene has been identified, a systematic review to correlate mutational genomic analysis with histology and immunophenotype of all lymphoproliferations in the Registry is planned.

THE GENE MUTATED IN XLP AND ITS PRODUCT

Without a clear idea concerning the nature of the biochemical defect in XLP, the initial efforts to find the gene were focused on mapping the genomic region of the disease. The inheritance pattern narrowed this to 160 cM, the size of the X chromosome.

Genetic linkage studies indicated that the *XLP* gene was linked to DXS42 and DXS37 of Xq25 *(38).* Subsequently, interstitial deletions involving Xq25 were identified by cytogenetic and molecular techniques *(39,40).* Haplotype analysis completed the fine genetic mapping of the *XLP* locus. In a large American family of four generations with 11 affected males, a double recombination event placed the *XLP* gene between DXS1001 and DXS8057, a region of 700 kb *(41).* Another breakthrough was the finding of a 250-kb interstitial deletion in an Italian XLP family *(41).*

Two genes were found by an International Consortium in the region corresponding to genomic sequences deleted in the Italian XLP family: a human homolog of the *Drosophila melanogaster* Tenascin gene (TNM) and an SH2-domain-containing gene *(42).* Only the SH2-domain-containing gene featured mutations in males with an XLP phenotype. The gene was designated *SH2D1A,* which encodes an SH2 domain 1A.

In parallel with the studies performed by the International Consortium, another collaborative effort, following a different strategy, independently succeeded in isolating the gene mutated in XLP. These investigators, led by C. Terhorse, were primarily interested in isolating novel proteins that interact with the T- and B-cell-specific molecule, signaling lymphocyte-activation molecule (SLAM). SLAM is a glycosylated type-I transmembrane protein present on the surface of B and T lymphocytes *(43)*. Activation of SLAM triggers T and B cell responses and is considered to be an important bidirectional T- and B-cell activator. The *XLP* gene was identified as a DNA sequence encoding a polypeptide of 128 amino acid (aa) residues that could interact with SLAM *(44)*. The corresponding cDNA was isolated and sequenced. Three unrelated XLP patients showed mutations in the coding region of the gene. The gene was named SLAM-associated protein (SAP). To avoid confusion, we will employ the name *SH2D1A* (AL023657) to refer to the gene mutated in XLP.

Shortly thereafter, a third group cloned the *XLP* gene. *(45)*.

The *SH2D1A* gene consists of four exons that encode an mRNA of 2530 nucleotides. The open reading frame (ORF) starts at nucleotide position 220 and ends at position 682. The translation initiation codon is 79 bp downstream from the start of the ORF. The gene is expressed in the thymus, spleen, peripheral blood, T-cell lines, concanavalin A (ConA) and anti-CD3 activated peripheral blood T cells, the T-cell (paracortical) nodal zone, and, to a lesser extent, the germinal centers of reactive lymph nodes *(42,44,45)*. It is undetectable in EBV immortalized B lymphoblasts and in most B-cell lines. Variable levels of expression are seen in Burkitt's lymphoma lines. *SH2D1A* is upregulated in T cells late in the immune response. The ORF is translated into a polypeptide of 128 aa that consists of a single SH2 domain flanked by a 5-aa amino and a 25-aa carboxy (C)-terminal sequence. The SH2D1A protein is cytoplasmic, as there is no amino (N)-terminal signal sequence. It is judged to represent a new type of SH2-domain-containing molecule that plays an important role in signal transduction, one unlikely to possess catalytic activity. It may function as a regulatory molecule in signal transduction, competing for phosphotyrosine binding with other SH2-domain-containing proteins.

One of the functions of *SH2D1A* is to bind SLAM, a cell-surface protein required for T–B cell interaction. Binding to SLAM inhibits the recruitment of SHP-2 *(44)*. It is also possible that *SH2D1A* plays a more general regulatory role in signal transduction by interactions with proteins other than SLAM upon T-cell activation.

SUMMARY

This review is based upon several elements: personal experiences with XLP boys and families, extensive research at the bench, review of the Registry material, and review of the literature. Most of us have been involved with the XLP project for quite some time. Over this time, the number of affected boys in the XLP Registry increased slowly, as did our understanding of the disease. The search for the gene alone consumed almost 7 yr, and in the end, required the efforts of an international consortium. Curiously, the same gene was discovered at the same time by a group of immunologists interested in elucidating genes involved in lymphocyte "cross-talk."

In 1995, we were invited to write a review of XLP for *Pediatric Research*. In the year preceding this invitation, the XLP Registry data had been entered on computer. Previously, the Registry data consisted, to a large extent, of David T. Purtilo's detailed knowledge of each affected child and their kindred. To our amazement, we discovered that 10% of boys with an established diagnosis of XLP were devoid of laboratory evidence for EBV infection. In the years since, these data have held firm. Hence, a new view appears to be emerging regarding the role of the virus in the disease.

The most common (63%) and devastating (7% survival) phenotype of XLP is fulminant IM with VAHS. In this state, an acute EBV infection clearly is the catalyst for the immunologic chaos that ensues. Since the *XLP* gene appears to be involved in T- and B-lymphocyte signaling, it seems reasonable to expect that a mutation of such a gene would convert a silent but efficient immune response to a banal viral infection into the immune anarchy of fulminant IM.

Turning to the other XLP phenotypes, one remains hard-pressed to postulate a pathogenic role for EBV, except to note that some of these boys subsequently develop EBV-driven fulminant IM from which they usually die, stemming from the basic molecular defect.

Perhaps, XLP stems from several genetic mutations. Our preliminary (unpublished) mutational analysis of 35 XLP boys reveals a spectrum of mutations in the *XLP* gene in all, even though diverse clinical phenotypes were represented. Clearly, the discovery of the *XLP* gene will enable us to better dissect this fascinating disease.

ACKNOWLEDGMENT

This work was supported by the William C. Havens Foundation, Omaha, NE and the Lymphoproliferative Research Fund.

REFERENCES

1. Purtilo DT, Yang JPS, Cassel CK, Harper R, Stephenson SR, Landing BH, Vawter GF. X-linked recessive progressive combined variable immunodeficiency (Duncan's disease). Lancet 1975; 1:935–941.
2. Harrington DS, Weisenburger DD, Purtilo DT. Epstein-Barr virus-associated lymphoproliferative lesions. Clin Lab Med 1988; 8:97–118.
3. Henle W, Henle G. The virus as the etiologic agent of infectious mononucleosis: In: Epstein MA, Achong BG (eds). The Epstein–Barr Virus. Berlin: Springer-Verlag, 1979, pp. 297–320.
4. Evans AS, Neiderman JC, McCollum RW. Seroepidemiologic studies of infectious mononucleosis with EB virus. N Engl J Med 1968; 279:1121–1127.
5. Fingeroth JD, Weis JJ, Tedder TF, Strominger JL, Biro PA, Fearon DT. Epstein-Barr virus receptor of human B lymphocytes is the C3d receptor CR2. Proc Natl Acad Sci USA 1984; 81:4510–4514.
6. Sixbey JW, Nedrud JG, Raab-Traub N, Hanes RA, Pagano JS. Epstein-Barr virus replication in oropharyngeal epithelial cells. N Engl J Med 1984; 310:1255–1230.
7. Tosato G, Steinberg AD, Yarchoan R, Heilman CA, Pike SE, DeSean V, et al. Abnormally elevated frequency of Epstein-Barr virus-infected B cells in the blood of patients with rheumatoid arthritis. J Clin Invest 1984; 73:1789–1795.
8. Gerber P, Nonyama M, Lucas S, Perlin E, Goldstein I. Oral excretion of Epstein-Barr virus by healthy subjects and patients with infectious mononucleosis. Lancet 1972; 2:988–989.
9. Tomkinson BE, Wagner DK, Nelson DL, Sullivan JL. Activated lymphocytes during acute Epstein-Barr virus infection. J Immunol 1987; 139:3802–3807.
10. Gross TG, Davis JR, Baker KS, Filipovich AH, Hinrichs SH, Pirruccello S, et al. Exaggerated IL-2 response to Epstein-Barr virus (EBV) in X-linked lymphoproliferative disease (XLP). Clin Immunol Immunopathol 1995; 75:280–281.

11. Paul JR, Brunell WW. The presence of heterophile antibodies in infectious mononucleosis. Am J Med Sci 1932; 183:90–104.

12. Bartley DC, Del Rio C, Shulman JA. Clinical complications. In: Schlossberg D (ed). Infectious Mononucleosis. Berlin: Springer-Verlag, 1989, pp. 35–48.

13. Wallace LE, Rickinson AB, Rowe M, Epstein MA. Epstein-Barr virus-specific cytotoxic T-cell clones restricted through a single HLA antigen. Nature 1982; 297:413–415.

14. Pearson GR, Orr TW. Antibody-dependent lymphocyte cytotoxicity against cells expressing Epstein-Barr virus antigens. J Natl Cancer Inst 1986; 56:485–488.

15. Blazar BA, Patarroyo M, Klein E, Klein G. Increased sensitivity of human lymphoid lines to natural killer cells after induction of the Epstein-Barr viral cycle by superinfection or sodium butyrate. J Exp Med 1980; 151:614–627.

16. Hasler F, Bluestein HG, Zvaifler NJ, Epstein LB. Analysis of the defects responsible for the impaired regulation of the Epstein-Barr virus-induced B cell proliferation by rheumatoid arthritis lymphocytes: I. Diminished gamma interferon production in response to autologous stimulation. J Exp Med 1983; 157:173–188.

17. Mathur A, Kamat DM, Filipovich AH, Steinbuch M, Shapiro RS. Immunoregulatory abnormalities in patients with Epstein-Barr virus-associated B cell lymphoproliferative disorders. Transplantation 1994; 57:1042–1045.

18. Papadopoulos EB, Ladanyi M, Emanuel D, Mackinnon S, Boulad F, Carabasi MH, et al. Infusions of donor leukocytes to treat Epstein-Barr virus-associated lymphoproliferative disorders after allogeneic bone marrow transplantation. N Engl J Med 1994; 330:1185–1191.

19. Weisenburger DD, Purtilo DT. Failure in immunological control of the virus infection: fatal infectious mononucleosis. In: Epstein MA, Achong BG (eds). The Epstein–Barr Virus—Recent Advances. London: William Heinemann, 1986, pp. 127–161.

20. Okano M, Gross TG. Epstein-Barr virus-associated hemophagocytic syndrome and fatal infectious mononucleosis. Am J Hematol 1996; 53:111–115.

21. Suyama CV. Epstein-Barr virus serologic testing: diagnostic indications and interpretations. Pediatr Infect Dis 1986; 5:337–342.

22. Greiner TC, Gross TG. Atypical immune lymphoproliferations. In: Hoffman (eds). Hematology: Basic Principles and Practice, 3rd edition Philadelphia: WB Saunders, 2000.

23. Hamilton JK, Paquin LA, Sullivan JL, Maurer HS, Cruzi PG, Provisor AJ, et al. X-linked lymphoproliferative syndrome registry report. J Pediatr 1980; 96:669–673.

24. Seemayer TA, Gross TG, Egeler RM, Pirruccello SJ, Davis JR, Kelly CM, et al. X-linked lymphoproliferative disease: twenty-five years after the discovery. Pediatr Res 1995; 38:471–478.

25. Seemayer TA, Grierson H, Pirruccello SJ, Gross TG, Weisenberger DD, Davis J, et al. X-linked lymphoproliferative disease. Am J Dis Child 1993; 147:1242–1245.

26. Gross TG, Filipovich AH, Conley ME, Pracher E, Schmiegelow K, Verdirame JD, et al. Cure of X-linked lymphoproliferative disease (XLP) with allogeneic hematopoietic stem cell transplantation (HSCT): report from the XLP registry. Bone Marrow Transplant 1996; 17:741–744.

27. Mroczek EC, Weisenburger DD, Grierson HL, Markin R, Purtilo DT. Fatal infectious mononucleosis and virus-associated hemophagocytic syndrome. Arch Pathol Lab Med 1987; 111:530–535.

28. Sullivan JL, Byron KS, Brewster FE, Baker SM, Ochs HD. X-linked lymphoproliferative syndrome: natural history of the immunodeficiency. J Clin Invest 1983; 71:1765–1778.

29. Steinherz R, Levy Y, Litwin A, Nitzan M, Friedman E, Levin S. X-linked lymphoproliferative syndrome. Am J Dis Child 1985; 139:191–193.

30. Grierson H, Purtilo DT. Epstein-Barr virus infections in males with the X-linked lymphoproliferative syndrome. Ann Intern Med 1987; 106:538–545.

31. Harrington DS, Weisenburger DD, Purtilo DT. Malignant lymphoma in the X-linked lymphoproliferative syndrome. Cancer 1987; 59:1419–1429.

32. Saemundsen AK, Purtilo DT, Sakamoto K, Sullivan JL, Synnerholm AC, Hanto D, et al. Documentation of Epstein-Barr virus infection in immunodeficient patients with life-threatening lymphoproliferative disease by Epstein-Barr virus complementary RNA/DNA and viral DNA/DNA hybridization. Cancer Res 1981; 41:4237–4242.

33. Falk K, Ernberg I, Sakthivel R, Davis J, Christensson B, Luka J, et al. Expression of Epstein-Barr Virus-encoded proteins and B-cell markers in fatal infectious mononucleosis. Int J Cancer 1990; 46:976–984.

34. Purtillo DT, Sakamoto K, Barnabei V, Seeley J, Bechtold T, Rogers G, et al. Epstein–Barr virus induced diseases in boys with the X-linked lymphoproliferative syndrome (XLP) Am J Med 1982; 73:49–56.

35. Egeler RM, de Kraker J, Slater R, Purtilo DT. Documentation of Burkitt lymphoma with t(8;14)(q24;q32) in X-linked lymphoproliferative disease. Cancer 1992; 70:683–687.

36. Williams LL, Rooney CM, Conley ME, Brenner MK, Krance RA, Heslop HE. Correction of Duncan's syndrome by allogeneic bone marrow transplantation. Lancet 1993; 2:587–588.

37. Turner AM, Berdoukas VA, Tobias VH, Ziegler JB, Toogood IR, Mulley JC, et al. Report on the X-linked lymphoproliferative disease in an Australian family. J Paediatr Child Health 1992; 28:184–189.

38. Skare JC, Grierson HL, Sullivan JL, Nussbaum RL, Purtilo DT, Sylla BS, et al. Linkage analysis of seven kindreds with the X-linked lymphoproliferative syndrome (XLP) confirms that the XLP locus is near DSX42 and DXS37. Hum Genet 1989; 82:354–358.

39. Sanger WG, Grierson HL, Skare J, Wyandt H, Pirruccello S, Fordyce R, Purtilo DT. Partial Xq25 deletion in a family with the X-linked lymphoproliferative disease. Cancer Genet Cytogenet 1990; 47:163–169.

40. Lanyi A, Li B, Ki S, Talmadge Cary Buresh, MD, Brichacek B, Davis JR, et al. A yeast artifical chromosome (YAC) contig encompassing the critical region of the X-linked lymphoproliferative disease (XLP). Genomics 1997; 39:55–65.

41. Bolino A, Yin L. Seri M. Cusano R, Cinti R, Coffey A, et al. A new candidate region for the positional cloning of the XLP gene. Eur J Hum Genet 1998; 6:509–517.

42. Coffey AJ, Brooksbank RA, Brandau O, Oohashi T, Howell GR, Bye JM, et al. Host response to EBV infection in X-linked lymphoproliferative disease results from mutations in an SH2-domain encoding gene. Nat Genet 1998; 20:129–135.

43. Cocks BG, Chang CC, Carballido JM, Yssel H, De Vries JE, Aversa G. A novel receptor involved in T-cell activation. Nature 1995; 376:260–263.

44. Sayos J, Wu C, Morra M, Wang N, Zhang X, Allen D, et al. The X-linked lymphoproliferative-disease gene product SAP regulates signals induced through the co-receptor SLAM. Nature 1998; 395:462–469.

45. Nichols KE, Harkin DP, Levitz S, Krainer M, Kolquist KA, Genovese C, et al. Inactivating mutations in an SH2 domain encoding-gene in X-linked lymphoproliferative syndrome. Proc Natl Scad Sci USA 1998; 95:13765–13770.

4

Posttransplant Lymphoproliferative Disorder

Lode J. Swinnen

INTRODUCTION

Recognized since the early days of organ transplantation, Epstein–Barr virus (EBV)-associated B-lymphoproliferative disorders remain a major complication of immunosuppression. Similar if not identical EBV-associated B-cell proliferations have since been described in congenital and in other acquired immunodeficiency states. Although the initial events in the course of viral lymphomagenesis appear to be unique to the setting of immunodeficiency, the subsequent evolution of lesions more closely resembles lymphomas seen in the general population.

The malignancies overrepresented in the organ transplant population are squamous skin and cervical carcinomas, B-cell lymphomas, and Kaposi's sarcoma *(1)*, all now known to be virally related. The malignancies most common in the general population, such as colon, lung, breast, and prostate cancer, do not appear to occur more frequently after organ transplantation. Failure of immune surveillance therefore does not result in a global increase in the incidence of malignancy, but appears to facilitate virally mediated oncogenesis. Posttransplant lymphoproliferative disorder is the most frequently fatal, and the most extensively studied, of these virally induced tumors.

INCIDENCE AND RISK FACTORS

The incidence of posttransplant lymphproliferative disorder (PTLD) varies according to the organ transplanted, the series reported, the immunosuppressive regimens used, and the age grouping of transplant recipients. Reviewing thoracic organ transplants over a 10-yr period at the University of Pittsburgh, Armitage et al. noted a 3.4% incidence following heart transplantation, and a 7.9% incidence following lung transplantation *(2)*. Determining the true incidence of PTLD has been difficult, as series have been small, the denominator from which registry cases were derived difficult to assess, and as length of follow-up often was not considered. In by far the largest analysis, using data collected by the multicenter European and North American Collaborative Transplant Study, Opelz et al. reported on PTLD incidence among 45,141 renal recipients and 7634 cardiac recipients. As had been noted in other series, incidence was highest in the first posttransplant year. During that first year, 0.2% of renal and 1.2% of cardiac recipients developed PTLD, rates that were calculated to be 20 and 120 times

From: *Infectious Causes of Cancer: Targets for Intervention*
Edited by: J. J. Goedert © Humana Press Inc., Totowa, NJ

Table 1
Risk Factors for Posttransplant Lymphoproliferative Disorder

- Pretransplant EBV seronegativity
- Pediatric age group
- Type of organ transplanted (nonrenal > renal)
- Monoclonal anti-lymphocyte antibody (OKT3)
- Mismatched or T-cell-depleted bone marrow transplant

higher than those seen in the general population. The incidence of PTLD in subsequent years was about 0.04% per year in renal and 0.3% per year in cardiac recipients *(3)*. In a subsequent report, analyzing 14,284 heart recipients and 72,360 kidney recipients, a cumulative incidence of 5000 per 100,000 by 7 yr of follow-up was noted in heart recipients, and slightly more than 1000 per 100,000 by 10 yr of follow-up in renal recipients *(4)*. This would imply a cumulative incidence of 5% for heart recipients and 1% for kidney recipients, numbers that are very much in keeping with what has been reported in smaller series.

The incidence of PTLD can, however, be much higher in patients who are EBV seronegative prior to transplant (Table 1) *(5,6)*. In a cohort of 154 cardiac recipients, a much higher proportion of patients who went on to develop PTLD were EBV seronegative prior to transplantation than were patients who did not develop the disease (30% vs 5%) *(7)*. The risk of PTLD in EBV-seronegative recipients in a series from the Mayo Clinic was determined to be 76 times that in seropositive recipients *(8)*. Most adults (90% or more) are EBV seropositive. The majority of seronegative patients are children, with a higher likelihood of seronegativity the younger the child is *(5,9)*. A series from the University of Pittsburgh identified a four times higher risk of PTLD for pediatric than for adult transplant recipients *(5)*. PTLD is therefore a particular problem among pediatric transplant recipients, and the risk has been considered to be sufficiently high as to preclude transplantation in some instances *(8)*.

The immunosuppressive regimen also significantly influences risk. A particularly high incidence of PTLD was noted following the introduction of cyclosporin A (CsA) *(10)*, which diminished when blood levels were monitored and lower doses of the drug were used *(11)*. The incidence of PTLD under FK 506 immunosuppression appears to be comparable to what has been seen with CsA *(12–14)*. PTLD incidence has typically been higher in nonrenal than in renal transplants. A possible reason is more intense immunosuppression in the vital organ recipients. Statistically significantly higher doses of cyclosporin and azathioprine were identified for heart than for kidney recipients on analysis of Collaborative Transplant Study data. A related observation was a statistically significant higher risk of PTLD among North American heart or kidney recipients than for such patients transplanted at European centers, amounting to a relative risk of 2.12. Correlation was made with higher immunosuppressive dosage among North American recipients *(3)*. Shortly after the introduction of the immunosuppressive antibody OKT3, a ninefold higher incidence of PTLD was noted among patients who had received induction therapy with OKT3 (11.4% vs 1.3%) in a Loyola University series of 154 consecutive cardiac transplants *(7)*. A strong dose–response effect was observed, in that 6.2% of patients who had received one course of the drug and 35.7% of patients who had received two courses developed PTLD. A murine monoclonal antibody directed against the human CD3 receptor–T-cell complex, OKT3 profoundly depletes circulating CD3⁺ T lymphocytes *(15)*, and has since been associated with a significant increase in the incidence of PTLD in several other series *(3,16,17)*. PTLD is relatively uncommon following allogeneic bone marrow transplantation (<1%) *(18)*, despite the severe immunodeficiency encountered, in the absence of certain risk factors. Use of a monoclonal anti-CD3 antibody known as 64.1 was found to be associated with a 14% incidence of PTLD, and T-cell depletion of donor marrow resulted in a 12% incidence *(19)*; in a separate series, T-cell depletion of mismatched donor marrow resulted in a 24% incidence of the disease *(20)*. All these observations underscore the fact that the intensity of immunosuppression, and particularly highly potent and selective anti-T-cell therapy, significantly increases the risk of PTLD.

ASSOCIATION WITH EBV

The EBV plays a central role in the pathogenesis of PTLD. Although EBV-negative PTLD has been demonstrated clearly, the vast majority of PTLDs are EBV associated. Clinical or serologic indications of a primary or reactivated EBV infection are often associated with the appearance of the disorder *(21)*. Tumor tissue has been found to contain EBV DNA and to actively express viral proteins *(22–24)*. T-cell deficiency or deliberate partial suppression of T-cell function to prevent graft rejection is believed to result in uncontrolled EBV-driven proliferation of B cells *(21–25)*. As proliferation continues, B-cell clones with a growth advantage presumably emerge, resulting in one or more clonal populations.

Although the exact mechanisms for the emergence of a clinical lymphoproliferative disorder remain unclear, this model is capable of explaining many of the unusual clinical and pathologic features of the disease. Tumor-associated EBV is clonal, further supporting an etiologic role for the virus rather than for subsequent infection of neoplastic B cells. The pattern of viral clones appears to correspond to B-cell clonality as determined by immunoglobulin gene rearrangement analysis. Lesions consisting of polyclonal or multiclonal B-cell proliferations contain multiple EBV clones, while monoclonal proliferations show evidence of a single infectious event *(26,27)*. Clonality of the virus is determined on the basis of the specific number of terminal repeat sequences formed when the linear EBV genome circularizes upon infection of a B cell.

Analysis of prior liver biopsy specimens in liver transplant recipients has shown the presence of EBV, as determined by polymerase chain reaction (PCR) or by *in situ* immunohistochemical staining for Epstein-Barr encoded RNA (EBER) expressing cells, in 70% of cases who subsequently developed PTLD. Only 10% of patients who did not go on to develop the disease had such findings *(24)*. A preclinical phase for PTLD is also suggested by observations that viral load, as determined in peripheral blood mononuclear cells, increases prior to the appearance of clinically detected disease *(28,29)*. It is not clear whether such rises in EBV load necessarily indicate EBV-driven neoplasia, or are reflective of severe immunodeficiency at the time. A study of EBV load in peripheral blood mononuclear cells conducted at the University of Edinburgh showed that rises in viral load occurred at some point in the posttransplant course of 73% of patients studied. Although the mean rise in patients with PTLD was

Table 2
EBV Latency Antigen Expression in EBV-Associated Malignancies

	Latency III	Latency II	Latency I
EBV genes expressed:	EBNA-1, EBNA-2 EBNA-3A, EBNA-3B EBNA-3C, EBNA LP LMP-1, LMP-2A	EBNA-1, LMP-1 LMP-2A, LMP-2B	EBNA-1
Phenotypes:	PTLD LCL AIDS NHL	HD NPC	BL

EBNA, Epstein–Barr nuclear antigen; PTLD, posttransplant lymphoproliferative disease; NHL, Non-Hodgkin's lymphoma; NPC, nasopharyngeal carcinoma; LMP, latent membrane protein; LCL, lymphoblastic cell line; HD, Hodgkin's disease; BL, Burkitt's lymphoma.

more than threefold higher, levels in patients who did not develop PTLD frequently equaled or exceeded the viral load seen in those who did *(30)*. It would appear from this and other studies that while sensitive to the presence of early PTLD, viral load as determined in circulating mononuclear cells may not be very specific, making screening problematic. Attempts at setting quantitative standards with predictive value are under way *(31)*. Interestingly, EBV DNA can be measured in serum from patients with PTLD, using very sensitive PCR techniques. In preliminary work, very high sensitivity and specificity for PTLD have been identified. It is not clear whether the presence of EBV DNA in serum reflects tumor metabolism or not, but this might explain the greater specificity of the EBV serum assay for PTLD *(32)*.

EBV infection of resting B cells in vitro results in immortalized lymphoblastoid cell lines that express the full range of latent viral cycle proteins (six nuclear antigens: EBNA-1, EBNA-2, EBNA-3A, -3B, -3C, EBNA-LP, and three membrane proteins: LMP-1, LMP-2A, LMP-2B), the so-called latency III pattern. The pattern of viral latency antigens differs among EBV-associated malignancies (Table 2). In the presence of adequate EBV-specific immunity in vivo, only the nonimmunogenic EBNA-1 is expressed (latency I) as exemplified in endemic Burkitt's lymphoma. Expression of viral latency proteins in PTLD resembles what is seen in lymphoblastoid cell lines, but a degree of restriction of expression has nonetheless been identified, possibly reflecting varying degrees of immune control *(33,34)*. Unlike oral hairy leukoplakia in immunodeficiency, PTLD has not been associated with fully productive viral lytic cycle *(33,35,36)*. Expression of normally highly immunogenic proteins might explain the reversibility of PTLD in some cases when immunosuppressives are reduced. In many instances, however, PTLD will not regress with such measures, despite expression of immunodominant EBNAs in the tumor. Chromosomal or structural gene alterations may sustain the growth of such lesions after an initial phase of EBV-dependent transformation and growth.

The mechanisms for EBV-driven neoplasia in PTLD remain unclear. Overexpression of bcl-2 might confer resistance to apoptosis. Such overexpression was identified in all PTLD tumors expressing LMP-1 in one series, while absence of LMP-1 expression was always associated with a lack of bcl-2 expression. Interestingly, the viral homolog of bcl-2, BHRF1, was not overexpressed in these tumors. Viral induction of human bcl-2 therefore appears to be the case *(36)*.

LMP-1 is the viral protein deemed to be of greatest importance for EBV-induced transformation of B cells, and it has been likened to an oncogene in that respect. In vitro LMP-1 mimics the effects of ligand-induced aggregation of CD40, activating the transcriptional activators nuclear factor-κ B (NF-κB) and activator protein 1 *(37,38)*. This activation is mediated by tumor necrosis factor-receptor associated (TRAF) signaling molecules, which interact directly with a portion of LMP-1 (*see also* Chapter 6) *(39)*. Recent work by Liebowitz has extended these observations to PTLD in vivo, by showing physical localization of LMP-1 and TRAF-1 and TRAF-3 *(40)*. This demonstration of LMP-1 as an effector of virus-induced B-cell transformation constitutes further indirect but compelling evidence for a causative role for EBV in PTLD *(41)*.

Cyclosporine has recently been directly linked to mechanisms for increased cell proliferation and invasiveness both in vitro and in severe combined immune deficiency (SCID) mice. Immune control would not play a role in those settings. Anti-transforming growth factor-β (TGF-β) antibodies prevented the in vitro phenotypic changes and the greater propensity for metastasis in SCID mice *(42)*. Although this provocative observation merits further investigation, it should be noted that the work was done with adenocarcinoma cells, that PTLD was recognized prior to the advent of cyclosporine, and is also seen in congenital immunodeficiency states.

HISTOPATHOLOGIC AND MOLECULAR FEATURES

The vast majority of PTLD lesions in solid organ recipients arise from recipient rather than from donor lymphocytes, the opposite of what is seen following allogeneic bone marrow transplantation. Three different techniques have been used to define the origin of PTLD. DNA restriction fragment length polymorphism analysis in one series found that the PTLD was of recipient origin in all of 16 solid organ recipients *(43)*. Similarly, recipient origin was found in 10 of 11 cases studied by genetic polymorphisms at several loci; and in 11 of 12 cases studied by microsatellite analysis *(44,45)*.

PTLD comprises a histologic spectrum extending from reactive or hyperplastic-looking morphologies to a picture indistinguishable from immunoblastic non-Hodgkin's lymphoma *(46–48)*. Thus, the question of whether PTLD is "malignant" or not has generated much controversy. Histologic features resembling a reactive process might be seen, with no monoclonal population detectable by immunophenotyping; nevertheless the disease ran a malignant, frequently lethal clinical course. It is now clear that most lesions found to be polyclonal by immunophenotyping contain one or more monoclonal subpopulations when studied by the much more sensitive technique of immunogenotyping on the basis of clonal gene rearrangements *(49,50)*. More than one clone may coexist within the same lesion ("oligoclonal" tumors), and both differing clones and differing histopathology may be seen in lesions at separate anatomic sites in the same patient *(49,51)*. Such clonal evolution and diversity contrasts sharply with the homogeneity seen in classic non-Hodgkin's lymphoma, and likely represents a very different mechanism for lymphoid neoplasia. If the conditions are conducive, EBV-driven lymphoproliferation seems to appear simultaneously at multiple sites in the body. The vast majority of PTLDs studied have been of B-cell origin; in a few cases the lesions have been of T-cell origin. EBV-negative aggressive T-cell lymphomas have

Table 3
Pathologic Classifications for PTLD

Frizzera *(46)*	Nalesnik *(52)*	Knowles *(48)*
• Polymorphic diffuse B-cell hyperplasia • Polymorphic diffuse B-cell lymphoma	• Polymorphic, nonclonal • Polymorphic, clonal by EBV and/or Ig gene analysis • Monomorphic • Mixed clonal and nonclonal	• Plasmacytic hyperplasia • Polymorphic B-cell hyperplasia and polymorphic B-cell lymphoma • Immunoblastic lymphoma or multiple myeloma

recently been identified by Hanson et al. as a rare, very late occurrence, presenting at a median of 15 yr following transplantation.

A pathologic classification system for PTLD was first described by Frizzera *(46)* and subsequently modified, including correlative molecular genetic analysis (Table 3) *(47,48)*. Plasmacytic hyperplasia is usually polyclonal, arises from the tonsils or cervical nodes, contains multiple EBV infection events, and lacks oncogene or tumor suppressor gene alterations. Polymorphic B-cell hyperplasia and polymorphic B-cell lymphoma were encountered at many sites in the body, were usually monoclonal, containing a single form of EBV, and lacked oncogene and tumor suppressor gene alterations. Immunoblastic lymphoma and multiple myeloma were monoclonal, contained a single form of EBV, and contained one or more structurally altered genes (N-*ras*, c-*myc*, *p53*, or others). Nalesnik and co-workers at the University of Pittsburgh have stressed polymorphism vs monomorphism in their approach to classification *(47,52)*. Controversies persist about the best way to classify PTLD. A recent Society of Hematopathology workshop on the subject recognized a number of other morphologies encountered among PTLDs *(53)*. At this point it is probably preferable to identify these tumors as PTLD, and to categorize them according to a PTLD classification, rather than to attempt to make these proliferations fit into a general non-Hodgkin's lymphoma classification.

EBV-negative PTLD remains poorly studied. Relatively rare, it may be becoming more frequent as a late complication of transplantation. The mechanisms for such tumors are unknown; interestingly, some have regressed with reduced immunosuppression *(54)*. T-cell PTLD is likewise a rare late event. Few cases have been investigated; about half of these have been peripheral T-cell lymphomas, some of which have been EBV positive *(55)*.

Data regarding cytogenetic abnormalities in PTLD have been sparse. Abnormalities have been identified, typically in tumors with monomorphic histology, but no distinct abnormality has been identified as being characteristic for PTLD. In a recent series of 28 patients, no clonal cytogenetic abnormalities were identified among 10 polymorphic tumors, all of which were polyclonal or oligoclonal. Analysis of 12 monomorphic cases revealed a variety of abnormalities in ten cases: chromosome 8 translocations involving the *myc* gene, trisomy 9, trisomy 11, and 11q27 *(40)*.

CLINICAL PRESENTATION

Patients may present with systemic effects of the disease, symptoms localized to anatomic sites of involvement, or with incidental clinical or radiologic findings while still asymptomatic. Although the disease is very heterogeneous, some clinical patterns have been identified. An infectious mononucleosis-like presentation, with prominent constitutional symptoms and rapid enlargement of the tonsils and cervical nodes, is often the case for PTLD presenting early after transplantation—less than about 6 mo to a year from the time of transplant *(50)*. In one series of renal transplant patients described by Hanto et al., this presentation accounted for approx 40% of patients. Patients tended to be young, present early after transplant, and have widespread disease *(56)*. Highly immunosuppressed patients may present with widespread disease, diffusely infiltrative multiorgan involvement, and systemic sepsis, within weeks of transplantation, and pursue a fulminant clinical course difficult to distinguish from sepsis alone *(57,58)*.

PTLD presenting later than about a year after transplantation is likely to be more circumscribed anatomically, manifest fewer systemic symptoms, and run a more gradual clinical course. Extranodal disease and visceral nodal involvement, often in the absence of superficial nodal involvement, is usually seen. Gastrointestinal involvement is a frequent finding in PTLD. Approximately 25% of patients in the University of Pittsburgh series presented with gastrointestinal disease, manifesting as acute abdomen, pain, obstruction, or hemorrhage *(57)*. The transplanted organ itself may be affected in up to 20% of cases, at times resulting in a mistaken diagnosis of rejection. Central nervous system involvement at presentation is mainly seen as part of very extensive disease. Multiple pulmonary nodules seem to be a particularly common presentation, and the lung may be the only site of disease *(58,59)*.

DIAGNOSIS AND TREATMENT

Early diagnosis and intervention are essential to the successful management of PTLD. A high index of suspicion is required, as the initial signs and symptoms of the disease may be relatively nonspecific. Although the EBV antibody titer often rises at or prior to the emergence of PTLD, that need not be the case. Conversely, a rise in EBV titer is not uncommon after transplantation, and need not imply the development of PTLD. The EBV titer is therefore of limited clinical utility. The diagnosis should be established histologically rather than cytologically, in view of the challenging morphology often encountered and the importance of ancillary studies (gene rearrangement analysis and evidence for EBV association) in such cases.

No uniform approach to the treatment of PTLD has been defined, and the literature on this subject has been largely anecdotal. However, certain observations can be generalized (Table 4). Treatment must be individualized to the specific clinical situation and to the type of organ transplanted. Reduction in immunosuppression can result in permanent resolution of PTLD. Unlike non-Hodgkin's lymphoma in general, PTLD can be eradicated by surgical resection or by irradiation of unresectable, strictly localized lesions. Chemotherapy has traditionally been viewed as a treatment of last resort owing to the very high morbidity and mortality reported in the past.

Starzl has long advocated the value of reduction in immunosuppression, which can result in complete and durable tumor regression *(57)*. The likelihood of response has

Table 4
Treatment Modalities for Posttransplant Lymphoproliferative Disorder

- Reduction in immunosuppression (± acyclovir)
- Surgical resection
- Limited field irradiation
- Interferon-α
- Cytotoxic chemotherapy
- Monoclonal anti-B-cell antibodies
- EBV-specific T cells

been linked to the interval since transplantation in the Pittsburgh series of heart recipients: more than 80% of patients presenting at less than 1 yr following transplantation responded to reduction in immunosuppression, while none presenting at more than 1 yr did so *(2)*. More variable results with reduced immunosuppression have been reported in other series: lower response rates and greater variability in terms of the interval since transplantation *(58,60)*. Attempts have been made at formulating a clinicopathologic classification (based on clinical features, histology, clonality, and the presence of oncogene alterations) that would be capable of predicting disease behavior and the likelihood of response to a reduction in immunosuppression *(46,48,50)*. Considerable overlap in categories exists, however, and the course of an individual patient remains difficult to predict. Patients classified as immunoblastic lymphoma or multiple myeloma by the Knowles–Frizzera classification system have been considered unresponsive to reduced immunosuppression, but these are retrospective data *(48)*.

A trial of reduced immunosuppression is therefore considered justified as the initial approach to all cases *(2,57)*. Rejection is a valid concern, and the extent and duration of a reduction in immunosuppression for recipients of a vital organ remains poorly defined and highly subjective. If complete remission is achieved by this means, immunosuppressives will need to be reinstituted before the onset of rejection. Based on the model of PTLD as a disease of overimmunosuppression, immunosuppressive agents have often been reinstituted at moderately reduced dosage. Data regarding the level of subsequent immunosuppression required remain anecdotal. Although the literature is sparse on this subject, partial responses tend to be transient. PTLD is an aggressive disease, and rapid progression is generally seen if eradication cannot be accomplished *(58)*.

A means for predicting whether any given PTLD will be responsive to reduced immunosuppression would be highly desirable. Rejection and rapid disease progression are both significant risks that might thereby be avoided. With this in mind, Cesarman et al. studied 36 PTLD patients for the presence of mutations in the *bcl-6* protooncogene, using single-strand conformation polymorphism and sequence analysis *(61)*. In 33 patients this could be related to clinical outcome. No *bcl-6* mutations were identified in cases classified as plasmacytic hyperplasia (Knowles–Frizzera classification). Mutations were found in 43% of polymorphic lesions and in 90% of PTLDs classified as immunoblastic lymphoma or multiple myeloma. *Bcl-6* mutations were predictive for lack of response to reduced immunosuppression. Although the association was statistically significant, the correlations were retrospective and treatment was variable. Nonetheless, this study represents the strongest data and the clearest predictor for response to reduced immunosuppressives to date. Unfortunately, the techniques used do not lend themselves to "real-time" clinical testing.

Local therapies such as resection or limited field irradiation have resulted in long-term remission in anatomically limited PTLD. That approach also has been used to remove a limited number of residual lesions after a partial response to reduced immunosuppression has been achieved (2,58).

Although regression of lymphoproliferations has been described following the use of high-dose acylovir in a small number of cases, the value of acyclovir remains unclear (59,62). Acyclovir, even at high doses, has proved to be ineffective as prophylaxis for PTLD in bone marrow transplant recipients (63). It is not known whether other drugs, such as ganciclovir or foscarnet, are of any greater efficacy. Uncontrolled studies have suggested possible prophylactic benefit (64), but firm conclusions cannot be drawn in the absence of a randomized, prospective study with a no-prophylaxis control arm. A course of full-dose intravenous acyclovir is viewed as relatively nontoxic, and has often been given simultaneously with reduction in immunosuppressives as initial management of PTLD.

Durable complete responses have been achieved with interferon-α-2b. Neither the response rate nor the mechanism of action is defined at this point. The drug might exert an antiviral and/or an antitumor effect; both early polyclonal proliferations and late-presenting monoclonal lesions have been reported to respond (63,65). In a series of 18 patients treated with interferon-α-2b and simultaneous reduction in immunosuppression, an overall response rate of 83% (77% complete response, 6% partial response) was reported. Rejection and life-threatening infection were noted in 50% of patients, and median survival was only 6 mo (66).

Chemotherapy has been viewed as a treatment of last resort for PTLD refractory to a reduction in immunosuppression. A mortality of 70% has been reported for patients presenting at more than 1 yr posttransplant (2,59). Septic and other complications of chemotherapy have been the major problem in some centers, while others have found refractory disease to be common (57,59,60). Those poor results have been obtained with a variety of regimens, frequently CHOP (*see* Chapter 8 for chemotherapy regiments). More encouraging results have been achieved in a series of cardiac recipients treated predominantly with ProMACE-CytaBOM (58). Mortality during chemotherapy was 25%, (sepsis, refractory disease); the surviving patients all achieved complete remission. No patient has relapsed, at a median follow-up of 64 mo. The factors responsible for this relatively favorable outcome are not clear. The regimen used may play a role, in that it allows the discontinuation of all other immunosuppressives for the duration of chemotherapy and minimizes exposure to doxorubicin in cardiac recipients. This approach is currently being tested in an intergroup study being conducted by the Southwest Oncology Group and the Eastern Cooperative Oncology Group (SWOG-9239). The advent of better supportive care measures, granulocyte colony-stimulating factor, and preventive antibiotics may further reduce the toxicity of chemotherapy in this patient population.

The therapeutic use of a mixture of anti-CD21 and anti-CD24 anti-B cell monoclonal antibodies was found to be effective in patients with polyclonal or oligoclonal disease in a European multicenter trial involving both organ and bone marrow transplant recipients with PTLD *(60,67)*. An update on this series of patients was recently reported *(68)*. Fifty-eight patients with PTLD (27 following bone marrow and 31 following organ transplantation) were treated. The overall complete response rate was 61%. The relapse rate was low at 8%. The long-term overall survival was 46% (bone marrow transplant, 35%; organ transplant, 55%) at a median follow-up of 61 mo. Complete remission was achieved in 46% of monoclonal and in 80% of oligoclonal cases ($p = .05$). Multivisceral disease, central nervous system (CNS) involvement, and late-onset PTLD (more than 1 yr posttransplant) were identified as predictive of poorer response on multivariate analysis. Only 29% of patients with CNS involvement and 22% of patients presenting later than 1 yr posttransplant achieved complete remission. Toxicity was mild, consisting of transient fever, hypotension, and neutropenia. The antibodies used are not currently clinically available. Anecdotal observations of efficacy for the humanized murine anti-CD20 antibody rituximab (Rituxan®) are being reported. This antibody is commercially available, and a prospective phase II study in adult and pediatric post-organ transplant lymphoproliferative disorder is currently in progress.

EBV-specific immunocompetence has been rapidly restored in T-cell-depleted allogeneic bone marrow recipients by the infusion of a limited number of peripheral blood leukocytes from the donor. PTLD was controlled in these cases without incurring graft-vs-host disease, presumably because of the high frequency of EBV-specific effector cells in the relatively small number of leukocytes transfused *(69)*. More recently, highly selective adoptive transfer of T-cell immunity has been achieved using in vitro expanded EBV-specific cytotoxic T cells as treatment and prophylaxis for PTLD in bone marrow transplant recipients *(70,71)*. Polyclonal T-cell lines containing both $CD4^+$ and $CD8^+$ cells were used, as it is not presently clear which antigens expressed by EBV-infected cells are important in generating an effector response. Adoptive transfer of EBV-specific T-cell immunity would clearly also lend itself to prophylactic measures against PTLD. Using such approaches in the organ transplant setting will require some adaptations, in view of the major histocompatibility complex (MHC)-restricted nature of the T-cell response, and the fact that the majority of PTLDs arise from recipient rather than from donor lymphocytes.

REFERENCES

1. Penn I. Cancer in the immunosuppressed organ recipient. Transplant Proc 1991; 23:1771–1772.
2. Armitage JM, Kormos RL, Stuart RS, et al. Posttransplant lymphoproliferative disease in thoracic organ transplant patients: ten years of cyclosporine-based immunosuppression. J Heart Lung Transplant 1991; 10:877–86.
3. Opelz G, Henderson R. Incidence of non-Hodgkin lymphoma in kidney and heart transplant recipients. Lancet 1993; 342:1514–1516.
4. Opelz G. Are post-transplant lymphomas inevitable? [editorial]. Nephrol Dialys Transplant 1996; 11:1952–1955.
5. Ho M, Jaffe R, Miller G, et al. The frequency of Epstein–Barr virus infection and associated lymphoproliferative syndrome after transplantation and its manifestations in children. Transplantation 1988; 45:719–727.
6. Cacciarelli TV, Esquivel CO, Moore DH, et al. Factors affecting survival after orthotopic liver transplantation in infants. Transplantation 1997; 64:242–248.

7. Swinnen LJ, Costanzo-Nordin MR, Fisher SG, et al. Increased incidence of lymphoproliferative disorder after immunosuppression with the monoclonal antibody OKT3 in cardiac-transplant recipients. N Engl J Med 1990; 323:1723–1728.

8. Walker RC, Paya CV, Marshall WF, et al. Pretransplantation seronegative Epstein–Barr virus status is the primary risk factor for posttransplantation lymphoproliferative disorder in adult heart, lung, and other solid organ transplantations. J Heart Lung Transplant 1995; 14:214–221.

9. Nalesnik MA, Rao AS, Furukawa H, et al. Autologous lymphokine-activated killer cell therapy of Epstein–Barr virus-positive and -negative lymphoproliferative disorders arising in organ transplant recipients. Transplantation 1997; 63:1200–1205.

10. Starzl TE, Nalesnik MA, Porter KA, et al. Reversibility of lymphomas and lymphoproliferative lesions developing under cyclosporin-steroid therapy. Lancet 1984; 1:583–587.

11. Beveridge T, Krupp P, McKibbin C. Lymphomas and lymphoproliferative lesions developing under cyclosporin therapy [letter]. Lancet 1984; 1:788.

12. Armitage JM, Fricker FJ, del Nido P, Starzl TE, Hardesty RL, Griffith BP. A decade (1982 to 1992) of pediatric cardiac transplantation and the impact of FK 506 immunosuppression. J Thorac Cardiovasc Surg 1993; 105:464–472.

13. Deschler DG, Osorio R, Ascher NL, Lee KC. Posttransplantation lymphoproliferative disorder in patients under primary tacrolimus (FK 506) immunosuppression. Arch Otolaryngol Head Neck Surg 1995; 121:1037–1041.

14. Cacciarelli TV, Esquivel CO, Cox KL, et al. Oral tacrolimus (FK506) induction therapy in pediatric orthotopic liver transplantation. Transplantation 1996; 61:1188–1192.

15. Bach JF, Chatenoud L. Immunologic monitoring of Orthoclone OKT3-treated patients: the problem of antimonoclonal immune response. Transplant Proc 1987; 19:17–20.

16. Walker RC, Marshall WF, Strickler JG, et al. Pretransplantation assessment of the risk of lymphoproliferative disorder. Clin Infect Dis 1995; 20:1346–1353.

17. Penn I. The changing pattern of posttransplant malignancies. Transplant Proc 1991; 23:1101–1103.

18. Zutter MM, Martin PJ, Sale GE, et al. Epstein–Barr virus lymphoproliferation after bone marrow transplantation. Blood 1988; 72:520–529.

19. Witherspoon RP, Fisher LD, Schoch G, et al. Secondary cancers after bone marrow transplantation for leukemia or aplastic anemia [see comments]. N Engl J Med 1989; 321:784–789.

20. Shapiro RS, McClain K, Frizzera G, et al. Epstein–Barr virus associated B cell lymphoproliferative disorders following bone marrow transplantation. Blood 1988; 71:1234–1243.

21. Purtilo DT. Epstein–Barr-virus-induced oncogenesis in immune-deficient individuals. Lancet 1980; 1:300–303.

22. Hanto DW, Frizzera G, Purtilo DT, et al. Clinical spectrum of lymphoproliferative disorders in renal transplant recipients and evidence for the role of Epstein–Barr virus. Cancer Res 1981; 41:4253–4261.

23. Young L, Alfieri C, Hennessy K, et al. Expression of Epstein-Barr virus transformation-associated genes in tissues of patients with EBV lymphoproliferative disease. N Engl J Med 1989; 321:1080–1085.

24. Randhawa PS, Jaffe R, Demetris AJ, et al. Expression of Epstein–Barr virus-encoded small RNA (by the EBER-1 gene) in liver specimens from transplant recipients with post-transplantation lymphoproliferative disease. N Engl J Med 1992; 327:1710–1714.

25. Klein G. Lymphoma development in mice and humans: diversity of initiation is followed by convergent cytogenetic evolution. Proc Natl Acad Sci USA 1979; 76:2442–2446.

26. Cleary ML, Nalesnik MA, Shearer WT, Sklar J. Clonal analysis of transplant-associated lymphoproliferations based on the structure of the genomic termini of the Epstein–Barr virus. Blood 1988; 72:349–352.

27. Kaplan MA, Ferry JA, Harris NL, Jacobson JO. Clonal analysis of posttransplant lymphoproliferative disorders, using both episomal Epstein–Barr virus and immunoglobulin genes as markers. Am J Clin Pathol 1994; 101:590–596.

28. Riddler SA, Breinig MC, McKnight JL. Increased levels of circulating Epstein–Barr virus (EBV)-infected lymphocytes and decreased EBV nuclear antigen antibody responses are associated with the development of posttransplant lymphoproliferative disease in solid-organ transplant recipients. Blood 1994; 84:972–984.

29. Rooney CM, Loftin SK, Holladay MS, Brenner MK, Krance RA, Heslop HE. Early identification of Epstein–Barr virus-associated post-transplantation lymphoproliferative disease. Br J Haematol 1995; 89:98–103.

30. Hopwood P, Brooks LA, MacCormac L, et al. Changes in Epstein–Barr virus load in the peripheral blood following cardiothoracic transplantation (abstr.). Eighth International Symposium on Tumor-Associated Herpesviruses, 1998, p. 5.

31. George D, Barnett L, Boulad F, et al. Semi-quantitative PCR analysis of genomic EBV DNA post BMT allows close surveillance of patients at risk for development of EBV-lymphoproliferative disorders (EBV-LPD) allowing prompt intervention (abstr.). Blood 1998; 92 (Suppl 1): 437a.

32. Swinnen LJ, Gulley ML, Hamilton E, Schichman SA. EBV DNA quantitation in serum is highly correlated with the development and regression of post-transplant lymphoproliferative disorder (PTLD) in solid organ transplant recipients (abstr.). Blood 1998; 92 (Suppl. 1): 314–315.

33. Cen H, Williams PA, McWilliams HP, Breinig MC, Ho M, McKnight JLC. Evidence for restricted Epstein–Barr virus latent gene expression and anti-EBNA antibody response in solid organ transplant recipients with post-transplant lymphoproliferative disorders. Blood 1993; 81:1393–1403.

34. Delecluse HJ, Kremmer E, Rouault JP, Cour C, Bornkamm G, Berger F. The expression of Epstein–Barr virus latent proteins is related to the pathological features of post-transplant lymphoproliferative disorders. Am J Pathol 1995; 146:1113–1120.

35. Rea D, Fourcade C, Leblond V, et al. Patterns of Epstein–Barr virus latent and replicative gene expression in Epstein–Barr virus B cell lymphoproliferative disorders after organ transplantation. Transplantation 1994; 58:317–324.

36. Murray PG, Swinnen LJ, Constandinou CM, et al. BCL-2 but not its Epstein–Barr virus-encoded homologue, BHRF1, is commonly expressed in posttransplantation lymphoproliferative disorders [see comments]. Blood 1996; 87:706–711.

37. Izumi KM, Kieff ED. The Epstein–Barr virus oncogene product latent membrane protein 1 engages the tumor necrosis factor receptor-associated death domain protein to mediate B lymphocyte growth transformation and activate NF-kappaB. Proc Natl Acad Sci USA 1997; 94:12592–12597.

38. Kieser A, Kilger E, Gires O, Ueffing M, Kolch W, Hammerschmidt W. Epstein–Barr virus latent membrane protein-1 triggers AP-1 activity via the c-Jun N-terminal kinase cascade. EMBO J 1997; 16:6478–6485.

39. Devergne O, Hatzivassiliou E, Izumi KM, et al. Association of TRAF1, TRAF2, and TRAF3 with an Epstein–Barr virus LMP1 domain important for B-lymphocyte transformation: role in NF-kappaB activation. Mol Cell Biol 1996; 16:7098–7108.

40. Liebowitz D. Epstein–Barr virus and a cellular signaling pathway in lymphomas from immunosuppressed patients. N Engl J Med 1998; 338:1413–1421.

41. Rickinson AB. Epstein–Barr virus in action in vivo. N Engl J Med 1998; 338:1461–1463.

42. Hojo M, Morimoto T, Maluccio M, et al. Cyclosporine induces cancer progression by a cell-autonomous mechanism. Nature 1999; 397:530–534.

43. Chadburn A, Suciu-Foca N, Cesarman E, Reed E, Michler RE, Knowles DM. Post-transplantation lymphoproliferative disorders arising in solid organ transplant recipients are usually of recipient origin. Am J Pathol 1995; 147:1862–1870.

44. Weissmann DJ, Ferry JA, Harris NL, Louis DN, Delmonico F, Spiro I. Posttransplantation lymphoproliferative disorders in solid organ recipients are predominantly aggressive tumors of host origin. Am J Clin Pathol 1995; 103:748–755.

45. Gulley ML, Schneider BG, Swinnen LJ. Origin of post-transplant lymphoproliferative disorder (PTLD) arising in solid organ recipients (abstr.). Eighth International Symposium on Tumor-Associated Herpesviruses 1998, p. 85.

46. Frizzera G, Hanto DW, Gajl-Peczalska KJ, et al. Polymorphic diffuse B-cell hyperplasias and lymphomas in renal transplant recipients. Cancer Res 1981; 41:4262–4279.

47. Nalesnik MA, Jaffe R, Starzl TE, et al. The pathology of posttransplant lymphoproliferative disorders occurring in the setting of cyclosporine A-prednisone immunosuppression. Am J Pathol 1988; 133:173–192.

48. Knowles DM, Cesarman E, Chadburn A, et al. Correlative morphologic and molecular genetic analysis demonstrates three distinct categories of posttransplantation lymphoproliferative disorders. Blood 1995; 85:552–565.

49. Cleary ML, Warnke R, Sklar J. Monoclonality of lymphoproliferative lesions in cardiac-transplant recipients. Clonal analysis based on immunoglobulin-gene rearrangements. N Engl J Med 1984; 310:477–482.

50. Hanto DW, Birkenbach M, Frizzera G, Gajl-Peczalska KJ, Simmons RL, Schubach WH. Confirmation of the heterogeneity of posttransplant Epstein–Barr virus-associated B cell proliferations by immunoglobulin gene rearrangement analyses. Transplantation 1989; 47:458–464.

51. Chadburn A, Cesarman E, Liu YF, et al. Molecular genetic analysis demonstrates that multiple posttransplantation lymphoproliferative disorders occurring in one anatomic site in a single patient represent distinct primary lymphoid neoplasms. Cancer 1995; 75:2747–2756.

52. Locker J, Nalesnik M. Molecular genetic analysis of lymphoid tumors arising after organ transplantation. Am J Pathol 1989; 135:977–987.

53. Harris NL, Ferry JA, Swerdlow SH. Posttransplant lymphoproliferative disorders: summary of Society for Hematopathology Workshop. Semin Diagn Pathol 1997; 14:8–14.

54. Nelson BP, Nalesnik MA, Locker JD. EBV negative post-transplant lymphoproliferative disorders: a distinct entity? (abstr.). Lab Invest 1996; 74:118A.

55. Van Gorp J, Doornewaard H, Verdonck LF, Klopping C, Vos PF, van den Tweel JG. Posttransplant T-cell lymphoma. Report of three cases and a review of the literature. Cancer 1994; 73:3064–3072.

56. Hanto DW, Gajl-Peczalska KJ, Frizzera G, et al. Epstein–Barr virus (EBV) induced polyclonal and monoclonal B-cell lymphoproliferative diseases occurring after renal transplantation. Clinical, pathologic, and virologic findings and implications for therapy. Ann Surg 1983; 198:356–369.

57. Nalesnik MA, Makowka L, Starzl TE. The diagnosis and treatment of posttransplant lymphoproliferative disorders. Curr Prob Surg 1988; 25:367–472.

58. Swinnen LJ, Mullen GM, Carr TJ, Costanzo MR, Fisher RI. Aggressive treatment for postcardiac transplant lymphoproliferation. Blood 1995; 86:3333–3340.

59. Morrison VA, Dunn DL, Manivel JC, Gajlpeczalska KJ, Peterson BA. Clinical characteristics of post-transplant lymphoproliferative disorders. Am J Med 1994; 97:14–24.

60. Leblond V, Sutton L, Dorent R, et al. Lymphoproliferative disorders after organ transplantation: a report of 24 cases observed in a single center. J Clin Oncol 1995; 13:961–968.

61. Cesarman E, Chadburn A, Liu YF, Migliazza A, Dalla-Favera R, knowles DM. BCL-6 gene mutations in posttransplantation lymphoproliferative disorders predict response to therapy and clinical outcome. Blood 1998; 92:2294–2302.

62. Hanto DW, Frizzera G, Gajl-Peczalska KJ, et al. Epstein–Barr virus-induced B-cell lymphoma after renal transplantation: acyclovir therapy and transition from polyclonal to monoclonal B-cell proliferation. N Engl J Med 1982; 306:913–918.

63. Filipovich AH, Mathur A, Kamat D, Kersey JH, Shapiro RS. Lymphoproliferative disorders and other tumors complicating immunodeficiencies. [Review]. Immunodeficiency 1994; 5:91–112.

64. McDiarmid SV, Jordan S, Lee GS, et al. Prevention and preemptive therapy of postransplant lymphoproliferative disease in pediatric liver recipients. Transplantation 1998; 66:1604–1611.

65. Shapiro RS, Chauvenet A, McGuire W, et al. Treatment of B-cell lymphoproliferative disorders with interferon alfa and intravenous gamma globulin [letter]. N Engl J Med 1988; 318:1334.

66. Liebowitz D, Anastasi J, Hagos F, LeBeau MM, Olopade OI. Post-transplant lymphoproliferative disorders (PTLD): clinicopathologic characterization and response to immunomodulatory therapy with interferon-alpha (abstr.). Ann Oncol 1996; 7:28.

67. Fischer A, Blanche S, Le Bidois J, et al. Anti-B-cell monoclonal antibodies in the treatment of severe B-cell lymphoproliferative syndrome following bone marrow and organ transplantation. N Engl J Med 1991; 324:1451–1456.

68. Benkerrou M, Jais JP, Leblond V, et al. Anti-B-cell monoclonal antibody treatment of severe posttransplant B-lymphoproliferative disorder: prognostic factors and long-term outcome. Blood 1998; 92:3137–3147.

69. Papadopoulos EB, Ladanyi M, Emanuel D, et al. Infusions of donor leukocytes to treat Epstein–Barr virus-associated lymphoproliferative disorders after allogeneic bone marrow transplantation. N Engl J Med 1994; 330:1185–1191.

70. Rooney CM, Smith CA, Ng CY, et al. Use of gene-modified virus-specific T lymphocytes to control Epstein–Barr-virus-related lymphoproliferation. Lancet 1995; 345:9–13.

71. O'Reilly RJ, Small TN, Papadopoulos E, Lucas K, Lacerda J, Koulova L. Biology and adoptive cell therapy of Epstein–Barr virus-associated lymphoproliferative disorders in recipients of marrow allografts. Immunol Rev 1997; 157:195–216.

5

Epstein–Barr Virus and Burkitt's Lymphoma

Guy de Thé

INTRODUCTION

In 1958, little attention was paid to Denis Burkitt's report in the *British Journal of Surgery* of a tumor involving the jaws of Ugandan children *(1)*. It was not totally neglected, however. Gregory O'Conor, a pathologist from the U.S. National Cancer Institute, traveled to Kampala and found that this tumor represented not only a clinical syndrome but also a distinct pathologic entity *(2)*.

Burkitt, a surgeon without formal scientific training but with an endless curiosity and determination, opened a new field in cancer research. He not only described the original cases, but also reported (through letters sent to colleagues in hospitals all over Africa) that the jaw tumor occurred from East to West Africa between 10° North and 10° South of the Equator, with a tail from East Africa toward South Africa. Later, through a medical safari during which he visited many hospitals from East to South Africa *(3)*, he observed that the jaw tumor, to be named Burkitt's lymphoma (BL), was dependent upon climatic factors such as temperature, humidity, and altitude *(4)*, which suggested the role of a transmissible, insect-borne oncogenic agent. He and Kafuko further suggested that holo- or hyperendemic malaria best reflected the African distribution of the tumor—rare if not absent in the arid Sahelic regions of Africa but the most frequent childhood tumor in the warm, humid lowlands of East Africa *(5)*. The hypothesis of a vector-borne agent aroused the interest of many tumor virologists working with mice or chickens in the United States, United Kingdom, and France, many of whom rushed to East Africa in a vain search for an oncogenic arbovirus in tumor specimens.

The light came when Denis Burkitt was invited to London to described this strange, climate-dependent childhood cancer. Anthony Epstein, a pathologist with expertise in electron microscopy, heard Burkitt's presentation and proposed a collaboration, leading to the shipment of tumor biopsies from Uganda. When the tumor cells were cultured for a few days in vitro, on electron microscopy they exhibited viruslike particles resembling Herpes simplex virus *(6)*. Henle and Henle *(7)* then showed that this agent was a new member of the human herpesviruses, and proposed to name it after its discoverers, Epstein and Barr.

The term endemic Burkitt's lymphoma refers to this historical discovery in Africa and is the primary focus of this chapter. Histologically similar tumors were later

From: *Infectious Causes of Cancer: Targets for Intervention*
Edited by: J. J. Goedert © Humana Press Inc., Totowa, NJ

described in temperate climates with no particular geographic distribution and named sporadic BL.

THE PATHOLOGIC, CLINICAL, AND EPIDEMIOLOGIC ENTITY

A malignancy is best defined by its histopathology, then by its localization in the body, and eventually by its epidemiologic characteristics. As mentioned earlier, the histopathology of Burkitt's jaw tumor was characterized initially by Gregory O'Conor *(2),* then by Denis Wright *(8),* and finally through an international consensus as an undifferentiated monomorphic lymphoma, with a characteristic starry sky pattern, in which lymphoblasts containing multinucleolar nuclei and cytoplasmic vacuoles were infiltrated with macrophages giving a typical pattern *(9).*

Subsequently, these high-grade lymphomatous cells were shown to be of B-cell lineage and to synthesize immunoglobulin M (IgM) at their cell surface *(10),* with immunophenotypic characteristics of a subset of germinal center cells that do not express deoxyribonucleotide transferase. The surface markers CD19, CD20, CD22, and CD79 are regularly present; CD10 and CD77 are frequently detectable; and CD23 and CD5 are characteristically undetectable *(11).* HLA class I, adhesion, and activation molecules—CD54 (ICAM-1), CD11a/18 (LFA-1), and CD58—are detectable at low levels on the cell surface *(12,13).*

Clinically, the most frequently involved sites are the jaws in endemic BL as seen in equatorial Africa and in Papua–New Guinea *(1,14,15).* Interestingly, very young children tend to have orbital or maxillar tumor *(16)* whereas jaw involvement is the rule in children developing molar tooth buds *(17).* Abdominal tumors with ascites are seen in about 50% of African BL cases and in 80% of sporadic BL in temperate climates *(18).* Bone marrow is invaded in 8% of the African Burkitt's tumors. In contrast, involvment of the central nervous system, including cerebrospinal fluid pleocytosis, cranial nerve palsy, and paraplegia is common in Africa but rare elsewhere *(18,19).* Other sites include the breast in pubertal girls, the testis in adolescent boys, and also salivary and thyroid glands, bone, pleura, and pericardium *(17–19).* The absence of involvement of the nasopharyngeal mucosa (a target for Epstein-Barr virus (EBV)-associated cancer of the nasopharynx; *see* Chapter 6), spleen, and peripheral lymph nodes is noteworthy.

The high prevalence of BL in tropical Africa probably dates back centuries, as attested by ancient masks depicting orbital tumors. The first described case was noted during the mission of Sir Albert Cook to Uganda in 1897 *(20).* Incidence data prior to the HIV/AIDS epidemic, reported by Edington and MacLean *(21),* found an annual rate of 5–10 cases per 100,000 children below 16 yr, with a peak between 5 and 10 yr of age, making BL the most frequent childhood cancer.

The ecologic risk factors for BL in East Africa—temperature, humidity, and altitude—were mainly investigated in Uganda but refined in the North Mara district of Tanzania, where the BL territory and the holo- or hyperendemic malaria area were sharply demarcated by an abrupt change in altitude to 1350 m above sea level *(22).*

Time–space clustering of BL first reported by Pike et al. in the West Nile District of Uganda was not observed by Brubaker et al. in the North Mara district of Tanzania *(23,24).* Familial clustering of BL has been reported in both African and Papua–New Guinean endemic areas *(25,26),* but genes linked to an increased risk of BL have not been identified. It is, however, highly probable that genetic determinants play a critical role in controlling the immune response to malaria and to primary EBV infection (such as the X-linked lymphoproliferative syndrome of Purtillo; *see* Chapter 4 [27]).

SPORADIC BL IN TEMPERATE CLIMATES

Young and Miller and then Levine et al. showed that non-Hodgkin's lymphomas (NHL) histopathologically similar to BL as described in Africa also occurred in the United States, with a yearly incidence rate averaging 0.06–0.10/100,000 children *(28,29)*. International registry data showed that Iraq, Israel, and Algeria were intermediate risk areas for BL incidence *(30–32)*. In these areas, the predominant clinical feature is abdominal involvement. On a global scale, the association with EBV appears to depend upon the socioeconomic level, ranging from a weak association (10–15%) in BL arising in European children (Lenoir, *unpublished data*) to 85% in Algerian cases *(32)* and 98% in Uganda *(see below* and refs. *41,42)*. These international patterns suggested a critical role of breast feeding and saliva in the transmission of EBV from a mother to her young infant.

THE EPSTEIN-BARR VIRUS

The DNA-enveloped virus uncovered by Epstein, Achong, and Barr in 1964 *(6)* is a member of the *Herpesviridae,* with 162 capsomers arranged as dodecahedron enclosing a linear, double-stranded DNA of about 172 kb. The complete genomic sequence of EBV was reported in 1982 by Kieff et al. *(33)*. The genomic structure of EBV is that of a γ herpesvirus (group C), with both terminal and internal repeats, dividing the genome into both short and long unique sequences that contain tandem repeat elements. Such nucleotide repeats are reflected in proteins by amino acid repeat domains that can be used to characterize EBV strain isolates *(34)*. Furthermore, the characteristic number of terminal repeats enabled the description of the monoclonality of EBV-associated tumors *(35)*. In infected B cells, the viral genome is episomal, intranuclear, and circular, essentially as an extra chromosome that is anchored at the nuclear membrane. In latent EBV infection, replication of episomal EBV occurs during the S phase of the cell cycle using cellular DNA polymerases and yielding EBV-infected daughter cells (not extracellular virions). Whether EBV sequences integrate into the chromosomes of tumor cells is still a matter of debate *(36–39)*.

In vivo, the level of host-cellular control over the latent EBV genes varies in different EBV-associated diseases. Table 1 shows that there are three types of EBV latency; the tightest control is type I, as seen in BL tumor cells. The cellular control of latency appears to operate mostly through methylation of the corresponding viral genes. At the host level, the critical mechanism involved in controlling latency is cell-mediated immunity.

Most latent antigens induce both humoral and, except for Epstein–Barr nuclear antigen 1 (EBNA-1), cell-mediated immune responses. IgG to viral capsid antigens (VCAs) is a useful prevalence marker for EBV infection. Anti-EBNA-1 antibodies are thought to reflect the level of cellular immunity, which is paradoxical given that EBNA-1 is not recognized by cytotoxic T-lymphocytes (CTLs). CTL activity against EBV epitopes is highly HLA restricted, including EBNA-2 with HLA-B51 and -A2; EBNA-3a with HLA-B8, -A2, and -B7; EBNA-3b with HLA-B7 and -B11; and EBNA-3c with HLA-B27 and -B44 *(40)*.

Table 1
Latent Viral Genes Expressed in Tumor Cells

Gene functions	Gene products	Type of latency	EBV-associated diseases
Unknown EB plasmid maintenance	EBERs EBNA-1	I	Burkitt's lymphoma
Transformation and maintenance of latency	EBERs EBNA-1 LMP-1 LMP-2A,-2B	II	Nasopharyngeal carcinoma and Hodgkin's disease
Transactivate cellular genes	Idem II + EBNA-2,-3 + LP	III	Infectious mononucleosis Posttransplant lympho- proliferative disease Lymphoblastoid cell lines

THE RELATIONSHIP BETWEEN EBV AND BURKITT'S LYMPHOMA

Nearly all, that is, up to 98%, of the biopsies of African BL tumors contain EBV genomes *(41,42)*. In contrast, only 20% of the biopsies of sporadic European or American BL cases, as determined by histopathology, contain EBV sequences *(43)*. In the tumor cells, EBV DNA remains episomal, as superhelically twisted circular molecules, with six to more than 100 copies per cell *(44)*. RNA transcripts from various EBV genes, representing 3–6% of the EBV genome, can be detected in tumor cells. Cultured BL biopsies regularly lead to the establishment of EBV-positive permanent tumor cell lines exhibiting type III latency *(see* Table 1 and Chapter 4). Besides EBV, these cell lines secrete intracytoplasmic and surface IgG.

Soon after its discovery, seroepidemiologic surveys showed that EBV infection was ubiquitous the world over. However, by comparing populations in which EBV-associated diseases differed drastically, we observed significant differences in the age at acquisition of EBV infection *(45)*. EBV infection occurred very early in life in Uganda, an area with a very high rate of BL; somewhat later in early childhood in Singapore and Hong Kong, where there are very high rates of EBV-associated nasopharyngeal carcinoma (NPC); and during late adolescence in socioeconomically developed countries, where infectious mononucleosis is frequent but BL and NPC are very rare *(45)*. Such age differences in the spread of EBV reflect socioeconomic status. By age 18 mo, more than 80% were infected by EBV in rural Uganda *(45)*, compared to 30% in low socioeconomic and 7% in high socioeconomic children in the United States *(46)*. After 18 mo of age, the rate of EBV infection among susceptible infants in Uganda is about 37% between 6 and 10 yr of age, and virtually nil thereafter.

In Africa, practically all pregnant women have been infected by EBV, and 66% of them shed EBV in their saliva. Their newborns are temporarily protected by maternal antibodies, which disappear within 6 mo. They can become infected soon after or even during that period by maternal saliva or breast milk. It is of interest that early primary infections in tropical Africa are clinically silent, with transient early antigen-restricted (EA-R) antibodies *(47)*, in contrast to infectious mononucleosis with transient EA-diffuse (EA-D) antibodies that occurs in European and American adolescents *(48).*

Given the ubiquity of EBV in Africa, the prevalence of infection does not differ between African BL patients and their age- and sex-matched controls. However, the geometric mean titers (GMTs) of VCA antibodies are significantly higher in African BL patients, with a GMT of 1:275, than in African control children with a GMT of 1:37 *(46).* Evans *(49)* estimated that 80% of the American lymphomas that fulfilled the clinical and histopathologic criteria of BL had high EBV antibody titers. EBV DNA and EBNA were found in the tumor cells of 80% of BL cases in Algeria but in only 24% of those in France *(50).*

THE UGANDAN BL PROSPECTIVE STUDY

In the late 1960s we sought to clarify whether an ubiquitous virus such as EBV could have an etiologic role in the development of a geographically and climatically restricted cancer, such as BL. Werner Henle postulated that BL represented a malignant form of infectious mononucleosis, that is, an acute syndrome occurring soon after a massive primary EBV infection in a very few susceptible African children who, for unknown reasons, had escaped earlier infection *(see also* Chapter 3). This hypothesis was in line with the recently discovered relationship between delayed EBV infection and infectious mononucleosis and with the known relationship between a late primary infection with poliovirus and the risk of paralytic polio. For viral-induced neoplasia in animals, however, oncogenic viruses must infect newborns to exhibit their oncogenic potential. Thus, I proposed an alternative hypothesis that EBV could be oncogenic and cause BL with a massive infection during the newborn period.

To test these hypotheses, in 1970 our team at the International Agency for Research on Cancer, under the auspices of the Virus Cancer Program of the U.S. National Cancer Institute, launched a prospective, population-based study in the West Nile district of Uganda. The specific aim of the study was to determine the viral profile in pre-BL sera of children who were going to develop the tumor *(51).*

Within 3 yr and with parents' consent, venous blood samples were drawn from 42,000 children, representing 85% of the eligible children aged 0–8 yr in selected parishes around Arua, an area endemic for BL. Nearly 90% of the enrolled children were followed during the next 5–8 yr, which represented an incredible challenge during Idi Amin Dada's dictatorial regime in Uganda. During this study period, 14 BL cases occured among enrolled children *(51),* giving a BL incidence rate of approx 7 per 100,000 per year, which was lower than expected but in parallel with the overall decline of BL incidence then observed in Uganda.

As shown in Fig. 1, 7–54 mo prior to clinical onset of the disease, the "pre-BL" sera had significantly higher IgG antibody titers to EBV VCA compared to sera from age-, sex-, and locality-matched controls *(51).* The level of antibodies in pre-BL sera was *not* related to the proximity of disease onset, in contrast to the case of infectious mononucleosis. When comparing pre- and post-BL sera, VCA titers did not increase (Fig. 2), indicating that the high VCA titers regularly observed in BL patients did not result from their disease process. Rather, high titers represented a risk marker for the disease reflecting a longstanding situation.

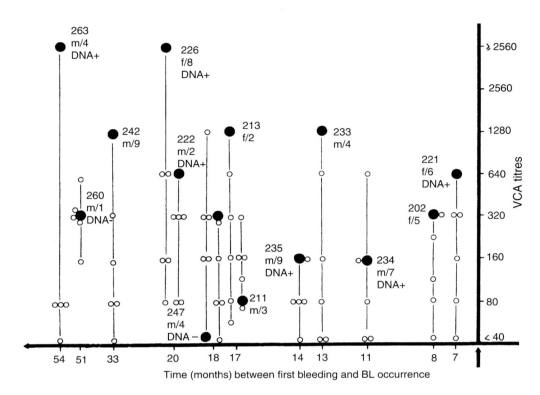

Fig. 1. EBV/VCA antibody titers of 14 children at various times prior to the development of BL in the prospective Ugandan study. (●), BL cases; (○), sex-, age-, and locality-matched controls; DNA +, EBV DNA detected in BL cases. (From de Thé et al., Nature, 1978; 274:756–761 with permission.)

Tumor DNA could be obtained for 10 BL cases, and EBV DNA could be detected in nine of them *(51)*. Worth noting here was the EBV-DNA negative case 247, with a low VCA titer 18 mo prior to disease onset, probably representing a rare EBV-unrelated case of BL.

Antibodies to EBNA followed the VCA pattern with unchanged titers between pre- and post-BL sera. In contrast, EA titers increased after tumor onset in seven BL cases but without a change in VCA titers *(51)*. Antibodies to other common viruses such as measles, herpes simplex, and cytomegalovirus were also unchanged in pre- and post-BL sera. The final result, with two additional BL cases detected later on, showed a strong correlation ($p = 0.002$) between VCA titers in pre-BL sera as compared to control sera. This pattern was not dependent upon the length of time between phlebotomy and onset of the disease *(51,52)*.

Children with the highest 10–25% of VCA antibody titers in tropical Africa are at highest risk for BL. With a BL yearly incidence, approx 20/100,000 in Uganda, it can be estimated that 0.2% of 5- to 9-yr-old children with high VCA titers will develop the tumor, thus emphasizing the need of critical cofactors in the etiology of BL.

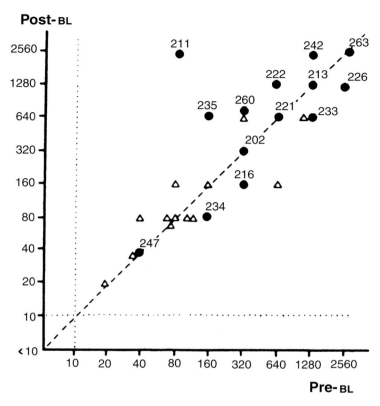

Fig. 2. EBV/VCA antibody titers at before and after the clinical onset of the tumor in children with BL (identified by code number) (●) as compared to sex-, age-, and locality-matched controls (△) bled on the same dates. (From de Thé et al., Nature, 1978; 274:756–761, with permission.)

COULD A SPECIFIC STRAIN OF EBV BE LINKED TO BL?

Bhatia *(53)* recently identified different amino acid sequences characterizing subtypes of EBNA-1, the only viral protein expressed in BL tumor cells, and showed that the subtype with alanine at position 487, commonest in normal individuals, was very rare in BL tumors. In contrast, the subtype V-leu (leucine at 487) with additional amino acid substitutions, was frequently associated with BL *(54)*. Such data suggest that specific mutations in EBNA-1 may be relevant to BL pathogenesis.

THE ROLE OF MALARIA IN BL PATHOGENESIS

There is a striking correspondence in the geographic distribution of BL and the areas with the highest transmission rate of falciparum malaria. This ecologic correlation is seen worldwide and on a microscale within Uganda *(55)*. Because sickle-cell trait (AS hemoglobin) is known to protect against severe complications of *Plasmodium falciparum* infection *(56)*, several studies investigated whether AS hemoglobin affected the risk of BL development *(57–59)*. The results suggested a possible protective effect but not at a significant level, owing to the small numbers of individuals studied.

An intervention study carried out in the North Mara district of Tanzania in the late 1970s was aimed at evaluating the impact of chloroquine distribution on BL incidence in children less than 10 yr of age. This trial confirmed the relationship between malaria and BL, as the BL incidence fell transiently during and shortly after the chloroquine administration period (1977–82) but increased later to a higher level *(60)*. Of note, BL incidence in the North Mara district was low before the trial, and chloroquine resistant strains of *P. falciparum* were detected as early as 1982, suggesting an epidemiologically more complex situation than originally thought *(61)*.

Of further interest for the pathogenesis of BL in relation to malaria, the experimental data indicated that two plasmodium species, *P. berghei* and *P. yeollii,* are mitogenic for the immature B cells *(62,63)*. With a high burden of plasmodium parasitemia, children up to age 5 have hyperactive B cells secreting high levels of IgG and IgM *(64)*. Furthermore, like human immunodeficiency virus (HIV), chronic malaria favors a shift toward Th2 helper cells producing IL-10, which depresses CTL functions and facilitates the outgrowth of EBV-infected B cells *(65–67)*. A plausible hypothesis is that primary EBV infection very early in life, when the immune system is immature, with a simultaneous heavy malaria burden could have multiplicative effects that further BL development *(68)*.

CHROMOSOMAL TRANSLOCATION, ONCOGENE ACTIVATION, AND BL DEVELOPMENT

A major breakthrough came from the observation that the majority of B-cell malignancies, and for that matter all BL tumors, exhibit chromosomal changes, the most common being a reciprocal chromosomal translocation of the immunoglobulin heavy-chain sequences of chromosome 8q to chromosome 14q, as detected in 75% of BL cases *(69)*. These chromosome alterations are not dependent on EBV infection. The translocation between chromosomes 8 and 2, observed in 16% of BL cases, involves the λ light-chain sequence, whereas that between chromosomes 8 and 22, observed in 9% of BL, involves the κ light-chain sequences on chromosome 22 *(69)*. One of these translocations is regularly present in 100% of BL cases, irrespective of the endemicity level or geographic location *(70)*. An exception is the BJAB line derived from an EBV negative African BL, which does not exibit any translocation involving chromosome 8. It is unclear whether BJAB was a true BL case or not, since its clinical, morphologic, and surface markers do not fit the characteristic BL pattern.

Of interest to understanding the interplay between the environmental and genetic events, Magrath and colleagues found that the breakpoints of the chromosomal translocations vary by geographic areas *(71)*. In 92 BL from different parts of the world, 75% of BL tumors from equatorial Africa, mainly Ghana, but in only 9% of BL tumors from the United States had break points in the far 5′ region of chromosome 8 *(71)*. Different break points in chromosome 8 were found in BL cases from Brazil, Argentina, and Chile.

Because these translocations involve genes related to immune responses, it has been suggested that they could be involved directly in BL pathogenesis *(69)*. Such translocations, however, are not exclusively associated with BL, as Sigaux et al. *(72)* showed that rearrangement of 8q24 relates to other malignant proliferations of the B-cell lineage. Furthermore, such chromosomal translocations, when occurring in lymphoblastoid cell lines, were not sufficient to make them fully malignant *(73)*.

The major oncogene involved in BL is indeed c-*myc,* which is translated in juxtaposition to the immunoglobulin locus, the cross over occuring 5' (upstream) of the c-*myc* gene and affecting its promoter/leader sequence *(74).* The c-*myc* oncogene has three exons, separated by two introns that include two promoters that are separated by 160 basepairs. The breakpoints occur often within the first intron, activating a cryptic promoter. Of importance for understanding BL pathogenesis, the c-*myc* product, regardless of rearrangements, is identical to and has the same functional activity as the normal c-*myc* product. The key seems to be deregulation of the c-*myc* transcript, enhancing or altering the promoter involved in its transcription *(74,75).* Croce *(69)* showed that, whereas on a normal chromosome 8, c-*myc* is not transcribed, it becomes constitutively transcribed at a high level on a translocated chromosome. This event apprears to be B-cell specific and is consistant with the hypothesis that there is tissue specificity for c-*myc* deregulation. Furthermore, Lombardi et al. (76) gave evidence that c-*myc* activation in vitro, obtained by introduction of activated c-*myc* genes into a lymphoblastoid line, was sufficient for tumorigenic conversion of B-cells.

As previously mentioned, geographic variations in the breakpoints on chromosome 8 have been observed *(69).* In most African BL, the break is 5' of the c-*myc* sequence, whereas in sporadic BL it is within the first intron. Other oncogenes such as B-*lym* or c-*fdgr* have been proposed as involved BL pathogenesis, but the data here are minimal.

BL IN AIDS

Extranodal non-Hodgkin's lymphomas (NHL) are very common in HIV infected individuals, developing often as primary tumors in the central nervous system *(77,78)* (*see also* Chapter 8). AIDS-related NHL comprise two distinct histopathologic types—diffuse large B-cell lymphomas, that often exhibit a dominant immunoblastic component, and BLs. In AIDS, 35–40% of BL tumors and most of those developing in the central nervous system are EBV associated *(79,80).*

HIV may contribute to NHL development through its severe dysregulation of EBV and chronic stimulation of the B-cell system. It appears that BL cases with c-*myc* translocations generally occur in AIDS patients who have a relatively conserved immune system, as compared to diffuse large cell NHL cases, which typically develop in patients with advanced immunodeficiency disease *(81).* Besides chromosomal translocations, mutations in the *p53* gene have been detected in 60% of BL in AIDS patients *(82).*

Diffuse large B-cell lymphomas resemble the posttransplant lymphoproliferative disorder with c-*myc* or *bcl-6* rearrangments *(83).* In contrast, AIDS-associated BL may be pathogenetically similar to sporadic BL, with chronic stimulation of the B-cell compartment of the immune system playing a critical role.

PATHOGENESIS

Sir Richard Doll and Richard Peto proposed that, on epidemiologic grounds, most cancers arise as a result of a multistep process, each step being causally related to an independent factor. In this model, Burkitt's lymphoma could be regarded as a Rosetta stone for oncogenesis, as three independent factors play an etiologic role in the pathogenesis of endemic BL, namely the EBV, a severe malaria burden, and last but not least c-*myc* oncogene activation linked to a specific chromosomal translocation. Severe EBV infection very early in life appears to act as the initiator, with very early infection in

Table 2
Incidence of BL in Children 4–14 yr of Age in Different Geographical Areas[a]

	Incidence NHL[b]	Proportion of BL	% EBV pos. BL	Incidence of BL
Uganda Early EBV infection + malaria	9–15	95%	97%	12
Algeria Early EBV infection, no malaria	2–4	47%	85%	1–2
France, USA Delayed EBV infection, no malaria	1–2	30%	10–15%	0.04–0.08

[a] Adapted with permission from de Thé *(68)*.

[b] NHL, Non-Hodgkin's lymphomas, per 100,000 per year.

immunologically immature children resulting in a large EBV infected B- or pre-B-cell population, which may be poorly controlled in the setting of malaria-related immuo-depressed cell-mediated immunity *(68)*.

A number of specific scenarios have been proposed in the interplay of these three factors. Based on the preliminary data of the Ugandan BL prospective study we proposed that perinatal infection by EBV could initiate BL pathogenesis *(84)*. Depressed EBV-specifc cell-mediated immunity, caused by falciparum malaria, would result in a rapid expansion of an EBV-infected B-cell subpopulation, this in turn favoring a random event resulting in chromosomal translocation *(68)*.

An interesting alternative hypothesis was proposed by Lenoir and Bornkamm in 1987 *(85)* in which they proposed that malaria could act first, rendering the later EBV infection more severe. As low socioeconomic status is a critical factor for BL development, viral and parasite infections could often occur nearly simultaneously. If so, the priority of one versus the other would be very difficult to investigate epidemiologically and possibly may not be essential.

By comparing the situation in three different geographical areas exhibiting large differences in BL incidence, namely East Africa, North Africa, and two Western countries (France and the United States), we were able to assess the respective weight of the two environmental etiologic factors, EBV and malaria. As seen in Table 2, perinatal mother-to-child infection by EBV appears to increase the risk of BL by a factor of about 20-fold, whereas a heavy malaria burden would further increase the risk by 10-fold, giving a 200-fold difference between Europe and East Africa *(68)*.

PREVENTION AND VACCINATION STRATEGIES

Knowing the different etiologic factors associated with BL, one is confronted with the best strategy to propose to control the disease. On a worldwide scale, endemic BL could be prevented to a certain extent by a better control of hyperendemic malaria, a longstanding priority of World Health Organization. But the continuing inability to develop a safe and effective malaria vaccine and the merely transient benefit of chemoprevention does not give much hope for the near future. The malaria intervention project of the International Agency for Research on Cancer in the North Mara district of Tanzania in the early 1980s showed that chemoprevention could have an effect in decreasing BL incidence *(60)*, but at the same time showed its limit by the emergence of chloroquine-resistant falciparum malaria in the treated population *(61)*.

As early as 1976, Epstein proposed that an EBV vaccine be developed *(86)* and to that end a colony of susceptible experimental animals (the cottontop marmoset) was developed in the United Kingdom. The EBV-membrane glycoprotein gp340 was selected as immunogen, inserted in various viral carriers *(87,88)*, and tested with various adjuvants and modes of presentation in the experimental animal model. The gp340 immunogen was found effective, and human trials were considered *(89)*. But which populations should be targetted?

The easiest and most justifiable target would be to prevent infectious mononucleosis in high risk groups, that is, to vaccinate students in high socioeconomic groups in the United States or Europe *(90)*. But for endemic BL in African children, it would be difficult, if not impossible, to propose a vaccine for all the children to prevent a tumor, that fortunately remains a low killer (0.1%) as compared to malaria (about 20%) in children below age 10. The present HIV epidemic in subSaharan Africa makes an EBV vaccine a low priority.

Although nasopharyngeal carcinoma (NPC) is a leading cancer in males in large parts of southern China and Southeast Asia, a preventive EBV vaccine is similarly difficult to propose, as no one can predict that a simple delay in primary infection by EBV in Chinese children would decrease the incidence of NPC after 40 or more yr. By contrast, a therapeutic vaccine for individuals who have EBV IgA antibodies, known to be at highest risk to develop NPC, could be considered and possibly successful in preventing the clinical onset of the tumor *(90)* (*see also* Chapter 6).

TREATMENT OF BL

Dennis Burkitt in Uganda and Peter Clifford in Nairobi explored the activity of a broad array of cytotoxic drugs and showed that the tumor responds very well to many, among the more effective being cyclophosphamide, methotrexate, vincristine, and cytarabine *(91–93)*. Using either cyclophosphamide as the sole systemic agent or using sequential delivery of cyclophosphamide and additional agents, up to 40% of patients can be cured *(94,95)*. It is also essential to use intrathecal therapy if relapse in the central nervous system is to be avoided *(96)*.

Unfortunately, although in the early days of chemotherapy better results were being achieved in African patients with BL than in patients in Europe and the United States, this is no longer the case. Approximately 90% of patients with BL in the Western world are cured while the majority in equatorial Africa either receive no treatment, or are given whatever drug happens to be available, with predictably poor results. Whether the African tumor is more responsive to treatment is not known, but the rarity of bone marrow involvement, an indicator of high risk for treatment failure in the West, suggests that it ought to be possible to cure at least 80% of patients with a relatively inexpensive and well tolerated treatment protocol. In a disease that accounts for half of all childhood neoplasms in an area of the world where half the population is less than 15 yr old, BL is a much more important public health problem than it is in Europe or the United States. It would seem that this tumor, which has provided so many insights into the role of viruses in human oncogenesis and the treatment of cancer, deserves more attention, at least to provide proper chemotherapy to all children with BL in Africa.

ACKNOWLEDGMENTS

I am grateful to Dr. Ian Magrath, National Cancer Institute, National Institutes of Health, for advice on the chemotherapy of BL and to Ms. L. Mauguin for help in preparing the manuscript with support from the VIRUS-CANCER-PREVENTION Fund.

REFERENCES

1. Burkitt DP. A sarcoma involving the jaws in Africa children. Br J Surg 1958; 46:218–223.
2. O'Conor GT. Malignant tumors in African children. II. A pathological entity. Cancer 1961; 14:270–283.
3. Burkitt DP. A children's cancer dependent on climatic factors. Nature 1962; 194:232–234.
4. Burkitt DP. Determining the climatic limitations of a childrens tumor common in Africa. Br Med J 1962; 2:1019–1023.
5. Kafuko GW, Burkitt DP. Burkitt lymphoma and malaria. Int J Cancer 1970; 6:1–9.
6. Epstein MA, Achong BG, Barr YM. Virus particles in cultured lymphoblasts from Burkitt's lymphoma. Lancet 1964; 1:702–703.
7. Henle G, Henle W. Immunofluorescence in cells derived from Burkitt's lymphoma. J Bacteriol 1966; 91:1248–1256.
8. Wright BH. Cytology and histochemistry of the Burkitt lymphoma. Br J Cancer 1963; 17:50–55.
9. Berard CW, O'Conor GT, Thoma LB, Torloni H (eds). Histological definition of Burkitt's tumor. Bull WHO 1969; 41:601–607.
10. Klein E, Klein G, Nadkarm JS, Wigzill H, Clifford P. Surface IgM-kappa specificity on cells derived from a Burkitt's lymphoma. Lancet 1967; 2:1068–1070.
11. Harris NL, Jaffe ES, Stein H, Banks PM, Chan JKC, Cleary ML, et al. A revised European-American classification of lymphoid neoplasms: a proposal from the International Lymphoma Study Group. Blood 1994; 84:1361–1392.
12. Masucci MG, Torsteinsdottir S, Colombani J, Brautbar C, Klein E, Klein G. Down-regulation of class I HLA antigens and of the Epstein–Barr virus-encoded latent membrane protein in Burkitt lymphoma lines. Proc Natl Acad Sci USA 1987; 84:4567–4571.
13. Andersson ML, Stam NJ, Klein G, Ploegh HL, Masucci MG. Aberrant expression of HLA class-I antigens in Burkitt lymphoma cells. Int J Cancer 1991; 47:544–550.
14. Seldam REJ, Cooke R, Atkinson L. Childhood lymphoma in the territories of Papua and New Guinea. Cancer 1966; 19:437–446.
15. Magrath I, Jain V, Bhatia K. Epstein-Barr virus and Burkitt's lymphoma. Semin Cancer Biol 1992; 3:285–295.
16. Olurin O, Williams AO. Orbito-ocular tumors in Nigeria. Cancer 1972; 30:580–587.
17. Burkitt DP. General features and facial tumours. In: Burkitt DP, Wright DH, (eds). Burkitt's Lymphoma. Edinburgh: E & S Livingstone, 1970, pp. 6–15.
18. Magrath IT. African Burkitt's lymphoma. History, biology, clinical features, and treatment. Am J Pediatr Hematol Oncol 1991; 13:222–246.
19. Ziegler JL, Bluming AZ, Morrow RH, Fass L, Carbone PP. Central nervous system involvement in Burkitt's lymphoma. Blood 1970; 36:718–728.
20. Davies JNP, Elmes S, Hutt MSR, Mtimavalye LAR, Owor R, Shaper L. Cancer in an African community, 1897–1956. An analysis of the records of Mengo Hospital, Kampala, Uganda: Part 1. Br Med J 1964; i:259–264. Part 2. Br Med J 1964; i:336–341.

21. Edington GM, MacLean CMU. Incidence of the Burkitt tumour in Ibadan, western Nigeria. Br Med J 1964; i:264–266.

22. Eshleman JL. A study of the relative incidence of malignant tumours seen at Shirati Hospital in Tanzania. E Afr Med J 1966; 43:274–283.

23. Pike MC, Williams EH, Wright B. Burkitt's tumour in the West Nile District, Uganda, 1961-65. Br Med J 1967; ii:395–399.

24. Brubaker G, Geser A, Pike MC. Burkitt's lymphoma in the North Mara district of Tanzania 1964-70: Failure to find evidence of time-space clustering in a high risk isolated rural area. Br J Cancer 1973; 28:469–472.

25. Brubaker G, Levin AG, Steel CM, Creasey G, Cameron HM, Linsell CA, et al. Multiple cases of Burkitt's lymphoma and other neoplams in families in the North Mara district of Tanzania. Int J Cancer 1980; 26:165–170.

26. Winnett A, Thomas SJ, Brabin BJ, Bain C, Alpers MA, Moss DJ. Familial Burkitt's lymphoma in Papua New Guinea. Br J Cancer 1997; 75:757–761.

27. Purtilo DT. Pathogenesis and phenotypes of an X-linked recessive lymphoproliferative syndrome. Lancet 1976; ii:882–885.

28. Young JL, Miller RW. Incidence of malignant tumours in US children. J Pediatr 1975; 86:254–258.

29. Levine PH, Kamaraju LS, Connelly RR, Berard CW, Dorfman RF, Magrath I, et al. The American Burkitt's lymphoma Registry: Eight years' experience. Cancer 1982; 49:1016–1022.

30. Al Fouadi A, Parkin M. Cancer in Iraq: seven years' data from the Baghdad Tumour Registry. Int J Cancer, 1984; 34:207–213.

31. Steinitz R. Israël. In: Waterhouse J, Muir C, Correa P, Powell J (eds). Cancer Incidence in Five Continents, Vol. III (IARC Scientific Publications No. 15), Lyon, International Agency for Research on Cancer, 1976:248–267.

32. Aboulola M, Boukheloua B, Ladjadj Y, Tazerout FY. Burkitt's lymphoma in Algeria. In: Lenoir GM, O'Conor GT, Olweny CLM (eds). Burkitt's Lymphoma: A Human Cancer Model, Vol. 60. Lyon, France: IARC, 1985, pp. 97–106.

33. Kieff E, Dambaugh T, Heller M, King W, Cheung A, Van Santen V, et al. The biology and chemistry of Epstein–Barr virus. J Infect Dis 1982; 146:506–517.

34. Gratama JW, Oosterveer MAP, Klein G, Ernberg I. EBNA size polymorphism can be used to trace Epstein–Barr virus spread within families. J Virol 1990; 64:4703–4708.

35. Raab-Traub N, Flynn K. The structure of the termini of the Epstein–Barr virus as a marker of clonal cellular proliferation. Cell 1986; 47:883–889.

36. Henderson A, Ripley S, Heller M, Kieff E. Chromosome site for Epstein–Barr virus DNA in a Burkitt tumor cell line and in lymphocytes growth-transformed *in vitro.* Proc Natl Acad Sci USA 1983; 80:1987–1991.

37. Lawrence JB, Villnave CA, Singer RH. Sensitive, high-resolution chromatin and chromosome mapping *in situ:* presence and orientation of two closely integrated copies of EBV in a lymphoma line. Cell 1988; 52:51–61.

38. Hurley EA, Agger S, McNeil JA, Lawrence JB, Calendar A, Lenoir G, et al. When Epstein–Barr virus persistently infects B-cell lines, it frequently integrates. J Virol 1991; 65:1245–1254.

39. Delecluse HJ, Bartnizke S, Hammerschmidt W, Bullerdiek J, Bornkamm GW. Episomal and integrated copies of Epstein–Barr virus coexist in Burkitt lymphoma cell lines. J Virol 1993; 67:1292–1299.

40. de Campos-Lima PO, Leviskaya J, Frisan T, Masucci MG. Strategies of immunoescape in Epstein–Barr virus persistence and pathogenesis. Semin Virol 1996; 7:75–82.

41. Nonoyama M, Huang CH, Pagano JS, Klein G, Singh S. DNA of Epstein–Barr virus detected in tissue of Burkitt's lymphoma and nasopharyngeal carcinoma. Proc Natl Acad Sci USA 1973; 70:3265–3268.

42. Zur Hausen H, Schulte-Holthausen H, Klein G, Henle W, Henle G, Clifford P, et al. EB-virus DNA in biopsies of Burkitt tumors and anaplastic carcinomas of the nasopharynx. Nature 1970; 228:1056–1057.

43. Ziegler JL, Andersson M, Klein G, Henle W. Detection of Epstein–Barr virus in American Burkitt's lymphoma. Int J Cancer 1976; 17:701–706.

44. Kaschuka-Dierich C, Adams A, Lindahl T, Bornkamm G, Bjursell G, Klein G, et al. Intracellular forms of Epstein-Barr virus DNA in human tumor cells *in vivo*. Nature 1976; 260:302–306.

45. De Thé G, Day NE, Geser A, Lavoue MF. Seroepidemiological of the Epstein–Barr virus: preliminary analysis of an international study. In: De Thé G, Epstein MA, Zur Hausen (eds). Oncogenesis and Herpes-Viruses., Vol. II Lyon, France: IARC, 1975, pp. 3–16.

46. Henle G, Henle W, Cliford P, Diehl V, Kafuko GW, Kirya BG, et al. Antibodies to Epstein–Barr virus in Burkitt's lymphoma and control groups. J Natl Cancer Inst 1969; 43:1147–1157.

47. Biggar RJ, Henle W, Fleisher G, Procker J, Lennette ET, Henle G. Primary Epstein–Barr virus infections in African infants. I. Decline of maternal antibodies and time of infection. Int J Cancer 1978; 22:239–243.

48. Biggar RJ, Henle G, Bocher J., Lennette ET, Fleischer G, Henle W. II. Clinical and serological observations during seroconversion. Int J Cancer 1978; 22:244–250.

49. Evans AS. Epidemiology of Burkitt's lymphoma: other factors. In: Lenoir GM, O'Conor GT, Olweny CLM (eds). Burkitt's Lymphoma: A Human Cancer Model. Lyon, France: IARC, 1985, pp. 197–204.

50. Philip T. Burkitt's lymphoma in Europe. In: Lenoir GM, O'Conor GT, Olweny CLM (eds). Burkitt's Lymphoma: A Human Cancer Model. Lyon, France: IARC, 1985, pp. 107–118.

51. De Thé G, Geser A, Day NE, Tukei PM, Williams EH, Beri DP, et al. Epidemiological evidence for a causal relationship between Epstein–Barr virus and Burkitt's lymphoma: Results of the Ugandan prospective study. nature 1978; 274:756–761.

52. Geser A, de Thé G, Lenoir G, Day NE, Williams EH. Final case reporting from the Ugandan prospective study of the relationship between EBV and Burkitt's lymphoma. Int J Cancer 1982; 29:397–400.

53. Bhatia K, Raj A, Guitiérrez MI, Judde JG, Spangler G, Venkatesh, H, Magrath IT. Variation in the sequence of Epstein–Barr virus nuclear antigen 1 in normal peripheral blood lymphocytes and in Burkitt's lymphomas. Oncogene 1996; 13:177–181.

54. Gutiérrez MI, Raj A, Spangler G, Sharma A, Hussain A, Judde JG, et al. Sequence variations in EBNA-1 may dictate restriction of tissue distribution of Epstein–Barr virus in normal and tumour cells. J Gen Virol 1997; 78:1663–1670.

55. Morrow RH Jr. Epidemiological evidence for a role of falciparum malaria in the pathogenesis of Burkitt's lymphoma. In: Lenoir GM, O'Conor GT, Olweny CLM, (eds). Burkitt's Lymphoma: A Human Cancer Model. Lyon, France: IARC, 1985, pp. 177–186.

56. Allison AC. Inherited factors in blood conferring resistance to protozoa. In: Garnham PCC, Pierce AE, Roitt I (eds). Immunity to Protozoa. Oxford: Blackwell, 1963, p. 109.

57. Williams AO. Haemoglobin genotypes, ABO blood groups and Burkitt's tumour. J Med Genet 1966; 3:177–179.

58. Pike MC, Morrow RH, Kisuule A, Mafigiri J. Burkitt's lymphoma and sickle cell trait. Br J Prev Soc Med 1970; 24:39–41.

59. Nkrumah FK, Perkins IV. Sickle cell trait, hemoglobin C trait, and Burkitt's lymphoma. Am J Trop Med Hyg 1976; 25:633–636.

60. Geser HM, Brubaker G, Drapper CC. Effect of a malaria suppression program on the incidence of African Burkitt's lymphoma. Am J Epidemiol 1989; 129:740–752.

61. Draper CC, Brubaker G, Geser A, Kilimali BVAEB, Wernsforfer WH. Serial studies on the evolution of chloroquine resistance in an area of East Africa receiving intermittent malaria chemosuppression. Bull World Health Org 1985; 63:109–118.

62. Jerusalem C. Relationship between malaria infection *(Plasmodium berghei)* and malignant lymphoma in mice. Z Tropenmed Parasitol 1968; 19:94–108.

63. Osmond DG, Priddle S, Rico-Vargas S. Proliferation of B cell precursors in bone marrow of pristane-conditioned and malaria-infected mice. Implications for B cell oncogenesis. Curr Top Microbiol Immunol 1990; 166:149–157.

64. Cohen S, McGregor IA. Gamma-globulin and acquired immunity to malaria. In: Garnam PCC, Pierce AE, Roitt I (eds). Immunity to Protozoa. Oxford: Blackwell, 1963, pp. 123–159.

65. Moss DJ, Burrows SR, Castelino DJ, Kane RG, Pope JH, Rickinson AB, et al. A comparison of Epstein–Barr virus-specific T-cell immunity in malaria-endemic and nonendemic regions of Papua New Guinea. Int J Cancer 1983; 31:727–732.

66. Whittle HC, Brown J, Marsh K, Greenwood BM, Seidelin P, Tighe H, et al. T-cell control of Epstein–Barr virus infected B-cells in lost during *P. falciparum* malaria. Nature 1984; 312:449–450.

67. Lam KM, Syed N, Whittle H, Crawford DH. Circulating Epstein–Barr virus carrying B cells in acute malaria. Lancet 1991; 337:876–878.

68. De Thé G. Epstein–Barr virus and Burkitt's lymphoma world-wide. The causal relationship revisited. In: Lenoir GM, O'Conor GT, Olweny CLM (eds). Burkitt's Lymphoma: A Human Cancer Model. Lyon, France: IARC, 1985, pp. 165–176.

69. Croce CM. Chromosome translocations and human cancer. Cancer Res 1986; 46:6019–6023.

70. Lenoir GM, Philip T, Sohier R. Burkitt-type lymphoma: EBV association and cytogenetic markers in cases from various geographic locations. In: McGrath IT, O'Conor GT, Ramot B (eds). Pathogenesis of Leukemias and Lymphomas. New York: Raven Press, 1984, pp. 283–295.

71. Shiramizu B, Barriga F, Neequaye J, Jafri A, Dalla-Favera R, Guttierez M, et al. Patterns of chromosomal breakpoint locations in Burkitt's lymphoma: relevance to geography and EBV association. Blood 1991; 77:1516–1526.

72. Sigaux F, Berger R, Bernheim A, Valensi F, Daniel MT, Flandrin G. Malignant lymphoma with band 8q14 chromosome abnormality: a morphologic continuum extending from Burkitt's lymphoma to immunoblastic lymphoma. Br Med J 1984; 57:393–405.

73. Steel CM, Morten JEN, Foster E. the cytogenetics of human lymphoid malignancy: studies in Burkitt's lymphoma and Epstein–Barr virus transformed lymphoblastoid cell lines. In: Lenoir GM, O'Conor GT, Olweny CLM (eds). Burkitt's Lymphoma: A Human Cancer Model. Lyon, France: IARC, 1985, pp. 265–292.

74. Leder P. Translocations among antibody genes in human cancer. In: Lenoir GM, O'Conor GT, Olweny CLM (eds). Burkitt's Lymphoma: A Human Cancer Model. Lyon, France: IARC, 1985, pp. 341–358.

75. Leder P. The state and prospect for molecular genetics in Burkitt's lymphoma. In: Lenoir GM, O'Conor GT, Olweny CLM (eds). Burkitt's Lymphoma: A Human Cancer Model. Lyon, France: IARC, 1985, pp. 465–468.

76. Lombardi L, Newcomb E, Dalla-Favea R. Pathogenesis of Burkitt's lymphoma: expression and activated c-*myc* oncogene cancer tumorigenic conversion of EBV infected human B lymphocytes. Cell 1987; 49:161–170.

77. Goplen AK, Dunlop O, Liestol K, Lingjaerde OC, Bruun JN, Maehlen J. The impact of primary central nervous system lymphoma in AIDS patients: a population-based autopsy study from Oslo. J Acquir Immune Defic Synd Hum Retrovirol 1997; 14:351–354.

78. Beral V, Peterman T, Berkelman R, Jaffe H. AIDS-associated non-Hodgkin lymphoma. Lancet 1991; 337:805–809.

79. MacMahon EME, Glass JD, Hayward SD, Mann RB, Becker PS, Charache P, et al. Epstein–Barr virus in AIDS-related primary central nervous system lymphoma. Lancet 1991; 338:969–973.

80. Hamilton-Dutoit SJ, Pallesen G, Franzmann MB, Karkov J, Black F, Skinhoj P, et al. AIDS-related lymphoma: histopathology, immunophenotype, and association with Epstein–Barr virus as demonstrated by in situ nucleic and hybridization. Am J Pathol 1991; 138:149–163.

81. Bhatia K, Spangler G, Gaidano G, Hamdy N, Dalla-Favera R, Magrath I. Mutations in the coding region of c-*myc* occur frequently in acquired immunodeficiency syndrome-associated lymphomas. Blood 1994; 84:883–888.

82. Bhatia K, Guitiérrez MI, Huppi K, Siwarski D, Magrath IT. The pattern of p53 mutations in Burkitt's lymphoma differs from that of solid tumors. Cancer Res 1992; 52:4273–4276.

83. Gaidano G, Dalla-Favera R. Molecular pathogenesis of AIDS-related lymphomas. Adv Cancer Res 1995; 67:113–153.

84. De Thé G. Is Burkitt's lymphoma related to perinatal infection by Epstein–Barr virus? Lancet 1977; i:335–337.

85. Lenoir GM, Bornkamm GW. Burkitt's lymphoma, a human cancer model for the study of the multistep development of cancer: proposal for a new scenario. Adv Viral Oncol 1987; 7:173–206.

86. Epstein MA. Epstein–Barr virus—is it time to develop a vaccine program? J Natl Cancer Inst 1976; 56:697–700.

87. Epstein MA, Morgan AJ. Prevention of endemic Burkitt's lymphoma. In: Lenoir GM, O'Conor GT, Olweny CLM (eds). Burkitt's Lymphoma: A Human Cancer Model. Lyon, France: IARC, 1985, pp. 293–302.

88. Morgan AJ. Epstein–Barr virus vaccines. Vaccine 1992; 10:563–571.

89. Evans AS. EBV vaccine: use in infectious mononucleosis. In: Tursz T, Pagano JS, Ablashi DV, De Thé G, Lenoir G, Pearson GR, (eds). Vth International Symposium on Epstein–Barr Virus and Associated Diseases, Annecy, France. London: John Libby Eurotext, 1992, pp. 593–598.

90. Zeng Y, Hong D, Jianming J, Naiquin H, Pingjun L, Wenjun P, et al. A 10-year prospective study on nasopharyngeal carcinoma in Wuzhou City and Zangwu County, Guangxi, China. In: Tursz T, Pagano JS, Ablashi DV, De Thé G, Lenoir G, Pearson GR (eds). Vth International Symposium on Epstein-Barr Virus and Associated Diseases (Colloque INSERM 225). Paris: INSERM/John Libbey Eurotext, 1993, pp. 735–741.

91. Burkitt D. The African lymphoma. Preliminary observations on response to therapy. Cancer 1965; 18:399–410.

92. Clifford P. Long-term survival of patients with Burkitt's lymphoma: an assessment of treatment and other factors which may relate to survival. Cancer Res 1967; 27:2578–2615.

93. Ziegler JL, Morrow RH Jr, Fast L, et al. Treatment of Burkitt's tumor with cyclophosphamide. Cancer 1970; 26:474–484.

94. Ziegler, JL Magrath IT, Olweny CLM. Cure of Burkitt's lymphoma: 10 year follow-up of 157 Uganda patients. Lancet 1979; ii:936–938.

95. Olweny CLM, Katongole-Mbidde E, Otim D, et al. Long-term experience with Burkitt's lymphoma in Uganda. Int J Cancer 1980; 26:261–266.

96. Ziegler JL, Bluming AZ. Intrathecal chemotherapy in Burkitt's lymphoma. Br Med J 1971; 508–512.

6

Epstein–Barr Virus and Nasopharyngeal Carcinoma

Nancy Raab-Traub

PATHOLOGY OF NASOPHARYNGEAL CARCINOMA AND ASSOCIATION WITH EPSTEIN–BARR VIRUS

The Epstein–Barr virus (EBV) is associated with malignancies that arise in both B lymphocytes and epithelial cells, including Burkitt's lymphoma, immunodeficiency-related lymphoma, and nasopharyngeal carcinoma (NPC) *(1,2)*. The malignancies associated with EBV develop years postinfection, suggesting that they represent some form of reactivated infection.

Nasopharyngeal carcinoma is an unusual tumor with intriguing epidemiologic and biologic characteristics. The tumor occurs worldwide but with exceptionally high incidence in particular populations in specific geographic regions *(3,4)*. The incidence is highest among the Cantonese in Southern China, and in Hong Kong and Singapore Chinese. It occurs with intermediate incidence in Mediterranean Arabs and in Malays in Singapore. The incidence is quite low in American Caucasians and Europeans. The extraordinarily elevated NPC incidence in distinct populations suggests that environmental and genetic elements and viral infection contribute to the development of this disease *(1)*.

Most NPC tumors develop within the fossa of Rosenmuller, a region of the nasopharynx that is rich in lymphocytes. The primary tumor is frequently not identified and more than 50% of patients present with cervical lymph node metastases *(5)*. NPC is classified histopathologically by the degree of differentiation *(6)*. The classification system recommended by the World Health Organization classifies NPC as keratinizing squamous cell carcinoma (type 1), nonkeratinizing carcinoma (type 2), and undifferentiated carcinoma (type 3). The type 1 squamous cell carcinomas can be further divided into well, moderately, or poorly differentiated. Well-differentiated tumors display obvious intercellular bridges and keratin pearls, whereas poorly differentiated tumors have largely cytoplasmic keratin. Type 2 tumors may have organized cell growth patterns but lack keratinization under light microscopy. Undifferentiated NPC or type 3 was also frequently called lymphoepithelioma owing to the heavy infiltration of the primary tumor with lymphocytes. The cells are almost syncytial in appearance and are arranged in strands or connected with lymphoid stroma. The large nuclei are irregular with prominent nucleoli *(5)*.

From: *Infectious Causes of Cancer: Targets for Intervention*
Edited by: J. J. Goedert © Humana Press Inc., Totowa, NJ

Serologic Association with EBV

The first association of NPC with EBV was revealed in seroepidemiologic data in which patients with NPC had elevated immunoglobulin G (IgG) and IgA antibody titers to the EBV viral capsid antigen (VCA) and to an antigen associated with replication, called early antigen (EA). Henle et al. showed that these titers correlated with tumor burden, remission, and recurrence *(7)*. Elevation of IgA antibodies can precede tumor development by 1–2 yr, suggesting that EBV infection has reactivated *(7)*. In addition, antibodies to the EBV nuclear antigen (EBNA) also were elevated in NPC, and elevated total serum immunoglobulins were indicative of clinical stage *(8)*. In other studies of Alaskan Eskimos, North American patients, and Asian Americans, titers were not consistently elevated prior to diagnosis and were not predictive of prognosis *(9)*. Overall, however, the data suggest that reactivation and replication of EBV may precede and denote the development of NPC, and that continued antibody response may reflect the presence of tumor.

Several studies have indicated that EBV serology also differs among the histologic subsets of NPC. In one of the first studies of the histologic subsets of NPC, patients with type 1 NPC had lower EBNA titers but similar IgG levels to the viral capsid and early antigens *(6)*. Among American cases, the nonkeratinizing, undifferentiated forms (type 2 and 3) had elevated IgG and IgA EBV titers whereas patients with well-differentiated carcinomas had EBV serologic profiles similar to those of control groups *(9)*. In contrast, in a study of Malaysian patients comprising Chinese, Malay, and other ethnic groups, those with all three forms of NPC had elevated IgA titers to the viral capsid *(10)*.

Titers to other replicative proteins including thymidine kinase, DNase, ribonucleotide reductase, and the EBV replication activator protein, ZEBRA, are also elevated in NPC *(11,12)*. The accurate quantitation of antibodies with enzyme-linked immunosorbent assays (ELISAs) using recombinant proteins may provide additional useful clinical tests.

Detection of Viral Nucleic Acid and Protein in Tumors

It was initially shown using hybridization kinetic analyses that the EBV DNA in Burkitt's lymphoma was homologous to that in NPC and that NPC had a relatively high copy number of EBV genomes *(13)*. Subsequent studies revealed that viral DNA and EBNA were present in the malignant NPC epithelial cells rather than in the infiltrating lymphoid cells *(14)*. Unlike the situation in Burkitt's lymphoma, EBV DNA was detected across the spectrum of endemicity from areas of high incidence to those of low incidence *(15,16)*. The detection of EBV DNA or the abundant, nonpolyadenylated EBV-encoded RNAs (EBERs) has been useful for identifying NPC that has metastasized to lymph nodes in the absence of identification of the primary tumor *(17)*.

Squamous cell carcinomas of the nasopharynx (type 1) are rare in all populations and even in areas of high incidence comprise <1% of the NPC tumors *(9)*. With the availability of cloned probes, EBV genomes have been detected in the squamous cell type 1 NPC *(16)*. However, other studies using *in situ* hybridization have not detected the viral genome in squamous cell carcinomas in European populations *(18)*. In all type 1 NPC samples from Malaysia, EBV DNA was detected on Southern blots; the EBERs were detected by *in situ* hybridization; and latent membrane protein 1 (LMP)-1 was detected by immunohistochemistry *(19)*. In areas of differentiation, the EBERs were usually not detected, and LMP-1 expression was considerably decreased *(19)*. This downregulation of EBV expression in differentiated cells may account for some of the variability in detection of EBV in the differentiated form of NPC. The difference in association with type 1 squamous cell NPC may also reflect differences in the sample populations, as most studies in Oriental populations, in which undifferentiated NPC is the prevalent type, have detected EBV in all forms of the tumor while studies of European or American NPC samples have had less consistent detection of EBV DNA in differentiated NPC.

DIAGNOSTIC CRITERIA FOR NPC

Cervical lymphadenopathy is the most common clinical presentation of NPC, with unilateral or bilateral nodal involvement in 50–70% of patients. The jugulodigastric lymph nodes are the most commonly affected *(20)*. Nasal symptoms may affect more than half of patients, with blood-stained nasal discharge in one-third of patients. Nasal obstruction is a late finding indicating a large tumor. Hearing loss is due to tumor obstruction of the eustachian tube, and tinnitus occurs in one-third of patients. Blood-stained sputum is common and in endemic areas warrants a thorough head and neck exam *(20)*. Neurologic symptoms may include cranial nerve paralysis that most frequently involves cranial nerves V and VI. Headache is a frequent occurrence and may be unilateral, central, or retroorbital. Headache may be due to erosion of the base of the skull or cranial nerve irritation.

EBV serology is an important tool in diagnosis of NPC, with elevated anti-IgA VCA in 95% of patients. These titers are useful in the identification of patients with occult NPC.

Clinical diagnosis is confirmed by nasopharyngeal biopsy, which may be performed in the outpatient clinic with local anesthesia. In an endemic area, biopsy is indicated by cervical lymphadenopathy, elevated EBV titers, cranial nerve paralysis involving nerves V and VI, and radiologically demonstrated lesions. When NPC is strongly suspected despite negative biopsy, computerized tomography or magnetic resonance imaging should be performed and can be used to guide an endoscopic biopsy in the suspicious area. As a final resort to make the diagnosis, the patient should be reexamined under general anesthesia with curettage of the nasopharynx *(20)*.

EBV INFECTION IN NPC

Clonality of EBV in NPC

Nasopharyngeal carcinoma cells cannot be cultivated in vitro, and it is a rare tumor that can be transplanted into nude mice *(21)*. Therefore EBV infection in NPC has been primarily characterized through analyses of viral nucleic acids and proteins in samples obtained at biopsy *(16,22,23)*. In latent infection, EBV DNA is detected as an extrachromosomal, circular episome. In permissive infection (also called replicative or lytic infection), linear DNA is packaged into virions *(24)*. In NPC samples, EBV episomes have been detected by electron microscopy *(25)*. Identification of the restriction enzyme fragments that represent the ends of the EBV genome on Southern blots has been particularly informative *(23)*. Within the virion, EBV DNA is a double-stranded linear molecule with homologous direct, tandemly repeated (TR) sequences of approx 500 basepairs at both ends of the linear genome *(26)*. The number of TR sequences is quite variable and differs among individual DNA molecules. The terminal restriction enzyme fragments of virion DNA are heterogeneous in size and, when identified on Southern blots, form a ladder array representing molecules that have differing numbers of the TR element. After entry into the cell, the DNA circularizes through the TR to form the intracellular, extrachromosomal episome. This circularization produces a fused restriction enzyme fragment that can be identified with DNA probes for either end of the linear genome. In monoclonal EBV-positive lymphomas and in NPC samples, a single fused restriction enzyme fragment is usually detected *(23)*. This suggests that every copy of the viral genome within each cell is identical with regard to the number of TR sequences and that the EBV episomes in every cell within the tumor are identical. This clonality of the viral genome suggests by extension that the NPC tumors are also clonal. The detection of homogeneous EBV molecules also suggests that the tumor cells are a clonal expansion of a single cell that was infected with EBV prior to clonal expansion.

Integration of EBV into the NPC Genome

EBV episomes are present in multiple copies in NPC and have obscured the detection of integrated forms of EBV. Using pulse field analysis, possible integrated forms of EBV were detected in 4 of 17 NPC samples *(27)*. The sites of integration were not determined, and it is unknown whether these integration events affect cellular expression or contribute to tumor development. However, integration is probably not a necessary event for the development of NPC.

EBV Expression in NPC

EBV gene expression differs by type of disease, and its expression in NPC is distinct from that detected in transformed lymphocytes. The initial studies of viral expression in NPC identified the regions of the viral genome that were transcribed, and these now are known to encode latent membrane protein 1 (LMP-1) and the EBV nuclear antigen, EBNA-1 *(22)*. The sequences that encode EBNA-2, a viral protein essential for transformation of lymphocytes, and EBNA-3A, -3B, and -3C were not transcribed in NPC. Northern blot analyses, cDNA cloning, and polymerase chain reaction (PCR) amplification have shown that the EBERs, the spliced mRNAs that encode LMP-1, latent membrane protein 2 (LMP-2), and the *BamHI* A fragment are consistently transcribed in NPC *(28–33)*.

These findings have been confirmed through identification of specific viral proteins with monoclonal antibodies. LMP-1 and EBNA-1 have been detected while EBNA-2, -3A, -3B, and -3C, and leader protein (LP) (also referred to as EBNA-2, -3, -4, -6, and -5, respectively) are usually not found *(34,35)*. Detection of the LMPs is not consistent. LMP-1 is not always detected in all cells or in all tumors on immunoblots; and the LMP-2 protein, which is difficult to detect in cell lines, has not yet been identified in tumor samples *(36)*. The ZEBRA protein has been detected in a few cells in some NPC, and the spliced ZEBRA mRNA and other replicative mRNAs can be detected using reverse transcriptase-based PCR *(37)*. A new protein encoded by the *BamHI* A RNAs was found in most NPC samples *(38)*.

These findings suggest that NPC represents a latent EBV infection with consistent expression of specific viral genes with an expression pattern distinct from that found in transformed B lymphocytes. This unique state of latency, termed latency II, is also found in several other malignancies linked to EBV, including Hodgkin's disease and T-cell lymphoma and in some lymphoid cell lines (*see also*, Chapter 7) *(2)*. These differences in expression indicate that regulation of viral expression is distinct in this form of latency and that different viral promoters may be active.

In B-lymphoid cell lines, the EBNA-2 and EBNA-3 proteins are two key regulators of viral transcription. EBNA-2 autoregulates the major promoter for transcription of the EBNAs, Cp, and a bidirectional promoter for LMP-1 and LMP-2 *(39–41)*. The promoter for LMP-1 is quite complex, and multiple binding proteins and *cis* elements have been identified *(24)*. This activation of the LMP-1 promoter by EBNA-2 is further modulated by EBNA-3C and LP *(42,43)*. EBNA-3C also binds one of the same cellular proteins, RBPJk, through which EBNA-2 binds DNA and affects EBNA-2 transactivation *(43)*. The restricted expression of RBPJk is responsible for some of the cell type specific differences that have been observed with EBNA-2-responsive promoters. EBNA-3A and -3B (EBNA-3 and -4) also bind this same protein and also are likely to regulate transcription *(24)*. In addition, leader protein (LP or EBNA-5) interacts with EBNA-2 to affect transcription *(42)*.

As the mRNAs that encode EBNA-1 to -6 all initiate at promoters within *BamHI* W (Wp) or *BamHI* C (Cp) in lymphocytes, it was of interest to determine the structure of the EBNA-1 mRNA in NPC. Intriguingly, the EBNA-1 mRNA was shown to initiate from sequences within *BamHI* Q *(44)*. This same transcription initiation site for EBNA-1 was identified in Burkitt's lymphoma *(45,46)*. Interestingly, this promoter appears to be autoregulated by EBNA-1 as there is an EBNA-1 binding site immediately 3′ to the start site.

In NPC, EBNA-2 to -6 are not expressed, yet the promoters for LMP-1 and LMP-2 are apparently active, as the genes are transcribed. It is presently unclear how expression of these genes is regulated in the absence of the EBNA-2 and EBNA-3 proteins. Recent studies suggest that the *BamHI* A RNAs may encode proteins that affect EBV expression.

Several studies have shown that methylation of the viral genome is an important regulatory element, as expressed genes are usually not methylated whereas regulatory elements for nonexpressed genes are frequently methylated *(47)*. In NPC, the LMP-1 coding exons were shown to be methylated in all tumors whereas the promoter region was methylated only in those tumors in which the LMP-1 protein was not detected. An additional difference in NPC is that two different mRNAs encode LMP-1. In addition to the well-characterized 2.8-kb LMP-1 mRNA, a second 3.7-kb mRNA has been detected *(29)*. This mRNA initiates from a promoter within the terminal repeat unit that in vitro is transactivated by the SP-1 transcription factor *(48)*.

MOLECULAR PROPERTIES OF THE VIRAL PROTEINS EXPRESSED IN CANCER

EBNA-1

The EBNA-1 protein binds to the origin of replication for the plasmid form of the viral genome (orip) and enables the viral episome to be replicated by the host DNA polymerase *(24).* Orip also contains a transcriptional enhancer element, composed of 30-basepair tandem repeats, that is activated by EBNA-1 binding *(24).* In the presence of EBNA-1, EBV episomal replication is believed to be blocked at the repeat element such that the episome is replicated primarily unidirectionally. It is presently unknown if EBNA-1 also binds and activates specific cellular enhancers. Several studies indicate that EBNA-1 has additional important properties that may contribute to tumorigenesis.

EBNA-1 has the ability to bind RNA in vitro, through potential arginine/glycine (RGG) motifs. EBNA-1 also activates expression of the lymphoid recombinase *RAG* genes through an as yet unidentified mechanism *(49).* Activation of the *RAG* genes could promote chromosomal rearrangement and translocations and possibly also facilitate viral integration. In addition, EBNA-1 transgenic mice have an increased incidence of lymphoma *(50).* This may indicate that EBNA-1 can activate expression of critical cellular genes and affect cellular growth control. EBNA-1 also is expressed in the permissive EBV infection, hairy leukoplakia, indicating that it contributes to replicative EBV infection *(51).*

Interestingly, EBNA-1 is apparently not recognized by cytotoxic lymphocytes (CTLs), and EBNA-1 specific T cells have not been identifed. One study has shown that EBNA-1 is not processed and presented in class I major histocompatibility complex (MHC) molecules *(52).* The EBNA-1 protein contains a simple repeat of glycine and alanine that is homologous to some cellular proteins. Transfer of this repeat element to a heterologous protein sequesters the protein from processing and expression within class I. This unique property would allow an EBV-infected cell that expressed only EBNA-1 to escape immune recognition.

LMP-1

LMP-1 is a transmembrane protein that is essential for the EBV-induced transformation of B lymphocytes in vitro *(24,53).* It is the only gene expressed during latency that is capable of transforming established cell lines in vitro *(54).* Expression in rodent fibroblasts induces focus formation, growth in soft agar, and tumorigenicity in nude mice. In lymphocytes, expression of LMP-1 induces expression of multiple cellular genes including B lymphocyte activation antigens, adhesion molecules, vimentin, HLA class II, transferrin receptor, and the anti-apoptotic genes, *bcl2* and *A20 (24).* *A20* expression blocks tumor necrosis factor-induced cell death and inhibits p53-mediated apoptosis *(55).* Transgenic mice that express LMP-1 under the control of the heavy chain immunoglobulin promoter and enhancer develop B-cell lymphomas *(56).* This study reveals that LMP-1 without expression of other EBV proteins is oncogenic in vivo.

Expression of many markers usually expressed in B cells has been described in primary NPC samples. These include CD23, CD24, Ia antigen, and Cdw 70 *(1,2).* Expression of adhesion molecules also is altered with elevated expression of ICAM-1 (CD54) and reduced expression of LFA-3 (CD58). These effects are likely due to expression of LMP-1.

In some epithelial cell lines, LMP-1 inhibits differentiation and causes morphologic transformation with decreased cytokeratin expression *(57).* Epithelial lines expressing LMP-1 have decreased expression of E-cadherin and increased invasive ability *(58).* In transgenic mice, in which LMP-1 was expressed in skin, the mice had epithelial hyper-

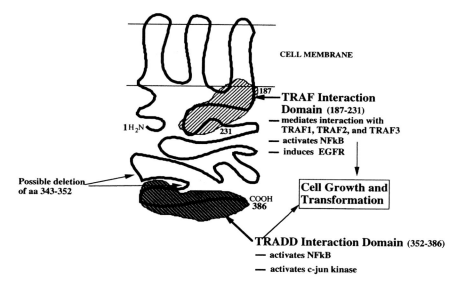

Fig. 1. Structure and functions of the latent membrane protein 1 (LMP-1) of Epstein–Barr virus (EBV).

plasia and altered expression of keratin 6 *(59)*. LMP-1 expression induces expression of the epidermal growth factor receptor, and elevated epidermal growth factor receptor is also detected in NPC *(60)*. A clinical analysis of NPC with or without detectable LMP-1 suggested that LMP-positive tumors grew more rapidly but that LMP-1 negative tumors had a greater chance of recurrence and increased tendency to metastasize *(61)*.

LMP-1 has a complex molecular structure with a cytoplasmic amino (N)-terminus, six transmembrane domains, and a long cytoplasmic carboxy (C)-terminal portion (Fig. 1). Within LMP-1 there is an 11-amino-acid repeat element and 10 amino acids that are deleted in some strains of EBV *(62)*. The C-terminal portion of LMP-1 interacts with cellular proteins that transduce signals from the tumor necrosis factor family of receptors *(63)*. The signaling molecules, termed TRAFs for tumor necrosis factor receptor associated factors, and a TRAF adaptor protein (TRADD) are activated by the receptor clustering that occurs after ligand binding. LMP-1 apparently acts as a constitutively activated member of this receptor family. Activation of these receptors activates the NFκB transcription factors and in some cases may induce apoptosis. Two domains have been identified in the C-terminus of LMP-1 that bind TRAF or TRADD, and both can activate NFκB *(64)*. The TRADD binding domain has been shown to also activate the c-*jun* terminal kinase *(65)*. Activation of NFκB is responsible for many of the cellular phenotypic changes that are induced by LMP-1. LMP-1 activates NFκB in both lymphocytes and epithelial cells and induces some of the same cellular genes in both cell types *(60,66)*. Induction of epidermal growth factor receptor (EGFR) expression requires the TRAF interacting domain but not the TRADD interacting domain *(67)*. Mutational analysis revealed that binding of TRAFs 1, 2, and 3 are required for induction of epithelial growth factor receptor *(67)*. This suggests that LMP-1 activates two distinct signaling pathways: one that activates NFκB and a second pathway mediated by TRAF activation that induces expression of genes such as the epidermal growth factor receptor.

LMP-2

The LMP-2 gene is expressed from a highly spliced mRNA that contains exons located at both ends of the linear EBV genome *(24)*. There are two differently spliced mRNAs for the two forms of *LMP-2*. The mRNA for *LMP-2A* (also called TP-1) has an exon that is lacking in the *LMP-2B* mRNA and that encodes a hydrophilic domain at the N-terminus of the protein *(24)*. The *LMP-2* mRNAs can be transcribed only across the fused termini of the episome or from rare integration events of two tandem copies. In NPC, consistent transcription of *LMP-2* has been detected by Northern blot analyses and PCR *(28)*. Antibodies to LMP-2 are highly specific for patients with NPC *(68)*. However, the protein is difficult to detect and has not yet been identified in NPC biopsy samples. LMP-2 is not required for lymphocyte transformation although it is consistently expressed during transformation and is coordinately regulated with LMP-1 *(24,69)*. LMP-2 is an integral membrane protein that has been shown to interfere with signal transduction from the activated immunoglobulin receptor *(70)*. The hydrophilic cytoplasmic domain of LMP-2 binds the cellular tyrosine kinases fyn and lyn *(24)*. This binding blocks subsequent signal transduction from the immunoglobulin receptor and inhibits B-cell activation that would initiate the viral replicative cycle *(70)*. In epithelial cells, LMP-2 becomes phosphorylated upon binding, possibly mediated by integrin binding *(71)*. LMP-2 becomes phosphorylated after plating of epithelial cells on extracellular matrix proteins such as fibronectin, although it presently is unclear how LMP-2 affects the biologic properties of epithelial cells.

BamHI A RNAs

In addition to the RNAs described above that are known to encode protein, a family of intricately spliced mRNAs were originally identified in examples of nasopharyngeal carcinoma *(29–31)*. Sequence analysis of cDNAs has revealed that the RNAs are 3′ coterminal but differentially spliced *(32,33)*. The various RNAs contain different exons forming novel open reading frames (ORFs). At least one of these ORFs has been shown encode protein *(30,38)*. Although these RNAs are most abundant in NPC, they have also been identified in transformed lymphocytes and in Burkitt's lymphoma *(2,72)*.

EBER RNAs

The most abundant RNAs in EBV-infected cells are small nuclear RNAs transcribed by RNA polymerase III *(73)*. These RNAs called EBERs are present at approx 10^6 copies per cell but are not necessary for lymphocyte transformation *(74)*. However, they are expressed in all of the malignancies associated with EBV and presumably contribute in some way to the maintenance of latency in vivo. Interestingly, expression of the EBER RNAs seems to be downregulated during differentiation, resulting in little or no EBER expression in differentiated regions of NPC tumors *(19)*. An extensive screening of EBER expression identified EBERs in 80% of type 1 NPC, in 98% of type 2, and in 97% of type 3. In the type 1 NPC, EBER expression was largely confined to the basal area and not detected in regions of differentiation *(75)*. The EBER RNAs are not detected in the permissive EBV infection, hairy leukoplakia *(76)*.

VIRAL INFECTION AND COFACTORS FOR THE DEVELOPMENT OF NPC

Strain Variation in NPC

As NPC occurs with high incidence in distinct ethnic populations and geographic locations, it is possible that its development is influenced by specific variants of EBV that are more prevalent in distinct geographic locations. The question of EBV strain variation has been examined in multiple ways *(16,77)*. The virus strains used for most studies of EBV have been obtained from lymphoid cell lines from Burkitt's lymphoma (HR1, W91, Akata, AG876) or the marmoset cell line infected with virus from a patient with infectious mononucleosis (B95) *(24)*. Virus has been obtained from NPC and used to transform lymphocytes, indicating that the virus in NPC is both replication and transformation competent *(2)*. Hybridization kinetic analyses and electron microscopy suggested similarity in genetic complexity of the viral genome in NPC and Burkitt's lymphoma; and restriction enzyme analysis of two NPC isolates, MABA and NPC-KT, indicated near identity to EBV strains from infectious mononucleosis and Burkitt's lymphoma *(13,77,78)*. EBV DNA within NPC biopsy samples was also shown to be similar to that in laboratory strains *(16)*.

Two types of EBV, referred to as EBV-1 and EBV-2, are distinguished by highly divergent sequences that encode the *EBNA-2* and *EBNA-3* genes *(24,79,80)*. EBV-2 has been detected in central Africa and is frequently detected in patients with human immunodeficiency virus (HIV), but neither type has been specifically associated with any pathologic phenotype *(2,81)*.

Restriction enzyme analyses have suggested that EBV strains may differ in prevalence in different populations. A common Chinese variant was initially described that was marked by the loss the *BamHI* site between the W1' and I1' fragments and frequently had an additional *BamHI* site in the *BamHI* F fragment *(82)*. A polymorphism in an *XhoI* site within the *LMP-1* gene also was detected in most Chinese samples *(83,84)*. A study of epithelial and lymphoid malignancies from endemic and nonendemic regions including Chinese, Mediterranean, and American populations determined the restriction enzyme polymorphisms and EBV type. This study identified the prevalent strain in Southeast Asia as a variant of EBV-1 with the *BamHI* and *XhoI* polymorphisms described previously *(83)*. An EBV-1 subtype similar to the MABA strain was found in NPC from areas of middle or low incidence. A new variant of EBV-2, with the polymorphisms from the right end of the genome similar to the Chinese EBV-1 strain, was identified in NPC and carcinoma of the parotid gland from Alaska *(83)*.

As EBV *LMP-1* is essential for transformation and is considered the EBV oncogene, recent studies have focused on strain variation in the *LMP-1* gene. The sequence of a Chinese isolate revealed several amino acid changes and deletion of 10 amino acids within *LMP-1 (84)*. Comparison of the *LMP-1* coding sequences in the prototype EBV-1 and EBV-2 strains revealed that the *LMP-1* sequences were nearly identical *(85)*. A comprehensive analysis of *LMP-1* sequence variation in NPC isolates from several geographic regions indicated that consistent sequence variation, including the 10 amino acid deletion, marked the Chinese strain *(62)*. In contrast, the Alaskan variant had many of these changes, but it was undeleted and represented EBV-2.

Many studies have focused on the small deletion in *LMP-1* and its prevalence in various pathologies associated with EBV *(86)*. One study analyzed the effect of the deletion on transformation ability by producing chimeric proteins. The data indicated that the enhanced transforming ability of the Chinese strain in BalbC 3T3 cells was transferred with the C-terminus that included the 10 amino acid deletion *(87)*. Deletion of the 10 amino acids in the B95 *LMP-1* resulted in the ability to induce transformation and tumorgenicity, while insertion of the 10 amino acids into the Chinese strain eliminated transformation and tumorigenicity. A similar study found that the differing ability of a deleted strain from NPC or the undeleted B95 *LMP-1* to activate NFκB or induce the epidermal growth factor receptor mapped to the transmembrane domain *(88)*. Several detailed studies of LMP-1 variation have now identified multiple strains that can be distinguished by phylogenetic trees, and at least six distinct variants of *LMP-1* can be identified *(89,90)*.

These studies indicate that certain EBV strains may be more prevalent in specific geographic regions. It is presently unknown whether certain variants may be linked to the development of NPC. The ability to distinguish strains may reveal epithelial trophic strains or identify strains with forms of *LMP-1* that have increased transforming properties that contribute to increased pathogenicity.

EBV INFECTION AND TRANSFORMATION OF EPITHELIAL CELLS IN VITRO

Although EBV readily infects and transforms B lymphocytes, it has been difficult to infect or transform human epithelial cells. Evidence of EBV infection of epithelial cells in vitro could be detected with wild-type strains obtained directly from throat washings but not laboratory isolates *(91)*.

The difficulty of infecting epithelial cells may be due to differences in expression of the EBV receptor, CD21 or CR2. There is conflicting evidence for expression of the receptor, dependent on the monoclonal antibody used and the source of epithelium *(2)*. Transfection of CD21 into an epithelial cell line facilitated infection, but the viral genome was rapidly lost from these cells and some cells spontaneously entered the replicative cycle *(92)*. Cell clones could be established that retained the EBV genome in episomal form and expressed EBNA-1 and LMP-1. These stably infected clones were impaired in the ability to differentiate, and viral replication could not be induced. This suggested that perhaps impairment in differentiation could influence the ability of EBV to establish a latent, transforming infection. A recent study showed that EBV infection of epithelial cells was greatly enhanced by cocultivation and did not require CD21 expression *(93)*. The binding of EBV to secretory IgA also facilitated EBV entry into epithelial cells that expressed the secretory component *(94)*. In polarized, stratified epithelial cultures, EBV was transcytosed through the epithelium without viral expression, while in unpolarized cultures, EBV replicative gene products were detected *(95)*.

Several EBV replicative proteins affect cellular cycle progression and apoptosis. The immediate early protein, ZEBRA, has been shown to interact with *p53* and interfere with *p53* transactivation while the EBV early gene, *BHRF1,* which is homologous to the *bcl2* gene, can block apoptosis induced by various agents *(2,96)*. Another early gene encoded by the BARF1 ORF can transform rodent fibroblasts and induce tumorigenicity in the EBV-negative Louckes Burkitt's lymphoma cell line *(97)*.

EBV INFECTION IN NORMAL AND PREMALIGNANT NASOPHARYNGEAL TISSUES

Several studies have attempted to ascertain the site and state of infection in the nasopharynx of normal populations and those at high risk to develop NPC. In patients with infectious mononucleosis, EBV DNA and viral antigens were detected in sloughed epithelial cells *(98,99)*. This suggested that the nasopharyngeal epithelial cells were the source of infectious virus that is detected in saliva during infectious mononucleosis. Evidence of EBV replication has been detected in epithelial cells in parotid tissue in which high copy numbers of EBV genomes were detected by *in situ* hybridization *(100)*. A recent study also showed evidence of EBV replication in epithelial cells adjacent to an EBV positive T-cell lymphoma *(101)*. The epithelial cells had high copy numbers of EBV DNA and were ZEBRA positive but EBER negative, while the malignant lymphocytes were positive for EBER and LMP-1 expression. Studies of normal nasopharyngeal mucosa have detected evidence of EBV only in lymphocytes in which EBER- and ZEBRA-positive cells were occasionally detected *(102)*. In nasal polyps, EBV-infected lymphocytes were detected, and some were positive for ZEBRA expression. This suggests that lymphocytes may be the source of virus secreted in the nasopharynx in reactivated infection.

A comprehensive screening of a large Chinese population identified 1267 individuals with IgA to VCA. Of the 203 who were biopsied, 46 had early NPC and an additional 12 had detectable NPC within 12 mo. In 14 samples from individuals without detectable NPC, a few cells were identifed as EBNA-positive or EBV DNA-positive by *in situ* hybridization *(103)*. In samples from patients with histologic evidence of NPC, EBV markers for EBNA or latent or replicative genes were not detected in normal tissue but only in samples with nests of tumor cells. A subsequent screen of biopsy samples regularly detected EBV in all examples of NPC but detected the genome only in a subset of cells displaying carcinoma *in situ (104)*. Carcinoma *in situ* with microinvasion had a higher proportion of EBV-positive cells. An extensive screening of 5326 biopsy samples from the ENT clinic at the University of Malaya, detected NPC or carcinoma *in situ* in 1811 samples. Remarkably, only 11 samples contained dysplasia or carcinoma *in situ* without adjacent invasive carcinoma. In the samples with relatively early disease, that is dysplasia or carcinoma *in situ,* EBER and LMP-1 were detected in all cells and analysis of the EBV termini revealed clonal EBV *(105)*. The very rare detection of dysplasia or carcinoma *in situ* suggests that in the development of NPC, dysplasia and carcinoma *in situ* rapidly develop into invasive carcinoma.

These studies in combination indicate that EBV infection in epithelial cells is rare. It occurs in primary infection, but in normal asymptomatic infection, EBV is harbored in lymphoid cells. The development of NPC may depend on the ability of EBV to establish a latent infection in epithelium. The changes that predispose the cells to this event may have already induced changes in growth properties. It is possible that the combination of prexisting cellular changes with EBV oncogene expression results in the rapid expansion of an infected cell that rapidly develops into malignant, invasive carcinoma *(1)*.

GENETIC CHANGES IN NPC

Although EBV infection is clearly an important factor in the development of NPC, the extraordinary differences in incidence indicate that other factors influence the development of NPC. Multiple dietary and environmental exposures have been linked to the development of this tumor *(3,4)*. Evidence suggests that consumption of salted fish is a contributing factor *(4,106,107)*. Carcinogenic compounds such as nitrosamine have been identified in salted fish and in food products consumed by other high-risk populations such as Tunisian stews and pepper mixtures *(108)*. In addition to dietary and environmental components that could affect cellular expression or EBV infection, genetic differences may exist in the high-risk populations. The putative genetic changes could work in concert with the viral oncogenic proteins to induce cancer.

An early investigation explored the relationship between HLA type and the development of NPC *(109,110)*. Several HLA types have been associated with development of the disease, and familial aggregation has been linked to the HLA region *(110)*. A recent study revealed that the cytotoxic T-cell presentation of LMP-2 was restricted to HLA A2.1 *(111)*. As LMP-2 is expressed in NPC, this restriction may be related to the lower incidence of NPC in people with HLA-A2 *(112)*. It has also been suggested that patients with NPC have impaired T-cell immunity to EBV in general. However, if impaired T-cell immunity and HLA-restricted presentation contributes to the development of NPC, one might anticipate elevated incidence of NPC in patients with AIDS, which has not been observed to date.

Genetic changes characteristic of other malignancies such as c-*myc* rearrangement, *p53* mutation, retinoblastoma deletions, or *ras* mutations have not been detected in NPC from Chinese, American, or Arab populations *(113–115)*. However, the unmutated p53 protein is detected at high levels in NPC, and p53 expression has been shown to be induced by NFκB, a transcription factor that is activated by LMP-1 *(116)*. Several studies have investigated whether an EBV protein possibly interferes with p53 function and eliminates a selection for inactivating mutations. The EBV ZEBRA protein binds p53 and inhibits p53 transcriptional transactivation, but ZEBRA is expressed in only rare NPC cells and would be unlikely to influence a selection for inactivating mutations in p53 in the majority of NPC cells *(96)*. In latent infections, EBV does not interfere with the ability of p53 to arrest cells in G_1 after DNA damage by inducing expression of the p21 cyclin kinase inhibitor, although two studies have shown that LMP-1 inhibited p53-mediated apoptosis induced by serum withdrawal *(55,117)*. This property could be due to induction of *bcl2*, which has been described in lymphoid cell lines *(118)*. However, elevated *bcl2* expression is not linked to EBV infection in epithelial tumors, and *bcl2* was not induced in epithelial cell lines expressing LMP-1 that were protected from apoptosis *(55,119)*. Inhibition of p53-mediated apoptosis was conferred by the A20 protein, which is induced by LMP-1 expression and blocks apoptosis induced by tumor necrosis factor or serum withdrawal. This inhibition of p53-mediated apoptosis is likely to be responsible for the lack of p53 mutations in EBV-associated cancers *(55)*.

Recent studies have identifed areas of loss of heterozygosity on several chromosomes including regions on chromosome 3p24 and 9p21 *(120,121)*. Although *p16* is not deleted in the C15 tumor passaged in nude mice, the gene is not expressed *(115)*. The *p16* gene is a critical regulator of cell cycle progression through G_1. Multiple genes that regulate cell cycle progression including the retinoblastoma gene, *cyclin D*, and cyclin-dependent kinases are mutated in cancers. Deletion of *p16* and repression of *p16* expression in NPC suggests that cell cycle regulation is also affected in NPC as it is many other tumors. The identification of other specific genes in the regions displaying chromosomal loss may identify critical cellular genes that are affected by mutagenic environmental factors or contribute to the development of NPC in high-risk populations.

SUMMARY

EBV infection is an etiologic and major contributing factor to the development of NPC. EBV is detected in the great majority of tumors and evidence of infection is usually detected in every malignant cell. EBV has consistent expression of specific viral genes in NPC with expression of *EBNA-1*, *LMP-1*, *LMP-2*, and *BamHI A* transcripts, similar to the latency II pattern described in lymphoid cell lines. In some cells the EBERs may not be detected and LMP-1 is not always detected in all tumors. These variations may reflect differences in viral expression dependent on the cell's state of differentiation or indicate that during tumor progression continued expression of the viral transforming functions may be subjected to immune selection.

It seems that the virus enters epithelial cells from permissively infected lymphocytes trafficking through lymphoid-rich areas of epithelium. Evidence of latent infection in normal epithelium has not been detected. In normal epithelial tissue, a permissive infection may occur or the virus may be transported through the epithelium via viral specific IgA. The tissue organization or genetic background of the cells may influence this process such that the virus does not replicate in the cells destined to develop into NPC, but rather a latent infection is established and viral transforming genes are expressed. Factors that could influence the outcome of infection could be the route of entry (IgA vs receptor mediated), the strain variant, or environmentally induced changes in the basal epithelium. This establishment of a predominantly nonpermissive infection could be the major event that leads to development of NPC. The expression of viral genes would then promote cellular proliferation and the rapid progression from dysplasia to cancer. Additional genetic changes may then contribute to the predominance of a specific clone or to tumor progression.

REFERENCES

1. Raab-Traub N. Epstein–Barr virus and nasopharyngeal carcinoma. In: Rickinson A (eds). Seminars in Cancer Biology. Saunders Scientific Publishers, Academic Press, London, 1993, pp. 297–303.
2. Rickinson AB, Kieff E. In: Fields BN, Knipe DM, Howley PM (eds). Fields Virology, 3rd edit., Vol. 2. Philadelphia: Lippincott-Raven, 1996, pp. 2397–2476.
3. de Thé G. Epidemiology of Epstein–Barr virus and associated diseases. In: Roizman B(eds). The Herpesviruses. New York: Plenum Press, 1982, pp. 25–87.
4. Ho JHC. Epidemiology of nasopharyngeal carcinoma (NPC). In: Ablashi DV, Huang AT, Pagano JS, Pearson GR, Yang CS (eds). Epstein–Barr virus and Human Disease. Humana Press, Totowa, NJ, 1990, pp. xli–xliv.
5. Pathmanathan R. Pathology. In: Chong VFH, Tsao SY (eds). Nasopharyngeal Carcinoma. Singapore: Armour, 1997, pp. 6–13.
6. Shanmugaratnam K, Chan SH, de Thé G, et al. Histopathology of nasopharyngeal carcinoma. Cancer 1979; 44:1029–1044.
7. Henle G, Henle W. Epstein–Barr virus-specific IgA serum antibodies as an outstanding feature of nasopharyngeal carcinoma. Int J Cancer 1976; 17:1–17.

8. Baskies AM, Chretien PB, Yan CS, et al. Serum glycoproteins and immunoglobulins in nasopharyngeal carcinoma: correlations with Epstein–Barr virus associated antibodies and clinical tumor stage. Am J Surg 1979; 138:478–488.

9. Pearson GR, Weiland LH, Neel HB. Application of Epstein–Barr virus (EBV) serology to the diagnosis of North American nasopharyngeal carcinoma. Cancer 1983; 51:260–268.

10. Sam CK, Prasad U, Pathamanathan R. Serological markers in the diagnosis of histopathological types of nasopharyngeal carcinoma. Eur J Surg Oncol 1989; 15:357–360.

11. Chen JY, Chen CJ, Liu MY et al. Antibodies to Epstein–Barr virus-specific Dnase in patients with nasopharyngeal carcinoma and control groups. J Med Virol 1987; 23:11–21.

12. Littler E, Newman W, Arrand JR. Immunological response of nasopharyngeal carcinoma patients to the Epstein–Barr virus coded thymidine kinase expressed in *Escherichia coli*. Int J Cancer 1990; 45:1028–1032.

13. Nonoyama M, Pagano, J. Homology between Epstein–Barr virus DNA and viral DNA from Burkitt's lymphoma and nasopharyngeal carcinoma determined by DNA-DNA reassociation kinetics. Nature 1973; 242:44–47.

14. Wolf H, zur Hausen H, Becker Y. EBV viral genomes in epithelial nasopharyngeal carcinoma cells. Nat Biol 1973; 244:245–267.

15. Desgranges C, Wolf H, de The G, et al. Nasopharyngeal carcinoma X. Presence of Epstein–Barr virus genomes in epithelial cells of tumors from high and medium risk areas. Int J Cancer 1975; 16:7–15.

16. Raab-Traub N, Flynn K, Pearson G, et al. The differentiated form of nasopharyngeal carcinoma contains Epstein–Barr virus DNA. Int J Cancer 1987; 39:25–29.

17. Chao TY, Chow KC, Chang JY, et al. Expression of Epstein–Barr virus-encoded RNAs as a marker for metastatic undifferentiated nasopharyngeal carcinoma. Cancer 1996; 78:24–29.

18. Niedobitek G, Hansmann MI, Herbst H, et al. Epstein–Barr virus and carcinomas: undifferentiated carcinomas but not squamous cell carcinomas of the nasopharynx are regularly associated with the virus. J Pathol 1991; 165:17–24.

19. Pathmanathan R, Prasad U, Chandrika G, et al. Undifferentiated, nonkeratinizing, and squamous cell carcinoma of the nasopharynx. Variants of Epstein–Barr virus-infected neoplasia. Am J Pathol 1995; 146:1355–1367.

20. Stanley R. Clinical presentation and diagnosis. In: Chong VFH, Tsao SY (eds). Nasopharyngeal Carcinoma. Singapore, Armour, 1997.

21. Busson P, Ganem G, Flores P, Mugneret F, Clausse B, Caillou B, Braham K, Wakasugi H, Lipinski M, Tursz T. Establishment and characterization of three transplantable EBV-containing nasopharyngeal carcinomas. Int J Cancer 1988; 42:599–606.

22. Raab-Traub N, Hood R, Yang CS, et al. Epstein–Barr virus transcription in nasopharyngeal carcinoma. J Virol 1983; 48:580–590.

23. Raab-Traub N, Flynn K. The structure of the termini of the Epstein–Barr virus as a marker of clonal cellular proliferation. Cell 1986; 47:883–889.

24. Kieff E. Epstein–Barr virus and its replication. In: Fields BN, Knipe DM, Howley PM, Chanock RM, Melnick JL, Monath TP, Roizman B, Straus SE (eds). Virology. Philadelphia: Lippincott-Raven, 1996, pp. 2343–2396.

25. Kaschka-Dierich C, Adams A, Lindahl T, et al. Intracellular forms of Epstein–Barr virus DNA in human tumor cells in vivo. Nature 1976; 260:302–306.

26. Given D, Yee D, Griem K, Kieff, E. DNA of Epstein–Barr virus. V. Direct repeats at the ends of Epstein–Barr virus DNA. J Virol 1979; 30:852–862.

27. Kripalani-Joshi S, Law HY. Identification of integrated Epstein–Barr virus in nasopharyngeal carcinoma using pulse field gel electrophoresis. Int J Cancer 1994; 56:187–192.

28. Busson P, McCoy R, Sadler R, et al. Consistent transcription of the Epstein–Barr virus LMP2 gene in nasopharyngeal carcinoma. J Virol 1992; 66:3257–3262.

29. Gilligan K, Sato H, Rajadurai P, et al. Novel transcription from the Epstein–Barr virus terminal *EcoR1* fragment, *DIJhet,* in a nasopharyngeal carcinoma. J Virol 1990; 64:4948–4956.

30. Gilligan K, Rajadurai P, Lin JC, et al. Expression of the Epstein–Barr virus *BamHI* A fragment in nasopharyngeal carcinoma: evidence for a viral protein preferentially expressed in epithelial cells. J Virol 1991; 65:6252–6259.

31. Hitt MM, Allday MJ, Hara T, Karran L, Jones MD, Busson P, Tursz T, Ernberg I, Griffin BE. EBV gene expression in an NPC-related tumor. EMBO J 1989; 8:2639–2651.

32. Sadler RH, Raab-Traub N. Structural analyses of the Epstein–Barr virus *BamHI* A transcripts. J Virol 1995; 69:1132–1141.

33. Smith PR, Gao Y, Karran L, et al. Complex nature of the major viral polyadenylated transcripts in Epstein–Barr virus-associated tumors. J Virol 1993; 67:3217–3225.

34. Fahraeus R, Fu JL, Ernberg I, Finke I, Rowe M, Klein G, Falk K, Nilsson E, Yadav M, Busson P, Tursz T, Kallin B. Expression of Epstein–Barr virus-encoded proteins in nasopharyngeal carcinoma. Int J Cancer 1988; 42:329–338.

35. Young L, Dawson C, Clark D, et al. Epstein–Barr virus expression in nasopharyngeal carcinoma. J Gen Virol 1988; 69:1051–1065.

36. Stewart JP, Arrand JR. Expression of the Epstein–Barr virus latent membrane protein in nasopharyngeal carcinoma biopsy specimens. Hum Pathol 1993; 24:239–242.

37. Cochet C, Martel-Renoir D, Grunewald V, et al. Expression of Epstein–Barr virus immediate early gene, *BZLF1,* in nasopharyngeal carcinoma tumor cells. Virology 1993; 197:358–365.

38. Fries KL, Sculley TB, Webster-Cyriaque J, et al. Identification of a novel protein encoded by the *BamHI* A region of the Epstein–Barr virus. J. Virol 1997; 71:2765–2771.

39. Laux G, Dugrillon F, Eckert C, et al. Identification and characterization of an Epstein–Barr virus nuclear antigen 2-responsive *cis* element in the bidirectional promoter region of latent membrane protein and terminal protein 2 genes. J Virol 1994; 68:6947–6958.

40. Sung NS, Kenney S, Gutsch D, et al. EBNA2 transactivates a lymphoid-specific enhancer in the *BamHI* C promoter of Epstein–Barr virus. J Virol 1991; 65:2164–2169.

41. Wang F, Tsang SF, Kurilla M, et al. Epstein–Barr virus nuclear antigen 2 transactivates latent membrane protein LMP1. J Virol 1990; 54:3407–3416.

42. Harada S, Kieff E. Epstein–Barr virus nuclear protein LP stimulates EBNA-2 acidic domain-mediated transcriptional activation. J Virol 1997; 71:6611–6618.

43. Robertson ES, Grossman S, Johannsen E, et al. Epstein–Barr virus nuclear protein 3C modulates transcription through interaction with the sequence-specific DNA binding protein, Jk. J Virol 1995; 69:3108–3116.

44. Smith PR, Griffin BE. Transcription of Epstein–Barr virus gene EBNA-1 from different promoters in nasopharyngeal carcinoma and B-lymphoblastoid cells. J Virol 1992; 66:706–714.

45. Sample J, Brooks L, Sample C, et al. Restricted Epstein–Barr virus protein expression in Burkitt lymphoma is due to a different Epstein–Barr nuclear antigen 1 transcriptional initiation site. Proc Natl Acad Sci USA 1991; 88:6343–6347.39.

46. Schaeffer BC, Woisetschlaeger M, Strominger JL, et al. Exclusive expression of Epstein–Barr virus nuclear antigen 1 in Burkitt lymphoma arises from a third promoter, distinct from the promoters used in latently infected lymphocytes. Proc Natl Acad Sci USA 1991; 88:6550–6554.

47. Ernberg I, Falk K, Minarovits J, et al. The role of methylation in the phenotype-dependent modulation of Epstein–Barr nuclear antigen 2 and latent membrane protein genes in cells latently infected with Epstein–Barr virus. J Virol 1989; 70:2989–3002.

48. Sadler RH, Raab-Traub N. The Epstein–Barr virus 3.5 kilobase latent membrane protein 1 mRNA initiates from a TATA-less promoter within the first terminal repeat. J Virol 1995; 69:4577–4581.

49. Srinivas SK, Sixbey J. Epstein–Barr virus induction of recombinase-activating genes *RAG1* and *RAG2.* J Virol 1995; 69:8155–8158.

50. Wilson J, Bell JL, Levine AJ. Expression of Epstein–Barr virus nuclear antigen-1 induces B cell neoplasia in transgenic mice. EMBO J 1996; 15:3117–3126.

51. Webster-Cyriaque J, Raab-Traub N. Transcription of Epstein–Barr virus latent cycle genes in oral hairy leukoplakia. Virology 1998; 248:53–65.

52. Levitskaya J, Coram M, Levitsky V, et al. Inhibition of antigen processing by the internal repeat region of the Epstein–Barr virus nuclear antigen-1. Nature 1995; 375:685–688.

53. Kaye K, Izumi K, Kieff E. Epstein–Barr virus latent membrane protein 1 is essential for B-lymphocyte growth transformation. Proc Natl Acad Sci USA 1993; 90:9150–9154.

54. Wang D, Liebowitz D, Kieff E. An EBV membrane protein expressed in immortalized lymphocytes transforms established rodent cells. Cell 1985; 43:831–840.

55. Fries K, Miller WE, Raab-Traub N. Epstein–Barr virus latent membrane protein 1 blocks p53-mediated apoptosis through the induction of the *A20* gene. J Virol 1996; 70:8653–8659.

56. Kulwichit W, Edwards RH, Davenport E, et al. Expression of the Epstein–Barr virus latent membrane protein 1 induces B-cell lymphoma in transgenic mice. Proc Natl Acad Sci USA 1998; 95:11963–11968.

57. Dawson CW, Rickinson AB, Young LS. Epstein–Barr virus latent membrane protein inhibits human epithelial cell differentiation. Nature 1990; 344:777–780.

58. Fahraeus R, Chen W, Trivedi P, et al. Decreased expression of E-cadherin and increased invasive capacity in EBV-LMP-transfected human epithelial and murine adenocarcinoma cells. Int J Cancer 1992; 52:834–838.

59. Wilson JB, Weinberg W, Johnson R, et al. Expression of the *BNLF-1* oncogene of Epstein–Barr virus in the skin of transgenic mice induces hyperplasia and aberrant expression of keratin 6. Cell 1990; 61:1315–1327.

60. Miller WE, Earp HS, Raab-Traub N. The Epstein–Barr virus latent membrane protein 1 induces expression of the epidermal growth factor receptor. J Virol 1995; 69:4390–4398.

61. Hu LF, Chen F, Zhen QF, et al. Differences in growth pattern and clinical course of EBV-LMP1 expressing and non-expressing nasopharyngeal carcinomas. Eur J Cancer 1995; 31:658–660.

62. Miller WE, Edwards RH, Walling DM, et al. Sequence variation in the Epstein–Barr virus latent membrane protein 1. J Gen Virol 1993; 75:2729–2740.

63. Mosialos G, Birkenbach M, Yalamanchili R, et al. The Epstein–Barr virus transforming protein LMP1 engages signaling proteins for the tumor necrosis factor receptor family. Cell 1995; 80:389–399.

64. Huen DS, Henderson SA, Croom-Carter D, et al. The Epstein–Barr virus latent membrane protein 1 (LMP1) mediates activation of NFkB and cell surface phenotype via two effector regions in its carboxy terminal cytoplasmic domain. Oncogene 1995; 10:549–560.

65. Eliopoulos AG, Young LS. Activation of the cJun N-terminal kinase (JNK) pathway by the Epstein–Barr virus-encoded latent membrane protein 1 (LMP1). Oncogene 1998; 16:1731–1742.

66. Paine E, Scheinman RI, Baldwin Jr AS, et al. Expression of LMP1 in epithelial cells leads to the activation of a select subset of NF-κB/Rel family proteins. J Virol 1995; 69:4572–4576.

67. Miller WE, Cheshire JL, Raab-Traub N. Interaction of Tumor Necrosis factor signaling proteins with the latent membane protein PxQxt motif is essential for induction of epidermal growth factor receptor expression. Mol Cell Biol 1998; 18:2835–2844.

68. Frech B, Zimber-Strobl U, Yip TTC, et al. Characterization of the antibody response to the latent infection terminal proteins of Epstein–Barr virus in patients with nasopharyngeal carcinoma. J Gen Virol 1993; 74:811–818.

69. Longnecker R, Kieff E. A second Epstein–Barr virus membrane protein (LMP2) is expressed in latent infection and colocalizes with LMP1. J Virol 1990; 64:2319–2326.

70. Miller CL, Lee JH, Kieff E, et al. An integral membrane protein (LMP2) blocks reactivationof Epstein–Barr virus from latency following surface immunoglobulin crosslinking. Proc Natl Acad Sci USA 1994; 91:772–776.

71. Scholle F, Longnecker R, Raab-Traub N. Epithelial cell adhesion to extracellular matrix proteins induces tyrosine phosphorylation of the Epstein–Barr virus latent membrane protein 2: a role for C-terminal src kinase. J Virol 1999; 73:4767–4775.

72. Brooks L, Yao QY, Rickinson AB, Young LS. Epstein–Barr virus latent gene expression in nasopharyngeal carcinoma cells: coexpression of EBNA1, LMP1, and LMP2 transcripts. J Virol 1992; 66:2689–2697.

73. Arrand JR, Rymo L. Characterization of the major Epstein–Barr virus-specific RNA in Burkitt lymphoma-derived cells. J Virol 1982; 41:376–389.

74. Swaminathan S, Tomkinson B, Kieff E. Recombinant Epstein–Barr virus deleted for small RNA (EBER) genes transforms lymphocytes and replicates in vitro. Proc Natl Acad Sci USA 1991; 88:1546–1550.

75. Tsai ST, Jin YT, Su IJ, Expression of EBER1 in primary and metastatic nasopharyngeal carcinoma tissues using in situ hybridization: a correlation with WHO histologic subtypes. Cancer 1996; 77:231–236.

76. Gilligan K, Rajadurai P, Resnick L, et al. Epstein–Barr virus small nuclear RNAs are not expressed in permissively infected cells in AIDS-associated leukoplakia. Proc Natl Acad Sci USA 1990; 87:8790–8794.

77. Raab-Traub N, Pritchett R, Kieff E. DNA of Epstein–Barr virus. III. Identification of restriction enzyme fragments which contain DNA sequences which differ among strains of EBV. J Virol 1978; 27:388–398.

78. Sato H, Takimoto T, Hatano M, et al. Epstein–Barr virus with transforming and early-antigen inducing ability originating from nasopharyngeal carcinoma. J Gen Virol 1989; 70:717–727.

79. Rowe M, Young L, Cadwallader K, et al. Distinction between Epstein–Barr virus type-A (EBNA-2A) and type-B (EBNA-2B) isolates extends to the EBNA-3 family of nuclear proteins. J Virol 1989; 63:1031–1039.

80. Sample J, Young L, Martin B, et al. Epstein–Barr virus type 1 and type 2 differ in their *EBNA-3A, EBNA-3B* and *EBNA-3C* genes. J Virol 1990; 64:4084–4092.

81. Walling D, Edmiston SN, Sixbey, JW, et al. Coinfection with multiple strains of the Epstein–Barr virus in human immunodeficiency virus-associated hairy leukoplakia. Proc Natl Acad Sci USA 1992; 89:6560–6564.

82. Lung M, Chang R, Huang M, et al. Epstein–Barr virus genotypes associated with nasopharyngeal carcinoma in southern China. Virology 1990; 177:44–53.

83. Abdel-Hamid M, Chen JJ, Constantine N, et al. EBV strain variation: geographical distribution and relation to disease state. Virology 1992; 190:168–175.

84. Hu LF, Zabarovsky ER, Chen F, et al. Isolation and sequencing of the Epstein–Barr virus BNLF-1 (LMP1) from a Chinese nasopharyngeal carcinoma. J Gen Virol 1991; 72:2399–2409.

85. Sample J, Kieff EF, Kieff ED. Epstein–Barr virus types 1 and 2 have nearly identical LMP-1 transforming genes. J Gen Virol 1994; 75: 2741–2746.

86. Knecht H, Bachmann E, Brousset P, et al. Deletions within the LMP1 oncogene of Epstein-Barr virus are clustered in Hodgkin's disease and identical to those observed in nasopharyngeal carcinoma. Blood 1993; 82:2937–2942.

87. Li SN, Chang YS, Liu ST. Effect of a 10 amino acid deletion on the oncogenic activity of latent membrane protein 1 of Epstein Barr virus. Oncogene 1996; 12:2129–2135.

88. Miller WE, Cheshire JL, Baldwin AS, et al. The NPC derived C15 LMP1 protein confers enhanced activation of NF-κB and induction of the EGFR in epithelial cells. Oncogene 1998; 16:1869–1877.

89. Edward RH, Seillier-Moiseiwitsch F, Raab-Traub N. Signature amino acid changes in LMP1 distinguish Epstein–Barr virus strains. Virology 1999; 261:79–95.

90. Walling DM, Shebib N, Weaver SC, et al. The molecular epidemiology and evolution of Epstein-Barr virus: sequence variation and genetic recombination in the latent membrane protein 1. J Infect Dis 1999; 179:763–774

91. Sixbey J, Vesterinen EH, Nedrud JG, et al. EBV replication in human epithelial cells infected in vitro. Nature 1983; 306:480–483.
92. Li QX, Young LS, Niedobitek G, et al. Epstein–Barr virus infection and replication in a human epithelial cell system. Nature 1992; 356:347–350.
93. Imai, S, Nishikawa, J, Takada, K. Cell-to-cell contact as an efficient mode of Epstein–Barr virus infection of diverse human epithelial cells. J Virol 1998; 72:4371–4378.
94. Sixbey JW, Yao QY. Immunoglobulin A-induced shift of Epstein–Barr virus tissue tropism. Science 1992; 255:1578–1580.
95. Gan YJ, Chodosh J, Morgan A, et al. Epithelial cell polarization is a determinant in the infectious outcome of immunoglobulin A-mediated entry by Epstein–Barr virus. J Virol 1997; 71:519–526.
96. Zhang Q, Gutsch D, Kenney S. Functional and physical interaction between *p53* and *BZLF1*: implications for Epstein–Barr virus latency. Mol Cell Biol 1994; 14:1929–1938.
97. Wei MX, Moulin JC, Decaussin G, et al. Expression and tumorigenicity of the Epstein–Barr virus *BARF1* gene in human Louckes B-lymphocyte line. Cancer Res 1994; 54:1843–1848.
98. Lemon SM, Hutt LM, Shaw JE, et al. Replication of EBV in epithelial cells during infectious mononucleosis. Nature 1977; 268:268–270.
99. Sixbey J, Nedrud JG, Raab-Traub N, et al. Detection of Epstein–Barr virus DNA and RNA in human pharyngeal epithelial cells. N Engl J Med 1984; 310:1225–1230.
100. Wolf H, Haus M, Wilmes E. Persistence of Epstein–Barr virus in the parotid gland. J Virol 1984; 51:795–798.
101. Wen S, Mizugaki Y, Shinozaki F, et al. Epstein–Barr virus (EBV) infection in salivary gland tumors: lytic EBV infection in non-malignant epithelial cells surrounded by EBV-positive T-lymphoma cells. Virology 1997; 227:484–487.
102. Tao Q, Srivastava G, Chan ACL. Evidence for lytic infection by Epstein–Barr virus in mucosal lymphocytes instead of nasopharyngeal epithelial cells in normal individuals. J Med Virol 1995; 45:71–77.
103. Desgrange C, Bornkam GW, Zeng Y, et al. Detection of Epstein–Barr viral DNA internal repeats in the nasopharyngeal mucosa of Chinese with IgA/EBV-specific antibodies. Int J Cancer 1982; 29:87–91.
104. Yeung WM, Zong YS, Chiu CT, et al. Epstein–Barr virus carriage by nasopharyngeal carcinoma in situ. Int J Cancer 1993; 53:746–750.
105. Pathmanathan R, Prasad U, Sadler RH, Flynn K, Raab-Traub N. Preinvasive neoplasia of the nasopharynx: a clonal proliferation of EBV-infected cells. N Engl J Med 1995; 333:695–698.
106. Armstrong RW, Armstrong MH, Yu MC, et al. Salted fish and inhalants as risk factors for carcinoma in Malaysian Chinese. Cancer Res 1983; 43:2967–2970
107. Ning JP, Yu MC, Wang QS, Henderson BE. Consumption of salted fish and other risk factors for nasopharyngeal carcinoma in Tianjink, a low risk region of China. J Natl Cancer Inst 1990; 82:291–296.
108. Poirier S, Ohshima H, De The G, Hubert A, Bourgade MC, Bartsch H. Volatiale nitrosamine levels in common foods from Tunisia, South China, and Greenland, high risk areas for nasopharyngeal carcinoma (NPC). Int J Cancer 1987; 39:292–296.
109. Lanier AP, Henle W, Bender TR, et al. Nasopharyngeal carcinoma in Alaskan Eskimos, Indians, and Aleuts: a review of cases and study of Epstein–Barr virus, HLA, and environmental risk factors. Cancer 1980; 46:2100–2106.
110. Lu SJ, Degos NE, Lepage V, et al. Linkage of a nasopharyngeal susceptibility locus to the HLA region. Nature 1990; 346:470–471.
111. Murray PG, Niedibitek G, Kremmer E, et al. Identification of target antigens for the human cytotoxic T-cell response to Epstein–Barr virus (EBV): implications for the immune control of EBV-positve malignancies. J Exp Med 1992; 176:157–168.

112. Burt RD, Vaughan TL, Nisperos B, et al. A protective association between the HLA-A2 antigen and nasopharyngeal carcinoma in US Caucasians. Int J Cancer 1994; 56:465–467.

113. Effert P, McCoy R, Abdel-Hamid M, Flynn K, et al. Alterations of the *p53* gene in nasopharyngeal carcinoma. J Virol 1992; 66:3768–3775.

114. Sun Y, Hegameyer G, Colburn N. Nasopharyngeal carcinoma shows no detectable retinoblastoma susceptibility gene alterations. Oncogene 1993; 8:791–795.

115. Sun Y, Hildesheim A, Lanier AP, et al. No point mutation but decreased expression of the p16/MTS1 tumor suppressor gene in nasopharyngeal carcinoma. Oncogene 1995; 10:765–788.

116. Niedobitek G, Agathanggelou A, Barber P, et al. Overexpression and Epstein–Barr virus infection in undifferentiated and squamous cell nasopharyngeal carcinomas. J Pathol 1993; 170:457–461.

117. Okan I, Wang Y, Chen F, et al. The EBV-encoded LMP1 protein inhibits p53-triggered apoptosis but not growth arrest. Oncogene 1995; 11:1027–1031.

118. Henderson S, Rowe M, Gregory C, et al. Induction of *bcl-2* expression by Epstein–Barr virus latent membrane protein 1 protects infected B cells from programmed cell death. Cell 1991; 65:1107–1115.

119. Lu QL, Elia G, Lucas S, et al. *Bcl-2* proto-oncogene expression in Epstein–Barr-virus-associated nasopharyngeal carcinoma. Int J Cancer 1993; 53:29–35.

120. Huang D, Lo KW, Choi PHK, et al. Loss of heterozygosity on the short arm of chromosome 3 in nasopharyngeal carcinoma. Cancer Genet Cytogenet 1991; 54:91–99.

121. Huang D, Lo KW, van Hasselt A, et al. A region of homozygous deletion on chromosome 9p21–22 in primary nasopharyngeal carcinoma. Cancer Res. 1994; 54:4003–4006.

7
Hodgkin's Disease

Paula G. O'Connor and David T. Scadden

OVERVIEW

Sir Thomas Hodgkin first described Hodgkin's disease (HD) in 1832 as a physician in training. This was followed by the description of the Hodgkin and Reed–Sternberg cells by multiple researchers between 1878 and 1902. The Lukes & Butler, Rye, and REAL classifications of HD were devised in the 1960s, 1980s, and 1990s, respectively. Yet, despite our longstanding ability to identify HD, the etiology of the disease has remained obscure.

Clinical and epidemiologic characteristics of HD including fever, night sweats, lymphadenopathy, bimodal age incidence, and case clustering prompted the search for an infectious etiology of the disease. The observation of a threefold increase in the incidence of HD in those with a history of mononucleosis focused the search on Epstein–Barr virus (EBV). Subsequent serologic, pathologic, and virologic evaluations support the idea that EBV plays a significant if not causative role in the development of subtypes of HD.

Seventy to eighty percent of all patients presenting with HD regardless of histologic subtype will be cured with combination chemotherapy and/or radiotherapy. These cures do not occur without risk—risk of sterility, second malignancy, severe organ toxicity, and infectious death. Targeting the viral antigens of EBV-associated HD using adoptively transferred virus-specific cytotoxic lymphocytes may provide an adjunctive or alternative therapy for those patients not cured or those unwilling to take the risks associated with conventional therapy.

EPIDEMIOLOGY OF HODGKIN'S DISEASE

Multiple Disease Hypothesis

The epidemiology of HD is complex. There is significant variation in HD incidence worldwide when analyzed by age, gender, ethnicity, geography, economic development, and histologic subtype.

MacMahon was the first to describe the bimodal age incidence of HD when he noted a first peak of disease in young adults between ages 15 and 35 and a second peak of disease in those over 50 (1). This observation was confirmed in other Western industrial nations but not in less developed nations (2). There, the first peak of disease was seen

From: *Infectious Causes of Cancer: Targets for Intervention*
Edited by: J. J. Goedert © Humana Press Inc., Totowa, NJ

earlier, in children between ages 5 and 9. The adult peak, however, remained in those over 50.

HD is divided into five disease types based upon histology. They are nodular scle-rosing HD (NSHD), mixed cellularity HD (MCHD), lymphocyte predominant HD (LPHD), nodular lymphocyte predominant HD (NLPHD), and lymphocyte depleted HD (LDHD). In the REAL classification scheme NSHD, MCHD, LPHD, and LDHD are referred to as classic HD while NLPHD, which has a greater association with non-Hodgkin's lymphoma (NHL), is set apart *(3)*. Studies before 1994 used the Lukes & Butler or Rye classification in which HD was divided into the four disease types of classic HD alone.

MacMahon and his colleagues noted international variance in the histology of HD in addition to age variation. Whereas MCHD was the predominant histologic subtype seen in the adult peak worldwide, NSHD was more frequently encountered in the first disease peak in Western industrial nations and MCHD more frequently seen in the first peak in less developed nations *(4)*. These observations led to the "two disease" or mul-tiple etiology hypothesis of HD. This hypothesis proposes at least two different etiolo-gies for HD, one being responsible for the young adult peak and the other(s) for the early childhood and adult peaks *(5)*.

Search for an Infectious Etiology

The patterns of HD in developing nations and young adult HD in the United States prompted the search for an infectious etiology. Shifting patterns of HD incidence in developing nations, coincident with socioeconomic change, were believed to be consis-tent with an alteration in the infective pattern of a possible transmissible agent *(6)*. Studies in the United States revealed case clustering, increased disease risk in those with small family size, early birth order, and high socioeconomic status *(7)*, features considered to be consistent with a late host response to a common infectious agent, and EBV was one of the first agents considered.

The link between EBV and HD began with the observation of similarities in the clin-ical presentation of infectious mononucleosis (IM) and HD, with fever, lymphadenopa-thy, and organomegaly. This was followed by the description of Reed–Sternberg-like cells in patients with IM, and the observation of increased HD incidence in those with a previous history of IM *(8–10)*. The link between EBV and HD was strengthened by subsequent evaluations revealing increased EBV titers in patients presenting with HD *(11)* and prospective data showing altered EBV serology in patients prior to the diagno-sis of HD *(8)*. In 1987, the EBV genome was found in Reed–Sternberg cells using Southern blot hybridization. Subsequent evaluations demonstrated the EBV genome in 40–50% of HD cases in the West. Eighty percent of the MCHD cases and 20% of the NSHD cases contained EBV, but it was rarely found in LPHD cases. Although not proving causality, these findings suggested a role for EBV in the pathogenesis of some cases of HD.

Genetics and Immunodeficiency

The question of genetic predisposition to HD was raised by accounts of increased rates of HD among children with immunodeficiency disorders such as ataxia telangiec-tasia and Wiskott–Aldrich's and Bloom's syndromes but not in children with other types of congenital immune deficiency or in those chronically immunosuppressed following organ transplantation. Given the current experience with increased HD in patients with human immmunodeficiency virus (HIV) infection, it is more likely that the increased rates of HD seen in some childhood immunodeficiency states has more to with the type and duration of immunodeficiency than with a specific genetic predisposition, defined by the underlying abnormality in these congenital syndromes. However, there is some evidence to suggest a genetic interplay with risk. An increased frequency of the major histocompatibility complex (MHC) class II allele *HLA-DPB1*0301* has been reported in patients with NSHD *(12)*. Since HLA type governs host–antigen interaction, HLA genotype may dictate the effectiveness of immunologic control of infectious agents participating in HD generation.

HD was noted in homosexual and bisexual men in San Francisco as early as 1984 *(13)*. However, definition of increased HD incidence in HIV-positive individuals did not come until 1992. Researchers examined the rates of HD in 6704 HIV-positive homosexual men, enrolled in the S.F. City Clinic HIV Cohort, and compared them with age-adjusted data from the Surveillance, Epidemiology, and End Results (SEER) registry *(14)*. An excess risk of 19.3 cases of HD per 100,000 patient-years was noted in the study cohort. This result was confirmed by multiple investigators *(15,16)*, including a group at the National Cancer Institute (NCI), which performed a linkage analysis of cancer surveillance and AIDS surveillance data collected by registries in several regions of the United States *(17)*. AIDS-related cancers were defined as those statistically increased after an initial AIDS diagnosis, with increasing prevalence from 5 yr before the diagnosis of AIDS through 2 yr after the diagnosis. The results were notable for a 7.6-fold increased relative risk of HD in patients with AIDS. A similar study in Australia revealed an 18.3-fold increase in the relative risk of HD in AIDS patients *(18)*. The risk in this study was limited to the 2 yr around the AIDS diagnosis and the period after diagnosis, suggesting that HD is a late manifestation of HIV infection, occurring in the setting of significant immunocompromise.

Several small studies from Italy, France, and Spain raise the question of an increased association between HD and HIV secondary to intravenous drug use (IVDU) *(19–21)*. In these studies patients with a history of IVDU were noted to have increased rates of HD relative to their homosexual counterparts. The cause for these findings is unclear—whether it be secondary to another biologically transmitted agent, a reflection of relative degrees of immunocompromise, or a reflection of ascertainment bias. Subsequent U.S. evaluations of cancer risk in hemophilic and homosexual individuals with AIDS show equivalent HD risk, suggesting that intravenous vs sexual risk factors do not enhance the HD risk already seen with HIV infection. Further evaluation, however, will be necessary to accurately define the relationship between HIV secondary to IVDU and HD.

PATHOGENESIS OF HD

Cell of Origin

The malignant cells of HD are the Hodgkin (H) cell, a mononuclear giant cell, and the Reed–Sternberg (RS) cell, its multinucleated variant. Their presence is necessary for the diagnosis of HD, yet cells similar to H–RS cells have been seen in other conditions such as non-Hodgkin lymphomas (NHLs), IM, and melanoma *(22)*. The diagnosis of HD requires the presence of H–RS cells in a background of reactive cells including lymphocytes, plasma cells, eosinophils, monocytes, and fibroblasts *(23)*. H–RS cells comprise < 2% of the tumor mass seen in most HD cases *(24,25)*. The paucity of H–RS cells in HD tumors has complicated efforts to define the pathogenesis of the disease. Their small number and difficulty in separating them from their surrounding cells has made clear assignment of their biologic characteristics difficult.

The cellular origin of the H–RS cell has been attributed at various points to lymphocytes, monocytes/macrophages, and dendritic and granulopoietic cells. Recent immunophenotyping and molecular studies, however, have identified the H–RS cell as a B cell *(24)*.

Immunohistochemical studies provided the first evidence of H–RS cell lineage *(26,27)*. They demonstrated the presence of B-cell antigens CD 19, 20, 22, 23, and 79a. However, no immunoglobulin mRNA or protein was identified. Subsequent analysis of the H–RS cells of LPHD revealed CD 20, 22, 75, and 79a on 70–90% of cases. Kappa and lambda light chain mRNA and protein were also identified in > 50% of cases, supporting the classification of the H–RS cell as a B cell in LPHD *(28)*. Other antigens noted on H–RS cells during these immunophenotyping studies included CD 15, 25, 30, 40, 54, 71 and MHC class II *(23)*. T-cell markers, including CD3 and the β-subunit of the T cell receptor, were also noted *(23,29)*. These markers were most consistent with a lymphoid origin for the H–RS cell although the specific lineage relationships were controversial based upon these conflicting results.

With evidence to suggest that H–RS cells were derived from specific lymphoid cells, studies to determine the H–RS cell lineage in the mid- to late 1980s utilized "whole tissue" samples and Southern blot techniques to identify clonal rearrangements of immunoglobulin or T-cell receptor genes *(30,31)*. More sensitive techniques isolating individual H–RS cells were developed in the early 1990s. Subsequent analyses of individual H–RS cells for immunoglobulin (Ig) rearrangement utilizing multiple polymerase chain reaction (PCR) primers identified clonal IgH gene rearrangements in the majority of H–RS cells *(32,33)*. Polyclonal Ig rearrangements were also noted, but only in a minority of cases, supporting the idea that H–RS cells in the majority of classic HD cases are clonal and B cell derived *(32,33)*.

Normal germinal center B cells undergo Ig variable region mutations to improve antibody affinity. B cells with productive rearrangements leave the germinal center and become memory cells. Cells with nonproductive rearrangements are selected to die by T-cell-mediated apoptosis. Analysis of the variable region of H–RS cell Ig gene rearrangements identify them as arrested germinal or postgerminal center B cells by their degree of homology with germline Ig sequences *(24)*.

H–RS Cell Function

H–RS cells are transformed postgerminal center B cells that have escaped T-cell-mediated destruction. The cause for this transformation, the process by which it occurs, how these cells elude immune detection, and how they bring about the HD phenotype is not completely clear. What is known about these processes has come from cytogenetic analysis of the H–RS cell and examination of H–RS cell markers and cytokine production, as an indicator of cell function and activity.

Meta- and interphase chromosomal analyses of HD specimens have revealed recurring aberrations in cells presumed to be H–RS cells. These include aneuploidy and deletions of 1p, 4q, 6q, 7q, and 14q *(34)*. The 4q25 deletion appears to be specific for HD, as it has not been described elsewhere *(34)*. The 6q deletion is seen frequently in NHLs and the 7q in a number of malignancies. The 14q deletion has been inconsistently found at 14q32, the *bcl2* breakpoint commonly seen in B cell lymphomas, and mutations associated with other common oncogenes such as *myc* have only sporadically been found. The most frequent finding during chromosomal analysis of HD tumor specimens is a normal karyotype *(29)*.

Recent data suggest that the H–RS cell may function as a rogue antigen presenting cell stimulating an immune response that is supportive, rather than destructive, of its presence. Among the panel of H–RS surface markers are antigen presenting molecules (MHC II, CD 80 and 86), adhesion molecules (CD 54 and 58), and tumor necrosis factor (TNF) family receptor molecules (CD 27, 30, 40 and 95) *(35)*. The antigen presenting molecules, CD 80 and 86, stimulate T-cell proliferation and lymphokine production. The adhesion molecules, CD 54 and 58, ensure attachment between H–RS and T cells. Cultured H–RS cells adhere to T cells and do not spontaneously detach *(36)*. This attachment likely enhances the cytokine-mediated interactions of H–RS cells and their surrounding T cells. The TNF receptor molecules, CD 30, 40 and 95, activate factors and pathways to alter cell growth and differentiation and block apoptosis *(37)*. How H–RS cells modulate TNF receptor signaling to favor their own survival and cytokine secretion over apoptosis is unclear *(24)*.

The cell surface markers and cytokines expressed by H–RS cells participate in the clinical and pathologic characteristics that are associated with HD. T cells, clustered around H–RS cells as part of the reactive infiltrate, participate in a pattern of stimulatory and costimulatory cytokine secretion that is thought to support the H–RS cell and cause the HD phenotype. The cytokines interleukin (IL)-1, IL-4, IL-6, IL-7, IL-9, IL-10, IL-12, TNF, lymphotoxin-α, interferon-γ, leukemia inhibitory factor (LIF), granulocyte-macrophage colony stimulating factor (GM-CSF), platelet-derived growth factor (PDGF), and ligands (L) for CD 30, 40 and 95 are elaborated as a result of this H–RS–T-cell cross talk *(24)*. Secretion of IL-1, IL-6, and TNF may contribute to the "B" symptoms of HD. Transforming growth factor-β (TGF-β), LIF, and PDGF are correlated with tissue sclerosis, while IL-3, 5, and GM-CSF are correlated with blood and tissue eosinophilia. IL-4, IL-10, and TGF-β are associated with reduced immune response *(23)*. Although these associations provide an intriguing link between cell physiology and clinical characteristics, their actual participation in the manifestations of HD is still conjectural.

HD elicits a significant immune response. H–RS cells, however, are thought to modify that response to favor their own survival by selectively expressing cell surface markers and cytokines. Perhaps one example of this selectivity is the increased expression of membrane-bound and soluble CD30 by H–RS cells. The increased expression of membrane-bound CD30 molecules may promote H–RS cell growth by mediating induction of IL-6 which has been shown to act as an autocrine growth factor for EBV-infected B lymphocytes *(24)*. Alternatively, the increased expression of soluble CD30 blocks T-cell activation by actively competing for CD30 ligand that might otherwise bind to the CD30 on T-cell surfaces.

Immunodeficiency and HD Pathogenesis

Increased rates of HD are seen in those with congenital and acquired cellular defects, most commonly involving the T cell. At the same time, in vivo and in vitro analyses of immune function in patients with HD have revealed abnormalities of cell-mediated immune function in early and late stage disease even prior to chemotherapy *(3,38,39)*. These abnormalities, including anergy to delayed hypersensitivity testing and decreased mitogenic response to known mitogenic stimulants, persist many years after the onset of remission *(3,40)*. The quality and degree of T-cell defect at which the risk for HD increases is not clear, nor is the interplay of preexisting immunodeficiency and HD-induced immunodeficiency.

Patients with HIV are at increased risk for HD. Data suggest that this risk increases with advancing disease *(41)*. However, multiple analyses of CD4 levels in HIV-infected patients reveal counts ranging from <10 to 1300 cells/µL, with median counts between 120 and 250 cells/µL *(19,20,42)*.

When HD occurs in patients with HIV, it is typically advanced, associated with B symptoms, and of the mixed cellularity or lymphocyte-depleted subtype *(41)*. This is irrespective of geography. Serrano *(42)* noted stage III or IV disease in 91% of his patients with HIV-associated HD, as compared to 46% in his patients without HIV. HIV-associated HD is commonly extranodal. Among the sites reported are the tongue, rectum, skin, and lungs *(41)*. The most common extranodal site, however, is bone marrow, which is involved in 41–50% of patients at presentation, and may be the only site of disease *(19,20,42)*.

The clinical pattern of HIV-associated HD with advanced stage, often extranodal tumor *(41)* is likely multifactorial in nature, in part reflecting late diagnosis, as patients with HIV frequently have "B" symptoms and lymphadenopathy without HD, and different HD biology in the immunocompromised. The EBV genome has been uniformly noted in the biopsy specimens of patients with HIV-associated HD *(43)*. EBV likely contributes to increased risk for HD but its impact on disease presentation and progression is unclear.

EBV

Infection to Latency

EBV is a lymphotropic γ-herpes virus. It is almost ubiquitous, with evidence of infection in approx 95% of the adult population worldwide. Infection is typically asymptomatic and occurs in childhood. Delayed EBV infection is manifest as the IM syndrome in up to 50% of those infected

EBV is spread by contact with oral secretions. The virus infects the epithelium of the oropharynx and salivary glands. Tonsillar crypt lymphocytes become infected and the virus then disseminates throughout the body. EBV establishes a latent viral infection in B cells, which may then become immortalized.

The EBV genome is a 172-kb double-stranded DNA molecule capable of encoding more than 100 genes. It enters B cells and epithelial cells using the CD21 receptor, which also serves as the receptor for the C3d component of complement. In acute B-cell infection, the EBV genome circularizes, forming an episome and expresses two nuclear proteins, Epstein–Barr nuclear antigen (EBNA)-2 and EBNA-LP *(44)*. These proteins in turn activate a series of genes and upregulate their own promoter and an upstream promoter, increasing the transcription of four other nuclear protein mRNAs (EBNA-3A, -3B, -3C, and EBNA-1) and three integral membrane protein mRNAs, latent membrane protein (LMP)-1, -2A, and -2B *(44)*.

Acute EBV infection is accompanied by polyclonal activation of B cells, natural killer (NK) cells, and cytotoxic lymphocytes. This cellular immune response is critical for controlling infection. The EBNAs and LMP molecules have multiple epitopes recognized in the context of MHC class I determinants, permitting specific cytotoxic lymphocyte killing. The cytocidal effects of these T cells are further enhanced by EBNA- and LMP-1-mediated production of adhesion molecules. These molecules increase the interaction between T cells and infected B cells. The immune response to EBV infection decreases the number of virally infected cells from the 1 in 1000, seen during acute IM, to the 1 in 1 million seen in latent infection *(45)*. Yet, complete eradication of EBV-infected cells does not occur for reasons that will be discussed later.

Oncogenesis

The differential expression of EBV-encoded proteins during latent infection enables EBV-infected cells to avoid T-cell-mediated killing and contributes to the oncogenicity of the virus. The proteins expressed during latency include those noted previously as well as small nuclear RNAs, EBER-1, and -2 *(46)*. Three patterns of latent protein expression have been identified utilizing cell culture systems and by analyzing EBV-associated tumor specimens. In latency pattern 1, EBNA-1 and the EBERs are expressed. In pattern 2, EBNA-1, the EBERs, LMP-1, -2A and -2B are expressed, and in pattern 3, EBNA-1, 2, 3A, 3B, 3C, the EBERS, LMP1, -2A, and -2B are expressed.

Each of the EBV latency patterns is associated with a specific tumor type. Pattern 1 is seen in Burkitt's lymphoma (BL); pattern 2 is seen in HD, nasopharyngeal carcinoma (NPC), and some peripheral T-cell lymphomas. Pattern 3 is seen in immunoblastic lymphomas in the immunocompromised and in post-transplant lymphoproliferative disorders (PTLPD, *see also* Chapters 4–6).

Of the EBV latency proteins, only LMP-1 is a proven viral oncogene *(47)*. The mechanism by which LMP-1 causes transformation is not completely understood but is intricately tied to its ability to mimic an activated tumor necrosis factor receptor (TNFR), thereby affecting signals for cell growth, differentiation, and death of the cell *(48)*. LMP-1 is an integral membrane protein, with six transmembrane domains, and a long cytoplasmic carboxy (C)-terminus. Aggregation of the cytoplasmic domains of LMP-1 molecules next to the plasma membrane appears to imitate the cytoplasmic domains of a growth receptor that has encountered ligand; thus LMP-1 mimics a constitutively activated receptor *(44)*.

The C-terminus of LMP-1 is divided into two parts, proximal and distal. They appear to interact with tumor necrosis factor receptor II associated factors (TRAFs) to activate NFκB, SAPK, and c-*jun*, transcription factors important for cell activation and growth stimulation *(44,49)*. IL-6 and IL-10 are among the gene products transcribed by these factors. BCL2 transcription may also be enhanced by NFκB activation. The TRAF-mediated pathway for transcription factor activation is similar to that used by activated CD 30 and 40, known TNFRs. The C-terminus of LMP-1 also interacts with the TNF receptor death domain protein (TRADD) *(44)*. Whether this interaction is capable of altering sensitivity to cell death signals is at this point not clear.

The transformation trigger for cells infected with EBV is unknown. It has been suggested, however, that viral evolution may lead to transformation and/or alter immunogenicity by modifying the epitopes presented to cytotoxic lymphocytes (CTLs). For example, base pair deletions in LMP-1, altering the C-terminus of the protein, have been identified in clinically and histologically aggressive cases of HD, NPC, and a few cases of angioimmunoblastic lymphadenopathy. This observation has been supported by finding greater tumorigenic capacity in cells transfected with deleted LMP-1 as compared to cells with a full-length gene (*see also* Chapter 6). In a murine carcinoma model, LMP-1 deletion mutants have also been shown to be less immunogenic than their intact counterparts *(40)*. These findings may partially explain why some individuals develop EBV-related disease while others do not.

LMP-1 is the only proven EBV oncogene, but must act in concert with EBNA-1, -2, -3A, -3C or LP to bring about stable cell transformation. For example, EBNA-2 is a known transitional activator of LMP-1 and interacts strongly with RBP-Jκ a transcription factor implicated in notch-mediated signaling *(50)*. Notch is an important mediator of cell fate decisions that induces proteins that block cell differentiation and has been shown to cause some T-cell leukemias *(51)*. In this fashion, EBNA-2 alters key regulatory pathways in infected cells and may contribute to stable cell transformation.

The initial studies defining the action of LMP-1 were performed in vitro. However, a recent examination of the interaction between LMP-1 and TRAF proteins in tumor specimens, from patients with EBV-positive HIV-associated NHL and posttransplant lymphoproliferative tumors, showed that LMP-1 functions as a signaling protein in vivo as well as in vitro *(52)*.

EBNA-1 and the EBERs are the only EBV gene products expressed in all of the latency patterns. The role of the EBERs in oncogenesis is unknown. EBNA-1 enables the EBV episome to replicate and persist in primate cells *(53)* and may also actively participate in cell transformation *(54)*. It binds RNA and DNA and has recently been shown to enhance both CD 25 expression and tumorgenicity of an HD cell line *(55)*.

Evasion of the Immune Response

The EBV gene products EBNA-3A, -3B, and -3C are highly immunogenic, eliciting exuberant CTL responses when presented in the context of MHC class I *(56)*. LMP-1, -2A, and -2B are also capable of eliciting a CTL response when presented in the context of class I MHC, yet patients with EBV-associated HD do not develop an immune response capable of containing their disease *(56)*. EBV gene products may contribute to the ability of the H–RS cell to evade immune detection.

EBNA-1 has a *cis*-acting glycine alanine repeat sequence that alters its processing through proteosomes and appears to allow it to escape immune surveillance. EBV-infected cells that express EBNA-1 in the absence of other EBNA and LMP transcripts are not recognized by cytotoxic lymphocytes *(40)*. This may account for the inability of immunocompetent hosts to eradicate EBV infection, as EBNA-1 alone has been detected in the B cells of EBV carriers.

Oudejans and his colleagues *(57)* assessed the expression of MHC-I, MHC-II, and transporter protein associated with antigen presentation 1 (TAP-1) in EBV-associated

HD tumors. They found higher levels of MHC class I expression and greater numbers of activated CTLs in the EBV-positive HD tumors compared to EBV-negative tumors. No differences were noted in MHC class II expression. Their findings suggest that mechanisms other than the downregulation of class I MHC and TAP-1 expression must explain the ineffective CTL response mounted against EBV-associated HD tumors, but the details regarding this are not known.

EBV Infection in HIV-Positive Patients

EBV infection is usually asymptomatic except when it is delayed or occurs in the setting of immunosuppression. In these cases infection can be overwhelming, producing the IM syndrome in the immunocompetent or lymphoproliferative disorders in the immunocompromised. Oral hairy leukoplakia due to EBV-stimulated epithelial cell overgrowth is also seen in those with HIV.

Two distinct strains of EBV have been identified based upon differences in the genomic regions encoding EBNA-2, -3, -4, and -6, permitting epidemiologic assessment of HIV patients with HD (40). Type 1 EBV is widespread in Western populations and is the more potent transforming virus in vitro, while type 2 is most commonly seen in equatorial Africa and is present in <10% of the population except in the HIV infected. Among HIV-seropositive individuals the prevalence is at least 30% (58–60). HIV-positive patients infected with type 2 EBV are usually coinfected with type 1 and HIV-seropositive hemophiliacs have been reported to have an almost 30% rate of infection with multiple strains of type 1 EBV (61). Patients with HIV may therefore be infected with multiple subspecies of EBV or coinfected with virus types 1 and 2, although no association with disease has been clearly shown. As more viral epidemiologic data become available, it may be possible to address the question of whether specific types of coinfection increase the risk for malignant transformation or influence the type of malignancy patients develop.

IMMUNOTHERAPY WITH EBV AS A THERAPEUTIC TARGET

HD is curable in 80% of cases with combination chemotherapy and/or radiation therapy. In those cases where cure is not achieved or patients are unable or unwilling to accept the risks associated with standard therapy, immunotherapy may provide an alternative therapeutic option.

Immunotherapy is any treatment that exploits the specificity of the immune system to limit disease progression or effect cure. It may be active as in the case of vaccines or passive as in the case of infused CTLs. Its toxicity generally does not overlap that caused by standard therapies. EBV, which is present in 40% of HD cases in the West and virtually all HIV-associated HD cases, is an attractive immunotherapy target given its immunogenicity, genetic stability, and constant presence within H–RS cells.

Vaccines

Vaccination therapies for HD have been considered but not extensively developed because of disease heterogeneity and its relative rarity. In 1991 the incidence of HD in the United States was 2.8 per 100,000 individuals; of these fewer than half were likely EBV associated (62). Although the incidence of EBV-associated HD is rare, the spectrum of disease related to EBV is quite large. This has led those interested in vaccine development to target primary EBV infection for vaccine therapy rather than EBV-related HD *(63)*.

Two vaccine strategies have been developed. The first utilizes glycoprotein (gp) 350/220, a viral envelope glycoprotein that induces neutralizing antibodies during EBV infection *(64)*. The second utilizes peptides from latent EBV proteins to stimulate EBV-specific CTLs *(65)*. The first has been tested in a small study in China, where EBV seroconversion takes place in 90% of children by age 3. It was given to nine EBV-negative 1-yr-old children, who were then followed for 30 mo. All developed antibodies to the gp 350/220 but only three developed antibodies to EBV virus capsid antigen (VCA), which was used as a marker of EBV infection. All of the children in the control group had VCA antibodies. At first glance these results are promising, but their true value, especially in regard to cancer prevention (HD, BL, or NPC), remains unclear *(see also* Chapter 5). This vaccine may simply delay primary infection. In the case of HD, it has been hypothesized that this might increase incidence rates rather than decrease them.

The second vaccine strategy, utilizing peptides from latent EBV proteins to stimulate EBV-specific CTLs in patients already infected with EBV, is currently being developed. Its success as an HD vaccine may be limited by the ability of patients with HD to activate T cells in vivo. Patients with HD have defects in cell-mediated immunity that have been shown to precede disease diagnosis. The utility of this vaccine to prevent HD in patients at high risk for the disease, such as those with Bloom's syndrome or ataxia telangiectasia, may also limited by their coexistent T-cell defects.

The spectrum and severity of disease caused by EBV makes development of a vaccine an attractive endeavor. However, vaccine development is limited by our ability to identify patients at risk and knowledge of how to modify the mediators of that risk.

Adoptive Immunotherapy

Cellular immune responses are the key to limiting primary and latent EBV infection. When that control is lost lymphoproliferative states such as HD may occur.

Adoptive immunotherapy, the transfer of activated autologous or allogeneic CTLs to induce or enhance an immune response to a specific target, was considered as a treatment strategy for EBV-associated HD, after observing regression of posttransplant lymphoproliferative tumors in response to the withdrawal of immunosuppression *(see* Chapter 4). This regression was interpreted as a response to reconstitution of CTL-mediated immune surveillance.

PTLD tumors express immunogenic EBV latency proteins that are processed via class I MHC for presentation to CTLs *(66)*. In the absence of EBV-specific CTLs, these tumor cells are allowed to proliferate. In their presence, they are specifically targeted for cell death. This presentation of viral antigens by tumor, to activated antigen specific CTLs in the context of MHC class I, is the premise for adoptive immunotherapy and is necessary for its success.

EBV-associated HD tumors meet the criteria necessary for adoptive immunotherapy, expressing MHC class I, in 75% of cases, and the immunogenic EBV latency proteins LMP-1, -2A, and -2B consistently *(67)*. EBNA-1 is also expressed in EBV-associated HD tumors, it but cannot be used to generate a CTL response because it is not presented via class I MHC. LMP-1 cannot be used despite class I presentation, because of frequent mutation that might alter CTL recognition. LMP-2A and 2-B, on the other hand, appear to be reasonable candidates for generating CTL responses.

Five LMP-2 epitopes have been defined that are expressed by HD tumors across a range of HLA types and subtypes, including HLA-A2, which is carried by 45–55% of the world population *(68)*. These LMP-2 epitopes appear to be highly conserved among EBV genomes, suggesting that adoptive immunotherapy for EBV-associated HD may have a broad range of applicability.

EBV-specific CTLs have been isolated and used to treat patients with relapsed EBV-associated HD *(69)*. These CTLs, containing MHC class I and II restricted cells, were generated ex vivo from 9 of 13 patients. They were expanded slowly in comparison to those generated from normal donors, which was attributed to decreased TCR ζ chain expression. The TCR ζ chain mediates transduction of signals for activation and proliferation of T cells *(69,70)*. Decreased TCR ζ chain expression has been noted previously in patients with HD. Whether this is a reflection of previous chemotherapy or a predictor of disease is not clear.

These EBV-specific CTLs were genetically labeled and infused into three patients. They persisted up to 13 wk after infusion and were associated with significant decreases in EBV DNA levels, suggesting efficacy against circulating EBV-infected cells. No assessment of antitumor effect was made. However, an in vitro assessment of the ability of CTLs to recognize and kill fibroblasts expressing LMP-2A was successful.

These data suggest that adoptive immunotherapy for HD is feasible. Whether this approach will have any meaningful antitumor effect requires further evaluation. Clinical trials using viral load, disease stage, and survival as end points are currently in progress.

CONCLUSION

Significant strides have been made in the treatment of HD in the last 50 yr despite our limited understanding of HD pathogenesis. Eighty percent of patients may now be cured with combination chemotherapy and/or radiation therapy. Nevertheless the morbidity associated with the disease and its therapy remains high. Sterility, second malignancy, severe organ toxicity, and psychosocial dysfunction are among the byproducts of our curative strategies and have an impact greater than expected on society, given that a significant proportion of HD occurs in the young. Molecular understanding of the role EBV plays in HD pathogenesis offers the potential of novel therapeutic approaches targeting viral induced signaling pathways or altered immunologic reactivity. Adoptive immunotherapy directed against specific EBV latent genes expressed in HD may offer an attractive future therapeutic option to add to our current armamentarium.

Our understanding of the role of cellular immunity in controlling EBV infection has led to the development of an immunologically based approach to treat and prevent some EBV-related disease. New treatment strategies will depend upon further unraveling the specific interplay of EBV and HD and exploiting it for therapeutic purposes.

REFERENCES

1. MacMahon B. Epidemiology of Hodgkin's disease. Cancer Res 1966; 26:1189–1200.
2. Grufferman S, Delzell E. Epidemiology of Hodgkin's disease. Epidemiol Rev 1984; 6:76–106.

3. De Vita VT, Jr, Mauch PM, Harris NL. Hodgkin's disease. In: De Vita VT Jr, Hellman S, Rosenberg SA (eds). Cancer: Principles & Practice of Oncology. Philadelphia, New York: Lippincott-Raven, 1997, pp.2242–2283.

4. Armstrong AA, Alexander FE, Cartwright R, et al. Epstein–Barr virus and Hodgkin's disease: further evidence for the three disease hypothesis. Leukemia 1998; 12:1272–1276.

5. Cole P, MacMahon B, Aisenberg A. Mortality from Hodgkin's disease in the United States. Evidence for the multiple etiology hypothesis. Lancet 1968; 11:1371–1376.

6. Vianna NJ, Greenwald P, Davies JNP. Nature of Hodgkin's disease agent. Lancet 1971; 1:733–736.

7. Gutensohn N, Cole P. Childhood and social environment and Hodgkin's disease. N Engl J Medi 1981; 304:135–140.

8. Mueller N, Evans A, Harris NL, et al. Hodgkin's disease and Epstein–Barr virus. Altered antibody pattern before diagnosis. N Engl J Med 1989; 320:689–695.

9. Kvale G, Hoiby EA, Pederson E. Hodgkin's disease in patients with previous infectious mononucleiosis. Cancer 1979; 23:593–597.

10. Rosdahl N, Larsen SO, Clemmensen J. Hodgkin's disease in patients with previous infectious mononucleiosis: 30 years' experience. Br Med J 1974; 2:253–256.

11. Johansson B, Klein G, Henle W, Henle G. Epstein–Barr virus-associated antibody patterns in malignant lymphoma and leukemia. Hodgkin's disease. Int Cancer 1970; 6:450–462.

12. Taylor GM, Gokhale DA, Crowther D, et al. Increased frequency of HLA-DPB1*0301 in Hodgkin's disease suggests that susceptibility is HVR-sequence and subtype-associated. Leukemia 1996; 10:854–859.

13. Biggar RJ, Horm J, Goedert JJ, Melbye M. Cancer in a group at risk of acquired immunodeficiency syndrome (AIDS) through 1984. Am J Epidemiol 1987; 126:578–586.

14. Hessol NA, Katz MH, Liu JY, Buchbinder SP, Rubino CJ, Holmberg SD. Increased incidence of Hodgkin's disease in homosexual men with HIV infection. Ann Intern Med 1992; 117:309–311.

15. Lyter DW, Bryant J, Thackeray R, Rinaldo CR, Kingsley LA. Incidence of human immunodeficiency virus-related and nonrelated malignancies in a large cohort of homosexual men. J Clin Oncol 1995; 13:2540–2546.

16. Rabkin CS, Biggar RJ, Horm JW. Increasing incidence of cancers associated with human immunodeficiency virus epidemic. Int J Cancer 1991; 47:692–696.

17. Goedert JJ, Cote TR, Virgo P, et al. Spectrum of AIDS-associated malignant disorders. Lancet 1998; 351:1833–1839.

18. Grulich A, Wan X, Law M, Coates M, Kaldor J. Rates of non-AIDS defining cancers in people with AIDS. J AIDS Hum Retrovirol 1997; 14:A18.

19. Andrieu JM, Roithmann S, Burarie JM, et al. Hodgkin's disease during HIV-1 infection: The French Registry experience. French Registry of HIV Associated Tumors. Ann Oncol 1993; 4:635–641.

20. Monfardini S, Tirelli U, Vaccher E, Foa R, Gavosta F. Hodgkin's disease in 63 intravenous drug users infected with human immunodeficiency virus. Ann Oncol 1991; 2:201–205.

21. Rubio R. Hodgkin's disease associated with human immunodeficiency virus infection. A clinical study of 46 cases. Cooperative Study Group of Malignancies Associated with HIV Infection of Madrid. Cancer 1994; 73:2400–2407.

22. Herbst H, Stein H, Niedobitek G. Epstein–Barr virus and CD 30+ malignant lymphomas. Crit Rev Oncol 1993; 4:191–239.

23. Gruss H, Pinto A, Duyster J, Poppema S, Herrmann F. Hodgkin's disease: a tumor with disturbed immunological pathways. Immunol Today 1997; 18:156–163.

24. Cossman J, Messineo C, Bagg A. Reed-Sternberg cell: survival in a hostile sea. Lab Invest 1998; 78:229–235.

25. Niedobitek G. The role of Epstein–Barr virus in the pathogenesis of Hodgkin's disease. Ann Oncol 1996; 7:5–10.

26. Schmid C, Pan L, Diss T, Isaacson PG. Expression of B-cell antigens by Hodgkin's and Reed–Sternberg cells. Am J Pathol 1991; 130:701–708.

27. Poppema S, de Jong B, Atmosoerodjo J, Idenberg V, Visser L, de Ley L. Morphologic, immunologic, enzyme histochemical and chromosomal analysis of a cell line derived from Hodgkin's disease. Evidence for a B-cell origin of Sternberg-Reed cells. Cancer 1985; 55:683–690.

28. Mason DY, Banks PM, Chan J. Nodular lymphocyte predominance in Hodgkin's disease. A distinct clinicopathological entity. Am J Surg Pathol 1994; 18:526–530.

29. Stein H, Hummel M, Marafioti T, Anagnostopoulos I, Foss HD. Molecular biology of Hodgkin's disease. Cancer Surv 1997; 30:107–123.

30. Weiss LM, Strickler JG, Hu E, Warnke RA, Sklar J. Immunoglobulin gene rearrangements in Hodgkin's disease. Hum Pathol 1986; 17:1009–1014.

31. Knowles DM, Neri A, Pelicci PG. Immunoglobulin and T-cell receptor beta-chain gene rearrangement analysis of Hodgkin's disease: implications for lineage determination and differential diagnosis. Proc Nat Acad Sci USA 1986; 83:7942–7946.

32. Kuppers R, Zhao M, Hansmann ML, Rajewsky K. Tracing B-cell development in human germinal centres by molecular analysis of single cells picked from histological sections. EMBO J 1993; 12:4955–4967.

33. Kuppers R, Rajewsky K, Zhao M, et al. Hodgkin's disease: Hodgkin and Reed–Sternberg cells picked from histologic sections show clonal immunoglobulin gene rearrangements and appear to be derived from B cells at various stages of development. Proc Nat Acad Sci USA 1994; 91:10962–10966.

34. Atkin NB. Cytogenetics of Hodgkin's disease. Cytogenet Cell Genet 1998; 80:23–27.

35. Gruss HJ, Kadin ME. Pathophysiology of Hodgkin's disease: functional and molecular aspects. Bailléres Clin Hematol 1996; 9:417–446.

36. Stuart AE, Williams ARW, Habeshaw JA. Rosetting and other reactions of the Reed–Sternberg cell. J Pathol 1976; 122:81–90.

37. Gruss HG, Dower SK. Tumor necrosis factor ligand superfamily: involvement in the pathology of malignant lymphomas. Blood 1995; 85:3378–3404.

38. Eltringham JR, Kaplan HS. Impaired delayed-hypersensitivity responses in 154 patients with untreated Hodgkin's disease. J Natl Cancer Inst Monogr 1973; 36:107–115.

39. Kumar RK, Penny R. Cell mediated immune deficiency in Hodgkin's disease. Immunol Today 1982; 3:269–273.

40. Dolcetti R, Boiocchi M. Epstein–Barr virus in the pathogenesis of Hodgkin's disease. Biomed Pharmacother 1998; 52:13–25.

41. Levine AM. Hodgkin's disease in the setting of human immunodeficiency virus infection. J Nat Cancer Inst Monogr 1998; 23:37–42.

42. Serrano M, Bellas C, Campo E, et al. Hodgkin's disease in patients with antibodies to human immunodeficiency virus. A study of 22 patients. Cancer 1990; 65:2248–2254.

43. Uccini S, Monardo F, Stoppacciaro A, et al. High frequency of Epstein–Barr virus genome in Hodgkin's disease of HIV-positive patients. Int J Cancer 1990; 46:581–585.

44. Kieff E. Current perspectives on the molecular pathogenesis of virus-induced cancers in human immunodeficiency virus infection and acquired immunodeficiency syndrome. J Natl Cancer Inst Monogr 1998; 23:7–14.

45. Cohen J. Epstein–Barr virus infections, including infectious mononucleiosis. In: Fauci AS, Braunwald E, Isselbacher KJ, et al. (eds). Harrison's Principles of Internal Medicine. New York: McGraw-Hill, 1998, pp. 1089–1091.

46. Howe JG, Steitz JA. Localization of Epstein–Barr virus-encoded small RNA's by in situ hybridization. Proc Natl Acad Sci USA 1986; 83:9006–9010.

47. Wang D, Liebowitz D, Kieff ED. An EBV membrane protein expressed in immortalized lymphocytes transforms established rodent cells. Cell 1985; 43:831–840.

48. Mosialos G, Birkenbach M, Yalammanchii R, Van Arsdale T, Ware C, Kieff ED. The Epstein–Barr virus latent membrane protein-1 (LMP-1) engages signalling proteins for the tumor necrosis factor receptor family. Cell 1995; 80:389–399.

49. Huen DS, Henderson SA, Croom-Carter D, Rowe M. The Epstein-Barr virus latent membrane protein-1 (LMP-1) mediates activation of NF-kappa B and cell surface phenotype via two effector regions in its carboxy-terminal cytoplasmic domains. Oncogene 1995; 10:549–560.

50. Johannsen E, Miller CL, Grossman SR, Kieff ED. EBNA-2 and EBNA-3C extensively and mutually exclusively associate with RBPJkappa in Epstein–Barr virus-transformed B lymphocytes. J Virol 1997; 70:4179–4183.

51. Pear WS, Aster JC, Scott ML, et al. Exclusive development of T-cell neoplasms in mice transplanted with bone marrow expressing activated Notch alleles. J Exp Med 1996; 183:2283–2291.

52. Liebowitz D. Epstein–Barr virus and a cellular signaling pathway in lymphomas from immunosuppressed patients. N Engl J Med 1998; 338:1413–1421.

53. Kieff ED. Epstein–Barr virus and its replication. In: Fields B, Knipe D, Howley PM (eds). Field's Virology. Philadelphia: Lippincott-Raven, 1996, pp. 2343–2396.

54. Niedobitek G, Young LS, Herbst H. Epstein–Barr virus infection and the pathogenesis of malignant lymphomas. Cancer Surv 1997; 30:143–162.

55. Kube D, Vockerodt M, Weber O, et al. Expression of Epstein–Barr virus nuclear antigen-1 is associated with enhanced expression of CD 25 in the Hodgkin cell line L428. J Virol 1999; 73:1630–1636.

56. Khanna R, Burrows SR, Kurilla MG, et al. Localization of Epstein–Barr virus cytotoxic T-cell epitopes using recombinant vaccinia: implications for vaccine development. J Exp Med 1992; 176:169.

57. Oudejans JJ, Jiwa NM, Kummer JA, et al. Analysis of major histocompatibility complex class I expression on Reed–Sternberg cells in relation to the cytotoxic T-cell response in Epstein–Barr virus-positive and -negative Hodgkin's disease. Blood 1996; 87:3844–3851.

58. Sculley TB, Apollini A, Hurren L, Moss DJ, Cooper DA. Coinfection with A- and B-type Epstein–Barr virus in human immunodeficiency virus-positive subjects. J Infect Dis 1990; 162:643–648.

59. Walling DM, Edmistan SN, Sixbey JW, Abdel-Hamid M, Resnick L, Raab-Traub N. Co-infection of multiple strains of the Epstein–Barr virus in human immunodeficiency virus-associated hairy leukoplakia. Proc Natl Acad Sci USA 1992; 89:6560–6564.

60. Kyaw MT, Hurren L, Evans L, et al. Expression of B-type Epstein–Barr virus in HIV-infected patients and cardiac transplant recipients. AIDS Res Hum Retroviruses 1992; 8:1869–1874.

61. Yao QY, Croom-Carter DSG, Tierney RJ, et al. Epidemiology of infection with Epstein–Barr virus types 1 and 2: lessons from the study of a T-cell-immunocompromised hemophiliac cohort. J Virol 1998; 77:4352–4363.

62. SEER cancer statistics review, 1973–1991: tables and graphs. In: Ries LA, Miller BA, Hankey BF, Kosary CL, Harras A, Edwards BK (eds). Bethesda: National Institutes of Health, National Cancer Institute, 1994.

63. Spring SB, Hascall G, Gruber J. Issues related to the development of Epstein–Barr virus vaccines. J Natl Cancer Inst 1996; 88:1436–1441.

64. Gu SY, Huang TM, Ruan L, et al. First EBV vaccine trial in humans using recombinant vaccinia virus expressing the major membrane antigen. In: Tursz T, Pagano JS, Ablashi DV, de The G, Lenoir G, Pearson GR (eds). The Epstein–Barr virus and associated diseases. Montrouge, France: Colloque INSERM John Libbey: Eurotext, 1993, pp. 579–584.

65. Moss DJ, Schmidt C, Elliott S, Suhrbier A, Burrows S, Khanna R. Strategies involved in developing an effective vaccine to EBV-associated disease. Adv Cancer Res 1996; 69:213–245.

66. Murray R, J., Kurilla MG, Brooks M, et al. Identification of target antigens for the human cytotoxic T cell response to Epstein–Barr virus (EBV): implications for the immune control of EBV-positive malignancies. J Exp Med 1992; 176:157–168.

67. Sing AP, Ambinder RF, Hong DJ, et al. Isolation of Epstein–Barr virus (EBV)-specific cytotoxic lymphocytes that lyse Reed–Sternberg cells: implications for immune-mediated therapy of EBV+ Hodgkin's disease. Blood 1997; 89:1978–1986.

68. Lee SP, Tierney RJ, Thomas WA, Brooks JM, Rickinson AB. Conserved CTL epitopes within EBV latent membrane protein 2: a potential target for CTL-based therapy. J Immunol 1997; 158:3325–3334.

69. Roskrow AM, Suzuki N, Gan YJ, et al. Epstein–Barr virus (EBV) specific cytotoxic lymphocytes for the treatments of patients with EBV-positive relapsed Hodgkin's disease. Blood 1998; 91:2925–2934.

70. Renner C, Ohnesorge S, Held G, et al. T cells from patients with Hodgkin's disease have a defective T-cell receptor zeta chain expression that is reversible by T-cell stimulation with CD3 and CD28. Blood 1996; 88:236–241.

8
AIDS-Related Lymphoma

Alexandra M. Levine

EPIDEMIOLOGY OF AIDS-RELATED LYMPHOMA

Lymphoma appears to be a late manifestation of human immunodeficiency virus (HIV) infection, occurring in approx 3–4% of patients as the initial AIDS-defining condition (1), but serving as the cause of death in 16–20% of individuals (2). Because only initial AIDS-defining conditions are reported to the Centers for Disease Control and Prevention (CDC) in the United States, it has been difficult to ascertain the true number of lymphoma cases that have occurred later in the course of HIV infection, after another AIDS-defining illness has already been diagnosed. In an attempt to clarify this issue, Coté and colleagues linked AIDS and cancer registries in certain areas of the United States, comparing lymphoma cases in HIV-infected and uninfected individuals (3). The relative risk of lymphoma within 3.5 yr of another AIDS diagnosis was 165-fold higher than that observed in the general population, confirming the high likelihood of lymphoma as a later manifestation of HIV disease. Of interest, the relative risk of lymphoma varied among specific pathologic types, with a 652-fold increase for high-grade immunoblastic lymphomas, 261-fold increase for small noncleaved (Burkitt's or Burkitt-like) lymphomas, and 113-fold increase for intermediate grade, diffuse large cell lymphoma (3).

Recently, the use of highly active anti-retroviral therapy (HAART) has been associated with a change in the natural history of HIV infection, leading to a 49% decline in AIDS mortality in 1997–8, and a significant decrease in the incidence of Kaposi's sarcoma (KS) and various opportunistic infections. It remains unclear whether the use of HAART will lead to a decreased incidence of AIDS-related lymphoma. In the Multicenter AIDS Cohort Study (MACS), rates of lymphoma increased by 21% per year between 1989–94 and 1996–7, at the same time that rates of KS fell by 66% (4). In the San Francisco cohort study of men who have sex with men (MSM), no significant decrease in the incidence of lymphoma has been demonstrated, when 1993–5 was compared to 1996 (5). In the CDC-sponsored Spectrum of Disease Study, based upon case records from 89 hospitals and clinics in nine U.S. cities, the incidence of primary brain lymphoma decreased from 8.5 cases/1000 person-years in 1994 to 0.9 cases/1000 person-years in 1996 (6). In an evaluation of cancers developing in participants of various AIDS Clinical Trials Group (ACTG) studies (7), the incidence of KS fell by 72% from 1992–1995, and declined another 88% in 1996–7. While the incidence of lymphoma

From: *Infectious Causes of Cancer: Targets for Intervention*
Edited by: J. J. Goedert © Humana Press Inc., Totowa, NJ

fell by 81% in the first time period (1992–95), the incidence declined by only 26% in 1996–7. These data would indicate that HAART has substantially decreased the risk of KS and primary brain lymphoma in HIV-infected individuals, while the incidence of systemic lymphoma has decreased to a much lesser extent. Further time will be required to ascertain the true impact of effective anti-retroviral therapy on the incidence of AIDS-related lymphoma. One may theorize that improved immune function and reduced B-cell stimulation in patients on HAART may reduce the risk of lymphoma. In contrast, because HAART-treated patients may survive longer with continued B-cell stimulation, dysregulation, and imperfect immune reconstitution, it is certainly plausible that the incidence of lymphoma will continue to increase in association with underlying HIV infection.

In contrast to KS, which occurs primarily in HIV-infected homosexual or bisexual men, the risk of lymphoma appears similar in all population groups at risk for HIV infection *(8)*. The vast majority of patients with AIDS-lymphoma have been men, consistent with the demographics of the epidemic of AIDS in the United States. Of interest, as the incidence of AIDS has increased among women in the United States, increasing numbers of women with AIDS-lymphoma are also being diagnosed *(9)*.

PATHOLOGIC TYPES OF AIDS-LYMPHOMAS

Certain pathologic features of AIDS-lymphomas are shared, while others are quite distinct. Essentially all AIDS-lymphomas are tumors of B lymphocytes, derived either from the germinal (follicular) center of lymph nodes, or from postfollicular B cells, in the process of terminal differentiation. Four distinct pathologic types of lymphoma comprise the vast majority of all AIDS-lymphomas *(8,10)*. Small noncleaved lymphomas, also termed Burkitt's or Burkitt-like lymphoma, tend to occur relatively early in the course of HIV infection, when CD4 cells are relatively high *(1)*. These comprise approx 30% of systemic AIDS-related lymphomas *(10)*. Diffuse large cell lymphoma and immunoblastic lymphomas are seen in another 30% of cases, respectively, and are often associated with lower CD4 cells in the blood, and more advanced HIV disease *(9,10)*. These lymphomas, comprised of germinal center and preterminally differentiated B lymphocytes, are the most common lymphomas confined to the brain, but are also seen with frequency in systemic AIDS-lymphoma. Recent classification systems of lymphoma have grouped both diffuse large cell and immunoblastic lymphomas within the same category, which is now termed diffuse large B-cell lymphomas *(11)*. As such, this group would constitute the largest number of AIDS-lymphoma cases. The last pathologic type of lymphoma associated with AIDS is primary effusion lymphoma (PEL), associated with infection by human herpesvirus type 8 (HHV-8) *(12)*. Although relatively uncommon, these lymphomas are of interest in terms of pathogenesis and clinical behavior (*see* Chapter 10).

ETIOLOGY AND PATHOGENESIS OF AIDS-LYMPHOMA

Common to all AIDS-related lymphomas is the concept that they arise in the setting of on-going B cell proliferation and stimulation. This B-cell hyperstimulation is partially due to HIV itself *(13)*, and may explain the polyclonal hypergammaglobulinemia characteristic of HIV infection, as well as the reactive lymphadenopathy, consisting of florid follicular (B-cell) hyperplasia. Aside from its direct effects on B lymphocytes,

HIV may also exert its effects indirectly, by inducing an inflammatory cytokine response from monocytes and T cells, leading to secretion of interleukin (IL)-6 and IL-10, both of which have been shown to induce B-cell proliferation *(14–18)*. Antigen-selected B-cell clones may be preferentially stimulated, as shown by the high rate of somatic mutations in the hypervariable regions of the immunoglobulin genes utilized by AIDS-lymphoma *(19,20)*, and by the fact that the repertoire of immunoglobulin genes utilized by AIDS-lymphoma show preferential usage of the V_H4 family, which have been implicated in the generation of B-cell autoreactive clones *(21,22)*.

In this setting of polyclonal B-cell proliferation, the progressive accumulation of mutational errors may predispose a given B-cell clone to a growth advantage, eventually leading to the development of monoclonal B-cell lymphoma. The specific genetic alterations leading to malignancy differ between the various pathologic types of AIDS-related lymphoma.

In AIDS-related Burkitt's lymphoma, a reciprocal chromosomal translocation between band 8q24 and one of the immunoglobulin gene loci (14q32, 2p11, or 22q11) leads to transcriptional deregulation of the c-*myc* protooncogene on chromosome 8 *(23,24)*. c-*myc* is a transcription factor that is involved in the entry of cells into the cell cycle (G_0/G_1). The deregulation of c-*myc* permits the transactivation of downstream immunoglobulin genes, with resultant monoclonal B-cell expansion. While Epstein–Barr virus (EBV) is present in approx 30% of AIDS-related Burkitt's lymphomas *(25)*, EBV transforming latent antigens are not expressed, suggesting that this virus is not intricately involved in the molecular pathogenesis of AIDS-related Burkitt's lymphoma. However, additional mutational errors, such as inactivating mutations and/or deletions of the *p53* tumor suppressor gene are present in approx 60% of AIDS-related Burkitt's lymphoma *(26)*, providing another mechanism for malignant outgrowth of clonal B lymphocytes. Mutations of *ras* genes have also been noted in occasional cases *(26)*.

The most common molecular aberrations described in AIDS-related diffuse large B-cell lymphoma and B-immunoblastic lymphoma include EBV infection and dysregulation of *bcl-6*. EBV infection is present in approx 70–80% of such cases *(27,28)*, with frequent expression of the EBV-encoded latent antigen LMP-1 *(28)*. Recent work by Liebowitz *(29)* has demonstrated the transforming ability of LMP-1, as it binds to TRAF molecules (TNF receptor associated factors), thereby activating NFκB, with further signaling serving to drive cell division. While EBV is not the only pathogenic factor in the development of AIDS-diffuse large-cell lymphoma, Kersten and colleagues have demonstrated that decreases of EBV-specific cytotoxic T-cell responses, with subsequent increased EBV viral load, correlate with development of large-cell lymphoma in HIV-infected patients *(30)*.

In addition to EBV, dysregulation of *bcl-6* has also been described in approx 70% of diffuse large B-cell lymphomas, in both HIV-infected and uninfected patients *(31)*. *Bcl-6* expression is restricted to B cells of the germinal center, and is essential for germinal center formation *(32)*. The protooncogene functions as a zinc-finger transcriptional repressor *(33)*. *Bcl-6* may be deregulated in lymphoma by means of chromosomal rearrangements or mutations of the 5′ regulatory sequences *(31,34)*. Although *bcl-6* deregulation appears to be the most common mutational aberration in AIDS-related diffuse large B-cell lymphoma, such deregulation is not common in

AIDS-related immunoblastic lymphoma, consistent with the postgerminal center derivation of these cells *(20)*.

The molecular pathogenesis of PEL has not yet been fully ascertained, although the tumor is clearly associated with infection by HHV-8 *(12)*. Of importance, the HHV8 genome carries structural and functional homologs of the human *bcl-2, IL-6,* and *cyclin D* genes, each of which may contribute to the development of lymphoid malignancy *(35)*. In addition, the majority of PEL cases are also infected with EBV, providing another potential mechanism for lymphomagenesis.

Hepatitis C (HCV) infection has been associated with a variety of lymphoproliferative disorders, and a high prevalence of HCV infection has been noted in HIV-negative patients with malignant lymphoma (*see also* Chapter 19) *(36)*. Because HCV has been demonstrated in as many as 40% of HIV-infected patients, Levine and colleagues studied the relationship, if any, between chronic HCV infection and the subsequent development of AIDS-related lymphoma *(37)*. Of interest, the study demonstrated no relationship between dual infection by HIV and HCV, and subsequent increased risk of lymphoma *(37)*.

In summary, essentially all AIDS-lymphomas develop in the setting of ongoing B-cell stimulation and proliferation. The development of specific mutational errors in these proliferating cells provides a mechanism for clonal selection, with evolution from polyclonal B-cell response to monoclonal B-cell lymphoma. The specific pathologic types of AIDS-lymphoma are associated with different genetic alterations, each of which may lead to malignant transformation.

CLINICAL PRESENTATION OF AIDS-RELATED LYMPHOMA

Between 80% and 90% of patients with AIDS-lymphoma complain of systemic "B" symptoms at initial diagnosis *(8,38,39)*, consisting of fevers, drenching night sweats, and/or ≥ 10% loss of normal body weight. Of importance, many opportunistic infections may present in similar fashion, including *Mycobacterium avium* complex (MAC), cytomegalovirus infection (CMV), *Cryptococcus,* and others. It is important for the clinician to consider lymphoma in the differential diagnosis of an HIV-infected patient with fever, weight loss, and/or night sweats.

Lymphomatous involvement of extranodal sites is very common in newly diagnosed patients with AIDS-lymphoma, with stage III or IV disease in approx 90% *(8,38,39)*. Visceral sites most often involved by lymphoma include the central nervous system (CNS) in approx 25%, bone marrow in 20–25%, gastrointestinal tract in approx 20%, and liver in 12% *(8)*. AIDS-lymphoma may also present in unusual sites, such as the rectum, oral cavity, gallbladder, heart, skin, earlobes, and others.

Aside from involvement of visceral organs, patients with AIDS-lymphoma also commonly present with peripheral and/or central lymphadenopathy. Peripheral lymph nodes may be extremely large, with a firm, rubbery consistency.

Specific symptoms of AIDS-lymphoma will depend upon the organ(s) involved. Patients with primary CNS lymphoma often complain of headache, seizures, focal neurologic defect, or altered mental status *(40)*. Headache or cranial nerve palsy may occur in patients with leptomeningeal involvement, although approx 20% of patients with lymphoma cells in the spinal fluid will be asymptomatic *(41)*. Gastrointestinal lymphoma may present with abdominal pain or distension, anorexia, nausea, or vomiting. Involvement of the rectum and/or perianal region often presents as a rectal mass, or pain upon defecation. Patients with bone marrow involvement have a statistically increased likelihood of leptomeningeal lymphoma *(42)*. Of interest, no specific symptom is associated with marrow involvement, and hematologic parameters are similar in the presence or absence of lymphoma, with the exception of thrombocytopenia <100,000/dL, seen more often in patients in whom the marrow is involved *(42)*.

DIAGNOSIS OF AIDS-LYMPHOMA

Biopsy of an abnormal area, either nodal or extranodal, is the "gold standard" for the diagnosis of lymphoma. Aside from morphologic assessment, additional immunophenotypic analyses are usually performed, to confirm the presence of monoclonality. Southern blot analysis may be performed to document genotypic monoclonality, although this technique is used only rarely for clinical purposes. Additional immunohistochemical analyses are usually performed, to document expression of other B-cell markers, such as CD20.

If an abnormal mass lesion is present in a relatively inaccessible site, such as the retroperitoneum, a fine needle aspiration (FNA) may be performed, in place of definitive biopsy. However, although the FNA may be helpful in the diagnosis of certain infections, the technique can lead to substantial error in patients with AIDS-lymphoma. At a minimum, an immunophenotypic study should be performed on cells obtained by FNA to confirm monoclonality, as a means of attempting to prove presence of lymphoma, as opposed to a reactive lesion of some type. In patients with known history of AIDS-lymphoma, an FNA is fully acceptable for diagnosis of relapsed disease.

STAGING WORKUP OF THE PATIENT WITH AIDS-LYMPHOMA

Routine evaluation of the patient with AIDS-lymphoma must include an assessment of the HIV disease, as well as the lymphoma. Because the level of CD4 cells will predict prognosis in such patients *(43,44)*, determination of CD4 and CD8 cell counts prior to therapy is indicated, as well as an assessment of HIV viral load. Because AIDS-related opportunistic infections are a common cause of death in patients with AIDS-lymphoma, every effort should be made to control the HIV infection.

Blood work is obtained at baseline, including assessment of renal and hepatic function, complete blood count, and level of lactate dehydrogenase (LDH). Elevated LDH levels have prognostic impact, portending a worse prognosis *(45)*. Uric acid levels may be elevated, owing to spontaneous tumor cell lysis. Hypercalcemia may also occur.

Computerized axial tomographic (CAT) scans are routinely performed in patients with known or suspected lymphoma. Mass lesions are expected in the organ(s) of involvement. Abdominal CAT scans reveal evidence of focal lymphomatous involvement, documented in 58 of 59 such patients who presented with predominant signs and symptoms related to the abdomen, and in 14 (26%) of 53 of those who had no specific abdominal symptoms *(46)*. Focal hepatic lesions are expected with liver involvement, varying from solitary to innumerable, and ranging from relatively small (1 cm) nodules to large masses, > 15 cm in diameter. Mass lesions in other extranodal sites are also routinely encountered. Involvement of the lung is associated with interstitial infiltrates, pulmonary nodules, and/or alveolar lung disease; pleural effusions may also be present. Generalized or localized lymphadenopathy is also expected on CAT scan.

Gallium-67 scanning can be particularly useful in patients with AIDS-lymphoma, and may differentiate malignant lymphoma from reactive lymphadenopathy *(47)*. High- and intermediate-grade lymphomas are almost always gallium avid, and the gallium scan may be useful in identifying lesions that have not yet caused specific organ or nodal enlargement on CAT scan. Aside from its known sensitivity and specificity in lymphoma, gallium-67 scanning may be particularly useful in the assessment of residual, stable masses after the completion of chemotherapy. These residual masses may occur in as many as 40% of patients with lymphoma who have been successfully treated, and are believed secondary to residual fibrosis in the area.

PROGNOSTIC FACTORS IN PATIENTS WITH AIDS-LYMPHOMA

In determining the prognosis of patients with AIDS-lymphoma, several issues must be considered, including factors related to HIV itself, those related to the patient, and those related to the lymphoma. In a large prospective study of 192 patients with newly diagnosed systemic AIDS-lymphoma, Straus and colleagues identified four characteristics that were independently associated with shorter survival: age >35 yr; CD4 cell counts < 100/μL; stage III/IV; and history of injection drug use *(44)*. The median overall survival for patients with none or one of these factors was 46 wk, vs 18 wk in the presence of three or four factors. Other factors that have been associated with poor prognosis in AIDS-lymphoma include elevated LDH, poor performance status, and history of AIDS prior to the onset of lymphoma *(43,45)*. Patients with primary CNS lymphoma have particularly short survival when compared to those with systemic AIDS-lymphoma *(8,40)*. It is unknown what impact HAART may have on these prognostic factors or on survival with AIDS-lymphoma overall.

TREATMENT OF PATIENTS WITH AIDS-LYMPHOMA

Systemic Chemotherapy for Newly Diagnosed Disease

AIDS-lymphoma is never considered truly localized, in terms of treatment decisions. The only exception is primary CNS lymphoma, which, by definition, is confined to the brain, and may be treated with local cranial radiation. In all other cases, despite what may appear to be localized disease, systemic chemotherapy is advocated, as opposed to local radiation or surgical excision alone.

At the outset of the AIDS epidemic in the early 1980s, the use of dose-intensive therapy was considered necessary for the achievement of complete remission and long-term survival in patients with *de novo* intermediate- or high-grade lymphoma, unrelated to HIV. Thus, regimens such as methotrexate, bleomycin, doxorubicin, cyclophosphamide, vincristine, dexamethasone (M-BACOD); prednisone, methotrexate, doxorubincin, cyclophosphamide, etoposide-cytosine arabinoside, bleomycin, vincristine, methotrexate (ProMACE-CytaBOM); methotrexate, doxorubicin, cyclophosphamide, vincristine, prendnisone, bleomycin (MACOP-B); and others were studied in single institutional trials, and found to be more effective when compared to older, less intensive regimens, such as doxorubicin, cyclophosphamide, vincristine, prednisone (CHOP) *(48,49)*. In the mid-1990s, a national high-priority trial was conducted in patients with *de novo* intermediate and high-grade lymphoma, in which patients were randomized between CHOP or one of the more intensive regimens. The results, pub-

Table 1
Low-Dose M-BACOD Regimen

Bleomycin	4 mg/m^2, d 1, iv
Doxorubicin	25 mg/m^2, d 1, iv
Cyclophosphamide	300 mg/m^2, d 1, iv
Vincristine sulfate	1.4 mg/m^2, d 1, iv (not to exceed 2 mg)
Dexamethasone	3 mg/m^2, d 1–5, po
Methotrexate (MTX)	500 mg/m^2, d 15, iv with folinic acid rescue, 25 mg po q6h × 4, beginning 6 h after completion of MTX
Cytosine arabinoside	50 mg, intrathecal, d 1, 8, 21, 28, cycle 1
Helmet-field radiotherapy	4000 cGy with known CNS involvement
Zidovudine	100 mg q4h for 1 yr, starting after chemotherapy
Total treatment	4–6 cycles, at 28-d intervals

See refs. *41* and *51* for further details.

lished in 1995, revealed that these newer regimens were not more effective than CHOP, and were associated with greater toxicity, even in these HIV-negative patients *(50)*. Nonetheless, at the outset of AIDS, these facts were not known. Various trials of high-dose intensive therapy were thus undertaken in HIV-infected patients, with poor results, especially in patients with poor prognostic indicators of disease *(8)*.

In an attempt to ascertain if lower doses of chemotherapy might be more effective in the setting of underlying HIV infection, Levine and colleagues *(41)* employed a low-dose modification of the M-BACOD regimen (Table 1). This low-dose regimen employed 50% dose levels of adriamycin and cyclophosphamide, along with early institution of CNS prophylaxis, and attenuation in the number of chemotherapy cycles actually administered. Patients were restaged after two cycles of therapy; if complete remission (CR) had been attained, two additional courses were given, with subsequent cessation of further chemotherapy, and institution of azidothymidine (the only anti-retroviral agent licensed in the United States for HIV disease at that time). In patients who had attained partial remission after two cycles (over 50% tumor reduction, with residual tumor remaining), an additional two cycles were given, followed by restaging again. If subsequent restaging demonstrated complete remission, these patients received two additional cycles, whereas those who failed to achieve CR were removed from protocol. The majority of patients thus received four to six cycles of dose-reduced therapy, in contrast to the 10 cycles that comprised the original M-BACOD protocol *(49)*. Complete remission was achieved in approx 50% of patients, and 70% of complete responders remained in continuous CR, without relapse. Although the median survival was only 6.5 mo in the group as a whole, a median survival of 15 mo was documented in patients who attained CR, most of whom eventually succumbed to AIDS-related complications.

However, the value of dose intensity remained somewhat controversial. Thus, in an attempt to clarify the value of such therapy, the AIDS Clinical Trials Group (ACTG) embarked upon a prospective, multicenter trial *(51)*. Patients were stratified by baseline prognostic indicators, and randomized to receive either the low-dose M-BACOD regimen discussed previously, or standard dose M-BACOD with hematopoietic growth fac-

Table 2
**Results of ACTG No. 142: Low-Dose vs Standard Dose M-BACOD in Newly
Diagnosed AIDS-Lymphoma (*N* = 192)**

	Low-dose	Standard dose	*p* Value
Complete remission	41%	52%	NS
Relapse rate	23%	40%	0.08
Median survival	35 wk	31 wk	NS
Grade 3, 4 toxicity	51%	70%	<0.008

See ref. *51* for further details.

tor support (GM-CSF). Patients randomized to low dose were allowed to receive GM-CSF if low granulocyte counts and/or febrile neutropenia had occurred in prior cycles. With 192 patients evaluable for response, no statistically significant difference was observed in response rates (Table 2). While patients with CD4 cells <100/µL did not respond as well as those with higher CD4 cells, the low-dose regimen appeared equivalent to standard dose M-BACOD in patients with either good risk or poor risk prognostic features. Although response rates were thus equivalent in the two dosing regimens, toxicity was significantly higher in those patients assigned to standard dose therapy, with ≥grade 3–4 toxicity in 70% of those assigned to standard dose, and 51% of those who received low dose therapy (*p.* <0.008). This large prospective trial would thus seem to indicate that low-dose chemotherapy is the current treatment of choice in patients with AIDS-related lymphoma *(51)*.

Additional studies have been conducted to explore the use of dose-intensive therapy, used specifically in patients with good risk AIDS lymphoma. The intensive LNH 84 regimen *(52)* consists of three cycles of adriamycin, cyclophosphamide, vindesine, bleomycin, and prednisone. This is followed by a consolidation phase of high-dose methotrexate plus leucovorin, ifosfamide, etoposide, asparaginase, and cytarabine. Intrathecal methotrexate is used in all patients as prophylaxis, and zidovudine maintenance therapy was employed after completion of chemotherapy. A complete remission rate of 63% was achieved. Median survival was 9 mo, while median disease-free survival for complete responders was 16 mo *(52)*. Although patients with good prognostic characteristics may be able to tolerate such a dose-intensive regimen, with a median survival of only 9 mo, it is still unclear whether such therapy is advantageous when compared to low-dose regimens.

A regimen of continuous infusion chemotherapy (CDE) was developed by Sparano and colleagues *(53)* with excellent results. This regimen consists of a 96-h continuous infusion of cyclophosphamide, doxorubicin, and etoposide (Table 3), which is repeated every 28 d until complete remission is achieved. When employed in 25 newly diagnosed patients, a complete remission rate of 58% was achieved, with a median duration of remission in excess of 18 mo, and a median overall survival of 18.4 mo. When subsequently used in conjunction with the anti-retroviral agent didanosine (ddI, Videx®), significantly less bone marrow toxicity was observed. Thus, when didanosine was added in alternate cycles of CDE, significantly less neutropenia, thrombocytopenia, and red cell transfusion requirement were found in the didanosine-containing cycles *(54)*. This regi-

Table 3
Infusional CDE Regimen

Drug	Dose/24 h	Total Dose per 96 h infusion
Cyclophosphamide	200 mg/m^2/d	800 mg/m^2/96 h
Doxorubicin	12.5 mg/m^2/d	50 mg/m^2/96 h
Etoposide	60 mg/m^2/d	240 mg/m^2/96 h

Daily dose of cyclophosphamide and doxorubicin are admixed in 1 L of fluid and infused through a central catheter. Etoposide is dissolved in a separate liter of intravenous fluid and given through a separate lumen of the central catheter or in a peripheral vein. *See* refs *53, 54, and 61* for further details.

men appears quite efficacious in patients with AIDS-lymphoma, including those with both poor and good prognostic characteristics at baseline.

Use of Hematopoietic Growth Factors with Chemotherapy

Neutropenia may occur as a consequence of HIV itself, or secondary to many of the anti-retroviral and other medications commonly used in HIV-infected patients. In both HIV-positive and HIV-negative individuals, absolute neutrophil counts < 500 or 1000/μL are associated with an increased risk of bacterial infection. In HIV-infected patients, serious bacterial infection is more likely to occur if the patient is also receiving cancer chemotherapy *(55)*. In this setting, both G-CSF (granulocyte colony stimulating factor) and GM-CSF (granulocyte-macrophage colony stimulating factor) have been shown to decrease the number of febrile episodes and hospitalizations, without significant toxicity, although no change in median survival has been reported *(56, 57)*.

Use of Anti-retroviral Agents with Combination Chemotherapy

Zidovudine (AZT, Retrovir®) has been used in conjunction with chemotherapy in patients with AIDS-lymphoma. However, zidovudine itself is associated with significant marrow suppression, and use of AZT, even with low-dose chemotherapy regimens, has been associated with severe bone marrow suppression. Thus, zidovudine should not routinely be used together with combination chemotherapy in patients with AIDS-lymphoma.

Both didanosine (ddI, Videx®) and dideoxycytadine (ddC, Hivid®) have been used at full dosage with various combination chemotherapy regimens for AIDS-lymphoma, resulting in no undue toxicity, and some evidence of increased efficacy. Thus, when ddI was combined with the infusional CDE regimen by Sparano and colleagues *(54)*, and when zalcitabine was added to the low-dose M-BACOD regimen by Levine and colleagues *(58)*, response rates were similar, while bone marrow toxicity was less than that observed with the chemotherapy regimen used alone. Furthermore, although zalcitabine has been associated with peripheral neuropathy, no increase in this toxicity was noted when used in combination with M-BACOD chemotherapy.

Recently, use of highly active anti-retroviral therapy (HAART) has been associated with a significant decrease in opportunistic infections, and improved survival in patients with HIV. The anti-retrovirals that comprise HAART regimens vary, and are usually comprised of three or four drugs, including a protease inhibitor. These drugs are complex, with multiple drug interactions, owing to their metabolism by the cytochrome P450 system. To evaluate the pharmacologic interactions with chemotherapy and HAART, Ratner and colleagues *(59)* have performed pharmacokinetic studies on 40 patients receiving low-dose CHOP, and 25 patients receiving full-dose CHOP along with stavudine (d4T, Zerit®), lamivudine (Epivir®, 3TC), and indinavir (Crixivan®). Of importance, either low-dose or full-dose CHOP delivered with HAART was found to be tolerable, and associated with minimal adverse drug interactions *(59)*.

Vaccher and colleagues also studied the use of CHOP chemotherapy, given in conjunction with various HAART regimens to 15 patients with AIDS-lymphoma *(60)*. Undue toxicity was not reported, although grade 4 anemia and grade 3–4 neurotoxicity was significantly higher in the patients receiving HAART, when compared to historical controls receiving CHOP alone *(60)*.

In an attempt to ascertain potential efficacy and/or toxicity of HAART with infusional chemotherapy, Sparano and colleagues *(61)* performed a feasibility trial, combining the infusional CDE regimen with G-CSF. All patients also received saquinavair (600 mg po TID), plus stavudine and didanosine. Patients were compared to a group of historical controls, who had been treated with the same CDE regimen with didanosine. A significant increase in grade 3 or 4 mucositis was seen in the CDE plus HAART patients, occurring in 67% (8/12) patients, vs 3/25 (12%) controls. The authors conclude that protease inhibitors may be associated with altered metabolism of chemotherapeutic drugs, leading to unexpected toxicity. However, this complication was not seen in the formal, prospective pharmacokinetic analyses performed by Ratner and colleagues in patients receiving CHOP plus HAART, which included indinivir (Crixivan®) as the protease inhibitor. It is possible that this discrepancy may be secondary to pharmacologic interactions occurring specifically with long-term (96 h) infusional chemotherapy, or it may reflect the different regimens and protease inhibitors that were studied. Further information is awaited.

Chemotherapy for Relapsed or Refractory AIDS-Lymphoma

While several agents and combinations of drugs have been tested in patients with relapsed or refractory AIDS-lymphoma, no real evidence of efficacy has emerged *(62,63)*. Additional trials are currently ongoing; results are awaited with interest.

PRIMARY CNS LYMPHOMA

The occurrence of lymphoma primary to the brain was one of the earliest reported manifestations of AIDS, and it remains a very difficult area in terms of therapy and survival. HIV-infected patients with primary CNS lymphoma present with severe immuodeficiency, and CD4 cell counts usually < 50/µl *(8,40)*. The majority have been diagnosed with another AIDS condition prior to the development of primary CNS lymphoma *(8)*. Pathologically, almost all such lymphomas are of diffuse large cell or immunoblastic subtypes, and are uniformly associated with EBV infection within malignant cells *(8,10,64)*. As such, presence of EBV DNA within spinal fluid may be used as a diagnostic criterion for primary CNS lymphoma *(65)*.

Altered mental status is the major symptom in approx 53% of patients, with profound abnormalities in the majority, although very subtle changes may also occur. Headache or other symptoms of increased intracranial pressure occur in approx 15% of patients, while focal neurologic defects occur in 51%, and seizures are reported in approx 27% *(40)*.

CAT scans or magnetic resonance imaging (MRI) scans of the brain reveal relatively large lesions (2–5 cm or more), which are relatively few in number (less than five). Gadolinium enhancement is expected, and ring enhancement (similar to that seen in toxoplasmosis) may be seen in as many as 50% of such cases *(8,66)*. However, no single finding on MRI or CAT scan proves that a patient has lymphoma vs other pathologic processes that frequently occur in the setting of HIV, such as toxoplasmosis, fungal infection, or others *(66)*. Use of positron-emission tomography (PET) scanning may be useful in differentiating cerebral lymphoma from toxoplasmosis *(67)*. Additionally, thallium-201 SPECT scanning may be useful, with median T1 uptake index of > 1.5, and a lesion size of >2.5 cm serving as independent predictors of primary CNS lymphoma *(68)*.

Optimal therapy for primary CNS lymphoma remains to be defined. Use of cranial radiation is associated with a complete remission rate of only 50% and median survival of only 2 or 3 mo. No specific regimen of chemotherapy has yet proven efficacious, perhaps owing to the serious level of immunocompromise in affected patients *(40)*.

Of interest, the incidence of primary CNS lymphoma appears to have decreased, coincident with the use of highly active anti-retroviral therapy *(6)*.

PRIMARY EFFUSION LYMPHOMA

Primary effusion lymphoma (PEL), originally termed body cavity based lymphoma, is uncommon, representing only a small fraction of all AIDS-lymphomas *(12)*. PEL is associated with a newly discovered human herpesvirus, termed Kaposi's sarcoma associated herpesvirus, or HHV-8 (*see also* Chapter 10) *(69,70)*. The disease has been reported in both HIV positive and HIV negative patients, although it appears more common in the former. Of interest, PEL has also been described in a cardiac transplant recipient, whose explanted heart was found, retrospectively, to be infected by HHV-8 *(71)*. Morphologically, the malignant cell is large, and appears anaplastic with immunoblastic features. The PEL cell usually lacks B-cell markers, but is B lymphoid in origin, based upon presence of immunoglobulin gene rearrangement on Southern blot analysis. HHV-8 is present, while the malignant cell often harbors EBV as well. Clinically, patients present with effusions, such as ascites, or effusions localized in the pleura or pericardium. Most patients do not have mass lesions at diagnosis, although this has been reported. Despite therapeutic intervention, survival is extremely short, in the range of approx 2 mo *(72)*.

REFERENCES

1. Beral V, Peterman T, Berkelman R, Jaffe H. AIDS associated non-Hodgkin lymphoma. Lancet 1991; 337:805–809.
2. Peters BS, Beck EJ, Coleman DG, Wadsworth MJH, McGuinness O, Harris JRW, et al. Changing disease patterns in patients with AIDS in a referral centre in the United Kingdom: the changing face of AIDS. Br Med J 1991; 302:203–207.
3. Cote TR, Biggar RJ, Rosenberg PS, Devesa SS, Percy C, Yellin FJ, et al. Non-Hodgkin's lymphoma among people with AIDS: incidence, presentation and public health burden. Int J. Cancer 1997; 73:645–650.

4. Jacobson LP. Impact of highly effective anti-retroviral therapy on the incidence of malignancies among HIV infected individuals. J AIDS Hum Retrovirol 1998; 17:A39, Abstr S5.

5. Buchbinder SP, Bittinghoff E, Colfax G, Holmberg S. Declines in AIDS incidence associated with highly active anti-retroviral therapy (HAART) are not reflected in KS and lymphoma incidence. J AIDS Hum Retrovirol 1998; 17:A39, Abstr S7.

6. Jones JL, Hanson DL, Ward JW. Effect of antiretroviral therapy on recent trends in cancers among HIV infected persons. J AIDS Hum Retrovirol 1998; 17:A38, Abstr S3.

7. Rabkin C, Testa MA, Fischl MA, Von Roenn J. Declining incidence of Kaposi's sarcoma in AIDS Clinical Trial Group trials. J AIDS Hum Retrovirol 1998; 17:A39, Abstr S4.

8. Levine AM. AIDS related lymphoma (review). Blood 1992; 80:8–20.

9. Seneviratne LC, Espina BM, Tulpule A, Dharmapala D, Sanchez M, Gill PS, et al. Evolving characteristics of AIDS-related lymphoma over time: a single institution study of 369 patients, in press.

10. Raphael M, Gentilhomme O, Tulliez M, Byron P-A, Diebold J. Histopathologic features of high-grade non-Hodgkin's lymphoma in acquired immunodeficiency syndrome. Arch Pathol Lab Med 1991; 115:15–20.

11. Harris NL, Jaffe ES, Stein H, Banks PM, Chan JKC, Cleary ML, et al. A revised European-American classification of lymphoid neoplasms: a proposal from the International Lymphoma Study Group. Blood 1994; 84:1361–1392.

12. Nador RG, Cesarman E, Chadburn A, Dawson DB, Ansari MQ, Said JW, et al. Primary effusion lymphoma: a distinct clinicopathologic entity associated with the Kaposi's sarcoma-associated herpes virus. Blood 1996; 88:645–656.

13. Schnittman SM, Lane HC, Higgins SE, Folks T, Fauci AS. Direct polyclonal activation of human B lymphocytes by the AIDS virus. Science 1986: 233:1084–1086.

14. Nakajima K, Martinez-Maza O, Hirano T, Breen EC, Nishanian PG, Salazar-Gonzalez JF et al. Induction of IL-6 production by human immunodefieicncy virus. J Immunol 1989; 142:531–536.

15. Tohyama N, Karasuyama H, Tada T. Growth autonomy and tumorigenicity of interleukin 6-dependent B cells transfected with interleukin 6 cDNA. J Exp Med 1990; 171:389–400.

16. Emilie D, Coumbaras J, Raphael M, Devergne O, Delecluse HG, Gisselbrecht C, et al. Interleukin-6 production in high grade B lymphoma: correlation with the presence of malignant immunoblasts in acquired immunodeficiency syndrome and in human immunodeficiency virus seronegative patients. Blood 1992; 80:498–504.

17. Masood R, Lunardi-Iskandar Y, Moudgil T, Zhang Y, Law RE, Huang C, et al. IL-10 inhibits HIV-1 replication and is induced by Tat. Biochem Biophys Res Commun 1994; 202:374–383.

18. Masood R, Zhang Y, Bond MW, et al. Interleukin 10 is an autocrine growth factor for AIDS related B cell lymphoma. Blood 1995; 85:3423–3430.

19. Jain R, Roncella S, Hashimoto S, Carbone A, Francia de Celle P, Foa R, et al. A potential role for antigen selection in the clonal evolution of Burkitt's lymphoma. J Imunol 1994; 153:45–52.

20. Gaidano G, Carbone A, Dalla-Favera R. Pathogenesis of AIDS-related lymphomas: molecular and histogenetic heterogeneity. Am J Pathol 1998; 152:623–630.

21. Bessudo A, Cherepakhin V, Johnson TA, Rassenti LZ, Feigal E, Kipps TJ. Favored use of immunoglobulin V_H4 genes in AIDS-associated B cell lymphomas. Blood 1996; 88:252–260.

22. Pascual V, Capra JD. V_H4-21, a human VH gene segment over represented in the autoimmune repertoire. Arthritis Rheum 1992; 35:11–18.

23. Chaganti RS, Jhanwar SC, Koziner B, Arlin Z, Mertelsmann R, Clarkson B. Specific translocations characterize Burkitt-like lymphoma of homosexual men with the acquired immunodeficiency syndrome. Blood 1983; 61:1265–1268.

24. Subar M, Neri A, Inghirami G, Knowles DM, Dalla-Favera R. Frequent c-*myc* oncogene activation and infrequent presence of Epstein–Barr virus genome in AIDS-associated lymphoma. Blood 1988; 72:667–671.

25. Shibata D, Weiss LM, Nathwani BN, Byrnes RK, Levine AM. Epstein Barr virus in benign lymph node biopsies from individuals infected with the human immunodeficiency virus is associated with concurrent or subsequent development of non-Hodgkin's lymphoma. Blood 1991; 77:1527–1533.

26. Ballerini P, Gaidano G, Gong JZ, Tassi V, Saglio G, Knowles DM, et al. Multiple genetic lesions in acquired immunodeficiency syndrome-related non-Hodgkin's lymphoma. Blood 1993; 81:166–176.

27. Hamilton-Dutoit SJ, Pallesen G, Granzmann MB, Karkov J, Black F, Pederson C. AIDS related lymphoma: histopathology, immunophenotype, and association with Epstein–Barr virus as demonstrated by *in situ* nucleic acid hybridization. Am J Pathol 1991; 138:149–163.

28. Hamilton-Dutoit SJ, Rea D, Raphael M, Sandvej K, Delecluse HJ, Gisselbrecht C, et al. Epstein–Barr virus latent gene expression and tumor cell phenotype in acquired immunodeficiency syndrome-related non-Hodgkin's lymphoma,. Am J Pathol 1993; 143:1072–1085.

29. Liebowitz D. Epstein-Barr virus and a cellular signaling pathway in lymphomas from immuno-suppressed patients. N Engl J Med 1998; 338:1413–1421.

30. Kersten MJ, Klein MR, Holwerda AM, Miedema F, van Oers MHJ. Epstein–Barr virus specific cytotoxic T cell responses in HIV-1 infection. J Clin Invest 1997; 99:1525–1533.

31. Gaidano G, Carbone A, Pastore C, Capello D, Migliazza A, Bloghini A, et al. Frequent mutation of the 5′ noncoding region of the *bcl-6* gene in acquired immunodeficiency syndrome-related non-Hodgkin's lymphomas. Blood 1997; 89:3755–3762.

32. Dent AL, Shaffer AL, Yu X, Allman D, Staudt LM. Control of inflammation, cytokine expression and germinal center formation by *bcl-6*. Science 1997; 276:589–592.

33. Ye BH, Lista F, Lo Coco F, Knowles DM, Offit K, Chaganti RSK, et al. Alterations of a novel zinc finger encoding gene, *bcl-6,* in diffuse large cell lymphoma. Science 1993; 262:747–750.

34. Gaidano G, Lo Coco F, Ye BH, Shibata D, Levine AM, Knowles DM, et al. Rearrangements of the *bcl-6* gene in AIDS associated non-Hodgkin's lymphoma: association with diffuse large-cell subtype. Blood 1994; 84:397–402.

35. Russo JJ, Bohenzky RA, Chien M-C, Chen J, Yan M, Maddalena D, et al. Nucleotide sequence of the Kaposi's sarcoma associated herpesvirus (HHV 8). Proc Natl Acad Sci USA 1996; 93:14862–14867.

36. Zuckerman E, Zuckerman T, Levine AM, et al. Hepatitis C virus infection in patients with B cell non-Hodgkin's lymphoma. Ann Intern Med 1997; 127:423–428.

37. Levine AM, Nelson R, Zuckerman E, et al. Lack of association between hepatitis C infection and development of AIDS related lymphoma. J Acquir Immune Defic Syndr Hum Retrovirol 1999; 20:255–258.

38. Ziegler JL, Beckstead JA, Volberding PA, Abrams DI, Levine AM, Lukes RJ, et al. Non-Hodgkin's lymphoma in 90 homosexual men: relation to generalized lymphadenopathy and the acquired immunodeficiency syndrome. N Engl J Med 1984; 311:565–570.

39. Kaplan LD, Abrams DI, Feigal E, McGrath M, Kahn J, Neville P, et al. AIDS associated non-Hodgkin's lymphoma in San Francisco. JAMA 1989; 261:719–724.

40. Baumgartner JE, Rachlin JR, Bechstead JH, et al. Primary central nervous system lymphoma: natural history and response to radiation therapy in 55 patients with AIDS. J Neurosurg 1990: 73:206–211.

41. Levine AM, Wernz JC, Kaplan L, et al. Low-dose chemotherapy with central nervous system prophylaxis and azidothymidine maintenance in AIDS-related lymphoma: a prospective multi-institutional trial. JAMA 1991; 266:84–88.

42. Seneviratne LC, Tulpule A, Mumanneni M, Espina BM, Wang G, Palmer M, et al. Clinical, immunological, and pathologic correlates of bone marrow involvement in 253 patients with AIDS-related lymphoma. Blood 1998; 92:244a.

43. Levine AM, Sullivan-Halley J, Pike MC, et al. Human immunodeficiency virus-related lymphoma: prognostic factors predictive of survival. Cancer 1991; 68:2466–2472.

44. Straus DJ, Huang J, Testa MA, Levine AM, Kaplan LD. Prognostic factors in the treatment of human immunodeficiency virus-associated non-Hodgkin's lymphoma: analysis of AIDS Clinical Trials Group protocol 142—low dose versus standard dose m-BACOD plus granulocyte-macrophage stimulating factor. J Clin Oncol 1998; 16:3601–3606.

45. Vaccher E, Tierlli U, Spina M, et al. Age and serum LDH level are independent prognostic factors in HIV related non-Hodgkin's lymphoma: a single institution study of 96 patients. J Clin Oncol 1996; 14:2217–2223.

46. Radin DR, Esplin JA, Levine AM, Ralls PW. AIDS-related non-Hodgkin's lymphoma: abdominal CT findings in 112 patients. Am J Radiol 1993; 160:1133–1139.

47. Podzamczer D, Ricat I, Bolao F, Romagosa V, Bonnin D, Guionnet N, et al. Gallium-67 scan for distinguishing follicular hyperplasia from other AIDS associated diseases in lymph nodes. AIDS 1990; 4:683–685.

48. McKelvy EM, Gottlieb JA, Wilson HE, et al. Hydroxydaunomycin (Adriamycin) combination chemotherapy in malignant lymphoma. Cancer 1982; 38:1484–1493.

49. Skarin AT, Canellos GP, Rosenthal DS, et al. Improved prognosis of diffuse histiocytic and undifferentiated lymphoma by use of high dose methotrexate alternating with standard agents (M-BACOD). J Clin Oncol 1983; 1:91–98.

50. Fisher RI, Gaynor ER, Dahlberg S, et al. Comparison of a standard regimen (CHOP) with three intensive chemotherapy regimens for advanced non-Hodgkin's lymphoma. N Engl J Med 1993; 238:1002–1006.

51. Kaplan LD, Straus DH, Testa MA, et al. Low dose compared with standard dose m-BACOD chemotherapy for non-Hodgkin's lymphoma associated with human immunodeficiency virus infection. N Engl J Med 1997: 336:1641–1648.

52. Gisselbrecht C, Oksenhendler E, Tirelli U, Lepage E, Gabarre J, Farcet JP, et al. HIV related lymphoma treatment with intensive combination chemotherapy. Am J Med 1993; 95:188–196.

53. Sparano JA, Wiernik PH, Strack M, Leaf A, Becker N, Valentine ES. Infusional cyclophosphamide, doxorubicin, and etoposide in HIV and HTLV-I related non-Hodgkin's lymphoma: a highly active regimen. Blood 1993; 81:2810–2815.

54. Sparano JA, Wiernik PH, Hu X, Sarta C, Schwartz EL, Soeiro R, et al. Pilot trial of infusional cyclophosphamide, doxorubicin and etoposide plus didanosine and filgrastim in patients with HIV associated non-Hodgkin's lymphoma. J Clin Oncol 1996; 14:3026–3035.

55. Meynard J-L, Guiguet M, Arsac S, et al. Frequency and risk factors of infectious complications in neutropenic patients infected with HIV. AIDS 1997; 11:995–998.

56. Kaplan L, Kahn J, Crowe S, Northfelt D, Neville P, Grossberg H, et al. Clinical and virologic effect of GM-CSF in patients receiving chemotherapy for HIV associated non-Hodgkin's lymphoma: results of a randomized trial. J Clin Oncol 1991; 9:929–940.

57. Keiser P, Rademacher S, Smith JW, Skiest D, Vadde V. Granulocyte colony stimulating factor use is associated with decreased bacteremia and increased survival in neutropenic HIV infected patients. Am J Med 1998; 104:48–55.

58. Levine AM, Tulpule A, Espina B, Boswell W, Buckley J, Rasheed S, et al. Low dose methotrexate, bleomycin, doxorubicin, cyclophosphamide, vincristine and dexamethasone with zalcitabine in patients with acquired immunodefieicncy syndrome related lymphoma: effect on HIV and serum IL6 levels over time. Cancer 1996; 78:517–526.

59. Ratner L, Redden D, Hamzeh F, Scadden D, Kaplan L, Ambinder R, et al. Chemotherapy for HIV-associated non-Hodgkin's lymphoma in combination with highly active antiretroviral therapy (HAART) is not associated with excessive toxicity. Fourth AIDS Malignancy Conference, Bethesda, MD, May, 1999.

60. Vaccher E, Spina M, Santarossa S, et al. Concomitant CHOP chemotherapy and highly active antiretroviral therapy in patients with HIV related non-Hodgkin's lymphoma. 12th World AIDS Conference, Geneva, Switzerland, 1998, Abstr 22289.
61. Sparano JKA, Wiernik PH, Hu X, Sarta C, Henry DH, Ratech H. Pilot trial of saquinavir and nucleoside analogues plus infusional cyclophosphamide, doxorubicin, and etoposide in patients with HIV associated non-Hodgkin's lymphoma. Second National AIDS Malignancy Conference, Bethesda, MD, 1998, Abstr 78.
62. Levine AM, Tulpule A, Tessman D, Kaplan L, Giles F, Luskey BD, et al. Mitoguazone therapy in patients with refractory or relapsed AIDS related lymphoma: results from a multicenter phase II trial. J Clin Oncol 1997; 15:1094–1103.
63. Tirelli U, Errante D, Spina M, et al. Second line chemotherapy in HIV related non-Hodgkin's lymphoma. Cancer 1996; 77:2127–2131.
64. MacMahon EME, Glass JD, Hayward SDC, Mann RB, Becker PS, Charache P, et al. Epstein Barr virus in AIDS related primary central nervous system lymphoma. Lancet 1991; 338:969–973.
65. Cinque P, Brytting M, Vago L, et al. Epstein Barr virus DNA in cerebrospinal fluid from patients with AIDS related primary lymphoma of the central nervous system. Lancet 1993; 342:398–401.
66. Ciricillo SF, Rosenblum MLP. Use of CT and MR imaging to distinguish intracranial lesions and to define the need for biopsy in AIDS patients. J Neurosurg 1990; 4:683–685.
67. Hoffman JM, Waskin HA, Schifter T, Hanson MW, Gray L, Rosenfeld S, et al. PDG-PET in differentiating lymphoma from nonmalignant central nervous system lesions in patients with AIDS. J Nucl Med 1993; 34:567–575.
68. Alcaide FG, Lomena F, Cruceta A, et al. Predictive value of thallium-201 SPECT in the diagnosis of primary central nervous system lymphoma in AIDS patients. 12th World AIDS Conference, Geneva, Switzerland, 1998, Abstr 22291.
69. Chang Y, Cesarman E, Pessin MS, Lee F, Culpepper J, Knowles DM, et al. Identification of herpesvirus-like DNA sequences in AIDS-associated Kaposi's sarcoma. Science 1994; 266:1865–1869.
70. Cesarman E, Chang Y, Moore PS, Said JW, Knowles DM. Kaposi's sarcoma associated herpesvirus like DNA sequences in AIDS-related body cavity based lymphomas. N Engl J Med 1995; 332:1186–1191.
71. Jones D, Ballestas ME, Kaye KM, Gulizia JM, Winters GL, Fletcher J, et al. Primary effusion lymphoma and Kaposi's sarcoma in a cardiac transplant recipient. N Engl J Med 1998: 339:444–449.
72. Komanduri KV, Luce JA, McGrath MS, Herndier BG, Ng VL. The natural history and molecular heterogeneity of HIV-associated primary malignant lymphomatous effusions. J Acquir Immune Defic Syndr Hum Retrovirol 1996; 13:215–226.

9
Leiomyoma and Leiomyosarcoma

Hal B. Jenson

INTRODUCTION

A relatively recent scientific finding over the past decade has been the chronicle of epidemiologic and virologic investigations that have documented the increased frequency of smooth muscle cell tumors in immunocompromised persons, and the unexpected association of these tumors with Epstein–Barr virus (EBV) infection of smooth muscle cells. In 1965, Nobel laureate Sir MacFarlane Burnet emphasized the critical role of immunosurveillance in limiting malignant transformation and development of cancer *(1)*. The acquired immunodeficiency syndrome (AIDS) epidemic, and also the development of powerful immunosuppressive drugs that have made organ transplantation possible, have validated the important role of tumor immunosurveillance. Immunocompromised individuals, whether the underlying cause is congenital, iatrogenic, or secondary to infection, have an approx 10–100-fold higher incidence of malignancies than immunocompetent individuals, with the frequent occurrence of unusual tumor types *(2)*.

Non-Hodgkin's lymphoma, Kaposi's sarcoma, and cervical cancer in women are considered AIDS-defining conditions *(3)*. Several other types of non-AIDS-defining cancers are also seen in human immunodeficiency virus type 1 (HIV-1)-infected patients, including Hodgkin's disease, squamous cell carcinoma, testicular neoplasms (particularly seminoma), and, as recently demonstrated, leiomyosarcoma. Many of the cancers associated with immunosuppression are also associated with specific viruses, including: some non-Hodgkin's lymphomas, which are associated with EBV; Kaposi's sarcoma, which is causally linked to Kaposi's sarcoma-associated herpesvirus (KSHV), also known has human herpesvirus type 8 (HHV-8); hepatocellular carcinoma, which is linked to hepatitis B and C viruses; cervical cancer, which is linked to human papillomaviruses types 16 and 18; and squamous cell carcinoma of the skin, which is linked to human papillomaviruses types 5 and 8 *(4,5)*. The association of EBV with leiomyosarcomas is a new addition to the list of tumors associated with immunosuppression that are also linked to a specific viral etiology.

HISTOPATHOLOGY

Tumors of smooth muscle may develop as hamartomas, leiomyomas, or leiomyosarcomas *(6)*. Hamartomas are disorganized overgrowth of mature cells with no malignant

From: *Infectious Causes of Cancer: Targets for Intervention*
Edited by: J. J. Goedert © Humana Press Inc., Totowa, NJ

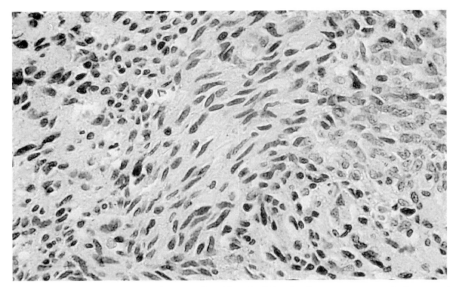

Fig. 1. Leiomyosarcomas are characterized by the histologic appearance of elongated, spindle-shaped cells with elongated, centrally placed nuclei and an eosinophilic cytoplasm. The cells tend to align in bundles or fascicles that intersect at right angles, which is demonstrated in this photomicrograph by the alignment of fusiform cells centrally surrounded by fascicles of cells sectioned at a perpendicular axis. (Photomicrograph courtesy of Vijay V. Joshi, MD, PhD)

potential. Leiomyomas are benign neoplasms of normal appearing cells that include primarily smooth muscle cells and occasionally some myofibroblasts, fibroblasts, and incompletely differentiated mesenchymal cells. Leiomyomas have little predilection for malignant transformation. Leiomyosarcomas are generally well-differentiated malignant neoplasms that are usually fairly well circumscribed. Myofibromas may also represent a portion of the spectrum of smooth muscle tumors, rather than being considered primarily fibroblastic tumors.

Smooth muscle cells have an elongated, fusiform, or spindle-shaped appearance with centrally placed nuclei and a fibrillary eosinophilic cytoplasm. Smooth muscle tumors are sometimes identified as spindle-cell tumors based on this morphology. Cells tend to align in bundles or fascicles that intersect at right angles or align in palisades (Fig. 1). Smooth muscle cells of leiomyomas and leiomyosarcomas usually express the smooth muscle cell form of calponin, which is restricted to smooth muscle cells in the adult but is also expressed in embryos in the early cardiac tube *(7);* smooth muscle α-actin, although its expression is also detected in skeletal and cardiac muscles to a lesser degree *(8);* and desmin. They do not express skeletal muscle myosin heavy chain, a skeletal muscle marker.

The histopathologic identification smooth muscle elements within a tumor is usually straightforward based on the typical morphology and identification of smooth muscle elements by immunohistochemical staining. However, the distinction between leiomyoma and leiomyosarcoma, and occasionally among other spindle-cell tumors, can be obscure *(6,9).* Poorly differentiated smooth muscle tumors may be difficult to distinguish from fibrosarcoma, neurogenic sarcoma, malignant fibrous histiocytoma, or undifferentiated sarcoma. Definitive histopathologic criteria defining benign (leiomyoma) and malignant (leiomyosarcoma) smooth muscle tumors are not well established. Increased tumor size, poorly differentiated cellularity, cytologic atypia, infiltration, necrosis, hemorrhage, and multifocal lesions roughly correlate with the malignant tendency for smooth muscle tumors. A frequently used objective criterion for malignancy is the level of mitotic activity. Even this, however, is not standardized, and several criteria have been recommended for various organs. Recommended criteria have included a mitotic index of ≥5 mitoses per 10 high-power microscope fields for uterine tumors *(10)*, ≥2 mitoses per 50 high-power fields for gastrointestinal tract tumors *(11,12)*, and ≥5 mitoses per 50 high-power fields for pulmonary tumors *(13)*. However, malignant behavior of smooth muscle tumors does not correlate well even with the degree of mitotic activity *(11,14,15)*. Some smooth muscle tumors with a histologic appearance of benign leiomyoma, even devoid of mitoses, behave clinically as malignant leiomyosarcoma *(11,15,16)*. Metastatic spread may be the only certain indicator of malignancy. The uncertainty of histologic definition of benign and malignant tumors has resulted in many reported cases of "smooth muscle tumors" without further subclassification. Capricious and unpredictable biological and clinical behavior characterize leiomyosarcomas.

EPIDEMIOLOGY

Leiomyosarcomas are uncommon tumors, with an overall incidence of one or two cases per million population *(17)*. Leiomyosarcomas are most frequently found in the uterus of adult women, but not of children, and less frequently in the gastrointestinal and hepatobiliary tracts. However, cases of smooth muscle tumors have been reported originating from every organ and appendage, reflecting the ubiquitous distribution of smooth muscle in blood vessels. Classifications based on anatomic location (i.e., superficial soft tissue, deep soft tissue, and visceral) appear to be rather arbitrary as all leiomyosarcomas are malignant.

Leiomyosarcomas are among the more common sarcomas of adults, and account for approx 2–9% of all soft tissue sarcomas in adults *(9,18–21)*, with a peak incidence in the fifth and sixth decades of life *(22–24)*. There is no sex difference, except for the obvious restriction of uterine leiomyosarcoma to women, or race difference *(9,11,17)*. Leiomyosarcomas have historically been rarely reported in children, accounting for only 2% of soft tissue sarcomas, which as a group are fifth in order of the most common types of tumors in children *(25,26)*. The three largest series of smooth muscle tumors in children reported only 10 original cases each *(26–28)*.

Perhaps because of their relative rarity, and perhaps because of the diversity of anatomic locations and clinical presentations, there are hundreds of individual cases of leiomyosarcomas described in the medical literature. However, their rarity and clinical diversity have impeded the advancement of understanding of their basic biology and pathogenesis.

Epidemiology in Immunocompromised Persons

Prior to 1985, leiomyosarcomas had been reported rarely in immunocompromised persons, including renal transplant recipients *(29,30)*, patients who received therapeutic gastric irradiation for peptic ulcer disease *(31)*, and in association with Alport's syndrome *(32)*. From 1985 to 1990, five cases of leiomyosarcoma associated with HIV-1 infection, all of which occurred in children, were reported *(33–35)*, including three cases by Chadwick et al. *(35)*, who suggested that this association indicated a direct or indirect role for HIV-1 infection in the development of leiomyosarcoma. Eleven additional cases of leiomyomas and leiomyosarcomas in HIV-1-infected persons were subsequently reported by others from 1991 through 1994 *(36–44)*, including nine children *(36,37,39–41,43,44)*, one adolescent *(38)*, and one adult *(42)*. (One case in the series by Chadwick et al. *[35]* was also in a separate report *[45,46]*; the imaging studies of the case reported by Sabatino et al. *[36]* were reported by Balsam and Segal *[47]*.)

During this period, leiomyoma and leiomyosarcoma were also being reported with increasing frequency in association with kidney or liver organ transplant *(2,48,49)*. Similar to leiomyosarcomas associated with HIV-1 infection, there was a surprisingly high proportion of cases in children, despite the fewer number of organ transplants in children. In a review of 8724 malignancies in 8191 organ allograft recipients, 5 of 15 (33%) leiomyosarcomas that were found had occurred in children *(2)*.

Association of EBV with Leiomyoma and Leiomyosarcoma

The identification of EBV infection of smooth muscle cells of leiomyosarcoma was first reported in a single case of an adult with HIV-1 infection, by Prévot et al. in 1994, and in two subsequent series published together in early 1995 of six HIV-1-infected persons *(50)*, and three organ transplant recipients *(51)*. These reports were substantiated by additional cases of EBV-associated leiomyomas and leiomyosarcomas (Table 1) in eight adults and three children with HIV-1 infection *(16,52–59)* and in six patients following organ transplants *(60–65)*, including three children *(60,64)*, one adolescent *(65)*, and two adults *(61–63)*. One peculiar aspect is the development of large cysts associated with hepatic leiomyosarcomas in the two adult patients following kidney transplant *(61–63)*.

All of the smooth muscle cells of the EBV-associated leiomyosarcomas harbor EBV. Using *in situ* hybridization for EBER (*EBV-encoded RNAs*), which is the most common method for detection of EBV in tissue, all reports document the presence of EBV EBER in all or > 90% of the smooth muscle cells of the tumor, but not in adjacent normal tissues. A series of seven smooth muscle cell tumors from four patients with AIDS near or at the time tumor diagnosis that were tested by semiquantitative polymerase chain reaction (PCR) amplification showed EBV levels from 170,442 to 659,668 EBV copies per 100,000 cells, with an average of 451,140 copies per 100,000 cells. If all cells are uniformly infected with EBV, as indicated by the uniform staining for EBER by *in situ* hybridization, there is an average of 4.5 EBV genome copies per cell *(56)*, consistent with the amounts of EBV in lymphoblastoid cell lines, which characteristically have 10 or fewer episomes per cell *(66)*. These results are also consistent with the semiquantitation of EBV reported in smooth muscle cell tumors from patients with organ transplant *(51)*. There are not lymphocytic infiltrates surrounding the tumors that might account for the high levels of EBV detected by PCR *(56,67)*. The extraordinarily high copy numbers of EBV in the tumor cells as determined by semiquantitative PCR are consistent with and supportive of the *in situ* hybridization results for the presence of EBV in all tumor cells. High levels of cell-free EBV present in plasma of three

Table 1
Summary of Cases of Documented EBV-Associated Smooth Muscle Tumors[a]

Report	Age	Sex	Tumor site(s)	Histology	Risk factors
Cases associated with HIV-1 infection					
Prévot et al., 1994 (90)	33 yr	Male	Liver	Leiomyosarcoma	HIV-1 infection (homosexual transmission, diagnosed at 31 yr of age)
McClain et al., 1995 (50) and Jenson et al., 1997 (56)	8 yr	Female	Lung Colon	Leiomyosarcoma Leiomyoma	HIV-1 infection (transfusion-associated, in the perinatal period, diagnosed at 4 yr of age)
	4 yr	Female	Stomach	Leiomyosarcoma	HIV-1 infection (perinatal transmission, diagnosed at 2 yr of age)
	7 yr	Female	Intestine	Leiomyosarcoma	HIV-1 infection (perinatal transmission, diagnosed at 2 yr of age)
	24 yr	Male	Liver	Leiomyosarcoma	HIV-1 infection (perinatal transmission, diagnosed at 18 yr of age)
	5 yr	Female	Colon tumor no. 1	Leiomyosarcoma	HIV-1 infection (perinatal transmission, diagnosed at 1 yr of age)
			Colon tumor no. 2 Colon tumor no. 3	Leiomyosarcoma Leiomyosarcoma	
	4 yr	Male	Lung	Leiomyoma	HIV-1 infection (transfusion-associated, in the perinatal period, diagnosed at 4 yr of age)
	29 yr	Female	Thoracic spine (with multifocal recurrences)	Leiomyosarcoma	HIV-1 infection (heterosexual transmission, diagnosed at 27 yr of age)
	7 yr	Female	Ethmoid sinus Colon	Leiomyosarcoma Leiomyosarcoma	HIV-1 infection (perinatal transmission, diagnosed at 1 yr of age)
Jimenez-Heffernan et al., 1995 (52)	2 yr	Male	Adrenal gland	Leiomyoma	HIV-1 infection (perinatal transmission, diagnosed at 1 yr of age)
Zetler et al., 1995 (53)	30 yr	Male	Adrenal gland	Leiomyosarcoma	HIV-1 infection (homosexual transmission, diagnosed at 22 yr of age)

Table 1
Continued

Report	Age	Sex	Tumor site(s)	Histology	Risk factors
Bluhm et al., 1997 (54)	35 yr	Male	Lung (multiple nodules)	"Smooth muscle tumor"	HIV-1 infection (illicit intravenous drug use, age at HIV-1 diagnosis not reported)
Boman et al., 1997 (55)	48 yr	Male	Lymph node, adrenal gland, pericardium	Leiomyosarcoma	HIV-1 infection (homosexual transmission, diagnosed at 43 yr of age)
	29 yr	Male	Adrenal gland	Leiomyosarcoma	HIV-1 infection (manner of transmission not reported, diagnosed at 20 yr of age)
Morgello et al., 1997 (57)	35 yr	Male	Cervical dura	Leiomyosarcoma	HIV-1 infection (bisexual transmission, age at HIV-1 diagnosis not reported)
Creager et al., 1998 (58)	33 yr	Male	Kidney	"Smooth muscle neoplasm"	HIV-1 infection (manner of transmission not reported, diagnosed at 25 yrs of age)
Kleinschmidt-DeMasters et al., 1998 (16)	34 yr	Female	Cavernous sinus	"Smooth muscle tumor"	HIV-1 infection (manner of transmission not reported, diagnosed at 27 yrs of age)
Krishnan et al., 1999 (59)	37 yr	Male	Kidney	Leiomyoma	HIV-1 infection (manner of transmission not reported, diagnosed for 8 yrs)
Cases associated with organ transplantation and immunosuppression					
Lee et al., 1995 (51)	4 yr	Female	Liver	"Smooth muscle tumor"	Liver transplantation 3 yr earlier (on immunosuppressive therapy with cyclosporine, azathioprine, corticosteroids)
	6 yr	Not reported	Lung, liver, stomach, colon	"Smooth muscle tumors"	Liver transplantation 5 yr earlier (on immunosuppressive therapy with cyclosporine, azathioprine, corticosteroids, and muromonab-CD3 (Orthoclone OKT3) for 1 mo after transplantation)
	2 yr	Female	Colon	"Smooth muscle tumors"	Liver and small bowel transplantation (on immunosuppressive therapy with tacrolimus, azathioprine, corticosteroids)
Timmons et al., 1995 (60)	9 yr	Male	Liver	Leiomyosarcoma (donor origin)	Liver transplantation 2 yr earlier (on immunosuppressive therapy with cyclosporine, azathioprine, corticosteroids)

Reference	Age	Sex	Site	Tumor	Clinical context
Davidoff et al., 1996 (64)	5 yr	Male	Liver	Leiomyoma	Heart transplantation 3 yr earlier (on immunosuppressive therapy with azathioprine, corticosteroids)
Le Bail et al., 1996 (61); Morel et al., 1996 (62)	53 yr	Female	Liver (with cyst formation), spleen	"Smooth muscle tumors" (host origin)	Kidney transplantation 2 yr earlier (on immunosuppressive therapy with cyclosporine, azathioprine, corticosteroids)
Sadahira et al., 1996 (63)	21 yr	Female	Liver (multiple nodules, with cyst formation)	"Smooth muscle tumor"	Kidney transplantation 5 yr earlier (on immunosuppressive therapy with azathioprine, corticosteroids)
Somers et al., 1998 (65)	15 yr	Male	Lung (>50 nodules in all lobes)	Leiomyosarcoma (donor origin)	Heart-lung transplantation 3 yr earlier (on immunosuppressive therapy with cyclosporine, azathioprine, corticosteroids)
			Liver	Leiomyosarcoma (host origin)	
	12 yr	Female	Liver	Leiomyosarcoma (host origin)	Liver transplantation 5 yr earlier (on immunosuppressive therapy with cyclosporine, corticosteroids)
Cases associated with other forms of immunosuppression					
Yunis, 1996 (72) (based on original case report by Shen and Yunis, 1976 [71])	5 yr	Male	Kidney	Leiomyosarcoma	Acute lymphocytic leukemia treated 6 wk earlier with chemotherapy and radiation therapy
Kleinschmidt-DeMasters et al., 1998 (16)	14 yr	Female	Transverse and sigmoid sinus	Leiomyosarcoma	Common variable immunodeficiency

[a] One leiomyosarcoma in an adult renal transplant recipient and one leiomyosarcoma in an adult heart transplant recipient that have been studied for the presence of EBV have been reported as negative, both by the same group (68,69). One leiomyosarcoma in a child with HIV-1 infection was tested for EBV in 1992 and reported as negative (40). Another leiomyosarcoma in a child with HIV-1 infection was reported but not tested for EBV infection (70).

patients tested (16,740 and 12,440, and 3973 genome copies per milliliter also support the hypothesis of high levels of EBV replication in immunosuppressed patients with EBV-associated leiomyosarcoma *(56)*. The presence of HIV-1 has been tested by *in situ* hybridization and by semiquantitative PCR and has not been found in the smooth muscle cells of HIV-1-associated leiomyosarcomas *(40,50,56)*.

One leiomyosarcoma in an adult renal transplant recipient and one leiomyosarcoma in an adult heart transplant recipient that have been studied for the presence of EBV have been reported as negative, in separate reports by the same group *(68,69)*. One leiomyosarcoma in a child with HIV-1 infection was tested for EBV in 1992 and reported as negative *(40)*. Another leiomyosarcoma in a child with HIV-1 infection was reported after the association with EBV was identified, but was not tested for EBV infection *(70)*.

Other forms of immunosuppression may also permit development of EBV-associated leiomyosarcoma. A leiomyosarcoma originally reported in 1976 *(71)*, in a 5-yr-old boy 3 yr after remission of acute lymphocytic leukemia that was treated with chemotherapy and radiation, was subsequently tested and found to contain EBV *(72)*. Another EBV-associated leiomyosarcoma was reported in a 14-yr-old girl with common variable immunodeficiency syndrome *(16,73)*.

The results of the EBV serologic testing are consistent with past EBV infection in all reported patients with smooth muscle cell tumors. There has not been a characteristic serologic profile such as that often found in nasopharyngeal carcinoma and Burkitt's lymphoma, which are also associated with EBV but that occur primarily in immunocompetent persons *(74)*.

Thus, the contribution of EBV to development of leiomyosarcomas appears to be limited to the milieu of the immunocompromised host, which may be congenital (e.g., common variable immunodeficiency) or acquired (e.g., HIV-1 infection, immunosuppressive therapy following organ transplant). EBV is not found in normal smooth muscle, and has not been found when tested in leiomyomas or leiomyosarcomas in the absence of HIV-1 infection or other immunocompromised conditions *(16,50,55,67)*. The absence of EBV in the leiomyosarcomas of immunocompetent persons, and its consistent presence in leiomyosarcomas of immunocompromised persons lends support to the hypothesis that EBV has an etiologic role in the increased incidence of soft tissue tumors in immunocompromised persons but that other mechanisms contribute to smooth muscle tumorigenicity.

PATHOGENESIS OF EBV-ASSOCIATED LEIOMYOSARCOMA

It is of note that presentation with multiple tumor nodules is common in immunocompromised persons who develop leiomyosarcomas. The most significant evidence of EBV infection of the muscle cells prior to malignant transformation is the finding of EBV monoclonality of leiomyosarcomas *(50,51,61)*. Of the tumors that have been tested, only monoclonal episomal EBV was found, indicating that EBV infection preceded malignant transformation; there was no viral integration into the cell genome to account for malignant transformation. The most striking case is that of a 5-yr-old female with two separate tumors biopsied at different times and from different sites, with each tumor demonstrating different EBV monoclonality, indicating that these two tumors developed independently *(50)*. A 15-yr-old male with multiple leiomyosarcomas following heart–lung transplant was found to have pulmonary tumors of donor origin and hepatic tumors of host origin *(65)*. A 24-yr-old male had equimolar biclonality of EBV in a leiomyosarcoma, consistent with dual EBV infection of tumor cells or a uniformly mixed cell population derived from two independent EBV infection events *(50)*. Either scenario is strong evidence of linkage of EBV to the tumor. Although metastases from a single tumor are possible, it appears that the primary factor that predisposes to leiomyosarcoma—impaired host immunosurveillance from impaired immunocompetence, resulting from either HIV-1 infection or from immunosuppressive therapy associated with organ transplant—facilitates the simultaneous development of multiple primary tumors.

The presence of EBV in both a leiomyoma and leiomyosarcoma occurring in an 8-yr-old girl *(50)* suggests that EBV infects the smooth muscle cells before they undergo malignant transformation and thus plays a pivotal role in the progression to malignancy. High levels of EBV as shown by *in situ* hybridization and semiquantitative PCR are indirectly indicative of such an scenario. Taken as a whole, the evidence of multiple discrete EBV cell infection events associated with the tumors of these patients demonstrates that EBV infection of smooth muscle cells and proliferation is probably not an infrequent occurrence under circumstances of impaired immunosurveillance.

The increased numbers of cases of leiomyomas and leiomyosarcomas in children compared to adults is even more remarkable considering the much greater number of adults compared to children with HIV-1 infection or organ transplant. After non-Hodgkin's lymphoma, leiomyosarcoma is the second leading cancer in children with HIV-1 infection *(75)*. Children may be more susceptible to developing EBV-associated tumors because primary EBV infection occurs in childhood *(76–78)*. The host may be less well prepared to limit primary EBV infection and the contribution of EBV to malignant transformation than under the typical scenario that is present in adults, with development of impaired immunosurveillance in the setting of previously established but well-controlled, latent EBV infection.

Entry of EBV into Smooth Muscle Cells

The presence of the EBV receptor (CD21, also known as CR2), which is also the receptor for the C3d component of complement *(79,80)*, on smooth muscle cells would appear to be a prerequisite for EBV infection of smooth muscle cells. The EBV receptor has been identified on striated muscle cells as well as a variety of nonlymphoid tissues including epithelium of the parotid gland, tonsil, skin, lung, esophagus, jejunum, colon, pancreas, kidney, and adrenal cortical cells and hepatocytes *(81)*.

The EBV receptor has been found to be present at relatively higher levels on the cells of both leiomyomas and leiomyosarcomas of HIV-1-infected patients but at lower levels in tumors from HIV-1-uninfected patients *(50,56)*. The receptor is detectable at much lower levels in normal smooth muscle tissues. The CD21 receptor is detected best with biotin-streptavidin procedures using the OKB7 *(82)* monoclonal antibody, and is undetectable using the HB5 *(83)* monoclonal antibody *(84)*, which may account for reported differences in identification of the CD21 on smooth muscle cells *(50,56,65)*. This also suggests that the CD21 antigen on smooth muscle cells *(84)* may not be identical to that found on epithelial cells or lymphocytes *(85,86)*.

Alternatively, the presence of CD21 may not be involved because the mechanism of EBV entry into different cell types may be by different routes *(87,88)*. It is possible that

that fusion of smooth muscle cells with EBV-infected lymphocytes could be the route of cell entry into nonlymphoid cells by EBV-induced formation of polykaryocytes of EBV-superinfected lymphoblastoid cells with cells devoid of EBV receptors *(89)*.

The presence of EBV in the leiomyomas and leiomyosarcomas from HIV-1-infected persons but not from immunocompetent persons suggests that entry of EBV into muscle cells is directly or indirectly affected by HIV-1 infection. In HIV-1-infected patients, EBV infection of smooth muscle cells may be facilitated by the increased expression of the EBV receptor and the higher circulating levels of EBV. However, given the increased incidence of leiomyosarcomas in organ transplant recipients as well as persons with AIDS, it is more likely that the contribution of HIV-1 to leiomyosarcoma is the result of decreased immunosurveillance rather than increased expression of EBV receptors. Although the CD21 receptor is present in low amounts on leiomyomas and leiomyosarcomas from immunocompetent children *(50,56)*, EBV infection is not found. This emphasizes the important role of immunosurveillance to eradicate virus or cells should EBV infection of smooth muscle cells occasionally occur. Under this scenario, persistent EBV infection is a prerequisite for malignant transformation and primarily the consequence of impaired immunosurveillance.

EBV Replication in Smooth Muscle Cells

The biology of EBV infection of smooth muscle cells has been studied best in explanted cells from a single leiomyosarcoma of a woman with HIV-1 infection *(84)*. The cells exhibited very slow growth in vitro with unusual elliptical and spindle-shaped morphology and fragmentation of the cytoplasm into long, tapering cytoplasmic processes. Greater than 90% of cells had diffuse expression of the smooth muscle isoform of actin by immunoperoxidase staining. Approximately 25% of cells expressed very bright fluorescence by immunostaining to the smooth muscle isoforms of calponin and actin. The majority of cells demonstrated a weak signal for CD21, and approx 5–10% of cells showed a strong signal confined to cell surfaces. The cultured cells harbored EBV, and infectious EBV continued to be detected by PCR and virus culture through several passages in vitro. Several EBV antigens were expressed including: latent antigen EBNA-1; immediate early antigen BZLF1; early antigen EA-D; and late antigens, including viral capsid antigen p160, gp125, and membrane antigen gp350. Human umbilical cord lymphocytes transformed with virus isolated from cultured cells yielded immortalized cell lines that expressed EBV antigens similar to other EBV-transformed lymphocyte cell lines. These findings confirm that EBV is capable of lytic infection of smooth muscle cells with expression of a repertoire of latent and replicative viral products and production of infectious virus, and may contribute to the oncogenesis of leiomyosarcomas.

The inability to derive immortalized, EBV-infected smooth muscle cell lines that are tumorigenic is, in many ways, similar to the inability to establish nonlymphoid cell lines from Kaposi's sarcoma harboring KSHV (*see* Chapter 10). The biology of these two gamma herpesviruses in these two tumors may have many similarities.

CONCLUSIONS

Leiomyoma and leiomyosarcoma expand the spectrum of EBV-associated malignancies, and also of AIDS- and organ transplant-related malignancies. The immune dysfunction of AIDS and the immunosuppression used following organ transplant appear to facilitate EBV infection of smooth muscle cells, malignant transformation, and subsequent proliferation. Further studies aimed at elucidating the molecular pathogenesis of these tumors may provide insight into the viral and cellular mechanisms that facilitate EBV infection of these cells, and the specific defects of immunosurveillance that permit EBV infection of smooth muscle cells and malignant transformation.

REFERENCES

1. Burnet M. Somatic mutation and chronic disease. Br Med J 1965; 1:338–342.
2. Penn I. Sarcomas in organ allograft recipients. Transplantation 1995; 60:1485–1491.
3. Centers for Disease Control and Prevention. 1993 revised classification system for HIV infection and expanded surveillance case definition for AIDS among adolescents and adults. MMWR Morb Mortal Wkly Rep 1992; 41:1–19.
4. Beral V, Newton R. Overview of the epidemiology of immunodeficiency-associated cancers. J Natl Cancer Inst Monogr 1998; 23:1–6.
5. Remick SC. Non-AIDS-defining cancers. Hematol Oncol Clin North Am 1996; 10:1203–1213.
6. Spencer JM, Amonette RA. Tumors with smooth muscle differentiation. Dermatol Surg 1996; 22:761–768.
7. Miano JM, Olson EN. Expression of the smooth muscle cell calponin gene marks the early cardiac and smooth muscle cell lineages during mouse embryogenesis. J Biol Chem 1996; 271:7095–7103.
8. Ruzicka DL, Schwartz RJ. Sequential activation of alpha-actin genes during avian cardiogenesis: vascular smooth muscle alpha-actin gene transcripts mark the onset of cardiomyocyte differentiation. J Cell Biol 1988; 107:2575–2586.
9. Cavazzana AO, Ninfo V, Tirabosco R, Montaldi A, Frunzio R. Leiomyosarcoma. Curr Top Pathol 1995; 89:313–332.
10. Christopherson WM, Williamson EO, Gray LA. Leiomyosarcoma of the uterus. Cancer 1972; 29:1512–1517.
11. Evans HL. Smooth muscle tumors of the gastrointestinal tract. A study of 56 cases followed for a minimum of 10 years. Cancer 1985; 56:2242–2250.
12. Morgan BK, Compton C, Talbert M, Gallagher WJ, Wood WC. Benign smooth muscle tumors of the gastrointestinal tract. A 24-year experience. Ann Surg 1990; 211:63–66.
13. Gal AA, Brooks JS, Pietra GG. Leiomyomatous neoplasms of the lung: a clinical, histologic, and immunohistochemical study. Mod Pathol 1989; 2:209–216.
14. Evans HL, Chawla SP, Simpson C, Finn KP. Smooth muscle neoplasms of the uterus other than ordinary leiomyoma. A study of 46 cases, with emphasis on diagnostic criteria and prognostic factors. Cancer 1988; 62:2239–2247.
15. Hashimoto H, Tsuneyoshi M, Enjoji M. Malignant smooth muscle tumors of the retroperitoneum and mesentery: a clinicopathologic analysis of 44 cases. J Surg Oncol 1985; 28:177–186.
16. Kleinschmidt-DeMasters BK, Mierau GW, Sze Cl, et al. Unusual dural and skull-based mesenchymal neoplasms: a report of four cases. Hum Pathol 1998; 29:240–245.
17. Polednak AP. Incidence of soft-tissue cancers in blacks and whites in New York State. Int J Cancer 1986; 38:21–26.
18. Myhre-Jensen O, Kaae S, Madsen EH, Sneppen O. Histopathological grading in soft-tissue tumours. Relation to survival in 261 surgically treated patients. Acta Pathol Microbiol Immunol Scand A Pathol 1983; 91:145–150.
19. Trojani M, Contesso G, Coindre JM, et al. Soft-tissue sarcomas of adults; study of pathological prognostic variables and definition of a histopathological grading system. Int J Cancer 1984; 33:37–42.

20. Enjoji M, Hashimoto H. Diagnosis of soft tissue sarcomas. Pathol Res Pract 1984; 178:215–226.
21. Markhede G, Angervall L, Stener B. A multivariate analysis of the prognosis after surgical treatment of malignant soft-tissue tumors. Cancer 1982; 49:1721–1733.
22. Hashimoto H, Daimaru Y, Tsuneyoshi M, Enjoji M. Leiomyosarcoma of the external soft tissues. A clinicopathologic, immunohistochemical, and electron microscopic study. Cancer 1986; 57:2077–2088.
23. Wile AG, Evans HL, Romsdahl MM. Leiomyosarcoma of soft tissue: a clinicopathologic study. Cancer 1981; 48:1022–1032.
24. Neugut AI, Sordillo PP. Leiomyosarcomas of the extremities. J Surg Oncol 1989; 40:65–67.
25. Young JLJ, Miller RW. Incidence of malignant tumors in U.S. children. J Pediatr 1975; 86:254–258.
26. Lack EE. Leiomyosarcomas in childhood: a clinical and pathologic study of 10 cases. Pediatr Pathol 1986; 6:181–197.
27. Yannopoulos K, Stout AP. Smooth muscle tumors in children. Cancer 1962; 15:958–971.
28. Botting AJ, Soule EH, Brown AL Jr. Smooth muscle tumors in children. Cancer 1965; 18:711–720.
29. Walker D, Gill TJI, Corson JM. Leiomyosarcoma in a renal allograft recipient treated with immunosuppressive drugs. JAMA 1971; 215:2084–2086.
30. Pritzker KPH, Huang SN, Marshall KG. Malignant tumours following immunosuppressive therapy. Can Med Assoc J 1970; 103:1362–1365.
31. Lieber MR, Winans CS, Griem ML, Moossa R, Elner VM, Franklin WA. Sarcomas arising after radiotherapy for peptic ulcer disease. Digest Dis Sci 1985; 30:593–599.
32. Cohen SR, Thompson JW, Sherman NJ. Congenital stenosis of the lower esophagus associated with leiomyoma and leiomyosarcoma of the gastrointestinal tract. Ann Otol Rhinol Laryngol 1988; 97:454–459.
33. Case records of the Massachusetts General Hospital. Weekly clinicopathological exercises. Case 9-1986. A 40-month-old girl with the acquired immunodeficiency syndrome and spinal-cord compression [published erratum appears in N Engl J Med 1986 Jun 5; 314(23):1523]. N Engl J Med 1986; 314:629–640.
34. Ninane J, Moulin D, Latinne D, et al. AIDS in two African children—one with fibrosarcoma of the liver. Eur J Pediatr 1985; 144:385–390.
35. Chadwick EG, Connor EJ, Guerra Hanson IC, et al. Tumors of smooth-muscle origin in HIV-infected children. JAMA 1990; 263:3182–3184.
36. Sabatino D, Martinez S, Young R, Balbi H, Ciminera P, Frieri M. Simultaneous pulmonary leiomyosarcoma and leiomyoma in pediatric HIV infection. Pediatr Hematol Oncol 1991; 8:355–359.
37. Mueller BU, Butler KM, Higham MC, et al. Smooth muscle tumors in children with human immunodeficiency virus infection. Pediatrics 1992; 90:460–463.
38. Orlow SJ, Kamino H, Lawrence RL. Multiple subcutaneous leiomyosarcomas in an adolescent with AIDS. Am J Pediatr Hematol Oncol 1992; 14:365–368.
39. Radin R, Kiyabu M. Multiple smooth muscle tumors of the colon and adrenal gland in an adult with AIDS. Am J Radiol 1992; 159:545–546.
40. Ross JS, Del Rosario A, Bui HX, Sonbati H, Solis O. Primary hepatic leiomyosarcoma in a child with the acquired immunodeficiency syndrome. Hum Pathol 1992; 23:69–72.
41. Challapalli M. Leiomyomata and leiomyosarcomata in HIV-infected children. [letter]. Diagn Cytopathol 1993; 9:366.
42. Steel TR, Pell MF, Turner JJ, Lim GH. Spinal epidural leiomyoma occurring in an HIV-infected man. Case report. J Neurosurg 1993; 79:442–445.
43. van Hoeven KH, Factor SM, Kress Y, Woodruff JM. Visceral myogenic tumors. A manifestation of HIV infection in children. Am J Surg Pathol 1993; 17:1176–1181.

44. Levin TL, Adam HM, van Hoeven KH, Goldman HS. Hepatic spindle cell tumors in HIV positive children. Pediatr Radiol 1994; 24:78–79.
45. McLoughlin LC, Nord KS, Joshi VV, DiCarlo FJ, Kane MJ. Disseminated leiomyosarcoma in a child with acquired immune deficiency syndrome. Cancer 1991; 67:2618–2621.
46. Murphy SB, Chadwick EG. HIV and smooth muscle tumors. [letter]. Pediatrics 1993; 91:1020–1021.
47. Balsam D, Segal S. Two smooth muscle tumors in the airway of an HIV-infected child. Pediatr Radiol 1992; 22:552–553.
48. Ha C, Haller JO, Rollins NK. Smooth muscle tumors in immunocompromised (HIV negative) children. Pediatr Radiol 1993; 23:413–414.
49. Danhaive O, Ninane J, Sokal E, et al. Hepatic localization of a fibrosarcoma in a child with a liver transplant. J Pediatr 1992; 120:434–437.
50. McClain KL, Leach CT, Jenson HB, et al. Association of Epstein–Barr virus with leiomyosarcomas in young people with AIDS. N Engl J Med 1995; 332:12–18.
51. Lee ES, Locker J, Nalesnik M, et al. The association of Epstein–Barr virus with smooth-muscle tumors occurring after organ transplantation. N Engl J Med 1995; 332:19–25.
52. Jimenez-Heffernan JA, Hardisson D, Palacios J, Garcia-Viera M, Gamallo, Nistal M. Adrenal gland leiomyoma in a child with acquired immunodeficiency syndrome. Pediatr Pathol Lab Med 1995; 15:923–929.
53. Zetler PJ, Filipenko D, Bilbey JH, Schmidt N. Primary adrenal leiomysarcoma in a man with acquired immunodeficiency syndrome (AIDS). Further evidence for an increase in smooth muscle tumors related to Epstein–Barr infection in AIDS. Arch Pathol Lab Med 1995; 119:1164–1167.
54. Bluhm JM, Yi ES, Diaz G, Colby TV, Colt HG. Multicentric endobronchial smooth muscle tumors associated with the Epstein–Barr virus in an adult patient with the acquired immunodeficiency syndrome. A case report. Cancer 1997; 80:1910–1913.
55. Boman F, Gultekin H, Dickman PS. Latent Epstein–Barr virus infection demonstrated in low-grade leiomyosarcomas of adults with acquired immunodeficiency syndrome, but not in adjacent Kaposi's lesion or smooth muscle tumors in immunocompetent patients. Arch Pathol Lab Med 1997; 121:834–838.
56. Jenson HB, Leach CT, McClain KL, et al. Benign and malignant smooth muscle tumors containing Epstein–Barr virus in children with AIDS. Leuk Lymphoma 1997; 27:303–314.
57. Morgello S, Kotsianti A, Gumprecht JP, Moore F. Epstein–Barr virus-associated dural leiomyosarcoma in a man infected with human immunodeficiency virus. Case report. J Neurosurg 1997; 86:883–887.
58. Creager AJ, Maia DM, Funkhouser WK. Epstein–Barr virus-associated renal smooth muscle neoplasm. Report of a case with review of the literature. Arch Pathol Lab Med 1998; 122:277–281.
59. Krishnan R, Freeman JA, Creager AJ. Epstein–Barr virus induced renal leiomyoma. J Urol 1999; 161:212.
60. Timmons CF, Dawson DB, Richards CS, Andrews WS, Katz JA. Epstein–Barr virus-associated leiomyosarcomas in liver transplantation recipients. Origin from either donor or recipient tissue. Cancer 1995; 76:1481–1489.
61. Le Bail B, Morel D, Merel P, et al. Cystic smooth-muscle tumor of the liver and spleen associated with Epstein–Barr virus after renal transplantation. Am J Surg pathol 1996; 20:1418–1425.
62. Morel D, Merville P, Le Bail B, Berger F, Saric J, Potaux L. Epstein–Barr virus (EBV)-associated hepatic and splenic smooth muscle tumours after kidney transplantation. Nephrol Dial Transplant 1996; 11:1864–1866.
63. Sadahira Y, Moriya T, Shirabe T, Matsuno T, Manabe T. Epstein–Barr virus-associated post-transplant primary smooth muscle tumor of the liver: report of an autopsy case. Pathol Int 1996; 46:601–604.

64. Davidoff AM, Hebra A, Clark BJ 3rd, et al. Epstein–Barr virus-associated hepatic smooth muscle neoplasm in a cardiac transplant recipient. Transplantation 1996; 61:515–517.

65. Somers GR, Tesoriero AA, Hartland E, et al. Multiple leiomyosarcomas of both donor and recipient origin arising in a heart-lung transplant patient. Am J Surg Pathol 1998; 22:1423–1428.

66. Kaschka-Dierich C, Adams A, Lindahl T, et al. Intracellular forms of Epstein–Barr virus DNA in human tumour cells in vivo. Nature 1976; 260:302–306.

67. Hill MA, Araya JC, Eckert MW, Gillespie AT, Hunt JD, Levine EA. Tumor specific Epstein–Barr virus infection is not associated with leiomyosarcoma in human immunodeficiency virus negative individuals. Cancer 1997; 80:204–2010.

68. Van Gelder T, Vuzevski VD, Weimar W. Epstein–Barr virus in smooth-muscle tumors. [letter]. N Engl J Med 1995; 332:1719.

69. van Gelder T, Jonkman FAM, Niesters HGM, et al. Absence of Epstein–Barr virus involvement in an adult heart transplant recipient with an epitheloid leiomyosarcoma. [letter]. J Heart Lung Transplant 1996; 15:650–651.

70. Dugan MC. Primary adrenal leiomyosarcoma in acquired immunodeficiency syndrome. [letter]. Arch Pathol Lab Med 1996; 120:797–798.

71. Shen SC, Yunis EJ. Leiomyosarcoma developing in a child during remission of leukemia. J Pediatr 1976; 89:780–782.

72. Yunis EJ. Role of Epstein–Barr virus in tumor development. J Pediatr 1996; 128:438.

73. Mierau GW, Greffe BS, Weeks DA. Primary leiomyosarcoma of brain in an adolescent with common variable immunodeficiency syndrome. Ultrastruct Pathol 1997; 21:301–305.

74. Jenson HB, Ench Y, Sumaya CV. Epstein–Barr virus. In: Rose NR, de Macario EC, Folds H, Lane HC, Nakamura RM (eds). Manual of Clinical Laboratory Immunology, 5 edit. Washington, DC: American Society for Microbiology Press, 1997, pp. 634–643.

75. Granovsky MO, Mueller BU, Nicholson HS, Rosenberg PS, Rabkin CS. Cancer in human immunodeficiency virus-infected children: a case series from the Children's Cancer Group and the National Cancer Institute. J Clin Oncol 1998; 16:1729–1735.

76. Evans AS. New discoveries in infectious mononucleosis. Mod Med 1974; 1:18–24.

77. Evans AS, Niederman JC, McCollum RW. Seroepidemiologic studies of infectious mononucleosis with EB virus. N Engl J Med 1968; 279:1123–1127.

78. Wang PS, Evans AS. Prevalence of antibodies to Epstein–Barr virus and cytomegalovirus in sera from a group of children in the People's Republic of China. J Infect Dis 1986; 153:150–152.

79. Jondal M, Klein G, Oldstone MB, Bokish V, Yefenof E. Surface markers on human B and T lymphocytes. VIII. Association between complement and Epstein–Barr virus receptors on human lymphoid cells. Scand J Immunol 1976; 5:401–410.

80. Hutt-Fletcher LM, Fowler E, Lambris JD, Feighny RJ, Simmons JG, Ross GD. Studies of the Epstein Barr virus receptor found on Raji cells. II. A comparison of lymphocyte binding sites for Epstein Barr virus and C3d. J Immunol 1983; 130:1309–1312.

81. Timens W, Boes A, Vos H, Poppema S. Tissue distribution of the C3d/EBV-receptor: CD21 monoclonal antibodies reactive with a variety of epithelial cells, medullary thymocytes, and peripheral T-cells. Histochemistry 1991; 95:605–611.

82. Nemerow GR, McNaughton ME, Cooper NR. Binding of monoclonal antibody to the Epstein Barr virus (EBV)/CR2 receptor induces activation and differentiation of human B lymphocytes. J Immunol 1985; 135:3068–3073.

83. Fingeroth JD, Weis JJ, Tedder TF, Strominger JL, Biro PA, Fearon DT. Epstein–Barr virus receptor of human B lymphocytes is the C3d receptor CR2. Proc Natl Acad Sci USA 1984; 81:4510–454.

84. Jenson HB, Montalvo EA, McClain KL, et al. Characterization of natural Epstein–Barr virus infection and replication in smooth muscle cells from a leiomyosarcoma. J Med Virol 1999; 57:36–46.

85. Sixbey JW, Davis DS, Young LS, Hutt-Fletcher L, Tedder TF, Rickinson AB. Human epithelial cell expression of an Epstein–Barr virus receptor. J Gen Virol 1987; 68:805–811.

86. Young L, Alfieri C, Hennessy K, et al. Expression of Epstein–Barr virus transformation-associated genes in tissues of patients with EBV lymphoproliferative disease. N Engl J Med 1989; 321:1080–1085.

87. Miller N, Hutt-Fletcher LM. Epstein–Barr virus enters B cells and epithelial cells by different routes. J Virol 1992; 66:3409–3414.

88. Yoshizaki T, Takimoto T, Takeshita H, et al. Epstein–Barr virus lytic cycle spreads via cell fusion in a nasopharyngeal carcinoma hybrid cell line. Laryngoscope 1994; 104:91–94.

89. Bayliss GJ, Wolf H. Epstein–Barr virus-induced cell fusion. Nature 1980; 287:164–165.

90. Prévot S, Néris J, de Saint Maur PP. Detection of Epstein Barr virus in an hepatic leiomyomatous neoplasm in an adult human immunodeficiency virus 1-infected patient. Virchows Arch 1994; 425:321–325.

10
Kaposi's Sarcoma and Other HHV-8 Associated Tumors

Chris Boshoff

INTRODUCTION

Kaposi's Sarcoma: History, Patterns and Pathology

As medical students in 1987 at Kalafong Hospital (Tembisa, South Africa) we were intrigued by a patient with tuberculosis and disseminated skin lesions. This was the first patient we had seen who was infected with the human immunodeficiency virus (HIV), and he had Kaposi's sarcoma (KS). We never imagined then that 10 yr later most patients at this hospital, as in many other South African hospitals, would have AIDS-related illnesses. One in eight South Africans is now HIV positive, compared with the nearly one in four adults in neighboring Botswana and Zimbabwe. No one anticipated then the enormous burden that HIV would have on southern Africa.

In 1981, when a few reports of *Pneumocystis carinii* pneumonia (PCP) and KS in young men from New York City and San Francisco heralded the acquired immunodeficiency syndrome (AIDS), few imagined that by the year 2000, 40 million people worldwide would be infected. In Africa, most HIV-positive patients still succumb to infectious causes, most notably tuberculosis. However, opportunistic neoplasms are also taking their toll and KS, for example, is now the most common tumor in men in Uganda (1).

In 1872, the Hungarian dermatologist Moriz Kaposi published the case histories of five middle-aged and elderly male patients in Vienna with *idiopathic multiple pigmented sarcomas* of the skin (2). For more than 100 yr, KS remained a rare curiosity to clinicians and cancer researchers, until it became highly significant as the sentinel of AIDS.

During that century, three clinical patterns of KS were described. *Classic KS* occurs predominantly in elderly male patients of Southern European and Middle Eastern origin (3). In some equatorial, eastern, and southern African countries, KS has existed for many decades, long preceding HIV and known as *endemic KS (4)*. Unlike classic KS, endemic KS also occurs in children, who present with lymphadenopathy rather than skin lesions. Endemic KS is generally a more aggressive disease than classic KS, although less so than AIDS-associated KS (5,6). The majority of African children with endemic KS die from the disease (7).

From: *Infectious Causes of Cancer: Targets for Intervention*
Edited by: J. J. Goedert © Humana Press Inc., Totowa, NJ

KS also is known to develop after an organ transplant and is designated *posttrans-plant or iatrogenic KS (8,9)*. Patients of Mediterranean, Jewish, or Arabian ancestry are clearly overrepresented among immunosuppressed patients who develop KS after a transplant *(3)*, indicating that those born in countries where classic KS occurs continue to be at risk of developing KS even if they migrate to low-risk countries. These data suggested that there is a genetic predisposition or environmental factor (possibly an infectious agent) responsible for KS development.

In 1981, the U. S. Centers for Disease Control and Prevention (CDC) became aware of an increased occurrence of two rare diseases, KS and PCP, among young homosexual men from New York City and California *(10)*. This was the beginning of the AIDS epidemic, and AIDS-KS is today the most common form of KS. In HIV-infected individuals the underlying immunosuppression leads to a fulminant disease that starts with a few skin lesions, but without treatment often develops into disseminated disease affecting various organs including lung, liver, gut, and spleen.

Histologically, KS is a complex lesion. In early (*patch* stage) KS lesions, there are a collection of irregular endothelial lined spaces that surround normal dermal blood vessels, and these are accompanied by a variable inflammatory infiltrate. This stage is followed by the expansion of a spindle-celled vascular process throughout the dermis. These spindle cells form slitlike, vascular channels containing erythrocytes (*plaque* stage KS). The later *nodular* stage KS lesions are composed of sheets of spindle cells, some of which are undergoing mitosis, and slitlike vascular spaces with areas of hemosiderin pigmentation. The spindle cells form the bulk of established KS lesions and are therefore thought to be the neoplastic component. Most of the spindle cells in KS lesions express endothelial markers, including CD31 and CD34. However, it was also shown that KS spindle cells express markers for smooth muscle cells, macrophages, and dendritic cells *(11,12)*, suggesting that spindle cells are either derived from pluripotent mesenchymal precursors or represent a heterogeneous population of cells. Circulating KS-like spindle cells have been isolated and cultured from patients with AIDS-KS and from those thought for other reasons to be at risk of AIDS-KS *(13)*. These circulating cells have an adherent phenotype and express markers of both macrophage and endothelial cells *(14)*. Recently, it was shown that all KS spindle cells express vascular endothelial growth factor receptor-3 (VEGFR-3) *(15,16)*. VEGFR-3 is usually expressed only by lymphatic endothelium *(15)* and by neoangiogenic vessels, but not by mature vascular endothelial cells, indicating that KS spindle cells probably belong to the endothelial cell lineage that can differentiate into lymphatic cells.

Early (patch stage) KS is probably a nonclonal proliferation of lymphatic endothelial cells or endothelial precursors (e.g., angioblasts) *(17)* with a prominent inflammatory and angiogenic response, whereas advanced disease can develop into a true clonal malignancy with metastases of clonally derived spindle cells to different sites *(18–21)*.

All known tumors produce cytokines, and their cells respond positively or negatively to cytokines in culture. KS is no exception and KS spindle cells or infiltrating CD8+ lymphocytes and macrophages express high levels of interleukin-6 (IL-6), basic fibroblast growth factor (bFGF), tumor necrosis factor α (TNF-α), Oncostatin M, and γ-interferon (γ-IFN) *(22–28)*. IL-6 is produced by KS spindle cells, and exogenous IL-6 enhances the proliferation of KS cells in culture *(25)*. γ-IFN also induces endothelial cells to acquire phenotypical features similar to those of KS spindle cells *(28)*. Because of the nature of KS lesions it has been suggested that these lesions are cytokine driven.

The more aggressive nature of HIV-associated KS has led to speculation that HIV-encoded proteins may enhance KS growth *(27)*. The HIV-1 Tat protein transactivates HIV viral genes and also some host cell genes *(29)*. Tat can be released by infected cells and can act extracellularly *(30,31)*. Tat induces a functional program in endothelial cells related to angiogenesis and inflammation including the migration, proliferation, and expression of plasminogen activator inhibitor-1 and E selectin *(32)*. Tat induces growth of KS spindle cells in vitro and is angiogenic in vivo and in transgenic mice *(27,31,33)*. The Tat basic domain contains an arginine- and lysine-rich sequence that is similar to that of other potent angiogenic growth factors including vascular endothelial growth factor-A (VEGF-A) and bFGF *(34)*. Tat specifically binds and activates the Flk-1/kinase domain receptor (Flk-1/KDR), a VEGF-A tyrosine kinase receptor *(35)*. Tat-induced angiogenesis can be inhibited by agents blocking this receptor *(35)*. The arginine, glycine, aspartic acid (RGD)-containing region of Tat also has been postulated to have a role in the pathogenesis of AIDS-KS, although baboons infected with HIV-2, which lacks an RGD sequence in Tat, can develop KS-like lesions, albeit of myofibroblast, rather than endothelial, origin *(27,36)*. AIDS-associated KS frequently is more aggressive than non-HIV-related KS, and it is possible that the angiogenic properties of Tat contribute to this phenomenon.

Studies of AIDS case surveillance support the pre-AIDS data on the existence of a sexually transmissible KS cofactor. KS occurs predominantly in homosexual and bisexual men with AIDS, less commonly in those acquiring HIV through heterosexual contact and rarely in AIDS patients with hemophilia or in intravenous drug users *(37,38)*.

A viral etiology for this tumor was suspected long before the onset of the AIDS epidemic *(4)*. In 1972, electron microscopy of KS tumor cells revealed herpesvirus-like particles that were attributed to cytomegalovirus (CMV) *(39,40)*. DNA sequences of CMV, human herpesvirus-6 (HHV-6), human papilloma viruses (HPV), BK virus (human polyoma virus), and other viral (including retroviral) or bacterial pathogens have all been detected in KS lesions and put forward as the suspected agents of KS *(41–43)*. However, these agents, including CMV, HHV-6, and papilloma viruses, are found only in some lesions, and BK virus is an ubiquitous agent present in many tumors and tumor cell lines *(41,43,44)*.

A NEW GAMMAHERPESVIRUS: HHV-8

herpein   Greek, to creep or crawl. Refers to the characteristic skin lesions caused by herpes simplex and herpes zoster infections.

> *O er ladies lips, who straight on kisses dream,*
> *Which oft the angry Mab with blisters plagues,*
> *Because their breaths with sweetmeats tainted are.*
>
> Shakespeare
> *Romeo and Juliet.* 1595

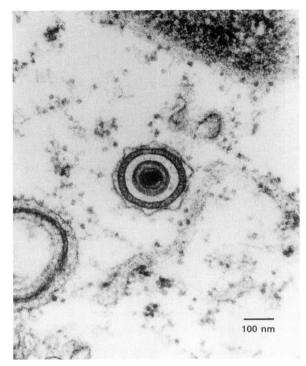

Fig. 1. Electron microscopy of a HHV-8 virion (kindly provided by Dharam Ablashi, ABI Inc). The dense herpesviral DNA core is seen, with surrounding capsid and envelope.

Discovery and Related Viruses

In 1994, the laboratory of Yuan Chang and Patrick Moore employed representational difference analysis (RDA) to identify sequences of a new herpesvirus in an AIDS-KS biopsy *(45)*. This virus is called human herpesvirus-8 (or KS-associated herpesvirus). RDA relies on cycles of subtractive hybridization and polymerase chain reaction (PCR) amplification to enrich and isolate rare DNA fragments that are present in only one of two otherwise identical populations of DNA *(46,47)*.

Nearly 100 herpesviruses have been identified and almost all mammal species have been shown to be infected by at least one member of the family. The known herpesviruses share a common virion architecture (Fig. 1) and four critical biological properties *(48):*

1. All herpesviruses encode enzymes involved in nucleic acid metabolism, DNA synthesis, and protein processing.
2. The synthesis of viral DNA and assembly of the capsid usually occur in the nucleus of infected cells.
3. Production of infectious virus progeny is generally accompanied by destruction of the infected cell (lytic infection).
4. Herpesviruses remain latent and persist for life in their hosts. Latent infection occurs in specific cell types, for example, the Epstein–Barr virus (EBV) persists in B lympho-

Table 1
Gammaherpesviruses Related to HHV-8

Virus	Acronym	Host
Epstein–Barr virus	EBV	Humans
Herpesvirus saimiri	HVS	Primates (NW)
Herpesvirus ateles	HVA	Primates (NW)
Alcelaphine herpesvirus	AHV-1	Domestic animals
Bovine herpesvirus-4	BHV-4	Cows
Equine herpesvirus-2	EHV-2	Horses
Murine herpesvirus-68	MHV-68	Rodents
Retroperitoneal fibromatosis herpesviruses	$RFHV_{Mn}$, $RFHV_{Mm}$	Primates (OW) *(230)*
Rhesus monkey rhadinovirus	RRV	Primates (OW) *(231)*

NW, New World primate; OW, Old World primate.

cytes. Latent herpesviral genomes persist as extrachromosomal circular episomes that express only a fraction of viral genes (the so-called latent genes).

The subfamily Gammaherpesvirinae includes the genera *Lymphocryptovirus* and *Rhadinovirus*. Viruses of this subfamily are characterized by their capacity to induce cell proliferation in vivo, resulting in transient or chronic lymphoproliferative disorders (Table 1).

DISEASES CAUSALLY LINKED TO HUMAN HERPESVIRUS-8

Kaposi's Sarcoma

HHV-8 DNA is present, by PCR, in all epidemiologic and clinical forms of KS, in all fresh biopsies tested, and in the vast majority of paraffin-embedded material (Table 2). The virus is rarely detectable in non-KS tissues (except blood) from the same individual, indicating that viral load is highest in KS lesions. This raised the question whether the cytokine-rich milieu of KS encourages HHV-8 replication or the proliferation of the cell type(s) harboring HHV-8, in which case HHV-8 is only a passenger in these lesions and does not necessarily cause them. However, HHV-8 is not present in other vascular tumors including angiomas and angiosarcomas, and it is only rarely detectable in other forms of skin tumors (including squamous carcinomas and melanomas) in immunosuppressed patients *(49–52)*. Furthermore, the detection of HHV-8 DNA by PCR in the peripheral blood of HIV-positive individuals is predictive of KS *(53,54)*, indicating that those at risk of KS have a higher viral load than those not at risk (Fig. 2).

To further strengthen the molecular epidemiologic association between HHV-8 and KS it was demonstrated by PCR *in situ* hybridization, RNA *in situ* hybridization, and immunohistochemistry that HHV-8 is present in nearly all spindle cells in KS lesions (Fig. 3) *(16,55–61)*. In early KS lesions, only a small proportion (< 10%) of spindle cells are positive for HHV-8, whereas VEGFR-3 is expressed by most cells *(16)*. This indicates that paracrine mechanisms are probably important in the initiation and progression of KS. In nodular lesions, >90% of the spindle cells contain HHV-8 latent

Table 2
Detection of HHV-8 DNA by PCR in KS Biopsies and Control Tissues

Type of lesion	Positive/no. tested (%)	
AIDS-KS	252/259 (97%)	
Classic KS	160/175 (91%)	
Iatrogenic KS	13/13 (100%)	
African endemic KS	71/80 (89%)	
HIV-negative homosexual men with KS	8/9 (89%)	
Control tissues	14/743 (1.8%)	$p < 0.0001$

Data compiled from refs. *45,142,* and *232–247.*

infection, suggesting that HHV-8 latent proteins provide a growth advantage to infected cells *(16)*.

Immunoblastic Variant Multicentric Castleman's Disease

As originally described by Castleman in 1956 *(62)*, Castleman's disease (CD) comprises a benign localized mass of lymphoid tissue. Histologically, the lesion is characterized by the presence of large follicles separated by vascular lymphoid tissue containing lymphocytes. This histologic form is known as the hyaline-vascular type of CD.

Subsequently, a variant that is distinguished by the presence of sheets of plasma cells in the interfollicular zone was described and is referred to as the plasma cell type of CD *(63)*. A more recently described multicentric form of the plasma cell variant of CD (MCD) is a systemic lymphoproliferative disorder often associated with immuno-logic abnormalities *(64)*. MCD is mainly of the plasma-cell type and has a poorer prognosis than the localized hyaline-vascular type *(65)*. MCD changes in lymph nodes are more commonly diagnosed in HIV-infected individuals.

Patients with MCD often develop secondary tumors such as KS, non-Hodgkin's lymphoma (NHL), and Hodgkin's disease *(66,67)*. Up to 25% of patients with MCD develop NHL *(64,68,69)*, and immunoblastic B-cell lymphoma is the most frequent subtype *(64,69,70)*.

Soulier and colleagues used PCR to identify HHV-8 DNA in CD biopsies *(70)*. Other groups have since confirmed this finding *(71,72)*. HHV-8 is present in immunoblasts (also called plasmablasts) in MCD (Fig. 4), and such immunoblasts are not present in HHV-8-negative MCD *(16,73)*. These HHV-8-positive immunoblasts belong to the B-cell lineage and express CD20. HHV-8-positive MCD is therefore a distinct disease entity and should be designated as an immunoblastic or plasmablastic variant of MCD *(74)*. Confluent clusters of HHV-8-positive immunoblasts also are present in biopsies of immunoblastic MCD, indicating that isolated HHV-8 immunoblasts can progress to form foci of microlymphoma *(74)*. HHV-8 also appears to be present in all tumor cells of immunoblastic lymphoma that develops in patients with the HHV-8-positive immunoblastic variant of MCD *(74)*. The development of immunoblastic lymphoma therefore represents a further evolution of this disorder (Fig. 5). Unlike HHV-8-positive primary effusion lymphoma cells (*see* next section), the immunoblasts in MCD are positive only for HHV-8 and not for EBV.

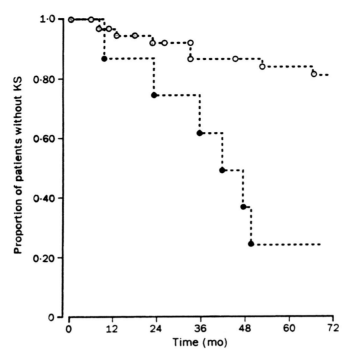

Fig. 2. Kaplan–Meyer curve, showing that the presence of HHV-8 in peripheral blood mononuclear cells by PCR is associated with the subsequent development of KS in a cohort of HIV-positive homosexual men. Proportion of individuals, in whose peripheral blood HHV-8 was (●) or was not (○) detected, and who remained free of KS after indicated time of follow-up.(From ref. *54* with permission.)

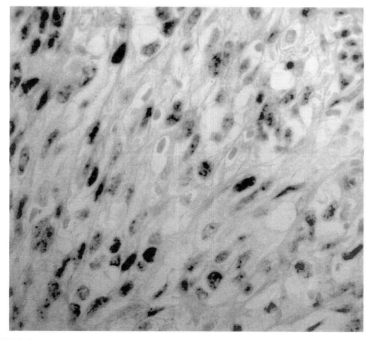

Fig. 3. HHV-8 latent nuclear protein (LNA/ORF 73) is expressed by the vast majority of spindle cells in KS lesions.

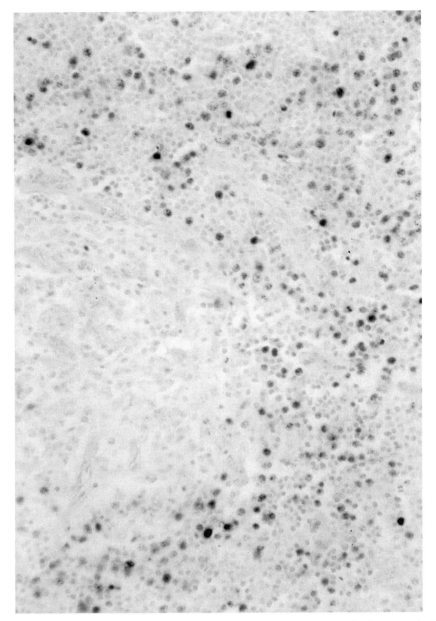

Fig. 4. HHV-8 LNA is expressed by immunoblasts surrounding germinal centers in MCD.

Whether occurring as isolated cells in the mantle zone, in small confluent clusters, or in the immunoblastic lymphomas, the HHV-8-positive immunoblasts in MCD invariably express cytoplasmic IgM λ, suggesting that these cells in all circumstances comprise a monoclonal population *(74)*.

Current studies suggest that HHV-8-positive MCD has a poorer prognosis than the HHV-8 negative cases *(16,73,75)*. A likely explanation is the presence of a monoclonal

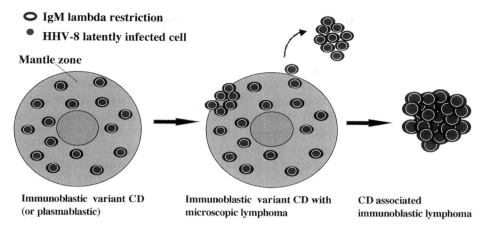

○ **IgM lambda restriction**

● **HHV-8 latently infected cell**

Mantle zone

| Immunoblastic variant CD (or plasmablastic) | Immunoblastic variant CD with microscopic lymphoma | CD associated immunoblastic lymphoma |

Fig. 5. Proposed involvement of HHV-8 in immunoblastic or plasmablastic Castleman's disease (CD).

lymphoma population of immunoblasts in the HHV-8-positive cases that can progress to an aggressive immunoblastic lymphoma (Fig. 5) *(74)*.

Primary Effusion Lymphoma

The emergence of primary effusion lymphoma (PEL, previously called body cavity based lymphoma) as a new disease entity is an intriguing story linked to the identification of HHV-8. Two groups initially recognized the unique aspects of some effusion-based lymphomas in patients with AIDS *(76,77)*. The lymphoma cells in these cases were negative for most lineage-associated antigens, although immunoglobulin (Ig) gene rearrangement studies indicated a B-cell origin. In 1992, Karcher et al. further demonstrated the distinctiveness of the syndrome, reporting a high prevalence of EBV, yet absence of c-*myc* rearrangements *(78)*. They also noted the tendency of the disease to remain confined to body cavities without further dissemination. In 1995, Cesarman and colleagues found that HHV-8 was specifically associated with PEL but not with other high-grade AIDS-related lymphomas *(79)*.

PEL possesses a unique constellation of features that distinguishes it from all other known lymphoproliferations. PEL presents predominantly as malignant effusions in the pleural, pericardial, or peritoneal cavities usually without significant tumor mass or lymphadenopathy. These lymphomas occur predominantly in HIV-positive individuals with advanced stages of immunosuppression *(80)*, but they are seen occasionally in HIV-negative patients *(81–83)*. More bizarre was the presentation of a PEL that persisted in the cavity created by a silicone breast implant *(83)*, which presumably is an immune privileged site. PEL and KS can occur in the same patient. Also, like KS, PEL occurs primarily in homosexual men and not in other HIV-positive risk groups *(81,84)*.

Most PELs do not express surface B-cell antigens. However, a B-cell lineage is indicated by the presence of clonal immunoglobulin gene rearrangement *(85,86)*, and the cells show morphologic features of plasmacytoid cells *(87)*. It still is unclear whether HHV-8 arrests cells at this stage of differentiation or infects and transforms these mature B cells. All PELs that lack c-*myc* rearrangments contain HHV-8 *(81)*. The majority, but not all, PELs are coinfected with EBV *(79,88)*, suggesting that the two viruses may cooperate in neoplastic transformation. Terminal repeat analysis indicates that EBV is monoclonal in most cases *(81,86)*, implying that EBV was present in tumor cells prior to clonal expansion. PEL cells consistently lack molecular defects commonly associated with neoplasia of mature B cells, including activation of the pro-tooncogenes *bcl-2, bcl-6,* c-*ras,* and K-*ras,* as well as mutations of *p53 (89,90).*

Southern blot analysis of PEL cells shows the presence of HHV-8 sequences in high copy number (50–150 viral episomes per cell). Cell lines from PEL have been established *(85,91–94)*. One HHV-8-positive, EBV-negative cell line also has been established from the peripheral blood of a patient with PEL *(87)*. Most but not all cell lines are coinfected with EBV. In the coinfected lines the expression of EBV latent proteins is restricted to Epstein–Barr nuclear antigen 1 (EBNA-1) and latent membrane protein-2 (LMP-2) *(87,95)*. Lines latently infected with HHV-8 can be induced with phorbol esters or *n*-butyrate to produce HHV-8 virions *(92,96)*.

It appears that HHV-8-positive PEL cells lack many adhesion molecules and homing markers present on other diffuse lymphomas. This may contribute to the peculiar effusion phenotype of these lymphomas and to the lack of macroscopic involvement of lymph nodes *(87)*.

Other

Confusion regarding the prevalence of HHV-8 was generated by reports that this virus is widespread in tissues affected by sarcoidosis *(97)* and in the bone marrow and circulating dendritic cells of patients with multiple myeloma (MM) *(98,99)*. We have not been able to detect HHV-8 in sarcoid tissues (Boshoff and Mitchell, *unpublished observations)*, and we consider this study as an example of contamination by using nested PCR, a technique that clearly requires confirmation of all positive amplicons by amplifying other nonoverlapping areas of the genome.

The reports of HHV-8 in the bone marrow and circulating dendritic cells of patients with MM are more intriguing. It is an attractive hypothesis because HHV-8 encodes a viral homolog of one of the cytokines, human interleukin 6 (huIL-6), that is involved in MM pathogenesis. The HHV-8-encoded IL-6 also can maintain the growth of huIL-6-dependent MM cell lines *(100,101)*. A further link might be that patients with MCD, the lymphoproliferation associated with HHV-8, often have immunoglobulin dyscrasias, and occasionally even develop MM. However, various groups, employing molecular and serologic techniques, have not been able to reproduce the findings that HHV-8 is associated with MM *(102–108)*. It also is clear that HHV-8 does not actually infect the myeloma cells themselves, but viral DNA has been proposed to be present in the dendritic cells in patients with MM. The role, if any, of HHV-8 in MM pathogenesis remains highly controversial.

Angioimmunoblastic lymphadenopathy with dysproteinemia (AILD) is a disorder occasionally associated with KS development. One study reported HHV-8 sequences in 20% of such lymphomas, but also in 17% of reactive lymphadenopathies from HIV-seronegative patients *(109)*. These were all Italian patients, perhaps reflecting a higher prevalence of HHV-8 in circulating B lymphocytes in this population, rather than an etiologic association.

SEROEPIDEMIOLOGY

Serologic Assays

Several HHV-8 serologic assays are currently available. The most widely used assays are based on detection of latent or lytic antigens in HHV-8-infected PEL cell lines, either by immunofluorescence *(110–112)* or enzyme immunoassay *(113)*. Assays also have been described that detect antibodies to recombinant HHV-8 latent and lytic proteins or synthetic peptides. Lytic proteins shown to be immunogenic include ORF (open reading frame) 65 *(112)*, ORF 26 *(114)*, and ORF K8.1 *(115,116)*. The only latent antigen thus far to be used in recombinant assays is ORF 73, which is the same antigen detected in latent immunofluorescence assays *(59,117,118)*. A study comparing various assays including recombinant proteins (ORFs 65 and K8.1) and immunofluorescence assays concluded that immunofluorescence assay (IFA) followed by confirmation with Western blot reactions with a panel of latent and lytic immunogenic antigens provide a reliable, sensitive, and specific method to detect HHV-8 antibodies *(119)*.

Seroprevalence

Northern Europe and North America

The seroprevalence of HHV-8 in the different HIV risk groups correlates with the incidence of KS. In Northern Europe and North America, HHV-8 is found predominantly in HIV-positive homosexual men *(110–112,120,121)* and not in HIV-positive patients with hemophilia, drug users, or heterosexuals.

In a cohort of men in San Francisco, it was shown that HHV-8 infection is associated with the number of homosexual partners and correlates with a previous history of a sexually transmitted disease (STD, such as gonorrhoea) and HIV infection *(122)*, suggesting that HHV-8 is sexually transmitted. In homosexual men attending the STD clinic at St. Thomas Hospital in London, in univariate analysis HHV-8 prevalence was correlated with a history of sex with an American, suggesting that HHV-8 was perhaps first introduced into the homosexual communities in the epicenters of HIV in the United States before spreading to Europe *(123)*. At the moment we can conclude that HHV-8 is transmitted among homosexual men during sex, although this does not necessarily imply sexual transmission.

Mediterranean Europe

The incidence of classic KS is significantly higher in Italy than in the United Kingdom or the United States *(3,124)*. Similarly, the prevalence of antibodies to HHV-8 in blood donors in Italy is significantly higher than rates reported in the United Kingdom or the United States *(125,126)*. Furthermore, the incidence of classic KS in Italy shows considerable regional variation *(124)* and the prevalence of HHV-8 in different regions correlates with this *(125,127)*. In addition, the geometric mean titer of anti-HHV-8 antibodies is highest in blood donors from the south, where the incidence of KS and the prevalence of HHV-8 is highest *(125)*. This is reminiscent of EBV infection, in which a high anti-EBV antibody titer correlates with an increased risk of developing Burkitt's lymphoma or nasopharyngeal carcinoma *(128,129)*.

Israel

The incidence of classic KS in Israel is among the highest in the world *(130)*. Similarly, the seroprevalence of HHV-8 among Israeli Jews is higher than that seen in the general populations of Western Europe and North America *(131)*. The incidence of classic KS is higher among North African (Sephardic) Jews than those of European descent (Ashkenazi), and the seroprevalence of HHV-8 among the different Jewish groups correlates with this *(131)*. Furthermore, mother-to-child transmission is important in the acquisition of HHV-8 in Israel *(131)*.

Africa

Endemic KS existed in Africa long before the AIDS epidemic; however, AIDS-KS is now one of the most common tumors in many parts of Africa. In Africa, where KS rates are relatively high among HIV-positive individuals, the prevalence of antibodies to HHV-8 is also higher than in North America and Northern Europe *(112,132–135)*. Early acquisition of HHV-8 in Africa is likely because KS is seen in African children *(7)*. Indeed, the prevalence of antibodies to HHV-8 increases steadily with age in Africa (Fig. 6) *(134,135)*, and this occurs even before puberty *(136–139)*. This indicates that HHV-8 is not predominantly transmitted during sex, as is seen among homosexual men in the West. Mother-to-child transmission and sibling-to-sibling transmission has been shown to occur in South Africa and in a Noir-Marron population living in French Guyana *(136,140)*. About one third of HHV-8 positive black mothers in South Africa transmit the virus to their children *(136)*. Interestingly, in contrast to mother-to-child transmission, father-to-child transmission does not appear to occur among the Noir-Marron population tested. In South Africa there is a significantly lower prevalence of anti-HHV-8 antibodies among whites than among blacks, and in black cancer patients the seroprevalence of HHV-8 declines with increasing education, suggesting that factors associated with poverty may contribute to the transmission of the virus *(135)*.

Transmission

Although one group reported the frequent detection of HHV-8 in the semen of healthy Italian donors *(141)*, in North America and the United Kingdom the current consensus is that HHV-8 is present only intermittently in the semen of patients with KS and sometimes in HIV-positive patients without KS, but only rarely in semen donors *(142–147)*. HIV-8 has also been found in prostate biopsies of HIV-positive men with or without KS *(148)*. HHV-8 shedding into semen from prostate fluid is therefore a possible mode of transmission. Infectious virus is also found in the saliva of HIV-positive individuals *(149)*. In patients with classic KS, HHV-8 DNA was shown to be present in tonsillar swabs and in saliva *(126)*. Although studies in homosexual men indicate that HHV-8 is transmitted during sex and the risk of having HHV-8 increases with the number of sexual partners, the exact mode and route are not known. Semen and saliva are possible routes of viral transmission, but their respective contribution to infection is still unknown. The role of breast milk, saliva, and other horizontal routes for mother-to-child and sibling-to-sibling transmission is also still unknown.

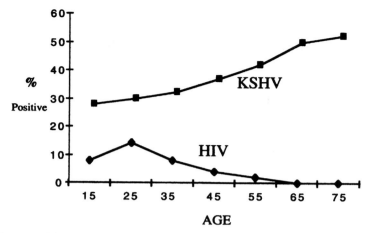

Fig. 6. Age-specific seroprevalence of HHV-8 and HIV in black South African patients with cancer. (From ref. *135* with permission.)

HHV-8 GENOME

Genomic Organization and Structure

The genome of HHV-8 was mapped and sequenced from cosmid and phage genomic libraries from a PEL cell line (BC-1, which also contains EBV) *(150)*. HHV-8 also was sequenced from a KS biopsy, and the genome was found to be almost identical to that in PEL *(151)*. The HHV-8 genome consists of an estimated 140.5-kb long unique coding region (LUR) flanked by approx 800-bp noncoding tandemly repeated units with an 85% G + C content. More than 80 ORFs have thus far been identified, including nearly 70 with sequence similarity to related gammaherpesviruses. Novel ORFs not present in other herpesviruses were designated *K1 – K15*, although many of these now appear to be present in related viruses.

Like other herpesviruses, HHV-8 encodes proteins involved in viral DNA replication including a DNA polymerase (Pol-8, *ORF 9*) and a polymerase processivity factor (PF-8, *ORF 59*) *(150,152)*. PF-8 complexes specifically with Pol-8 to synthesize HHV-8 DNA *(152)*. Other proteins involved in viral replication include helicase-primase proteins (ORFs 40, 41, and 44) and a single-stranded DNA (ssDNA) binding protein (*ORF 6*).

ORFs encoding proteins that could be targets for anti-herpesviral agents include thymidylate synthase (*ORF 70*) and thymidine kinase (*ORF 21*) homologs *(96)*.

Strain Variation: The Left- and Right-Hand Ends of the Genome

The left end of the genome of herpesvirus saimiri (HVS), the related New World primate gammaherpesvirus, is essential for HVS T-cell transformation. The first ORF of HHV-8, *K1*, has therefore demanded attention (Fig. 7). However, unlike the products of the first two ORFs of HVS (STP and Tip), K1 is an early lytic cycle transmembrane protein that does not seem to be expressed in latently infected PEL cells *(153)* and that has no sequence or structural similarity to HVS STP *(154)*. K1 is structurally similar to lymphocyte receptors and can transduce signals associated with B-cell activation

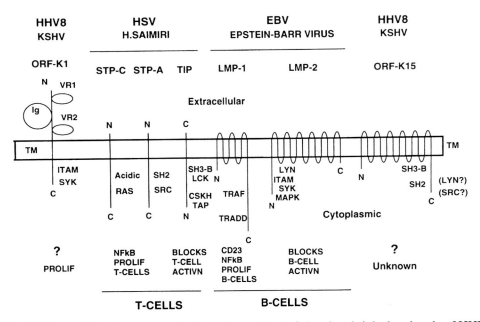

Fig. 7. The relative structure and orientations of the left-hand and right-hand ends of HHV-8 compared to HVS and EBV. (From ref. *159* with permission.)

(155). The role of K1 in KS spindle cell growth or B-cell transformation is therefore questioned. Nevertheless, expression of the *K1* gene in rodent fibroblasts produced morphologic changes and focus formation indicative of transformation *(154).* Furthermore, a recombinant herpesvirus, in which the *STP* oncogene of HVS was replaced with *K1*, immortalized primary T lymphocytes and induced lymphoproliferations in common marmosets *(154).*

Polymorphisms in *ORF K1* identified subtypes A, B, C, and D, which display 15–30% amino acid differences in their *ORF K1* coding regions *(156,157).* These subtypes have close associations with the geographic and ethnic background of individuals. Within these four subtypes, more than 13 clades have now been described *(158).* Subtype B is found almost exclusively in patients from Africa, subtype C in individuals from the Middle East and Mediterranean Europe, subtype A in Western Europe and North America, and subtype D so far has been described only in individuals from the Pacific Islands *(158,159).* No subtype yet appears to correlate with a specific disease or with a more aggressive course for KS. The unusually high genetic divergence identified in *ORF K1* reflects some unknown powerful biologic selection process acting specifically on this immunoglobulin receptor-like signal transducing protein *(157,159).* This could be related to evolving mechanisms of viral evasion from the immune system in different populations.

K15 is at the extreme right-hand side of the HHV-8 genome (Fig. 7). Two alternatively highly diverged forms of this complex spliced gene (P or M) exist. P is the predominant form; M (for minor) is seen in < 15% of viral isolates *(159).* K15 is a latent membrane protein related to both EBV LMP-1 and -2 *(159).* K15 has a tumor necrosis

Table 3
HHV-8 Immediate Early and Latent Proteins

Latent proteins	
Latent nuclear antigen	ORF 73
v-cyclin	ORF 72
v-FLIP	ORF71
Latent membrane protein	K15
Kaposin(s)	K12, 12.1, and 12.2
v-IL-6[a]	K2
Immediate early proteins	
HHV-8 Rta[b]	ORF 50

[a] Appears to be latently expressed only in hematopoietic, rather than mesenchymal, cells *(100,248)*.

[b] HHV-8 ORF 50 is homologous to EBV Rta (BRLF 1), a transcriptional transactivator that activates early lytic gene expression from the latent viral genome *(249,250)*.

factor receptor-associated (TRAF) binding domain, and like LMP-1 might therefore trigger the NF-κB pathway of signal transduction. The P and M subtypes appear unlinked to the *ORF K1* genotypes, suggesting that one of these two forms was introduced into the HHV-8 genome by recombination with a related but unidentified primate or human γ2-herpesvirus.

HHV-8 Latent Proteins

In EBV, the latent nuclear proteins (EBNA 1–6) and latent membrane proteins (LMP-1/-2A and -2B) are essential for persistence of the episomal genome, maintenance of latency, initiation of lytic viral infection, evasion or elicitation of antiviral immune responses, and driving cellular proliferation (and therefore tumorigenesis). These EBV proteins have been shown to interact or upregulate cellular proteins involved in transformation (including p53, pRb, cyclin D, histone deacetylase, and TRAF). A number of HHV-8 ORFs are transcribed during latency (Table 3) *(160,161)*.

LATENT NUCLEAR PROTEIN (ORF 73/LNA).

ORF 73 of HHV-8 encodes a latent immunogenic nuclear antigen (LNA) protein detected as nuclear speckling by immunofluorescence using HHV-8-positive sera on PEL cells *(59,117,118)*. HHV-8 LNA (ORF 73) has a long acidic repeat region containing a large leucine-zipper motif *(150)*, suggesting direct interaction with other viral or cellular proteins. *ORF 73* is transcribed with the viral cyclin and FLIP (*see* later) homologs *(117,162,163)*. LNA is expressed in all KS spindle cells latently infected with HHV-8, in all the immunoblasts in HHV-8-associated CD, and in all cells of PEL (Fig. 3 and 4) *(16)*. Like EBNA-1, LNA is essential to maintain the HHV-8 episome (extrachromosomal persistence) *(164)*. Furthermore, LNA tethers HHV-8 DNA to chromosomes during mitosis to allow the segregation of viral episomes to all progeny cells (Fig. 8) (*164* and Bourboulea and Boshoff, *unpublished observations*). LNA therefore maintains a stable episome during mitosis. An attractive application of this function of LNA would be to use HHV-8 LNA in vectors for gene therapy to allow stable transmission of the required genes to all progeny cells. Strategies including the development of small molecules that interfere with the func-

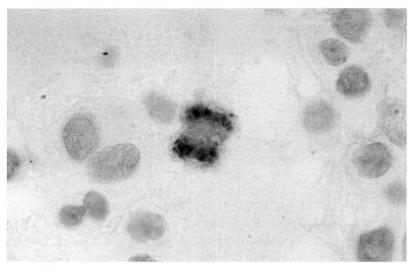

Fig. 8. An HHV-8 positive immunoblast in MCD undergoing mitosis, showing that LNA (encoded by ORF 73) associates with chromosomes.

tions of LNA should also be useful to abort latent HHV-8 infection and therefore prevent HHV-8-associated diseases.

v-Cyclin.

Cellular cyclins are critical components of the cell cycle. Cyclins are regulatory subunits of a specific class of cellular kinases. By physically associating with an inactive cyclin-dependent kinase (CDK) core, cyclins lead to the formation of active kinase holoenzymes that recognize and phosphorylate an array of cellular substrate molecules. The phosphorylating activity of these holoenzymes is responsible for regulating the passage of cells through the replication cycle. Cyclins associate with their partners (the CDKs) to be fully active. The HHV-8 cyclin has highest sequence similarity to the cellular D-type cyclins. The HHV-8 cyclin (ORF 72) is expressed during latency, inferring a possible role in tumorigenesis. The HHV-8 cyclin forms active kinase complexes with CDK6 *(165,166)* to phosphorylate the retinoblastoma protein (pRb) at authentic sites *(167)*. Furthermore, unlike cellular D cyclin/CDK6 complexes, HHV-8 cyclin/CDK6 activity is resistant to inhibition by CDK inhibitors (CKI) p16, p21, and p27 *(168)*. Ectopic expression of v-cyclin prevents arrest of the cell cycle normally imposed by each inhibitor, and it stimulates cell-cycle progression in quiescent fibroblasts *(168)*. HHV-8 cyclin/CDK6 also phosphorylates (inactivates) p27 *(169)*, the CKI known to be an effective inhibitor of cyclin E/CDK2 activity *(170)*. This suggests that this viral cyclin can activate both pathways necessary for progression from the G_1 into the S phase of the cell cycle (i.e., cyclin D/CDK6 and cyclin E/CDK2).

The expression of the HHV-8 cyclin in latently infected spindle and PEL cells *(58,171,172)* indicates a possible role in the proliferation of these cells or arrest of their differentiation. Cyclin D1 expression, not cyclins E or A, inhibits the differentiation of immature myoblasts *(173)*. HPV E7 also has been shown to uncouple cellular differentation and proliferation in human keratinocytes (*see also* Chapters 14 and 16) *(174)*. As KS spindle cells appear to represent undifferentiated endothelial cells *(16)*, this role for the HHV-8 cyclin is an attractive hypothesis.

v-FLIP.

ORF 71 (K13) of HHV-8 encodes a FLICE inhibitory protein (FLIP) homolog. Cellular FLIP interferes with apoptosis signaled through death receptors *(175)*. v-FLIPs are present in several viruses (including RRV, HVS, equine herpesvirus, and the human molluscipoxvirus) *(176,177)*. Cellular and viral FLIPs contain two death-effector domains that interact with the adaptor protein FADD *(178,179)*, and that inhibit the recruitment and activation of the protease FLICE *(178,180)* by the CD95 death receptor *(181)*. FLICE initiates proteolytic activation of other ICE protease family members, which in turn leads to apoptosis *(178,180)*. Cells expressing FLIPs are protected against apoptosis induced by CD95 or by TNF-R1 *(176,177)*. HHV-8 FLIP (ORF 71) is transcribed as a bicistronic transcript with HHV-8 cyclin (ORF 72) during latent infection, but no functional assays for the HHV-8 FLIP have yet been published. Like cellular FLIP, the v-FLIP encoded by HHV-8 might block one of the principal pathways by which immune mechanisms cause cell death, such as induction of apoptosis by the tumor necrosis factor family of receptors. The expression of HHV-8 FLIP during latency could therefore be one mechanism whereby HHV-8 latently infected cells escape apoptosis induced by cytotoxic T cells.

K12 (KAPOSIN).

K12 encodes an abundantly expressed latency-associated transcript, T0.7 (Kaposin), that is expressed in most KS spindle cells. K12 transforms rat fibroblasts in cluture, inferring a role in spindle and lymphoma cell proliferation *(57,182,183)*. K12 appears to be part of a complex spliced larger protein that is expressed in latency. The function of this latent viral protein is not yet known.

Captured Genes

A number of recognizable genes pirated from eukaryotic cellular DNA are encoded by HHV-8 and related viruses (Table 4) *(100)*. The structural proteins and viral enzymes that are common to most herpesviruses probably originated from an ancient progenitor of contemporary herpesviruses. In contrast, the recognizable cellular genes listed in Table 4 occur only sporadically in some herpesviruses, are probably more recent acquisitions from the host genome, and might support viral replication in a specific microenvironment, which for HHV-8 could be the microvasculature *(184)*. The captured eukaryotic genes have acquired unique properties that can give us insight into the biology of their cellular counterparts *(184)*, which is one reason they have been the most studied proteins encoded by HHV-8.

VIRAL CHEMOKINES, CYTOKINES, AND CYTOKINE RECEPTORS

The v-IL-6 (K2) is functional in preventing apoptosis of IL-6-dependent mouse and human myeloma cell lines in vitro *(100,185,186)*, indicating that it could also possibly play a role in maintaining the proliferation of HHV-8-positive hematopoietic cells, including circulating B cells, PEL cells, and immunoblasts. The v-IL-6 appears to be expressed during latency in these hematopoietic cells *(73,100)*. v-IL-6 activates JAK/STAT signaling via interactions with the gp130 subunit of the IL-6 receptor, but

Table 4
Cellular Genes Pirated by MHV-68, HVS, and HHV-8

MHV-68	HVS	HHV-8[a]
CCPH (ORF 4)	CCPH (ORF 4)	CCPH (ORF 4)
—	TS (ORF 70)	TS (ORF 70)
—	DHFR (ORF 2)	DHFR (ORF 2)
cyclin D (ORF 72)	cyclin D (ORF 72)	cyclin D (ORF 72)
GPCR (IL-8R) (ORF 74)	GPCR (IL-8R) (ORF 74)	GPCR (IL-8R) (ORF 74)
—	FLIP (ORF 71)	FLIP (ORF 71)
Bcl-2 (M11)	bcl-2 (ORF 16)	bcl2 (ORF 16)
	IL-17 (S13)	—
	CD 59 (S15)	—
	—	IRF I-III (K9, K10, K10.1)
	—	IL-6 (K2)
	—	MIP I–III (K4, K6, K4.1)
	—	OX-2 (K14)

[a] RRV also encodes all these cellular homologs

These gammaherpesviruses encode an array of cellular gene homologs that are involved in **viral DNA replication:** CCPH, complement control protein homolog; DHFR, dihydrofolate reductase; TS, thymidylate synthetase; **cellular proliferation:** cyclin D homolog; GPCR, G-protein coupled receptor/IL-8 receptor; **anti-apoptosis:** bcl-2 homolog; FLIP, FLICE inhibitory protein; IL-6, interleukin-6; and **escape from immune responses:** MIP, macrophage inhibitory proteins; IRF, interferon regulatory factor homologs; OX-2, a potential homolog of cellular OX-2 (function not clear).

unlike cellular IL-6 it does not require the α-subunit of this receptor *(187)*. In KS lesions, v-IL-6 is expressed only in the fraction of cells undergoing lytic infection *(100)*.

Chemokines (*chemo*attractant cyto*kines*) currently are hot topics because their receptors have been shown to be essential for HIV to enter cells (*see also* Chapter 11). CC and CXC chemokines also can block HIV infection of T cells, macrophages, and microglial cells. HHV-8 encodes three (possibly four) chemokine genes. Two of these genes *v-MIP-1* (*K6*) and *v-MIP-II* (*K4*), share extensive sequence identity (45%), while *v-MIP-III* (*K4.1*) is more distantly related. The chemokines encoded by HHV-8 (v-MIP-I–III*)* are more promiscuous than the cellular chemokines in binding to both CC and CXC receptors *(188,189)*. v-MIP-II activates the CCR3 receptor, which is involved in the trafficking of eosinophils and Th2 lymphocytes *(189,190)*. v-MIP-II and v-MIP-III also are chemoattractants for Th2 cells by way of CCR8 and CCR4 *(191,192)*. The principal function of HHV-8 chemokines could therefore be to switch an antiviral Th1 response to a Th2 environment which is more favorable for the virus.

vMIP-II blocks HIV-1 infection of CD4+/CCR3+ cells, which could have implications for progression of HIV disease. v-MIP-I and -II also block HIV infection of microglial cells in culture (Hibbitts and Clapham, *unpublished observations*). Various groups reported that patients with KS (and therefore high HHV-8 viral loads) *(54)* have a statistically significant lower incidence of developing HIV-related central nervous system (CNS) disease including encephalopathy (Fig. 9) *(155,193,194)*. Furthermore,

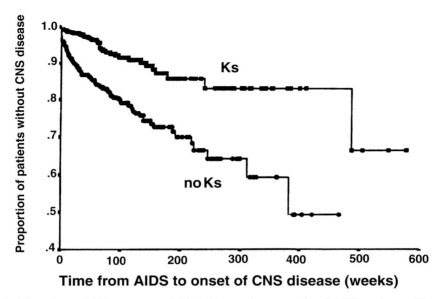

Fig. 9. Time from AIDS to onset of CNS disease in a sample of 1109 patients. (From ref. *194*.)

unlike the cellular CC chemokines MIP-1α and RANTES, the three HHV-8 chemokines induce angiogenesis and might therefore also play a direct paracrine role in tumorigenesis *(189,192).*

v-GPCR/ORF 74

Another HHV-8 protein that might be involved in cellular proliferation is the HHV-8 encoded G-protein-coupled receptor (v-GPCR). v-GPCR is fully active for down-stream signaling in the absence of chemokine ligands (constitutively active) *(195),* and it can transform fibroblasts *(196).* Cellular GPCRs that are constantly stimulated or that become constitutively active by mutation can transform cells, and they are involved in the pathogenesis of some human tumors *(197–200).* v-GPCR shows most sequence similarity to the human receptors for IL-8 (CXCR-1 and CXCR-2) *(171,201),* an endothelial cell chemokine and angiogenic factor. v-GPCR activates a mitogenic sig-naling pathway, the phosphoinositide pathway, in COS-1 cells, and in vitro transfection of rat fibroblasts with v-GPCR leads to cell proliferation *(195).* v-GPCR is able to trig-ger signaling cascades leading to activation of AP-1 *(195),* which is a transcription fac-tor involved in survival and proliferation of cells and in the activation of inflammatory and angiogenic growth factors *(202,203).* The GPCR-specific kinase-5 (GRK-5) inhibits v-GPCR-stimulated proliferation of rodent fibroblasts *(204).* v-GPCR does cause an angiogenic switch in cells expressing this protein *(196),* implying a potential role in upregulating VEGF in KS spindle cells. However, it is not clear whether v-GPCR is actually expressed in latently infected KS spindle cells.

v-IRFs

Interferons (IFNs) are a family of cytokines with antiviral activity. The interferon regulated factor (IRF) family of transcription factors positively or negatively regulate

IFN-stimulated response elements in the promoters of genes under IFN induction control. IRF-1 functions as an activator for IFN and IFN-inducible genes, whereas IRF-2 represses the action of IRF-1 *(205)*. In growing cells IRF-2 is more abundant than IRF-1, but after stimulation by IFN or viruses the amount of IRF-1 increases relative to IRF-2. This suggests that a transient decrease in the IRF-2/IRF-1 ratio may be a critical event in the regulation of cell growth by IFNs. Consistent with this hypothesis, IRF-1 has antiproliferative properties both in vitro and in vivo. Furthermore, IRF-1 and IRF-2 have antagonistic and prooncogenic activities, respectively, when overexpressed in NIH3T3 cells *(205)*.

HHV-8 encodes at least four ORFs with IRF sequence similarity. v-IRF-I was the first HHV-8-encoded protein found to transform NIH3T3 cells and to induce tumor formation *(206)*. v-IRF-I also was shown to inhibit responses of type I and type II IFNs and to block IRF-1-mediated transcription *(207,208)*. The HHV-8 IRFs (I–IV) are not expressed in latently infected spindle cells and therefore probably do not play a direct role in the proliferation of these cells *(206)*. It is still unclear whether low levels are expressed in latently infected hematopoietic cells *(100,206)*. v-IRF could be involved in evasion of immune responses of lytic infected cells by repressing cellular IFN-mediated signal transduction.

V-BCL-2

HHV-8 encodes a gene (ORF 16) with sequence similarity to cellular *bcl-2*, as do EBV and HVS *(209,210)*. The heterodimerization of cellular *bcl-2* with *bax* is important in overcoming *bax*-mediated apoptosis *(211)*. Whether HHV-8–*bcl-2* dimerizes with *bcl-2* family members in vivo is not yet clear *(209,210)*, although HHV-8–bcl-2 can overcome *bax*-mediated apoptosis. HHV-8–bcl-2 appears to be expressed only during lytic infection *(160)*, suggesting that this viral protein is expressed to prolong cell survival during lytic infection, until complete virions are released from the cell.

VIRAL PROPAGATION

In culture, HHV-8 is difficult to propagate. Only a few cells, including B cells *(96,212)*, endothelial cells *(213,214)*, and 293 cells *(214,215)*, support lytic infection, but not very efficiently. All currently available KS cell lines are negative for HHV-8 *(216)*. HHV-8-infected endothelial cells have a prolonged survival and grow in soft agar *(217)*. Although this suggests that HHV-8 induces transformation of these infected cells, only a fraction of cells in culture appear to be infected, implying that HHV-8 affects the growth of the surrounding uninfected cells via paracrine mechanisms *(217)*. There is no precedent for an oncogenic virus to transform cells in this manner. HHV-8 might not be a transforming virus in the classical sense.

HHV-8 IMMUNITY AND TREATMENT

The introduction of aggressive anti-HIV therapies has led to a decline in the incidence of KS in AIDS patients and also in the resolution of KS in those already affected *(218)*. This suggests that cellular immune responses, compromised in AIDS but recovering after highly active antiretroviral therapy (HAART), could be important in the control of HHV-8 infection and in the development of KS.

Like EBV, HHV-8 probably establishes a persistent infection that is normally controlled by the immune system, and the number of HHV-8-infected cells probably is under immunologic control. When this immune control declines due to acquired or iatrogenic immunosuppression, the number of HHV-8-infected cells increases with subsequent unchecked proliferation of virally infected cells and development of HHV-8-related tumors.

HHV-8, like other herpesviruses, is able to elicit HLA class I restricted cytotoxic T-cell (CTL) responses *(219)*. In particular, CTLs against HHV-8 proteins (K1, K8.1, and K12) without homology to EBV proteins have been found, thereby excluding cross-reactivity of CTLs with EBV.

K8.1 is a 228-amino-acid viral glycoprotein expressed during lytic viral replication *(116,220)*. K8.1 is highly immunogenic and therefore useful in measuring humoral immunity against HHV-8 *(116)*. K8.1 has no overt amino acid sequence similarity with any viral or cellular sequence currently available in databases. K8.1 localizes on the surface of cells and virions. The ORF in EBV that shares genomic position and orientation with K8.1 encodes gp350/220, which is known to bind to CR2 (CD21) on host cells *(221)*. K8.1 is involved in HHV-8 binding to cells *(220)*. gp350/220 of EBV evokes powerful humoral immune responses and is indeed being investigated as an EBV vaccine *(222)*.

CTL restricted by the HLA molecules HLA-A2, -A3, -B7, and -B8 were all shown to recognize at least one of these three HHV-8 proteins. HLA alleles were found to present epitopes from more than one viral protein. For example, HLA-A2 and -A3 restricted epitopes were demonstrated in K8.1 and K12, and HLA-B8 presented all three proteins. This suggests a broad repertoire of CTL responses to HHV-8 as seen in other viral infections.

In one pilot study, HHV-8-specific CTL responses were not present in most patients with KS, indicating that a decline in cellular immune responses against HHV-8 may be present in HIV-positive patients with KS and could contribute to KS pathogenesis *(219)*. This would be reminiscent of the lack of EBV-specific CTLs seen in immunosuppressed patients that correlates with the onset of EBV-driven lymphoproliferation.

The fact that in posttransplant KS, the lesions can regress when immunosuppressive therapy is stopped further suggests that immunosurveillance plays an important role in the maintenance of these lesions. It remains to be seen whether adoptive immunotherapy with cytotoxic T cells directed against HHV-8-encoded proteins will play a future role in the management of HHV-8-associated tumors.

KS is a complex tumor, and various immune responses could be involved in its pathogenesis *(223)*. The rapid resolution of KS in some HIV-positive patients started on HAART suggests that a small improvement in immunity might be important in disease control. CD4+ T helper responses, natural killer (NK), and leukocyte-activated killer cells (LAK) also could be involved to control the growth of HHV-8-positive cells. The rapid decline in viral load of HIV itself has also been suggested to play a role in the response of KS lesions to HAART *(223)*.

In vitro, HHV-8 replication is insensitive to ganciclovir and acyclovir, but is moderately sensitive to foscarnet (phosphonoacetic acid) and sensitive to cidofovir *(224)*. As these agents target lytic herpesviral infection, if lytic infection is necessary to drive tumor formation or to recruit inflammatory cells to form KS lesions, these drugs might prove useful in the future to manage KS. Foscarnet has been shown to induce KS lesion regression in one small study *(225)* and to reduce the onset of KS in other studies *(226,227)*. Foscarnet and cidofovir are, however, associated with significant toxicity and would seem to be inappropriate therapy for most KS patients. More recently and more encouraging, despite low in vitro sensitivity, intravenous or high-dose (4.5 g/d) oral ganciclovir reduced the occurrence of KS by 75% or more in a placebo-controlled randomized clinical trial *(228)*.

The complex histology and expression pattern of HHV-8 proteins in KS suggest that the role of HHV-8 in KS pathogenesis is not straightforward and the model of KS tumorigenesis might not be like any other viral induced malignancy *(229)*. A causal role for HHV-8 in immunoblastic CD and PEL also has not been confirmed. Sero- and molecular epidemiologic studies have shown that HHV-8 is the infective cause of KS, and molecular studies support a causal role for HHV-8 in the pathogenesis of immunoblastic CD and PEL. However, very little regarding the mechanisms of HHV-8-induced tumorigenesis is currently known.

ACKNOWLEDGMENT

The author's studies are supported by the Cancer Research Campaign, the Medical Research Council, and Glaxo Wellcome.

REFERENCES

1. Ziegler JL, Newton R, Katongole-Mbidde E, et al. Risk factors for Kaposi's sarcoma in HIV positive subjects in Uganda. AIDS 1997; 11:1619–1626.
2. Kaposi M. Idiopathisches multiples pigmentsarcom der haut. Arch Dermatol und Syphillis 1872; 4:265–273.
3. Franceschi S, Geddes M. Epidemiology of classic Kaposi's sarcoma, with special reference to Mediterranean population. Tumori 1995; 81:308–314.
4. Oettle AG. Geographic and racial differences in the frequency of Kaposi's sarcoma as evidence of environmental or genetic causes. In: Ackerman LV, Murray JF (eds). Symposium on Kaposi's sarcoma. Basel: Karger, 1962.
5. Bayley AC. Aggressive Kaposi's sarcoma in Zambia. Lancet 1984; i:1318.
6. Wabinga HR, Parkin DM, Wabwire-Mangen F, Mugerwa JW. Cancer in Kampala, Uganda in 1989–91: changes in incidence in the era of AIDS. Int J Cancer 1993; 54:23–36.
7. Ziegler JL, Katongole Mbidde E. Kaposi's sarcoma in childhood: an analysis of 100 cases from Uganda and relationship to HIV infection. Int J Cancer 1996; 65:200–203.
8. Penn I. Kaposi's sarcoma in immuno-suppressed patients. J Clin Lab Immunol 1983; 12:1–10.
9. Penn I. Kaposi's sarcoma in organ transplant recipients: report of 20 cases. Transplantation 1997; 27:8–11.
10. Service PH. Kaposi's sarcoma and *Pneumocystis* pneumonia among homosexual men in New York City and California. MMWR 1981; 30:305–308.
11. Nickoloff BJ, Griffiths CE. The spindle-shaped cells in cutaneous Kaposi's sarcoma. Histologic simulators include factor XIIIa dermal dendrocytes. Am J Pathol 1989; 135:793–800.
12. Sturzl M, Brandstetter H, Roth WK. Kaposi's sarcoma: a review of gene expression and ultrastructure of KS spindle cells in vivo. AIDS Res Hum Retrovir 1992; 8:1753–1764.
13. Browning PJ, Sechler JM, Kaplan M, et al. Identification and culture of Kaposi's sarcoma-like spindle cells from the peripheral blood of human immunodeficiency virus-1-infected individuals and normal controls. Blood 1994; 84:2711–2720.

14. Sirianni MC, Uccini S, Angeloni A, Faggioni A, Cottoni F, Ensoli B. Circulating spindle cells: correlation with human herpesvirus-8 (HHV-8) infection and Kaposi's sarcoma. Lancet 1997; 349:255.

15. Jussila L, Valtola R, Partanen TA, et al. Lymphatic endothelium and Kaposi's sarcoma spindle cells detected by antibodies against the vascular endothelial growth factor receptor-3. Cancer Res 1998,58:1599–1604.

16. Dupin N, Fisher C, Kellam P, et al. Distribution of HHV-8 positive cells in Kaposi's sarcoma, multicentric Castleman's disease, and primary effusion lymphoma. Proc Natl Acad Sci USA 1999; 96:4546–4551.

17. Risau W. Mechanisms of angiogenesis. Nature 1997; 386:671–674.

18. Rabkin CS, Bedi G, Musaba E, Biggar RJ. AIDS-related Kaposi's sarcoma is a clonal neoplasm. N Engl J Med 1995; 1:257–260.

19. Rabkin CS, Janz S, Lash A, et al. Monoclonal origin of multicentric Kaposi's sarcoma lesions. N Engl J Med 1997; 336:988–993.

20. Delabesse E, Oksenhendler E, Lebbe C, Verola O, Varet B, Turhan AG. Molecular analysis of clonality in Kaposi's sarcoma. J Clin Pathol 1997; 50:664–668.

21. Gill P, Tsai YC, Rao AP, et al. Evidence for multiclonality in multicentric Kaposi's sarcoma. Proc Natl Acad Sci 1998; 95:8257–8261.

22. Samaniego F, Markham PD, Gallo RC, Ensoli B. Inflammatory cytokines induce AIDS-Kaposi's sarcoma-derived spindle cells to produce and release basic fibroblast growth factor and enhance Kaposi's sarcoma-like lesion formation in nude mice. J Immunol 1995; 154:3582–3592.

23. Salahuddin SZ, Nakamura S, Biberfeld P, et al. Angiogenic properties of Kaposi's sarcoma-derived cells after long-term culture in vitro. Science 1988; 242:430–433.

24. Nair BC, DeVico AL, Nakamura S, et al. Identification of a major growth factor for AIDS-Kaposi's sarcoma cells as oncostatin M. Science 1992; 255:1430–1432.

25. Miles SA, Rezai AR, SalazarGonzalez JF, et al. AIDS Kaposi sarcoma-derived cells produce and respond to interleukin 6. Proc Natl Acad Sci USA 1990; 87:4068–4072.

26. Ensoli B, Salahuddin SZ, Gallo RC. AIDS-associated Kaposi's sarcoma: a molecular model for its pathogenesis. Cancer Cells 1989; 1:93–96.

27. Ensoli B, Gendelman R, Markham P, et al. Synergy between basic fibroblast growth factor and HIV-1 Tat protein in induction of Kaposi's sarcoma. Nature 1994; 371:674–680.

28. Fiorelli V, Gendelman R, Sirianni MC, et al. Gamma-interferon produced by CD8+ T cells infiltrating Kaposi's sarcoma induces spindle cells with angiogenic phenotype and synergy with human immunodeficiency virus-1 Tat protein: an immune response to human herpesvirus-8 infection Blood 1998; 91:956–967.

29. Vaishnaw YN, Wong-Staal F. The biochemistry of AIDS. Annu Rev Biochem 1991; 60:577–630.

30. Frankel AD, Pabo CO. Cellular uptake of the Tat protein from human immunodeficiency virus. Cell 1988; 55:1189–1193.

31. Ensoli B, Buonaguro L, Barillari G, et al. Release, uptake, and effects of extracellular human immunodeficiency virus type 1 Tat protein on cell growth and viral transactivation. J Virol 1993; 67:277–287.

32. Albini A, Barillari G, Benelli R, Gallo RC, Ensoli B. Angiogenic properties of human immunodeficiency virus type 1 Tat protein. Proc Natl Acad Sci USA 1995; 92:4838–4842.

33. Vogel J, Hinrichs SH, Reynolds RK, Luciw PA, Jay G. The HIV tat gene induces dermal lesions resembling Kaposi's sarcoma in transgenic mice. Nature 1988; 335:606–611.

34. Albini A, Benelli R, Presta M, et al. HIV-Tat protein is a heparin-binding angiogenic growth factor. Oncogene 1996; 12:289–297.

35. Albini A, Soldi R, Giunciuglio D, et al. The angiogenesis induced by HIV-1 Tat protein is mediated by the Flk-1/KDR receptor on vascular endothelial cells. Nat Med 1997; 2:1371–1375.

36. Barnett SW, Murthy KK, Herndier BG, Levy JA. An AIDS-like condition induced in baboons by HIV-2. Science 1994; 266:642–646.

37. Beral V, Peterman TA, Berkelman RL, Jaffe HW. Kaposi's sarcoma among persons with AIDS: a sexually transmitted infection Lancet 1990; 335:123–128.

38. Beral V. Epidemiology of Kaposi's sarcoma. In: Beral V, Jaffe HW, Weiss RA (eds). Cancer, HIV and AIDS, Vol. 10. New York: Cold Spring Harbor Laboratory Press, 1991:5–22.

39. Giraldo G, Beth E, Hagenau F. Herpes-type virus particles in tissue culture of Kaposi's sarcoma from different geographic regions. J Natl Cancer Inst 1972; 49:1509–1526.

40. Giraldo G, Kourilsky FM, Henle W, et al. Antibody patterns to herpesviruses in Kaposi's sarcoma: serological association of European Kaposi's sarcoma with cytomegalovirus. Int J Cancer 1975; 15:839–848.

41. Monini P, Rotola A, de Lellis, L. et al. Latent BK virus infection and Kaposi's sarcoma pathogenesis. Int J Cancer 1996; 66:717–722.

42. Rappersberger K, Tschachler E, Zonzits E, et al. Endemic Kaposi's sarcoma in human immunodeficiency virus type 1- seronegative persons: demonstration of retrovirus-like particles in cutaneous lesions. J Invest Dermatol 1990; 95:371–381.

43. Huang YQ, Li JJ, Rush MG, et al. HPV-16-related DNA sequences in Kaposi's sarcoma. Lancet 1992; 339:515–518.

44. Kempf W, Adams V, Pfaltz M, et al. Human herpesvirus type 6 and cytomegalovirus in AIDS-associated Kaposi's sarcoma: no evidence for an etiological association. Hum Pathol 1995; 26:914–919.

45. Chang Y, Cesarman E, Pessin MS, et al. Identification of herpesvirus-like DNA sequences in AIDS-associated Kaposi's sarcoma. Science 1994; 266:1865–1869.

46. Lisitsyn N, Lisitsyn N, Wigler M. Cloning the differences between two complex genomes. Science 1993; 259:946–951.

47. Lisitsyn NA, Lisitsina NM, Dalbagni G, et al. Comparative genomic analysis of tumors: detection of DNA losses and amplification. Proc Natl Acad Sci USA 1995; 92:151–155.

48. Roizman B. The family herpesviridae: a brief introduction. In: Roizman B, Whitley RJ, Lopez C (eds). The Human Herpesviruses. New York: Raven Press, 1993, pp. 1–9.

49. Adams V, Kempf W, Schmid M, Muller B, Briner J, Burg G. Absence of herpesvirus-like DNA sequences in skin cancers of non-immunosuppressed patients. Lancet 1995; 346:1715.

50. Lin BTY, Chen YY, Battifora H, Weiss LM. Absence of Kaposi's sarcoma-associated herpesvirus-like DNA sequences in malignant vascular tumors of the serous membranes. Mod Pathol 1996; 9:1143–1146.

51. Boshoff C, Talbot S, Kennedy M, O'Leary J, Schulz T, Chang Y. HHV8 and skin cancers in immunosuppressed patients. Lancet 1996; 348:138.

52. Uthman A, Brna C, Weninger W, Tschachler E. No HHV8 in non-Kaposi's sarcoma mucocutaneous lesions from immunodeficient HIV-positive patients. Lancet 1996; 347:1700–1701.

53. Moore PS, Kingsley LA, Holmberg SD, et al. Kaposi's sarcoma-associated herpesvirus infection prior to onset of Kaposi's sarcoma. AIDS 1996; 10:175–180.

54. Whitby D, Howard MR, Tenant Flowers M, et al. Detection of Kaposi sarcoma associated herpesvirus in peripheral blood of HIV-infected individuals and progression to Kaposi's sarcoma. Lancet 1995; 346:799–802.

55. Boshoff C, Schulz TF, Kennedy MM, et al. Kaposi's sarcoma-associated herpesvirus infects endothelial and spindle cells. Nat Med 1995; 1:1274–1278.

56. Li JJ, Huang YQ, Cockerell CJ, Friedman Kien AE. Localization of human herpes-like virus type 8 in vascular endothelial cells and perivascular spindle-shaped cells of Kaposi's sarcoma lesions by in situ hybridization. Am J Pathol 1996; 148:1741–1748.

57. Staskus KA, Zhong W, Gebhard K, et al. Kaposi's sarcoma-associated herpesvirus gene expression in endothelial (spindle) tumor cells. J Virol 1997; 71:715–719.

58. Davis MA, Sturzl MA, Blasig C, et al. Expression of human herpesvirus 8-encoded cyclin D in Kaposi's sarcoma spindle cells. J Natl Cancer Inst 1997; 89:1829–1831.

59. Rainbow L, Platt GM, Simpson GR, et al. The 222-234 kd nuclear protein (LNA) of Kaposi's sarcoma-associated herpesvirus (human herpesvirus 8) is encoded by orf 73 and a component of the latency-associated nuclear antigen. J Virol 1997; 71:5915–5921.

60. Sturzl M, Blasig C, Schreier A, et al. Expression of HHV-8 latency-associated T0.7 RNA in spindle cells and endothelial cells of AIDS-asssiated, classical and African Kaposi's sarcoma (KS). Int J Cancer 1997; 72:68–71.

61. Kellam P, Bourboulia D, Dupin N, Talbot S, Boshoff C, Weiss RA. Characterising monoclonal antibodies against KSHV latent nuclear antigen (LNA-1). J Virol 1999, 73:5149–5155.

62. Castleman B, Iverson L, Menendez VP. Localized mediastinal lymph-node hyperplasia resembling thymoma. Cancer 1956; 9:822–830.

63. Keller AR, Hochholzer L, Castleman B. Hyaline-vascular and plasma cell types of giant lymph node hyperplasia of the mediastinim and other locations. Cancer 1972; 29:670–683.

64. Frizzera G, Massarelli G, Banks PM, Rosai J. A systemic lymphoproliferative disorder with morphologic features of Castleman's disease. Am J Surg Pathol 1983; 7:211–231.

65. Herrada J, Cabanillas F, Rice L, Manning J, Pugh W. The clinical behavior of localized and multicentric Castleman's disease. Ann Intern Med 1998; 128:657–662.

66. Abdel-Reheim FA, Koss W, Rappaport ES, Arber DA. Coexistence of Hodgkin's disease and giant lymph node hyperplasia of the plasma-cell type (Castleman's disease). Arch Pathol Lab Med 1996; 120.

67. Frizzera G. Castleman's disease and related disorders. Semin Diagn Pathol 1988; 5:346–364.

68. Weisenburger DD, Nathwani BN, Winberg CD, Rappaport H. Multicentric angiofollicular lymph node hyperplasia: a clinicopathologic study of 16 cases. Hum Pathol 1985; 16:162–172.

69. Oksenhendler E, Duarte M, Soulier J, et al. Multicentric Castleman's disease in HIV infection: a clinical and pathological study of 20 patients. AIDS 1996; 10:61–67.

70. Soulier J, Grollet L, Oksenhendler E, et al. Kaposi's sarcoma-associated herpesvirus-like DNA sequences in multicentric Castleman's disease. Blood 1995; 86:1276–1280.

71. Barozzi P, Luppi M, Masini L, et al. Lymphotropic herpes virus (EBV, HHV-6, HHV-8) DNA sequences in HIV negative Castleman's disease. J Clin Pathol Mol Pathol 1996; 49:M232–M235.

72. Corbellino M, Poirel L, Aubin JT, et al. The role of human herpesvirus 8 and Epstein-Barr virus in the pathogenesis of giant lymph node hyperplasia (Castleman's disease). Clin Infect Dis 1996; 22:1120–1121.

73. Parravicini C, Corbellino M, Paulli M, et al. Expression of a virus-derived cytokine, KSHV vIL-6, in HIV seronegative Castleman's disease. Am J Pathol 1998; 6:1517–1522.

74. Dupin N, Diss T, Kellam P, et al. HHV-8 is associated with a plasmablastic variant of Castleman's disease that is linked to HHV-8 positive plasmablastic lymphoma. Blood 2000; 95, in press.

75. Chadburn A, Cesarman E, Nador RG, Liu YF, Knowles DM. Kaposi's sarcoma-associated herpesvirus sequences in benign lymphoid proliferations not associated with human immunodeficiency virus. Cancer 1997; 80:788–797.

76. Knowles DM, Inghirami G, Ubriaco A, Dalla-Favera R. Molecular genetic analysis of three AIDS-associated neoplasms of uncertain lineage demonstrates their B-cell derivation and the possible pathogenetic role of the Epstein–Barr virus. Blood 1989; 73:792–799.

77. Walts AE, Shintaku P, Said JW. Diagnosis of malignant lymphoma in effusions from patients with AIDS by gene rearrangement. Am J Clin Pathol 1990; 194:170–175.

78. Karcher DS, Dawkins F, Garrett CT. Body cavity-based non-Hodgkin's lymphoma (NHL) in HIV-infected patients: B-cell lymphoma with unusual clinical, immunophenotypic, and genotypic features. Lab Invest 1992; 92:80a.

79. Cesarman E, Chang Y, Moore PS, Said JW, Knowles DM. Kaposi's sarcoma-associated herpesvirus-like DNA sequences in AIDS-related body-cavity-based lymphomas. N Engl J Med 1995; 332:1186–1191.

80. Komanduri KV, Luce JA, McGrath MS, Herndier BG, Ng VL. The natural history and molecular heterogeneity of HIV-associated primary malignant lymphomatous effusions. J Acquir Immune Defic Syndr Hum Retrovirol 1996; 13:215–226.

81. Nador RG, Cesarman E, Chadburn A, et al. Primary effusion lymphoma: a distinct clinicopathologic entity associated with the Kaposi's sarcoma-associated herpes virus. Blood 1996; 88:645–656.

82. Strauchen JA, Hauser AD, Burstein DA, Jimenez R, Moore PS, Chang Y. Body cavity-based malignant lymphoma containing Kaposi's sarcoma-associated herpesvirus in an HIV-negative man with previous Kaposi's sarcoma. Ann Intern Med 1997; 125:822–825.

83. Said JW, Tasaka T, Takeuchi S, et al. Primary effusion lymphoma in women: report of two cases of Kaposi's sarcoma herpes virus-associated effusion-based lymphoma in human immunodeficiency virus-negative women. Blood 1996; 88:3124–3128.

84. Jaffe ES. Primary body cavity-based AIDS-related lymphomas. Am J Pathol 1996; 105:141–143.

85. Ansari MQ, Dawson DB, Nador R, et al. Primary body cavity-based AIDS-related lymphomas. Am J Clin Pathol 1996; 105:221–229.

86. Cesarman E, Nador RG, Aozasa K, Delsol G, Said JW, Knowles DM. Kaposi's sarcoma-associated herpesvirus in non-AIDS-related lymphomas occuring in body cavities. Am J Pathol 1996; 149:53–57.

87. Boshoff C, Gao S-J, Healy LE, et al. Establishment of a KSHV positive cell line (BCP-1) from peripheral blood and characterizing its growth in vivo. Blood 1998; 91:1671–1679.

88. Otsuki T, Kumar S, Ensoli B, et al. Detection of HHV-8/KSHV DNA sequences in AIDS-associated extranodal lymphoid malignancies. Leukemia 1996; 10:1358–1362.

89. Carbone A, Gloghini A, Vaccher E, et al. Kaposi's sarcoma-associated herpesvirus DNA sequences in AIDS-related and AIDS-unrelated lymphomatous effusions. Br J Haematol 1996; 94:533–543.

90. Nador RG, Cesarman E, Knowles DM, Said JW. Herpesvirus-like DNA sequences in a body-cavity-based lymphoma in an HIV-negative patient. N Engl J Med 1995; 333:943.

91. Cesarman E, Moore PS, Rao PH, Inghirami G, Knowles DM, Chang Y. In vitro establishment and characterization of two acquired immunodeficiency syndrome-related lymphoma cell lines (BC-1 and BC-2) containing Kaposi's sarcoma-associated herpesvirus-like (KSHV) DNA sequences. Blood 1995; 86:2708–14.

92. Renne R, Zhong W, Herndier B, et al. Lytic growth of Kaposi's sarcoma-associated herpesvirus (human herpesvirus 8) in culture. Nat Med 1996; 2:342–346.

93. Arvanitakis L, Mesri EA, Nador RG, et al. Establishment and characterization of a primary effusion (body cavity-based) lymphoma cell line (BC-3) harboring Kaposi's sarcoma- associated herpesvirus (KSHV/HHV-8) in the absence of Epstein–Barr virus. Blood 1996; 88:2648–2654.

94. Gaidano G, Cechova K, Chang Y, Moore PS, Knowles DM, Dalla Favera R. Establishment of AIDS-related lymphoma cell lines from lymphomatous effusions. Leukemia 1996; 10:1237–1240.

95. Horenstein MG, Nador RG, Chadburn A, et al. Epstein–Barr virus latent gene expression in primary effusion lymphomas containing Kaposi's sarcoma-associated herpesvirus/human herpesvirus-8. Blood 1997; 90:1186–1191.

96. Moore PS, Gao SJ, Dominguez G, et al. Primary characterization of a herpesvirus agent associated with Kaposi's sarcoma. J Virol 1996; 70:549–558.

97. Di Alberti L, Piattelli A, Artese L, et al. Human herpesvirus 8 variants in sarcoid tissues. Lancet 1997; 350:1655–1661.

98. Rettig MB, Ma HJ, Vescio RA, et al. Kaposi's sarcoma associated herpesvirus infection of bone marrow dendritic cells from multiple myeloma. Science 1997; 276:1851–1854.

99. Said JW, Rettig MR, Heppner K, et al. Localisation of Kaposi's sarcoma-associated herpesvirus in bone marrow biopsy samples from patients with multiple myeloma. Blood 1998; 90:4278–4282.

100. Moore PS, Boshoff C, Weiss RA, Chang Y. Molecular mimicry of human cytokine and cytokine response pathway genes by KSHV. Science 1996; 274:1739–1744.

101. Burger R, Neipel F, Fleckenstein B, et al. Human herpesvirus type 8 interleukin-6 homologue is functionally active on human myeloma cells. Blood 1998; 91:1858–1863.

102. Parravicini C, Lauri E, Baldini L, et al. Kaposi's sarcoma-associated herpesvirus infection and multiple myeloma. Science 1997; 278:1969.

103. Masood R, Zheng T, Tulpule A, et al. Kaposi's sarcoma-associated herpesvirus infection and multiple myeloma. Science 1997; 278:1969–1970.

104. MacKenzie J, Sheldon J, Morhan G, Cook G, Schulz TF, Jarrett RF. HHV-8 and multiple myeloma in the U. K. Lancet 1997; 350:1144–1145.

105. Marcelin A-G, Dupin N, Bouscary D, et al. HHV-8 and multiple myeloma in France. Lancet 1997; 350:1144.

106. Cull GM, Timms JH, Haynes AP, et al. Dendritic cells cultured from mononuclear cells and CD34 cells in myeloma do not harbour human herpesvirus 8. Br J Haematol 1998; 100:793–796.

107. Whitby D, Boshoff C, Luppi M, Torelli G. Kaposi's sarcoma-associated herpesvirus infection and multiple myeloma. Science 1997; 278:1971–1972.

108. Tarte K, Olsen SJ, Yang Lu Z, et al. Clinical grade functional dendritic cells from patients with multiple myeloma are not infected with Kaposi's sarcoma-associated herpesvirus. Blood 1998; 91:1852–1857.

109. Luppi M, Barrozi P, Maiorana A, et al. Human herpesvirus-8 DNA sequences in human immunodeficiency virus-negative angioimmunoblastic lymphadenopathy and benighn lymphadenopathy with giant germinal center hyperplasia and increased vascularity. Blood 1996; 87:3903–3909.

110. Gao SJ, Kingsley L, Li M, et al. KSHV antibodies among Americans, Italians and Ugandans with and without Kaposi's sarcoma. Nat Med 1996; 2:925–928.

111. Kedes DH, Operskalski E, Busch M, Kohn R, Flood J, Ganem D. The seroepidemiology of human herpesvirus 8 (Kaposi's sarcoma-associated herpesvirus): distribution of infection in KS risk groups and evidence for sexual transmission. Nat Med 1996; 2:918–924.

112. Simpson GR, Schulz TF, Whitby D, et al. Prevalence of Kaposi's sarcoma associated herpesvirus infection measured by antibodies to recombinant capsid protein and latent immunofluorescence antigen. Lancet 1996; 348:1133–1138.

113. Chatlynne LG, Lapps W, Handy M, et al Detection and titration of human herpesvirus-8-specific antibodies on sera from blood donors, acquired immunodeficiency syndrome patients, and Kaposi's sarcoma patients using a whole virus enzyme-linked immunosorbent assay. Blood 1998; 92:53–58.

114. Davis DA, Humphrey RW, Newcomb FM, et al. Detection of serum antibodies to a Kaposi's sarcoma-associated herpesvirus specific peptide. J Infect Dis 1997; 175:1071–1079.

115. Chandran B, Smith MS, Koelle DM, Corey L, Horvat R, Goldstein E. Reativities of human sera with human herpesvirus-8 infected BCBL-1 cells and identification of HHV-8-specific proteins and glycoproteins and the encoding cDNAs. Virology 1998; 243:208–217.

116. Raab M-S, Albrecht J-C, Birkmann A, et al. The immunogenic glycoprotein gp35-37 of human herpesvirus 8 is encoded by open reading K8.1. J Virol 1998; 72:6725–6731.

117. Kellam P, Boshoff C, Whitby D, Matthews S, Weiss RA, Talbot SJ. Identification of a major latent nuclear antigen (LNA-1) in the human herpesvirus 8 (HHV-8) genome. J Hum Virol 1997; 1:19–29.

118. Kedes DH, Lagunoff M, Renne R, Ganem D. Identification of the gene encoding the major latency-associated nuclear antigen of the Kaposi's sarcoma-associated herpesvirus. J Clin Invest 1997; 100:2606–2610.

119. Zhu L, Wang R, Sweat A, Goldstein E, Horvat R, Chandran B. Comparison of human sera reactivities in immunoblots with recombinant human herpesvirus (HHV)-8 proteins associated with the latent (ORF73) and lytic (ORFs 65, K8.1A, K8.1B) replicative cycles and in immunofluorescence assays with HHV-8-infected BCBL-1 cells. Virology 1999; 256:381–392.

120. Lennette ET, Blackbourn DJ, Levy JA. Antibodies to human herpesvirus type 8 in the general population and in Kaposi's sarcoma patients. Lancet 1996; 348:858–61.

121. Kedes DH, Ganem D, Ameli N, Bacchetti P, Greenblatt R. The prevalence of serum antibody to human herpesvirus 8 (Kaposi sarcoma-associated herpesvirus) among HIV-seropositive and high-risk HIV-seronegative women. JAMA 1997; 277:478–481.

122. Martin JN, Ganem DE, Osmond DH, Page-Shafer KA, Macrae D, Kedes DH. Sexual transmission and the natural history of human herpesvirus 8 infection. N Engl J Med 1998; 338:948–954.

123. Smith N, Sabin CA, Bourboulia D, et al. Serologic Evidence of Human Herpesvirus 8 transmission by homosexual but not heterosexual sex. J Infect Dis 1999; 480:600–606.

124. Geddes M, Franceschi S, Balzi D, Arniani S, Gafa L, Zanetti R. Birthplace and classic Kaposi's sarcoma in Italy. J Natl Cancer Inst 1995; 87:1015–1017.

125. Whitby D, Luppi M, Barozzi P, Boshoff C, Weiss RA, Torelli G. HHV-8 seroprevalence in blood donors and lymphoma patients from different regions of Italy. J Natl Can Inst 1998; 90:395–397.

126. Cattani P, Capuano M, Cerimele F, et al. Human herpesvirus 8 seroprevalence and evaluation of nonsexual transmission routes by detection of DNA in clinical specimens fom human immunodeficiency virus-seronegative patients from central and southern Italy, with and without Kaposi's sarcoma. J Clin Microbiol 1999; 37:1150–1153.

127. Calabro ML, Sheldon J, Favero A, et al. Seroprevalence of Kaposi's sarcoma-associated herpesvirus/human herpesvirus 8 in several regions in Italy. J Hum Virol 1998; 1:207–213.

128. de-The G, Geser A, Day NE, et al. Epidemiological evidence for causal relationship between Epstein-Barr virus and Burkitt's lymphoma from Ugandan prospective study. Nature 1978; 274:756–761.

129. de-The G, Lavoue MF, Muenz L. Differences in EBV antibody titres of patients with nasopharyngeal carcinoma originating from high, intermediate and low incidence areas. IARC Sci Publ 1978; 20:471–481.

130. Iscovich J, Bofetta P, Winkelmann R, Brennan P, Azizi E. Classic Kaposi's sarcoma in Jews living in Israel, 1961–1989: a population-based incidence study. AIDS 1998; 12:2067–2072.

131. Davidivici B, Karakis I, Bourboulea D, Ariad S, Sarov B, Boshoff C. The seroepidemiology of HHV-8 among Israeli Jews. 2000, unpublished.

132. Gao SJ, Kingsley L, Li M, et al. KSHV antibodies among Americans, Italians and Ugandans with and without Kaposi's sarcoma. Nat Med 1996; 2:925–928.

133. Ariyoshi K, Schim van der Loeff M, Cook P, et al. Kaposi's sarcoma in the Gambia, West Africa is less frequent in human immunodeficiency virus type 2 than in human immunodeficiency virus type 1 infection despite a high prevalence of human herpesvirus 8. J Hum Virol 1998; 1:192–199.

134. Olsen S, Chang Y, Moore P, Biggar R, Melbye M. Increasing Kaposi's sarcoma-associated herpesvirus seroprevalence with age in a highly Kaposi's sarcoma endemic region, Zambia in 1985. AIDS 1998; 12:1921–1925.

135. Sitas F, Carrara H, Beral V, et al. Antibodies against human herpesvirus-8 in black South African patients with cancer. NEJM 1999; 340:1863–1871.

136. Bourboulia D, Whitby D, Boshoff C, et al. Serological evidence for vertical transmission of KSHV/HHV-8 in healthy South African children. JAMA 1998; 280:31–32.

137. He J, Bhat G, Kankasa C, et al. Seroprevalence of human herpesvirus 8 among Zambian women of childbearing age without Kaposi's sarcoma (KS) and mother-child pairs with KS. J Infect Dis 1998; 178:1787–1790.

138. Gessain A, Mauclere P, van Beveren M, et al. Human herpesvirus 8 primary infection ocurs during childhood in Cameroon, Central Africa. Int J Cancer 1999; 81:189–192.

139. Mayama S, Cuevas LE, Sheldon J, et al. Prevalence and transmission of Kaposi's sarcoma-associated herpesvirus (human herpesvirus-8) in Ugandan children and adolescents. Int J Cancer 1998; 11:817–820.

140. Plancoulaine S, Abel L, van Beveren M, et al. Natural history of human herpesvirus 8 infection in an endemic population: evidence for mother-child and sib-sib transmission, but not for heterosexual transmission. 2000, in press.

141. Monini P, de Lellis L, Fabris M, Rigolin F, Cassai E. Kaposi's sarcoma-associated herpesvirus DNA sequences in prostate tissue and human semen. N Engl J Med 1996; 334:1168–1172.

142. Ambroziak JA, Blackbourn DJ, Herndier BG, et al. Herpes-like sequences in HIV-infected and uninfected Kaposi's sarcoma patients. Science 1995; 268:582–583.

143. Corbellino M, Bestetti G, Galli M, Parravicini C. Absence of HHV-8 in prostate and semen. N Engl J Med 1996; 335:1237.

144. Viviano E, Vitale F, Ajello F, et al. Human herpesvirus type 8 DNA sequences in biological samples of HIV-positive and negative individuals in Sicily. AIDS 1997; 11:607–612.

145. Tasaka T, Said JW, Koeffler HP. Absence of HHV-8 in prostate and semen. N Engl J Med 1996; 335:1237–1238.

146. Howard MR, Whitby D, Bahadur G, et al. Detection of human herpesvirus 8 DNA in semen from HIV-infected individuals but not healthy semen donors. AIDS 1997; 11:F15–F19.

147. Lin J-C, Lin S-C, Mar E-C, et al. Retraction: is KSHV in semen of HIV-infected homosexual men? Lancet 1998; 351:1365.

148. Daimond C, Brodie SJ, Krieger JN, et al. Human herpesvirus 8 in the prostate glands of men with Kaposi's sarcoma. J Virol 1998; 72:6223–6227.

149. Koelle DM, Huang M-L, Chandran B, Vieira j, Piepkorn M, Corey L. Frequent detection of Kaposi's sarcoma-associated herpesvirus (human herpesvirus-8) in saliva of human immunodeficiency virus-infected men: clinical and immunologic correlates. J Infect Dis 1997; 176:94–102.

150. Russo JJ, Bohenzky RA, Chien MC, et al. Nucleotide sequence of the Kaposi sarcoma-associated herpesvirus (HHV8). Proc Natl Acad Sci USA 1996; 93:14862–14867.

151. Neipel F, Albrecht JC, Ensser A, et al. Primary structure of the Kaposi's sarcoma associated human herpesvirus 8. Genbank accession no. U93872, 1997.

152. Lin K, Dai CY, Ricciardi RP. Cloning and functional analysis of Kaposi's sarcoma-associated herpesvirus DNA polymerase and its processivity factor. J Virol 1998; 72:6228–6232.

153. Lagunoff D, Ganem D. The structure and coding organization of the genomic termini of Kaposi's sarcoma-associated herpesvirus (human herpesvirus-8). Virology 1997; 236:147–154.

154. Lee H, Veazey R, Williams K, et al. Deregulation of cell growth by the K1 gene of Kaposi's sarcoma-associated herpesvirus. Nat Med 1998; 4:435–440.

155. Lee H, Guo J, Li M, et al. Identification of an immunoreceptor tyrosine-based activation motif of K1 transforming protein of Kaposi's sarcoma-associated herpesvirus. Mol Cell Biol 1998; 18:5219–5228.

156. Nicholas J, Jian-Chao Z, Alcendor DJ, et al. Novel organizational features, captured cellular genes, and strain variability within the genome of KSHV/HHV-8. J Natl Cancer Inst 1998; 23:79–88.

157. McGeoch DJ, Davidson AJ. The descent of human herpesvirus 8. In: Boshoff C, Weiss R (eds). Seminars in Cancer Biology: Kaposi's Sarcoma-Associated Herpesvirus. London: Academic Press, 1999.

158. Zong J-C, Ciufo DM, Alcendor DJ, et al. High level variability in the ORF-K1 membrane protein gene at the left end of the Kaposi's sarcoma-associated herpesvirus (HHV-8) genome defines four major virus subtypes and multiple clades in different human populations. J Virol 1999; 73:4156–4170.

159. Hayward GS. KSHV strains: the origins and global spread of the virus. In: Boshoff C, Weiss RA (eds). Seminars in Cancer Biology: Kaposi's Sarcoma-Associated Herpesvirus, Vol. 9. London: Academic Press, 1999, pp. 187–199.

160. Sarid R, Flore O, Bohenzky RA, Chang Y, Moore PS. Transcription mapping of the Kaposi's sarcoma-associated herpesvirus (human herpesvirus 8) genome in a body cavity-based lymphoma cell line (BC-1). J Virol 1998; 72:1005–1012.

161. Dittmer D, Lagunoff M, Renne R, Stastus K, Haase A, Ganem D. A cluster of latently expressed genes in Kaposi's sarcoma-associated herpesvirus. J Virol 1998; 72:8309–8315.

162. Sarid R, Wiezorek JS, Moore PS, Chang Y. Characterization and cell cycle regulation of the major Kaposi's sarcoma-associated herpesvirus (human herpesvirus 8) latent genes and their promoter. J Virol 1999; 73:1438–1446.

163. Talbot S, Weiss RA, Kellam P, Boshoff C. Transcriptional analysis of human herpesvirus-8 (HHV-8) open reading frames 71, 72, 73, K14 and 74 in a primary effusion lymphoma cell line. Virology 1999; 257:84–94.

164. Ballestas ME, Chatis PA, Kaye KM. Efficient persistence of extrachromosomal KSHV DNA mediated by latency-associated nuclear antigen. Science 1999; 284:641–644.

165. Godden-Kent D, Talbot SJ, Boshoff C, et al. The cyclin encoded by Kaposi s sarcoma-associated herpesvirus (KSHV) stimulates cdk6 to phosphorylate the retinoblastoma protein and Histone H1. J Virol 1997; 71:4193–4198.

166. Li M, Lee H, Yoon DW, et al. Kaposi's sarcoma-associated herpesvirus encodes a functional cyclin. J Virol 1997; 71:1984–1991.

167. Chang Y, Moore PS, Talbot SJ, et al. Cyclin encoded by KS herpesvirus. Nature 1996; 382:410.

168. Swanton C, Mann DJ, Fleckenstein B, Neipel F, Peters G, Jones N. Herpesviral cyclin/Cdk6 complexes evade inhibition by CDK inhibitor proteins. Nature 1997; 390:184–187.

169. Ellis M, Chew YP, Fallis L, et al. Degradation of p27KIP cdk inhibitor triggered by Kaposi's sarcoma virus cyclin-cdk6 complex. EMBO J 1999; 18:644–653.

170. Sheaff RJ, Groudine M, Gordon M, Roberts JM, Clurman BE. Cyclin E-CDK2 is a regulator of p27Kip1. Genes Dev 1997; 11:1464–1478.

171. Cesarman E, Nador RG, Bai F, et al. Kaposi's sarcoma-associated herpesvirus contains G protein-coupled receptor and cyclin D homologs which are expressed in Kaposi's sarcoma and malignant lymphoma. J Virol 1996; 70:8218–8223.

172. Reed JA, Nador RG, Spaulding D, Tani Y, Cesarman E, Knowles DM. Demonstration of Kaposi's sarcoma-associated herpesvirus cyclin D homolog in cutaneous Kaposi's sarcoma by colorimetric in situ hybridisation using a catalysed signal amplification system. Blood 1998; 91:3825–3832.

173. Skapek SX, Rhee J, Spicer DB, Lassar AB. Inhibition of myogenic differentiation in proliferating myoblasts by cyclin D1-dependent kinase. Science 1995; 267:1022–1024.

174. Jones DL, Alani RM, Munger K. The human papillomavirus E7 oncoprotein can uncouple cellular differentiation and proliferation pathways in human keratinocytes by abrogating p21 Cip1-mediated inhibition of cdk2. Genes Dev 1997; 11:2101–2111.

175. Irmler M, Thome M, Hahne M, et al. Inhibition of death receptor signals by cellular FLIP. Nature 1997; 388:190–195.

176. Bertin J, Armstrong RC, Ottilie S, et al. Death effector domain-containing herpesvirus and poxvirus proteins inhibit both Fas- and TNFR1-induced apoptosis. Proc Natl Acad Sci USA 1997; 94:1172–1176.

177. Thome M, Schneider P, Hofmann K, et al. Viral FLICE-inhibitory proteins (FLIPs) prevent apoptosis induced by death receptors. Nature 1997; 386:517–521.

178. Boldin MP, Varfolomeev EE, Pancer Z, Mett IL, Camonis JH, Wallach D. A novel protein that interacts with the death domain of Fas/APO1 contains a sequence motif related to the death domain. J Biol Chem 1995; 270:7795–7798.

179. Chinnaiyan AM, Tepper CG, Seldin MF, et al. FADD/MORT1 is a common mediator of CD95 (Fas/APO-1) and tumor necrosis factor receptor-induced apoptosis. J Biol Chem 1996; 271:4961–4965.

180. Muzio M, Chinnaiyan AM, Kischkel FC, et al. FLICE, a novel FADD-homologous ICE/CED-3-like protease, is recruited to the CD95 (Fas/APO-1) death-inducing signaling complex. Cell 1996; 85:817–827.

181. Nagata S. Apoptosis by death factor. Cell 1997; 88:355–365.

182. Zhong W, Wang H, Herndier B, Ganem D. Restricted expression of Kaposi sarcoma-associated herpesvirus (human herpesvirus 8) genes in Kaposi sarcoma. Proc Natl Acad Sci USA 1996; 93:6641–6646.

183. Muralidhar S, Pumfery AM, Hassani M, et al. Identification of Kaposin (ORF K12) as a human herpesvirus 8 (Kaposi's sarcoma-associated herpesvirus) transforming gene. J Virol 1998; 72:4980–4988.

184. Boshoff C. Coupling herpesvirus to angiogenesis: viral pirates on a cellular sea. Nature 1998; 391:24–25.

185. Neipel F, Albrecht JC, Ensser A, et al. Human herpesvirus 8 encodes a homolog of interleukin-6. J Virol 1997; 71:839–842.

186. Nicholas J, Ruvolo VR, Burns WH, et al. Kaposi's sarcoma-associated human herpesvirus-8 encodes homologues of macrophage inflammatory protein-1 and interleukin-6. Nat Med 1997; 3:287–292.

187. Molden J, Chang Y, You Y, Moore PS, Goldsmith MA. A Kaposi's sarcoma-associated herpesvirus-encoded cytokine homolog (vIL-6) activates signaling through the shared gp 130 receptor subunit. J Biol Chem 1997; 272:19625–19631.

188. Kledal TN, Rosenkilde MM, Coulin F, et al. A broad spectrum chemokine antagonist encoded by Kaposi's sarcoma-associated herpesvirus. Science 1997; 277:1656–1659.

189. Boshoff C, Endo Y, Collins PD, et al. Angiogenic and HIV inhibitory functions of KSHV-encoded chemokines. Science 1997; 278:290–293.

190. Sallusto F, Mackay CR, Lanzavecchia A. Selective expression of the eotaxin receptor CCR3 by human T helper 2 cells. Science 1997; 277:2005–2007.

191. Sozzani S, Luini W, Bianchi G, et al. The viral chemokine macrophage inflammatory protein-II is a selective Th2 chemoattractant. Blood 1998, 92:4036–4039.

192. Stine J, Wood C, Raport C, et al. The Kaposi's sarcoma-associated herpesvirus chemokine vMIP-III is a functional ligand for CCR4 and a selective chemoattractant for Th2 cells. 2000, unpublished.

193. Liestoel K, Goplen AK, Dunlop O, Bruun JN, Moehlen J. Kaposi's sarcoma and protection from HIV dementia. Science 1998; 280:361–362.

194. Baldeweg T, Catalan J, Gazzard BG, Weiss RA, Boshoff C. Kaposi's sarcoma and protection from HIV dementia. Science 1998; 280:361–362.

195. Arvanitakis L, Geras-Raaka E, Varma A, Gershengorn MC, Cesarman E. Human herpesvirus KSHV encodes a constitutively active G-protein-coupled receptor linked to cell proliferation. Nature 1997; 385:347–349.

196. Bais C, Santomasso B, Coso O, et al. Kaposi's sarcoma associated herpesvirus (KSHV/HHV-8) G protein-coupled receptor is a viral oncogene and angiogenesis activator. Nature 1998; 391:86–89.

197. Alblas J, Van Etten I, Moolenaar WH. Truncated, desensitization-defective neurokinin receptors mediate sustained MAP kinase activation, cell growth and transformation by a Ras-independent mechanism. EMBO J 1996; 15:3351–3360.

198. Coughlin SR. Expanding horizons for receptors coupled to G proteins: diversity and disease. Curr Opin Cell Biol 1994; 6:191–197.

199. Julius D, Livelli TJ, Jessell TM, Axel R. Ectopic expression of the serotonin lc receptor and the triggering of malignant transformation. Science 1989; 244:1057–1062.

200. Milano CA, Allen LF, Rockman HA, et al. Enhanced myocardial function in transgenic mice overexpressing the beta2- adrenergic receptor. Science 1994; 264:582–586.

201. Guo HG, Browning P, Nicholas J, et al. Characterization of a chemokine receptor-related gene in human herpesvirus 8 and its expression in Kaposi's sarcoma. Virology 1997; 228:371–378.

202. Karin M, Liu Z, Zandi E. AP-1 Function and regulation. Curr Opin Cell Biol 1997; 9:240–246.

203. Kolch W, Martiny-Baron G, Kieser A, Marme D. Regulation of the expression of the VEGF/VPS and its receptors: role in tumor angiogenesis. Breast Cancer Res Treat 1995; 36:139–155.

204. Geras-Raaka E, Arvanitakis L, Bais C, Cesarman E, Mesri EA, Gershengorn MC. Inhibition of constitutive signaling of Kaposi's sarcoma-associated gerpesvirus G protein-coyupled receptor by protein kineases in mammalian cells in culture. J Exp Med 1998; 187:801–806.

205. Taniguchi T, Harada H, Camphries M. Regulation of the interferon system and cell growth by the IEF transcription factors (review). J Cancer Res Clin Oncol 1995; 121:516–520.

206. Gao S-J, Boshoff C, Jayachandra S, Weiss RA, Chang Y, Moore PS. KSHV ORF K9 (vIRF) is an oncogene which inhibits the interferon signalling pathway. Oncogene 1997; 15:1979–1985.

207. Zimring JC, Goodbourn S, Offerman MK. Human herpesvirus 8 encodes an interferon regulatory factor (IRF) homolog that represses IRF-1-mediated transcription. J Virol 1998; 72:701–707.

208. Li M, Lee H, Guo J, et al. Kaposi's sarcoma-associated herpesvirus viral interferon regulatory factor. J Virol 1998; 72:5433–5440.

209. Cheng EHY, Nicholas J, Bellows DS, et al. A Bcl-2 homolog encoded by Kaposi sarcoma-associated virus, human herpesvirus 8, inhibits apoptosis but does not heterodimerize with Bax or Bak. Proc Natl Acad Sci USA 1997; 94:690–694.

210. Sarid R, Sato T, Bohenzky RA, Russo JJ, Chang Y. Kaposi's sarcoma-associated herpesvirus encodes a functional bcl-2 homologue. Nat Med 1997; 3:293–298.

211. Sato T, Hanada M, Bodrug S, et al. Interactions among members of the Bcl-2 protein family analyzed with a yeast two-hybrid system. Proc Natl Acad Sci USA 1994; 91:9238–9242.

212. Mesri EA, Cesarman E, Arvanitakis L, et al. Human herpesvirus-8/Kaposi's sarcoma-associated herpesvirus is a new transmissible virus that infects B cells. J Exp Med 1996; 183:2385–2390.

213. Panyutich EA, Said JW, Miles SA. Infection of primary dermal microvascular endothelial cells by Kaposi's sarcoma-associated herpesvirus. AIDS 1998; 12:467–472.

214. Renne R, Blackbourn D, Whitby D, Levy J, Ganem D. Limited transmission of Kaposi's sarcoma-associated herpesvirus in cultured cells. J Virol 1998; 72:5182–5188.

215. Foreman KE, Friborg J Jr, Kong WP, et al. Propagation of a human herpesvirus from AIDS-associated Kaposi's sarcoma. N Engl J Med 1997; 336:163–171.

216. Flamand L, Zeman RA, Bryant JL, Lunardi Iskandar Y, Gallo RC. Absence of human herpesvirus 8 DNA sequences in neoplastic Kaposi's sarcoma cell lines. J AIDS Hum Retrovirol 1996; 13:194–197.

217. Flore O, Rafii S, Ely S, O'Leary JJ, Hyjek EM, Cesarman E. Transformation of primary human endothelial cells by Kaposi's sarcoma-associated herpesvirus. Nature 1998; 394:588–592.

218. Jacobson LP, Yamashita TE, Detels R, et al. Impact of potent anti-retroviral therapy on the incidence of Kaposi's sarcoma and non-Hodgkin's lymphomas among HIV-1 infected individuals. J AIDS 1999, 21 Supp 1:538–541.

219. Osman M, Kubo T, Gill Y, et al. Identification of KSHV specific cytotoxic responses. J Virol 1999; 73:in press.

220. Li M, MacKey J, Czajak SC, Desrosiers RC, Lackner AA, Jung JU. Identification and characterization of Kaposi's sarcoma-associated herpesvirus K8.1 virion glycoprotein. J Virol 1999; 73:1341–1349.

221. Tanner J, Weis J, Fearon D, Whang Y, Kieff E. Epstein-Barr virus gp 350/220 binding to the B lymphocyte C3d receptor mediates adsorption, capping, and endocytosis. Cell 1987; 50:203–213.

222. Rickinson AB, Kieff E. Epstein–Barr virus. In: Fields BN, Knipe DM, Howley PM (eds). Fields Virology, Vol. 2. Philadelphia: Lippincott–Raven, 1996, pp. 2397–2447.

223. Gallo RC. The enigmas of Kaposi's sarcoma. Science 1998; 282:1837–1839.

224. Kedes DH, Ganem D. Sensitivity of Kaposi's sarcoma-associated herpesvirus replication to antiviral drugs. J Clin Invest 1997; 99:2082–2086.

225. Morfeldt L, Torsander J. Long-term remission of Kaposi's sarcoma following foscarnet treatment in HIV-infected patients. Scand J Infect Dis 1994; 26:749.

226. Jones J, Peterman T, Chu S, Jaffe H. AIDS-associated Kaposi' sarcoma. Science 1995; 267:1078–1079.

227. Mocroft A, Youle M, Gazzard B, Morcinek J, Halai R, Phillips AN. Anti-herpesvirus treatment and risk of ~Kaposi' sarcoma in HIV infection. AIDS 1996; 1996:1101–1105.

228. Martin DF, Kuppermann BD, Wolitz RA, Palestine AG, Li H, Robinson CA. Oral ganciclovir for patients with cytomegalovirus retinitis treated with a ganciclovir implant. Roche Ganciclovir Study Group. N Engl J Med 1999; 340:1063–1070.

229. Ganem D. KSHV and Kaposi's sarcoma: the end of the beginning. Cell 1997; 91:157–160.

230. Rose TM, Strand KB, Schultz ER, et al. Identification of two homologs of the Kaposi's sarcoma-associated herpesvirus (human herpesvirus 8) in retroperitoneal fibromatosis of different macaque species. J Virol 1997; 71:4138–4144.

231. Desrosiers RC, Sasseville VG, Czajak SC, et al. A herpesvirus of rhesus monkeys related to the human Kaposi's sarcoma-associated herpesvirus. J Virol 1997; 71:9764–9769.

232. Boshoff C, Whitby D, Hatziioannou T, et al. Kaposi's-sarcoma-associated herpesvirus in HIV-negative Kaposi's sarcoma. Lancet 1995; 345:1043–1044.

233. Dupin N, Grandadam M, Calvez V. Herpes-like DNA sequences in patients with Mediterranean Kaposi's sarcoma. Lancet 1995; 345:761–762.

234. Moore PS, Chang Y. Detection of herpesvirus-like DNA sequences in AIDS-associated Kaposi's sarcoma lesions from persons with and without HIV infection. N Engl J Med 1995; 332:1181–1185.

235. Lebbe C, de Cremonx P, Rybojad M, Costa da Cunha C, Morel P, Calvo F. Kaposi's sarcoma and new herpesvirus. Lancet 1995; 345.

236. Schalling M, Ekman M, Kaaya EE, Linde A, Biberfeld P. A role for a new herpes virus (KSHV) in different forms of Kaposi's sarcoma. Nat Med 1995; 1:705–706.

237. Chang Y, Ziegler J, Wabinga H, et al. Kaposi's sarcoma-associated herpesvirus and Kaposi's sarcoma in Africa. Arch Intern Med 1996; 156:202–204.

238. Chuck S, Grant RM, Katongole-Mbidde E, Conant M, Ganem D. Frequent presence of a novel herpesvirus genome in lesions of human immunodeficiency virus-negative Kaposi's sarcoma. J Infect Diseases 1996; 173:248–251.

239. O'Neil E, Henson TH, Ghorbani AJ, Land MA, Webber BL, Garcia JV. Herpes virus-like sequences are specifically found in Kaposi's sarcoma lesions. J Clin Pathol 1996; 49:306–308.

240. Buonaguro FM, Tornesello ML, Beth-Giraldo E, et al. Herpesvirus-like DNA sequences detected in endemic, classic, iatrogenic and epidemic Kaposi's sarcoma (KS) biopsies. Int J Cancer 1996; 65:25–28.

241. Cathomas G, McGandy CE, Terracciano LM, Itin PH, De Rosa G, Gudat F. Detection of herpesvirus-like DNA by nested PCR on archival skin biopsy specimens of various forms of Kaposi sarcoma. J Clin Pathol 1996; 49:631–633.

242. Gaidano G, Pastore C, Gloghini A, et al. Distribution of human herpesvirus-8 sequences throughout the spectrum of AIDS-related neoplasia. AIDS 1996; 10:941–949.

243. Jin YT, Tsai ST, Yan JJ, Hsiao JH, Lee YY, Su IJ. Detection of Kaposi's sarcoma-associated herpesvirus-like DNA sequence in vascular lesions. A reliable diagnostic marker for Kaposi's sarcoma. Am J Clin Pathol 1996; 105:360–363.

244. Dictor M, Rambech E, Way D, Witte M, Bendsoe N. Human herpesvirus 8 (Kaposi's sarcoma-associated herpesvirus) DNA in Kaposi's sarcoma lesions, AIDS Kaposi's sarcoma cell lines, endothelial Kaposi's sarcoma simulators, and the skin of immunosuppressed patients. Am J Pathol 1996; 148:2009–2016.

245. Luppi M, Barozzi P, Maiorana A, et al. Frequency and distribution of herpesvirus-like DNA sequences (KSHV) in different stages of classic Kaposi's sarcoma and in normal tissues from an Italian population. Int J Cancer 1996; 66:427–31.

246. McDonagh DP, Liu J, Gaffey MJ, Layfield LJ, Azumi N, Traweek ST. Detection of Kaposi's sarcoma-associated herpesvirus-like DNA sequence in angiosarcoma. Am J Pathol 1996; 149:1363–1368.

247. Lebbe C, Agbalika F, de Cremoux P, et al. Detection of human herpesvirus 8 and human T-cell lymphotropic virus type 1 sequences in Kaposi sarcoma. Arch Dermatol 1997; 133:25–30.

248. Staskus KA, Sun R, Miller G, et al. Cellular tropism and viral interleukin-6 expresion distinguish human herpesvirus 8 involvement in Kaposi's sarcoma, primary effusion lymphoma, and multicentric Castleman's disease. J Virol 1999; 73:4181–4187.

249. Sun R, Lin S-F, Gradoville, L., Yuan Y, Zhu F, Miller G. A viral gene that activates lytic cycle expression of Kaposi's sarcoma-asociated herpesvirus. Proc Natl Acad Sci 1998; 95:10866–10871.

250. Lukac D, Renne R, Kirshner JR, Ganem D. Reactivation of Kaposi's sarcoma-associated herpesvirus infection from latency by expression of the ORF50 transactivator, a homolog of the EBV R protein. Virology 1998; 252:304–312.

III
Retroviruses

11

Retroviruses and Cancer

Robin A. Weiss

INTRODUCTION

Retroviruses are relevant to oncologists in three distinct ways. First, human retroviruses as infectious pathogens lead to the development of cancer. Neoplasia may result from the direct infection and transformation of the precursor tumor cell by the retrovirus, as is evident in adult T-cell leukemia caused by the human T-cell lymphotropic virus type I (HTLV-I) (*see* Chapter 12). Neoplasia may also develop as an indirect consequence of retrovirus infection, as seen in acquired immune deficiency syndrome (AIDS) following infection by human immunodeficiency virus (HIV). In this case, the retroviral genome does not infect or persist in the tumor cells; rather immunodeficiency allows cells infected by oncogenic herpesviruses to proliferate as "opportunistic neoplasms" analogous to opportunistic infections. Secreted retroviral proteins, such as Tat, might also play a role in HIV oncogenesis.

The second reason why retroviruses are relevant to oncologists is the insight that retroviruses of animals has provided on general mechanisms of oncogenesis, including the majority of human cancers not caused by viruses. Thus many of the oncogenes found to be active in human tumors were first discovered in retroviruses of mice, cats, and chickens. In addition, the activation of cellular genes by retroviral insertion into chromosomal DNA provided a model of oncogenesis essentially similar in mechanism to gene rearrangement and chromosome translocation in human tumors. It is noteworthy that three Nobel Prizes in Medicine and Physiology have been awarded for salient discoveries in retrovirology: to Peyton Rous in 1966 for his demonstration in 1911 that a transmissible, filterable agent (now known as Rous sarcoma virus) can cause cancer (*see* Chapter 1); to Howard M. Temin and David Baltimore in 1975 for their discovery of reverse transcriptase (RT) in retroviruses, the enzyme that synthesizes DNA from RNA; and to J. Michael Bishop and Harold E. Varmus in 1989 for their elucidation and derivation of retroviral oncogenes from normal cellular genes.

The third reason why retroviruses demand attention from oncologists is their use as tools in diagnosis and therapy. Without reverse transcriptase, we would not be able to make complementary DNA (cDNA), which provides us indirectly with recombinant proteins such as interferon for cancer treatment, DNA arrays of expressed genes for cancer gene profiles, and reverse transcriptase-polymerase chain reaction (RT-PCR) for

From: *Infectious Causes of Cancer: Targets for Intervention*
Edited by: J. J. Goedert © Humana Press Inc., Totowa, NJ

diagnosis and prognosis. Moreover, recombinant retroviruses are the vectors commonly used for gene therapy in cancer. The concept of retroviral vectors arose from the demonstration that retroviruses can acquire and transduce cellular oncogenes. Because such viruses can carry genes with pathogenic consequences, it became apparent that specially constructed retroviruses should similarly be able to deliver therapeutic genes.

Retroviruses have been intensively studied over the past 30 yr, generating a vast literature of research papers. A recent textbook *(1)* contains all the basic biology and molecular biology for a modern understanding of retroviruses. An earlier comprehensive text *(2)* provides the historical background of retrovirology, including details of the discovery of human retroviruses and their link to malignant disease. In this chapter, a brief outline is given of retroviral replication, transmission, and oncogenesis, together with a discussion of the role of retroviruses in human cancer.

CLASSIFICATION OF RETROVIRUSES

Retroviruses (Family: *Retroviridae*) were taxonomically divided into three subfamilies: the *Oncovirinae,* which include those with oncogenic potential but also other virus strains; the *Lentivirinae,* including HIV, and the prototype, visna virus of sheep which causes slow, progressive degeneration of the central nervous system; and the *Spumavirinae,* or foamy viruses, which have not been shown to be pathogenic. More recently, retroviruses have been classified into seven distinct genera by dividing oncoviruses into five groups that are only distantly related by genome sequence and morphology (Table 1). More generally, retroviruses are divided into those with "simple" genomes, having *gag, pol,* and *env* genes and perhaps one other, and those with "complex" genomes, also possessing regulatory genes such as *tat* and *rev* of HIV and *tax* of HTLV, and accessory genes, such as *nef, vif,* and *vpr* of HIV.

RETROVIRUS REPLICATION AND TRANSMISSION

Replication Cycle

Retroviruses are so called because they go "backwards" in genetic information flow, that is, they synthesize DNA from an RNA template. This step occurs early in the replication cycle of retroviruses (Fig. 1). The extracellular, transmissible virus particles contain duplicate strands of RNA, with which the enzyme molecules of reverse transcriptase are already associated. After binding to cell surface receptors, fusion with the cell membrane and uncoating, reverse transcription is activated in the remaining core of the retrovirus in the cytoplasm of the infected host cell. The first DNA strand is copied from the RNA genome which is then removed by an RNase H function of reverse transcriptase, followed by synthesis of the second DNA strand to form a double-stranded DNA genome. The DNA from of the genome has extended sequences repeated at each end called long terminal repeats (LTR). The 5′ LTR has promoter and enhancer sequences that respond to cellular and viral proteins that regulate gene expression.

During the first step in this process, reverse transcriptase can switch between the two diploid viral RNA strands, leading to genetic recombination between one strand and the other. However, because the initial DNA strand is synthesized from single-stranded RNA which is then rapidly destroyed, any errors in the fidelity of DNA transcription

Table 1
New Classification of Retroviridae

Genus	Example	Morphology of virion[a]	Genome	Disease
Alpharetrovirus	Rous sarcoma virus	C-type	Simple	Sarcoma
	Avian leukosis virus	C-type		Leukemia
Betaretrovirus	Murine mammary tumor virus	B-type	Simple	Carcinoma
	Simian retrovirus 2	D-type		Immune deficiency
Gammaretrovirus	Murine leukemia virus	C-type	Simple	Leukemia
	Gibbon ape leukemia virus	C-type		Leukemia
Deltaretrovirus	Human T-cell lymphotropic virus	C-type	Complex	Leukemia
				CNS disease
	Bovine leukosis virus	C-type		Leukemia
Epsilonretrovirus	Fish dermal sarcoma virus	C-type	Simple	Sarcoma
Lentivirus	Human immunodeficiency virus	C-type	Complex	AIDS
	Sheep Maedi-Visna virus	C-type		CNS disease
				Pneumonia
Spumavirus	Simian foamy virus	C-type	Complex	None

[a] C-type virions, concentric core condenses under plasma membrane during the budding of virus particles; B-type, cytoplasmic core eccentric after budding; D-type, cytoplasmic core concentric cone-shaped cores. Lentiviruses have cone-shaped cores; spumaviruses have prominent envelope spikes.

are not recognized and repaired as happens during editing chromosomal DNA replication. The error-prone nature of reverse transcription, together with recombination between the two parental RNA genomes of the virus, accounts for viral variation. Thus viruses such as HIV-1, which undergo a high rate of replication throughout infection, generate many variants explaining the rapid evolution and diversification of the virus population. It allows drug-resistant mutations to occur, and selection and recombination of such mutants. Recombination also permits the much rarer emergence of onco-gene-bearing retroviruses, if RNA transcripts with cellular sequences are incorporated into viral particles.

Once the double-stranded DNA genome is formed in the "preintegration complex" of the virus, it migrates to the nucleus and becomes inserted into the DNA in the chromosomes of the host. With HIV and other lentiviruses, the preintegration complex can be translocated through pores in the nuclear membrane to gain access to chromosomal DNA in nondividing cells such as macrophages. In contrast, the majority of oncogenic retroviruses can gain access to the chromosomes only during mitosis, when the nuclear membrane disassembles. Such retroviruses therefore require at least one cell division including mitosis to achieve stable infection.

Insertion of the viral genome into chromosomal DNA is called integration. It is mediated by another viral enzyme, integrase, and this is an obligatory step in the viral life-cycle. It results in the viral genome, now called the DNA provirus, being contiguous with cellular DNA. This means that if the infected cell subsequently undergoes

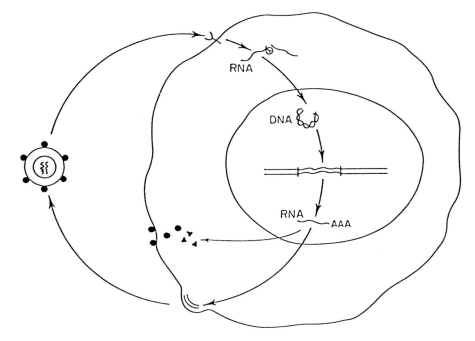

Fig. 1. Simplified replication cycle of retroviruses.

DNA synthesis and mitosis, the proviral DNA will be replicated as part of cellular DNA in the chromosomes. The linear sequence of the DNA provirus is the same as that of viral RNA in virus particles. Integration takes place almost anywhere in the cellular genome and on any chromosome, but usually is restricted to regions of actively transcribed chromatin. Nonetheless, the DNA provirus can remain latent for many cell generations.

Active transcription of integrated proviral DNA to produce RNA gives rise to two functional types of RNA. Full-length transcripts contain packaging sequence signals and are encapsidated into the next generation of virus particles; they can also be translated to synthesize the Gag proteins (core antigens) and the Pol proteins (protease, reverse transcriptase, and integase enzymes). The Env proteins forming the transmembrane (TM) and outer surface (SU) glycoproteins are translated from a spliced mRNA initiated from the 5′ LTR but spliced to the *env* gene transcript downstream from *gag* and *pol*. The mRNA of regulatory genes of complex retorviruses is also spliced.

The Gag and Pol proteins are translated as large precursor proteins that are cleaved by viral protease into component enzymes and structural proteins. This occurs late in the life cycle, often during the process of budding progeny particles. The Env glycoproteins are synthesized on the rough endoplasmic reticulum like host secretory and membrane-tethered proteins. Env is also produced as a precursor and is cleaved by cellular proteases such as furins into TM and SU components that remain associated together. Groups of three TM/SU molecules—or trimers—form the envelope spikes of the retrovirus particle. Epitopes on SU recognize specific cell surface receptors in the next round of infection.

Retroviral pathogenesis tends to be correlated with a high virus load and replication rate, so that reducing the viral burden should ameliorate or delay disease. Current anti-retroviral therapy is based on our understanding of retrovirus replication. Thus HIV treatment uses a combination of inhibitors of the early reverse transcription and the late proteolytic cleavage steps, targeting the viral enzymes and thus causing relatively few side effects in the infected person. In retroviral oncogenesis, however, once a clonal neoplasm has arisen anti-retroviral therapy is unlikely to be useful.

Retrovirus Genomes

All retroviruses share in common the following basic gene sequence shown in DNA with LTRs: 5′LTR-*gag-pol-env*-3′LTR. Retroviruses with only these three genes, or with one extra gene, are called simple retroviruses, whereas others such as HTLV and HIV, which have more than one gene extra to *gag, pol,* and *env,* are called complex. The extra genes may have regulatory functions, such as *tax* and *rex* of HTLV-I, and *tat* and *rev* of HIV. Both *tax* and *tat* serve as positive feedback controllers of viral transcription by interacting with the LTR, although they act via different molecular mechanisms. *Rex* and *rev* also have similar functions in aiding transport of long transcripts of viral RNA from the nucleus to the cytoplasm.

HIV and related lentiviruses also have so-called accessory genes that aid viral replication, particularly in nonproliferating macrophages. *Vif* encodes a protein that becomes incorporated into virus particles to make an early, ill-understood step in infection more efficient. *Vpr* guides the preintegration complex to the nucleus; it also arrests host cells in the G_2 phase of the cell cycle. *Vpu* function is unknown. *Nef* has multiple functions including downregulation of the CD4 cell surface receptor and signal transduction to activate transcription.

The mouse mammary tumor virus (MMTV) has a "simple" genome, but with one extra gene, to *gag, pol,* and *env* called *sag,* situated at the 3′ end of the genome and overlapping the 3′ LTR, the equivalent position to *nef* in HIV. The protein encoded by this gene acts as a superantigen by binding to Vβ molecules of host T lymphocytes and activating their proliferation. MMTV has probably evolved this mechanism to aid transmission in the milk. Because the virus can stably infect only cells undergoing mitosis, induction of cell division in immune cells by a superantigen permits infection of the gut lymphocytes in the infant mouse. The virus migrates to and infects the mammary gland only upon sexually maturity and estrogen stimulation. The LTR of MMTV has a glucocorticoid steroid responsive enhancer sequence as well as being responsive to female sex hormones. This is an example of tight regulation by host factors of a virus that is a vertically transmitted infection from mother to pup (*see also* Chapter 27).

Large DNA viruses such as pox viruses and herpesviruses have on occasion during evolution incorporated host genes into their genomes. These genes can help to evade immune responses, trigger cell proliferation, prevent apoptosis, and encode other functions that help the virus-infected cell to survive in the host. Because full viral replication is lytic, destroying the host cell, any delay in cell death helps viral replication. For example, human herpesvirus 8 (HHV-8 or KSHV) has acquired numerous cellular genes during its evolution and these may play a role in its oncogenic properties (*see* Chapter 10). Some oncogenic retroviruses with simple genomes also pick up cellular genes and incorporate them into the viral genome, where they are known as viral oncogenes *(onc).* In contrast to herpesviruses, however, the acquisition of host oncogenes by retroviruses is not part of their replication strategy. Rather, they represent rare events during oncogenesis. Indeed, such viruses are called acutely transforming retroviruses and they are usually defective, having lost parts of *gag, pol,* or *env* in gaining an *onc.*

Subsequent clonal development of the tumor allows the amplification of defective, *onc*-bearing retroviruses. They may also be transmitted from one host cell to another by a replication-competent "helper" retrovirus, which supplies the necessary Gag, Pol, and Env proteins for transmission. However, there are few cases of transmission of acutely transforming viruses from one host animal to another. The possession of a cyclin gene homolog by the Walleye dermal sarcoma virus of fish is one such example of transmission.

Retrovirus Transmission

Retroviruses are infectiously transmitted from one host to another by horizontal spread and by vertical transmission from mother to offspring. Retroviral genomes can also be transmitted noninfectiously as mendelian proviruses integrated in the germ line of the host. These inherited proviruses are known as endogenous retroviruses, in contrast to exogenous, infectiously transmitted retroviruses.

Infectious Transmission

Among the various retroviruses of animals and humans there are numerous routes of transmission. Indeed all the main modes of infection, bar aerosols, are recorded for one retrovirus or another. The enteric route has already been mentioned in regard to MMTV, for which the common mode of vertical transmission is via the mother's milk to suckling mice. The mammary gland secretes large amounts of MMTV particles, and infected cells may also be a source of seeding virus.

Milk transmission is also known for the human retroviruses HTLV-I and HIV *(3).* During primary infection of lactating mothers, before seroconversion, relatively high levels of HIV-1-infected cells are present in milk. Pediatric infection by this route was clearly shown before blood screening was introduced, when mothers who received HIV-contaminated postpartum blood transfusions tragically infected their infants. Vertical transmission of HIV-2 is less frequent. Milk is a common mode of passing HTLV-I in which transmission tends to increase with time of lactation after birth, possibly because maternal antibodies initially have a protective effect. HTLV-I transmission is cell associated. Maternal screening and counseling against breastfeeding is helping to reduce HTLV-I transmission in Japan *(4).*

Parenteral transmission occurs with most groups of retrovirus. This may be through biting and scratching among animals, such as transmission of feline leukemia virus among male cats. In humans, both HIV and HTLV are parenterally transmitted. In the case of HIV, cell-free virus in the blood is infectious, hence the contamination of pooled batches of unscreened plasma products such as clotting factors for the treatment of hemophilia. In the case of HTLV, transmission appears to be almost wholly cell associated, as removal of leukocytes and platelets from blood prevents transmission and no cases of HTLV-I infection have been linked to administration of acellular blood products *(3).*

Injection is a common mode of retrovirus transmission. Iatrogenic infection was common, as, for example, when syringes and needles common for immunising a whole herd against other infections allowed bovine leukemia virus (BLV) to spread from one contaminated animal to others. Nonsterile needles in medical use have similarly aided spread HIV and HTLV-I. However, the greatest risk has been among recreational and addictive injecting drug users. The second strain of HTLV (HTLV-II) also spread widely among injecting drug users in Western cities, whereas it is otherwise an extremely rare infection, although endemic among several native American communities and among certain African pygmy tribes *(5)*.

Sexual transmission is the commonest mode of HIV infection, from men to women, women to men, and homosexually between men. The United Nations Global Programme on AIDS estimates that approx 75% of the 38 million people currently infected with HIV worldwide acquired the virus heterosexually, 13% parenterally, 10% vertically as infants from mothers, and 3% homosexually. HTLV-I is also transmitted sexually, largely via infected leukocytes in semen, with a bias of male to female transmission. The risk of infection per sexual act is much lower for HTLV-I than for HIV.

Arthropod-borne retrovirus transmission is also known, althrough it has not been recorded with mosquitoes thus far. BLV can be transmitted via flies, and horseflies (clegs) are a frequent route of transmission of equine infectious anemia virus (EIAV). As BLV is closely related to HTLV, and EIAV is a lentivirus similar to HIV, we should not assume that the human retroviruses could not adapt to arthropod-borne transmission, if not by mosquitoes by, say, bed bugs and ticks. However, there are no epidemiologic data to suggest that this has occurred.

Mendelian Transmission

Most vertebrate species that have been studied carry numerous copies of integrated DNA proviruses in their chromosomes. These endogenous genomes arose when cells in the germ line, precursor cells to eggs and sperm became infected by exogenous viruses and the viral genome was passed on to the next generation. Hosts carrying viruses that are cytopathic in replication would naturally be at a selective disadvantage. For example, neither lentiviruses nor foamy viruses exist in endogenous form. Moreover, most endogenous viral genomes become defective over evolutionary time with deletions or stop codons in their genes, so that they cannot reemerge as infectious agents.

Some endogenous genomes, however, are potentially infectious. These have usually been acquired in the germ line of the host in recent evolutionary time. They occur, for example, in chickens, mice, cats, pigs, and baboons. They can be activated to produce experimentally infectious retrovirus. The host often has evolved mechanisms to prevent viremia or high virus load that result would from spontaneous production of virus from endogenous genomes, for example, by mutating or blocking cell surface receptors for the virus, thus preventing spread within the body from a few cells in which the virus was activated. The strains of mice in which endogenous MMTV or murine leukemia virus (MLV) become active tend to be laboratory strains specially selected to lack resistance genes and to have a high incidence of mammary tumors or thymic lymphomas, respectively.

Cross-species infection of retroviruses can be deduced from analyzing genome sequence relationships. Thus the endogenous retrovirus of cats known as RD114 is closely related to baboon endogenous virus (BaEV) and is absent from large cat species. HIV-1 probably crossed recently from chimpanzees to humans, and HIV-2 almost certainly came from sooty mangabey monkeys. We therefore need to be alert to new potential routes of retroviral zoonosis. A replication-competent recombinant stock of murine leukemia virus caused lymphomas in monkeys in a gene therapy trial. There is also concern that pig endogenous retroviruses might infect human recipients of porcine xenografts.

None of the human endogenous retroviral (HERV) genomes are known to be infective when activated from human cells in culture, although some have full-length viral genomes with open reading frames for each gene. Endogenous particles with Gag antigens and reverse transcriptase enzyme activity are produced, for instance, in the human placenta, and may be associated with disease, as discussed later.

MECHANISMS OF RETROVIRAL ONCOGENESIS

Oncogenesis is a multifactorial, multistep process requiring several genetic changes within a neoplastic cell lineage before malignancy becomes manifest. Retroviruses can play a role in these processes by a number of different mechanisms, some direct, some indirect.

Direct Oncogenesis

Directly acting oncogenic retroviruses are those in which the cancer cell precursor is infected by the virus that integrates into host DNA. Usually the viral genome persists and can be readily detected in the tumor tissue. Indeed, its integration site is a useful marker for determining the monoclonal status of the neoplastic cells. Figure 2 depicts three distinct ways in which a retrovirus may directly contribute toward malignant transformation.

Insertional Mutagenesis

Figure 2A shows the integration of the provirus adjacent to a cellular protooncogene. This leads to the ectopic activation of expression of that oncogene so that it is overexpressed or inappropriately expressed when there are no external signals to do so. Retroviral insertional mutagenesis is formally similar to oncogene activation resulting from chromosome translocation, such as activation of the c-*myc* oncogene by the promoter of an immunoglobulin gene in chromosome 8 translocations in Burkitt's lymphoma.

In the case of retroviruses, insertional gene activation is frequently driven by promoter sequences in the viral LTR, in which case the insertion must occur upstream of the oncogene to form a transcriptional unit with initiation of RNA within the LTR. This is commonly the situation in the formation of B-cell lymphoma in the bursa of Fabricius in chickens infected with avian leukosis virus (ALV). Among millions of bursal follicle cells infected, only a few with insertions before the c-*myc* gene will proliferate clonally.

Alternatively, enhancer sequences in the proviral LTR may allow the binding of transcriptionally active nuclear proteins without regard to being upstream or downstream of mRNA initiation. This situation is often seen in murine mammary tumors where MMTV inserts adjacent to the *wnt*-1 or *int*-2 oncogenes.

Retroviral tumors triggered by insertional mutagenesis often have a more complex, multiple stage course of tumorigenesis than simply integration of the proviral DNA

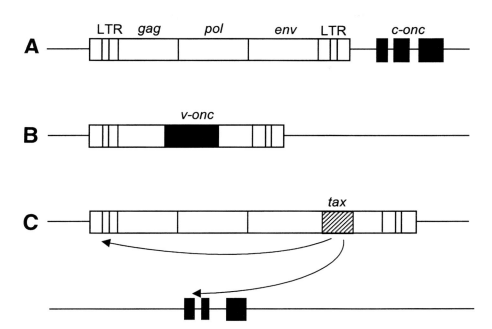

Fig. 2. Molecular mechanisms of retroviral oncogenesis. **(A)** Replication-competent virus integrates next to a cellular oncogene (c-*onc*) and activates it. **(B)** Acute transforming viruses carry a viral oncogene (v-*onc*) as part of their genome, which is usually defective and requires a helper virus. **(C)** Human and bovine leukemia viruses carry transactivating *(tax)* genes that upregulate both viral and cellular genes through protein expression. (Adapted from Weiss, ref. *20*.)

into a target cell, although infection of the bursa by ALV in newly hatched chickens may be sufficient to trigger clonal proliferation. In the case of murine and feline leukemia viruses causing T-cell (thymic) lymphomas, a series of recombination events occurs between the replicating retrovirus and endogenous proviruses, giving rise to recombinant viruses with modified tissue tropisms.

Acutely Transforming Retroviruses

Some retroviruses carry oncogenes as part of their own genome, as depicted in Fig. 2B. In this case, the oncogene is active irrespective of the integration site in the host genome because it is controlled by the promoter and enhancer sequences in the proviral LTR immediately upstream from the oncogene. Viral oncogenes are often further mutated within their coding sequence to give direct mitogenic effects; they may also be incorporated into an existing open reading frame of a viral gene to encode a chimeric, fusion protein, say, with part of a Gag or Env polypeptide.

Retroviruses bearing oncogenes as part of their own genome are usually defective for replication. But they can cause tumors within days of infection as each infected cell becomes transformed. If a "helper" virus providing all the replicative functions is also present, the acutely transforming virus can form progeny to infect and transform neighbouring cells forming a polyclonal neoplasm. Perhaps owing to their rapid oncogenicity, as well as their defectiveness, acutely transforming retroviruses are seldom

Table 2
Oncogenes Originally Identified Through Their Presence in Acutely Transforming Retroviruses

Oncogene	Protein	Source of virus	Tumor
abl	Kinase	Mouse, cat	Pre B-cell leukemia
akt	Kinase	Mouse	T-cell lymphoma
crk	Kinase activator	Chicken	Sarcoma
erb-a	TH-R	Chicken	Erythroleukemia
erb-b	EGF-R	Chicken	Erythroleukemia
ets	TF	Chicken	Myeloid leukemia
fes/fps	Kinase	Chicken, cat	Sarcoma
fgr	Kinase	Cat	Sarcoma
fms	Kinase	Cat	Sarcoma
fos	TF	Mouse	Osteosarcoma
jun	TF	Chicken	Fibrosarcoma
kit	Kinase	Cat	Sarcoma
mil/raf	Kinase	Chicken, mouse	Sarcoma
mos	Kinase	Mouse	Sarcoma
myb	TF	Chicken	Myeloid leukemia
myc	TF	Chicken	Myelocytoma, lymphoma, carcinoma
h-*ras*	G-protein	Rat	Sarcoma
k-*ras*	G-protein	Rat	Sarcoma
rel	TF	Turkey	Reticuloendotheliosis
ros	Kinase	Chicken	Sarcoma
sea	Kinase	Chicken	Sarcoma, leukemia
sis	PDGF	Monkey	Sarcoma
ski	TF	Chicken	Carcinoma
src	Kinase	Chicken	Sarcoma
yes	Kinase	Chicken	Sarcoma

Abbreviations: EGF-R, epidermal growth factor; PDGF, platelet-derived growth factor; TH-R, thyroid hormone receptor; TF, nuclear transcription factor.

Adapted from Weiss, 1998 *(20)*.

transformed from one infected host to another. Rather, they have been recognized by veterinary pathologists and propagated by experimental inoculation.

Retroviral oncogenes were first recognized before the discovery of their cellular counterparts. Table 2 lists some of the known viral oncogenes and the host animals in which they were first found. The proteins they encode act at multiple steps of cell growth or cell death signaling pathways: as extracellular growth factors or cytokines (e.g., *sis*), as spontaneously signaling receptors on the cell surface (e.g., c-*erb*B), as proteins further downstream in signal transduction pathways (e.g., *ras*), and as transcriptional regulators in the nucleus (e.g., *myc* and *fos*). Thus the study of oncogenic animal retroviruses has given great insight into molecular mechanisms of oncogenesis.

Because complex retroviruses such as HIV and foamy viruses also have strong promoter and enhancer elements in their LTR sequences, it remains a puzzle why they do not cause clonal cell proliferations as a result of integration. The explanation may be that the viruses are cytopathic. Moreover, transcription relies on viral proteins such as Tat (HIV) and Bel-1 (foamy virus) transactivating the LTR, and this is less likely to occur in clonally proliferating cells that need to survive the cytopathic effect of the virus. No tumors are known to result from integration of complex retroviruses into precursor tumor cells. However, McGrath et al. (Chapter 13) describe evidence of clonal integration of HIV in supporting antigen-presenting cells that are present in rare non-B-cell lymphomas in AIDS.

Transactivating Genes

When the human T-lymphotropic retrovirus (HTLV-I) was first identified and associated with adult T-cell leukemia/lymphoma (*see* Chapter 12), it was assumed that it exerted its oncogenic effect via insertional mutagenesis. However, it soon became apparent that clonal integrations occurred at completely different chromosomal sites in tumor cells from different patients with the same disease. HTLV-I is a complex retrovirus encoding several small proteins in addition to Gag, Pol, and Env. At least one of these, Tax, acts as a transcriptional control protein acting in positive control feedback on the virus's own LTR promoter. Tax will also transactivate a variety of cellular genes, including CD25, the β-chain of the interleukin 2 (IL-2) receptor, and may promote cell proliferation in this way (Fig. 2C).

Whereas both insertional mutagenesis and acutely transforming retroviruses exert their oncogenic effects as *cis*-acting elements, that is the promoter or enhancer must be in linear relation on the DNA to the oncogene, Tax works in *trans,* that is by encoding a protein that can diffuse to bind to numerous promoter elements throughout the cellular genome. There are animal models of HTLV-I Tax-mediated transformation. Many old world monkeys harbor HTLV-related viruses, and bovine leukosis virus (which causes B-cell rather than T-cell lymphomas) also is oncogenic via a Tax-related transactivating mechanism.

Indirect Oncogenesis

Certain virus infections may greatly increase the risk of cancer without directly infecting tumor cells or their precursors. This is probably the case with hepatitis C virus infection (*see* Chapters 17–19) and also for the retrovirus, HIV. HIV is considered oncogenic owing to the very high relative risk of certain cancers in AIDS, particular Kaposi's sarcoma (KS) and non-Hodgkin's lymphoma (NHL) which are associated with gammaherpesviruses (Chapters 8 and 10) *(3).* Some other viral cancers, such as human papilloma virus-related carcinoma *in situ* of the uterix cervix in women and anal neoplasia of homosexual men are also increased, although this is less marked for invasive carcinoma (*see* Chapter 15). Testicular tumors are elevated modestly in incidence in HIV infection, judged from cohort studies. All these cases may be a consequence of the immune deficiency caused by HIV.

It is notable that the major carcinomas seen in the Western world, such as cancer of the bowel, prostate, breast, and lung are not markedly increased in AIDS, although an increased risk of lung cancer and melanoma has been observed in some studies. Moreover, some virally induced cancers such as hepatocellular carcinoma or HTLV-I-related adult T-cell leukemia/lymphoma are not increased either. Thus Paul Erhlich's hypothesis 90 yr ago on immune surveillance of cancer, later championed by Lewis Thomas and McFarlane Burnet, does not appear to be upheld by an examination of cancer rates in AIDS or, indeed, in immunosuppressed transplant patients. It should be borne in mind, however, that such tumors usually occur later in life than the majority of AIDS and transplant patients. These tumors might require a greater number of somatic mutations than NHL or KS and having acquired them may then increase upon immunosuppression. An analysis of elderly immunodeficient persons could be informative.

The simplest model for HIV oncogenesis in KS and NHL is that HIV itself has an indirect effect through immune deficiency whereas the gammaherpesviruses have a direct oncogenic effect on infecting the tumor cells themselves. This notion is supported by the relative increase in these tumors in other immunsuppressed conditions, and because KS does not occur in AIDS patients who are not infected by HHV-8, such as most intravenous drug users and persons with hemophilia who received HIV-contaminated clotting factors. The apportionment of risk attributable to HIV and to HHV-8 is difficult to assess (*see* Chapter 10). A recent study of more than 3000 cancer patients in South Africa *(6)* showed a particularly strong risk of KS in HIV infection combined with high titer seroreactivity to HHV-8 latent nuclear antigen. Contrary to earlier suggestions, there was no specific serologic association of HHV-8 with multiple myeloma or prostate cancer *(6,7)*.

It has also been postulated that the Tat protein of HIV may play an indirect, paracrine role in KS *(8)*. Tat acts as a co-mitogen with basic fibroblast growth factor on certain HHV-8 cell lines derived from KS lesions. Some mice transgenic for Tat expression develop skin proliferations that bear a resemblance to KS. Tat of HIV-2 does not exhibit a mitogenic effect in vitro, and it is noteworthy that of the few KS cases among HIV-positive persons in The Gambia, West Africa, all except one were associated with HIV-1 although the majority of AIDS cases in The Gambia at the time of data collection were due to HIV-2 *(9)*.

HUMAN RETROVIRUSES

Five groups of retrovirus have been reported as human infections:

1. Human immunodeficiency viruses types 1 and 2 (HIV-1 and HIV-2) are the lentiviruses that cause acquired immune deficiency syndrome (AIDS). Before the term HIV was coined in 1986, HIV was called LAV or HTLV-III.
2. Human T-lymphotropic viruses, type I and type II (HTLV-I and HTLV-II), cause adult T-cell leukaemia and neurologic disease (*see* Chapter 12).
3. Human foamy virus (HFV) is a spumavirus originally detected in cultured nasopharyngeal carcinoma of a Kenyan patient. Because the HFV genome is indistinguishable from that of the simian foamy virus type 6 (SFV-6) of chimpanzees, it may represent a single case of zoonosis *(10)*. Serologic studies indicate that human populations are not infected by spumaviruses although they are endemic in many primate species. Zoonotic SFV infection without symptoms has been recorded in primate handlers who have suffered bites or deep puncture wounds *(11)*.
4. Human retrovirus 5 (HRV-5) is a retroviral genome occurring at very low viral load in normal subjects but particularly in patients with arthritis and systemic lupus erythematosus *(12)*. The virus has not yet been propagated in vitro; its genome is related to the B-type and D-type retroviruses (betaretrovirus).
5. Human endogenous retroviruses (HERV) are Mendelian loci in human chromosomes representing "fossil" infections of the germ line. These endogenous genomes derive from mammalian C-type and D-type (HERV-K) retroviruses *(13)*. No lentiviruses or

spumaviruses are known to have become endogenous. HERV genomes are defective, that is, human endogenous retroviral genomes have not been rescued in infectious form, in contrast to BaEV of baboons and PERV of pigs, which threaten the safety of human xenotransplantation from these sources *(14)*. Some HERV genomes, however, express envelope and other proteins, for example, ERV-3 in the human placenta *(15)*, HERV-K in type 1 diabetes *(16)*, and an HERV-W related C-type genome, MSRV, in multiple sclerosis *(17)*, but such findings remain controversial. Of greatest interest to oncology is the finding that HERV-K is expressed and produces particles in testicular germ cell tumors, both seminoma and teratocarcinoma *(13)*.

CONCLUSIONS AND PROSPECTS

Retroviruses have played an immensely informative role in elucidating the genetic basis of cancer. Animal retroviruses have arguably been more important for understanding nonretroviral human cancers than those caused by HTLV-I or HIV. These human pathogens, however, could not have been investigated so rapidly without a knowledge of animal retroviruses. For instance, both HTLV-I and HIV were initially discovered through assays in culture for reverse transcriptase, previously developed for animal retroviruses, and zidovudine was first shown to be an anti-retroviral drug long before HIV came to light in experiments with murine Rauscher leukemia virus.

Control of infection by human retroviruses may be achieved by screening of blood donations and pregnant women, by safer sexual practices in the case of HIV, and for those societies that can afford it, anti-retroviral therapy. A vaccine to protect against HTLV-I is achievable scientifically, but without the political or public health will to apply it. Genuinely efficacious, broad specturn HIV vaccines are barely on the horizon. Yet an effective, affordable HIV vaccine is the one factor that could halt the HIV pandemic.

As for the treatment of retrovirus-associated tumors once they have appeared, there is little improvement in sight for adult T-cell leukemia/lymphoma. KS responds to cytotoxic cancer therapy, to anti-retroviral therapy, and to some anti-herpesvirus drugs such as Forscarnet and Cidofovir (*see* Chapter 10). These observations suggest that continued HHV-8 replication might play a role in KS oncogenesis.

The recent likely origin of HIV-1 from chimpanzees *(18)* serves to remind us that retroviruses can jump host species. We therefore need to be mindful that we do not unwittingly introduce new animal retrovirus to humans via xenotransplantation *(14)*.

Finally, human kind's ingenuity is putting retroviruses to good use. Retroviruses are being harnessed as vectors to treat cancer by delivering gene therapy. Again, vigilance is needed to preclude the emergence of replication-competent recombinant retroviruses from vector packaging cells, as these can be oncogenic *(19)*.

REFERENCES

1. Coffin JM, Hughes SH, Varmus HE. Retroviruses. New York: Cold Spring Harbor Laboratory Press, 1997, pp. 1–843.
2. Weiss RA, Teich NM, Varmus HE, Coffin J. RNA Tumor Viruses. New York: Cold Spring Harbor Laboratory Press, 1985, pp. 1396, 1233.
3. IARC Working Group on the Evaluation of Carcinogenic Risks to Humans. Human immunodeficiency viruses and human T-cell lymphotropic viruses. Lyon, France, 1–18 June 1996. IARC Monogr Eval Carcinog Risks Hum 1996; 67:1–424.

4. Tajima K, Takezaki T. Human T cell leukaemia virus Type I. In: Newton R, Beral V, Weiss RA (eds). Infections and Human Cancer. New York: Cold Spring Harbor Laboratory Press, 1999, pp. 191–211.

5. Gessain A, Mahieux R. Genetic diversity and molecular epidemiology of primate T cell lymphotropic viruses. In: Dalgleish AG, Weiss RA (eds). HIV and the New Viruses. London: Academic Press, 1999, pp. 281–327.

6. Sitas F, Carrara H, Beral V, et al. Antibodies against human herpesvirus 8 in black South African patients with cancer. N Engl J Med 1999; 340:1863–1871.

7. Boshoff C, Weiss RA. Kaposi's sarcoma-associated herpesvirus. Adv Cancer Res 1998; 75:57–86.

8. Ensoli B, Gendelman R, Markham P, et al. Synergy between basic fibroblast growth factor and HIV-1 Tat protein in induction of Kaposi's sarcoma. Nature 1994; 371:674–680.

9. Ariyoshi K, Schim van der Loeff M, Cook P, et al. Kaposi's sarcoma in the Gambia, West Africa is less frequent in human immunodeficiency virus type 2 than in human immunodeficiency virus type 1 infection despite a high prevalence of human herpesvirus 8. J Hum Virol 1998; 1:193–199.

10. Rosenblum L, McClure MO. Non-lentiviral primate retroviruses. In: Dalgleish AG, Weiss RA (eds). HIV and the New Viruses. London: Academic Press, 1999, pp. 251–279.

11. Heneine W, Switzer WM, Sandstrom P, et al. Identification of a human population infected with simian foamy viruses. Nat Med 1998; 4:403–407.

12. Griffiths DJ, Cooke SP, Herve C, et al. Detection of human retrovirus 5 in patients with arthritis and systemic lupus erythematosus. Arthritis Rheum 1999; 42:448–454.

13. Lower R, Lower J, Kurth R. The viruses in all of us: characteristics and biological significance of human endogenous retrovirus sequences. Proc Natl Acad Sci USA 1996; 93:5177–5184.

14. Weiss RA. Science, medicine, and the future—xenotransplantation. Br Med J 1998; 317:931–937.

15. Venables PJ, Brookes SM, Griffiths D, Weiss RA, Boyd MT. Abundance of an endogenous retroviral envelope protein in placental trophoblasts suggests a biological function. Virology 1995; 211:589–592.

16. Conrad B, Weissmahr RN, Boni J, Arcari R, Schupbach J, Mach B. A human endogenous retroviral superantigen as candidate autoimmune gene in type I diabetes. Cell 1997; 90:303–313.

17. Perron H, Garson JA, Bedin F, et al. Molecular identification of a novel retrovirus repeatedly isolated from patients with multiple sclerosis. Proc Natl Acad Sci USA 1997; 94:7583–7588.

18. Gao F, Bailes E, Robertson DL, et al. Origin of HIV-1 in the chimpanzee *Pan troglodytes troglodytes*. Nature 1999; 397:436–441.

19. Donahue RE, Kessler SW, Bodine D, et al. Helper virus induced T cell lymphoma in nonhuman primates after retroviral mediated gene transfer. J Exp Med 1992; 176:1125–1135.

20. Weiss RA. The oncologist's debt to the chicken. Avian Pathol 1998; 27:S8–15.

12

Adult T-Cell Leukemia/Lymphoma

Masao Matsuoka

INTRODUCTION

Adult T-cell leukemia (ATL) is a neoplasm of activated helper T lymphocytes, which was the first human cancer found to be caused by a retrovirus, human T-cell lymphotropic virus type I (HTLV-I). It was around the year 1973 that ATL, previously an unknown disease entity, was first recognized in Japan *(1)*, and it was internationally acknowledged in 1977 *(2,3)*. HTLV-I was isolated from a cell line derived from a patient with aggressive cutaneous T cell lymphoma *(4)*. The disease in this patient was later considered to be ATL. ATL cells were first cultured successfully in vitro by Miyoshi et al. *(5)*, and these cell lines then were used to detect antibodies against virus-related antigens in ATL patients by an indirect immunofluorescence assay *(6)*. Sera from ATL patients reacted to these cells, showing a relationship between the virus and ATL. The entire structure of this virus was determined by Yoshida and his colleagues *(7)*. The discovery of ATL had far-reaching effects not only in medicine and virology, but also in oncology and biology. The presence of HTLV-I provirus enables us to analyze each step of leukemogenesis from infection to the highly aggressive acute or lymphoma types of ATL. Therefore, ATL is a good model to be analyzed to clarify the oncogenesis of lymphoid cells.

HTLV-I

The etiologic association between HTLV-I and ATL was based on the following observations *(8,9)*: (1) The areas of high incidence of ATL correspond closely with those of high prevalence of HTLV-I infection as extensively studied in Japan; (2) HTLV-I immortalizes human T cells in vitro; (3) monoclonal integration of HTLV-I proviral DNA was demonstrated in ATL neoplastic cells; and (4) all individuals with ATL have antibodies against HTLV-I. HTLV is therefore the first retrovirus directly associated with human malignancy.

HTLV-I belongs to Oncovirinae subfamily of retroviruses, which includes the bovine leukemia virus (BLV), the human T-cell lymphotropic virus type II (HTLV-II), and the simian T-cell leukemia virus (STLV). Like other retroviruses, the HTLV-I proviral genome has *gag, pol,* and *env* genes, flanked by long terminal repeat (LTR) sequences at both ends. A unique structure was found between *env* and the 3′-LTR,

From: *Infectious Causes of Cancer: Targets for Intervention*
Edited by: J. J. Goedert © Humana Press Inc., Totowa, NJ

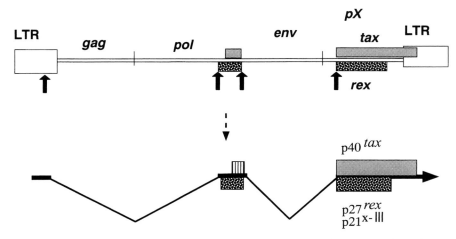

Fig. 1. Structure of HTLV-I. HTLV-I proviral genome has the *gag, pol,* and *env* genes, flanked by long terminal repeat (LTR) sequences at both sides. A unique structure was found between *env* and 3′-LTR, which was named the pX region that encodes the regulatory proteins, p40^*tax* (Tax), p27^*rex* (Rex), and p21.

denoted the pX region, that encodes the regulatory proteins, p40^*tax* (Tax), p27^*rex*, and p21 (Fig. 1). Among them, Tax protein is thought to play a central role in the leukemogenesis of ATL, because of its pleiotropic actions (Fig. 2) *(10,11)*. Tax does not bind to promoter or enhancer sequences by itself, but it interacts with cellular proteins that are transcriptional factors or modulators of cellular functions. By binding to various cellular factors, such NFκB, SRF, and CREB, Tax activates transcription of both viral and cellular genes. Conversely, Tax can transrepress the transcription of certain genes, such as *lck* and DNA polymerase β *(12,13)*. Activation of NFκB results in transcriptional activation of cellular genes such as interleukin 2, and interleukin 2 receptor genes. Tax can also bind IκB, promoting activation of NFκB *(14)*. Binding of Tax to CREB causes transcriptional activation of viral genes.

Tax also appears to allow dysregulated cell cycling by binding and thus inactivating p16^*INK4A*, a key inhibitor of cyclin-dependent kinases 4 and 6 *(15)*. Tax also has been reported to interact with *MAD1,* which acts as a mitotic checkpoint gene *(16)*. Disturbance of checkpoint genes might be associated with chromosomal instability, which is frequently observed in ATL cells. It is associated with leukemogenesis by generating chromosomal instability.

In HTLV-I transformed cell lines, the *p53* gene is highly expressed but is functionally impaired *(17)*. Phosphorylation of *p53* at Ser15 observed in HTLV-I transformed cell lines inactivates *p53* by blocking its interaction with basal transcription factors *(18)*. Inactivation of this major cancer suppressor gene, in cooperation with inactivation of p16^*INK4A*, is thought to contribute to HTLV-I-related leukemogenesis and ultimately ATL.

The pleiotropic functions of Tax are thought to contribute to the immortalization of HTLV-I infected cells, especially CD4^+ positive T lymphocytes (Fig. 2). Indeed, the proliferation of HTLV-I-infected cells in vivo is clonal, as detected by analysis of inte-

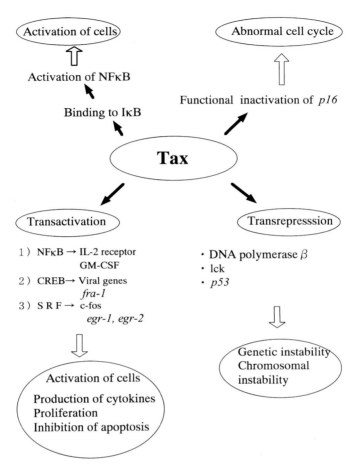

Fig. 2. Pleiotropic actions of Tax.

gration sites. As described later, persistent proliferation is observed in HTLV-I carriers *(19,20)*. After infection with HTLV-I, a very long latent period, about 50 yr in Japan, is present before the onset of ATL. Such a long latent period indicates that multistep tumorigenesis is necessary for the development of ATL. During this latent period, genetic and epigenetic mutations are thought to accumulate in infected cells.

EPIDEMIOLOGY OF ATL AND HTLV-I

Both HTLV-I and ATL have been shown to be endemic in some regions of the world, especially in southwest Japan *(21)*, the Caribbean islands, the countries surrounding the Caribbean basin *(22,23)*, and parts of Central Africa *(24)*. In addition, epidemiologic studies of HTLV-I revealed high seroprevalence rates in Melanesia, Papua–New Guinea *(25)*, the Solomon islands *(26)*, and among Australian aborigines. In the Middle East, a focus of HTLV-I was found in Iranian Jews who reside in the Mashad region *(27)*. Antibodies against HTLV-I have been found in approx 1.2 million individuals *(28)*, and more than 800 cases of ATL have been diagnosed each year in Japan alone.

The cumulative, 70-yr incidence of ATL among HTLV-I carriers in Japan is estimated at about 2.5% (3–5% in males and 1–2% in females) if competing risks for the other diseases are neglected *(29)*.

HTLV-I seroprevalence rises in an age-dependent manner, and it is higher in females than in males *(30)*. Three major routes of HTLV-I transmission have been identified: mother-to-infant, sexual, and parenteral. Mother-to-infant transmission occurs mainly via breast milk. HTLV-I-positive lymphocytes have been identified in the breast milk from a seropositive mother *(31)*. Intervention trials in Japan showed that breast-feeding accounts for most mother-to-infant transmission. Breast-fed infants showed a 13% seroconversion rate, whereas bottle-fed infants experienced a 3% seroconversion rate *(32)*. Prolonged breast-feeding is associated with a higher rate of seroconversion among infants—0% for < 6 mo, 28% for >6 mo of breast-feeding. Other mechanisms of HTLV-I transmission from mother to infant remain unknown. Studies of married couples and sexually active groups have shown that sexual transmission of HTLV-I occurs from male to female, from female to male, and from male to male. Studies in seropositive couples showed that male-to-female infection is more efficient than female-to-male infection, which may explain a part of higher HTLV-I seroprevalence among women. Transfusion with cellular components is associated with HTLV-I transmission *(33)*. Transfusion of plasma is not associated with transmission, showing that viable infected cells are necessary for transmission.

EVOLUTION OF ATL

It is important to analyze the natural course from infection with HTLV-I to the onset of ATL to clarify the mechanism of leukemogenesis. The natural course of HTLV-I infection to ATL is thought to be as follows. HTLV-I transmission is mainly from mother to infant by breast-feeding or male-to-female by sexual intercourse. HTLV-I can infect many kinds of cells in vivo, such as T-lymphocyte, B-lymphocyte, monocyte, and dendritic cells, revealing that HTLV-I may not need a specific receptor for infection *(34)*. Consistent with this finding, the heat shock cognate protein has been reported as a candidate generic receptor for HTLV-I *(35)*. HTLV-I provirus is detected mainly in CD4$^+$ memory T lymphocytes in healthy carriers *(36)*. Indeed, carriers with a high HTLV-I provirus load have an increased number of memory T lymphocytes, as do patients with the neurodegenerative disease called HTLV-I-associated myelopathy/tropical spastic paraparesis (HAM/TSP) *(our unpublished data)*. This suggests that viral proteins, especially Tax, promote the proliferation of CD4$^+$ memory T lymphocytes. HTLV-I provirus load, which is correlated with the number of HTLV-I infected cells, differed more than 100-fold among HTLV-I carriers *(37)*. It is important to study whether provirus load is constant or variable across time in individuals. To address this question, we analyzed sequential DNA samples from peripheral blood mononuclear cells of HTLV-I carriers who were followed in a Miyazaki cohort study for up to 7 yr *(19,38)*. It was revealed that provirus loads fluctuated only two- to fourfold in most carriers, showing that provirus loads were relatively constant over time for up to 7 yr in individual carriers.

What determines the provirus load in carriers? As shown in the previous studies *(37, 39,40)*, age and sex did not influence provirus load. It is assumed that immune responses, especially cytotoxic T lymphocytes (CTLs) against HTLV-I, control the number of HTLV-I-infected cells. In persons with a powerful CTL response to viral antigens, virus load might be limited to a low level. In patients with HTLV-associated myelopathy/tropical spastic paraparesis (HAM/TSP), a high frequency of CTLs against HTLV-I was reported *(41,42),* and specific HLA haplotypes were reported to be common in HAM/TSP patients compared to HTLV-I carriers *(43).* It is paradoxical that patients with HAM/TSP showed both high provirus load and a strong immune response against HTLV-I. Another explanation for differences in provirus load is that the capacity of viral replication itself is different with various virus strains or that cellular factors that interact with Tax may differ among carriers. It remains to be determined what kind of factors determine HTLV-I provirus load in the infected individuals.

The HTLV-I provirus is genetically very stable, especially compared with the other major human retrovirus, human immunodeficiency virus (HIV). It has been postulated that increased HTLV-I load is achieved not by replication of virus, but by clonal proliferation of infected cells. In HTLV-I carriers, HTLV-I provirus is randomly integrated in the host genome. In other words, the integration site is specific to each HTLV-I-infected cell. A part of LTR and flanking genomic DNAs were amplified by inverse polymerase chain reaction (PCR), with each detected band representing a clonal proliferation of HTLV-I infected cells. Using this assay to analyze clonal proliferation of HTLV-I-infected cells in HTLV-I carriers, some clones persisted over 7 yr in the same individuals *(19).* These persistent clones were CD4$^+$ lymphocytes, which is consistent with the fact that HTLV-I predominantly immortalizes CD4$^+$ T lymphocytes in vitro.

A long latent period of about 50 yr precedes the onset of ATL, suggesting the multistep mechanism of leukemogenesis (Fig. 3). Various mutations of oncogenes and tumor-suppressor genes have been demonstrated in cancers, and it has been established that multiple changes are necessary for the appearance of malignant disease. In ATL cells, mutations of *p53* have been detected in about 30% of patients examined *(44,45).* Such mutations were detected in the more aggressive disease state. In one patient, no mutation was detected in ATL cells in the chronic phase, but the mutation was demonstrated in the acute phase. Deletion or mutation of the *p16^{INK4A}* gene was also reported in ATL. Again, those abnormalities were observed in acute or lymphoma-type ATL, suggesting that somatic DNA changes in *p53* or *p16^{INK4A}* genes are associated with the progression of ATL *(46,47).* Mutations of the *Fas* gene are also reported in patients with ATL cells *(48).* Such findings indicate that multistep changes are required for leukemogenesis in ATL, and other genetic and epigenetic changes remain to be analyzed.

CLASSIFICATION OF ATL

ATL patients can be classified into four clinical subtypes according to the clinical features: acute, chronic, smoldering, and lymphoma type.

The diagnostic criteria for HTLV-I associated ATL have been defined as follows: (1) There is histologically and/or cytologically proven lymphoid malignancy with T-cell surface antigens. (2) Abnormal T lymphocytes are always present in the peripheral blood, except in the lymphoma type. These abnormal T lymphocytes include not only typical ATL cells, the so-called flower cells, but also the small and mature T lymphocytes with incised or lobulated nuclei that are characteristic of the chronic or smoldering type. (3) Antibody to HTLV-I is present in the sera at diagnosis. Shimoyama and

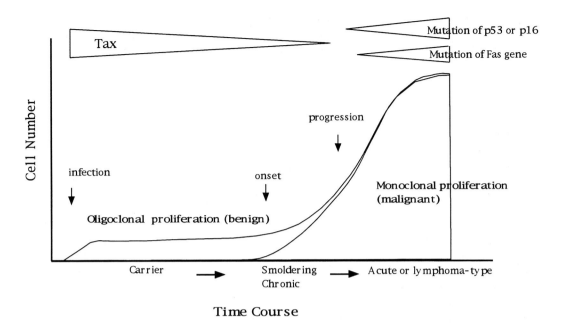

Fig. 3. Schema of natural course of HTLV-I infection leading to onset of ATL.

members of the Lymphoma Study Group (LSG)(1984–1987) proposed the following diagnostic criteria for classifying ATL into the four subtypes *(49)*:

1. Smoldering type, 5% or more abnormal lymphocytes of T-cell nature in the peripheral blood (PB); normal lymphocyte level ($< 4 \times 10^9$/L); no hypercalcemia; lactate dehydrogenase (LDH) value of up to 1.5 times the normal upper limit; no lymphadenopathy; no involvement of liver, spleen, central nervous system (CNS), bone, or gastrointestinal tract; and neither ascites nor pleural effusion. Skin or pulmonary lesions may be present. In patients with < 5% abnormal T lymphocytes in PB, at least one histologically proven skin or pulmonary lesion should be present.
2. Chronic type; absolute lymphocytosis of more than 3.5×10^9/L; LDH value up to twice the normal upper limit; no hypercalcemia; no involvement of CNS, bone, or gastrointestinal tract; and neither ascites nor pleural effusion. There may be histologically proven lymphadenopathy with or without extranodal lesions and there may be involvement of liver, spleen, skin, and lung, and 5% or more abnormal lymphocytes.
3. Lymphoma type; no lymphocytosis, 1% or fewer abnormal lymphocytes in PB; histologically proven lymphadenopathy with or without extranodal lesions.
4. Acute type; the most common form of presentation, highly aggressive malignancy that shows lymphadenopathy, hepatosplenomegaly, and skin lesions, but does not meet the criteria of the other types.

SEROLOGY OF HTLV-I

Anti-HTLV-I antibodies are positive in almost patients with ATL, although seronegative ATL cases have been reported *(50,51)*. There is no difference between ATL patients and HTLV-I carriers in the pattern of serum antibodies. The presence of serum antibodies to HTLV-I can be demonstrated by enzyme-linked immunosorbence, gelatin particle hemagglutination, indirect immunofluorescence, and Western blotting assays *(52)*. Carriers with a high level of anti-HTLV-I antibody and a low titer of anti-Tax antibody have recently been noted to be at high risk for ATL *(53)*.

HTLV-I PROVIRAL DNA

The definitive diagnosis of ATL requires the detection of the monoclonal integration of HTLV-I provirus in genomic DNA from peripheral blood mononuclear or lymph node cells. Monoclonal integration of the HTLV-I provirus is not detected in patients with other T-cell malignancies. The detection of HTLV-I proviral DNA is essential for the diagnosis of ATL, especially in endemic areas. This feature has contributed to the understanding of T-cell malignancies *(54)*. Monoclonal integration of HTLV-I provirus can be detected by the Southern blot method. Defective HTLV-I provirus was found in 56% of patients with ATL, and two different types of defective provirus were identified in ATL using Southern blot analysis. Type 1 defective provirus retains both LTRs, but lacks internal sequences, such as *gag, pol,* or *env.* Type 2 defective provirus lacks 5′-LTR and 5′ internal sequences *(55)*. Type 2 defective provirus is usually found in aggressive subtypes of ATL, namely acute and lymphoma types, and only one chronic ATL case has had type 2 defective provirus in its genome. This suggests that the genetic instability to generate type 2 defective provirus is associated with the progression of ATL. Because type 2 defective provirus cannot produce viral proteins including Tax, ATL cells with type 2 defective provirus can escape from immunosurveillance of the host. It is assumed that during the early stage of leukemogenesis, such as smoldering and chronic ATL, Tax plays a critical role. Later, Tax may not be necessary, as accumulated genetic or epigenetic changes cause the progression to acute or lymphoma types of ATL.

MORPHOLOGY OF ATL CELLS

Abnormal lymphocytes of various sizes and with cytoplasmic basophilia are seen in acute ATL. Most of the cells characteristically exhibit lobulated nuclei; most of them are bi- or multifoliate and separated by deep indentations. Cells with such a configuration are known as "flower cells" (Fig. 4a).

Cells from chronic ATL are relatively uniform in size and nuclear configuration (Fig. 4b), and are smaller than those seen in either acute or smoldering ATL. Chronic ATL cells rarely have small vacuoles and do not have azurophilic granules. Cells in this type of ATL also exhibit lobular division of the nuclei, which are usually bi- or trifoliate. The nuclear chromatin is in the form of coarse strands and is deeply stained. The nucleocytoplasmic ratio is larger than that in normal lymphocytes.

Cells in smoldering ATL are relatively large and do not have cytoplasmic granules or vacuoles (Fig. 4c). The lobulated nuclei are bi- or trifoliate. Some nuclei exhibit indentations or clefts, which appear as a ridge formation.

PHENOTYPIC MARKERS OF ATL CELLS

Immunophenotypic analyses of ATL cells with various monoclonal antibodies have revealed that ATL cells have the phenotype of activated helper/inducer T lymphocytes. Most ATL cells are positive for CD2, 3, 4, 25, and HLA-DR, and are negative for CD7 and 8 *(56)*. A characteristic feature of ATL cells is the decreased CD3/T cell receptor

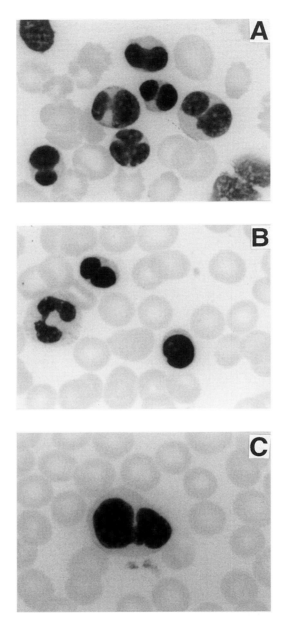

Fig. 4. Cell morphology of ATL cells. Leukemic cells are shown from acute **(a)**, chronic **(b)**, and smoldering **(c)** ATL.

(TCR) expression on their surfacs *(57,58)*. This is a phenomenon specific to ATL cells and is not observed in other T-cell malignancies. There are several reports of ATL cases with different leukemic cell phenotypes, for example, $CD4^+$ and $CD8^+$; $CD4^-$ and $CD8^-$; $CD4^-$ and $CD8^+$ *(59)*. Most of these variant forms are exhibited in acute ATL and indicate poor prognosis. Phenotypic changes in ATL cells have been observed in some patients during the clinical course of the disease. For example, typical CD4$^+$, CD8$^-$ ATL cells changed into CD4$^+$, CD8$^+$, perhaps indicating an exacerbation of ATL and analogous to the phenotypic change that occurs with in vitro activation of T cells. There have been several reports of double-negative ATL (CD4$^-$ and CD8$^-$). CD95 (Fas/ APO-1) antigen is positive in most of ATL patients, and CD95$^+$ ATL cells are highly susceptible to antibody against Fas antigen *(60)*.

CYTOGENETIC STUDY OF ATL

Karyotype analyses of 107 patients with ATL revealed various chromosomal abnormalities as follows *(61)*: (1) Trisomies of chromosome 3 (21%), 7 (10%), and 21 (9%); monosomy of X chromosome (38%) in females; and loss of a Y chromosome (17%) in males were frequent numerical abnormalities. (2) Frequent structural abnormalities were translocations involving 14q32 (28%) or 14q11 (14%), and deletion of 6q (23%). There was no chromosomal abnormality specific for ATL, but abnormalities were detected in the aggressive acute or lymphoma types of ATL rather than in the nonaggressive chronic or smoldering type *(62)*.

CLINICAL FEATURES OF ATL

One hundred eighty-seven patients with ATL were studied by Takatsuki and co-workers in Kyushu, Japan *(63)*. There were 113 males and 74 females (1.5:1), whose age at onset ranged from 27 to 82 yr, with a median age of 55 yr.

The predominant physical findings were peripheral lymph node enlargement (72%), hepatomegaly (47%), splenomegaly (25%), and skin lesions (53%). Various skin lesions, such as papules, erythema, and nodules were frequently observed in ATL patients. ATL cells densely infiltrate the dermis and epidermis, forming Pautrier's microabscesses in the epidermis (Fig. 5). Hypercalcemia (50%) was frequently associated with ATL. Other findings at onset of the disease were abdominal pain, diarrhea, pleural effusion, ascites, cough, sputum, and an abnormal shadow on chest X-ray films. The white blood cell count ranged from normal to 500×10^9/L. Leukemic cells resembled Sézary cells, having indented or lobulated nuclei. The typical surface phenotype of ATL cells characterized by monoclonal antibodies was CD3$^+$, CD4$^+$, CD8$^-$, and CD25$^+$. Anemia and thrombocytopenia were rare. Eosinophilia was frequently observed in ATL patients as well as in those with other T-cell malignancies *(64)*. Cytokines, such as interleukin-5 (IL-5), secreted by ATL cells, are considered to cause the eosinophilia. The presence of neutrophilia and eosinophilia indicates the highly aggressive acute or lymphoma types of ATL, rather than the chronic or smoldering types.

Serum LDH is elevated in most ATL patients, and higher LDH levels indicate an advanced or aggressive disease state. Hypercalcemia, a frequent complication in ATL patients, can be life threatening. Serum calcium and LDH levels reflect the extent of disease and are useful for monitoring tumor and disease activity. Hyperbilirubinemia, observed when ATL cells infiltrate the liver, indicates a poor prognosis. Hypergamma-globulinemia is very rare in ATL, which is consistent with the in vitro suppressor-inducer activity of ATL cells for immunoglobulin synthesis. β_2-Microglobulin is a component of class I HLA antigen, and serum levels of this component are correlated with the disease activity of non-Hodgkin's lymphoma or myeloma. Serum β_2-

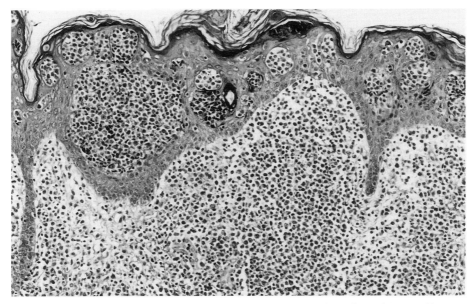

Fig. 5. Skin involvement of ATL. Histology of skin invasion of ATL cells.

microglobulin also is elevated in ATL patients and correlated with disease activity *(65)*. ATL cells express IL-2 receptor α-chain on their surfaces and secrete its soluble forms. Levels of soluble IL-2 receptors as well as levels of serum β₂-microglobulin are elevated in the sera of patients with ATL, and the levels of soluble IL-2 receptor are correlated with the tumor mass and clinical course *(66,67)*.

Familial occurrences of ATL have been reported. Three sisters, ranging in age from 56 to 59 yr, developed lymphoma-type ATL during a 19-mo period *(68)*. The patients were born in Kumamoto Prefecture, an endemic area of HTLV-I. As their lives and environments in adulthood were clearly different, HTLV-I infection may have occurred in childhood. The findings suggest that the disease developed after a long latent period following the first viral infection and that unidentified genetic factors are associated with its onset.

The survival time in acute and lymphoma-type ATL ranged from 2 wk to >1 yr, with a median of 8 mo. The causes of death were pulmonary complications including *Pneumocystis carinii* pneumonia, hypercalcemia, *Cryptococcus* meningitis, and disseminated herpes zoster. All patients were positive for anti-HTLV-I antibodies and HTLV-I proviral DNA in the leukemia/lymphoma cells.

These features and the clinical course, ATL subtype, frequency of hypercalcemia and opportunistic infections, cell morphology, phenotypic profile, and response to treatment appear to be the same for Japanese, Caribbean, and African ATL patients. The only difference is age at onset: the Japanese patients at diagnosis are older *(69)*. Blattner et al. *(22)* and Gibbs et al. *(70)* have reported that the mean ages of ATL patients in the United States and Jamaica were 43 and 40 yr, respectively.

COMPLICATIONS OF ATL

ATL cells infiltrate the spleen, skin, lung, gastrointestinal tract, CNS, kidney, and liver. Such invasions cause the various clinical manifestations (diarrhea, abdominal pain, cough, sputum). Because the immune system in ATL patients is severely compromised, and opportunistic infections such as cytomegalovirus pneumonia, disseminated fungal infections, bacterial sepsis, and bacterial pneumonia are frequent complications.

Pulmonary Complications

It is noteworthy that pulmonary infiltration may be the first symptom of ATL. Infiltration of ATL cells can be diagnosed by identification of ATL cells in the tissue from transbronchial lung biopsy, in bronchial lavage fluid, or occasionally in sputum. In some patients, the lung is the main organ of involvement, and respiratory symptoms (cough, dyspnea) are initial complaints. *Pneumocystis carinii,* viral, and fungal infections are often observed in ATL patients, with the immunodeficiency associated with ATL an important factor in the occurrence of these opportunistic infections. These infections and related pulmonary complications are the major causes of death in ATL patients. The frequency of *Pneumocystis carinii* pneumonia in ATL patients has recently been decreasing due to the prophylactic administration of sulfamethoxazole-trimethoprim.

Hypercalcemia

Since ATL was established as a clinical entity, it has been shown that hypercalcemia is one of the characteristic complications. The prevalence of hypercalcemia in ATL patients is 28% at admission and > 50% during the entire clinical course with or without lytic bone lesions *(71)*. Pathological analyses of bone from autopsy cases with hypercalcemia have disclosed osteoclast proliferation and bone resorption (Fig. 6). Thus, hypercalcemia associated with ATL has been shown to be humorally mediated hypercalcemia of malignancy (HHM), based on the observation of osteoclastic bone resorption and the biochemical characterization of the metabolic abnormalities. ATL was the first hematologic malignancy to be consistently associated with HHM, a condition previously been found in only a few patients with certain solid tumors. In HHM, certain factor(s) produced by tumor cells cause extensive bone resorption in the absence of direct invasion of tumor cells into bone. It has been reported that several factors with osteoclast activation activity are produced by ATL cells. Wano et al. reported the production of IL-1α and β by fresh ATL cells *(72)*. Expression of transforming growth factor-β (TGF-β) has also been detected in fresh ATL cells *(73)*. The parathyroid hormone related protein (PTHrP) gene has been isolated and identified as a causative factor in the HHM of solid tumors *(74)*. The similar pathophysiology of HHM and hypercalcemia of ATL indicates that PTHrP might be a causative factor in ATL hypercalcemia. The expression of the PTHrP gene has been demonstrated in HTLV-I infected T-cell lines. It was also shown that ATL cells expressed a large amount of PTHrP mRNA in all samples tested. These findings suggest that PTHrP might be an important factor in causing the hypercalcemia of ATL in cooperation with IL-1 or TGF-β. Indeed, HTLV-I infection itself induced PTHrP expression *(75)*.

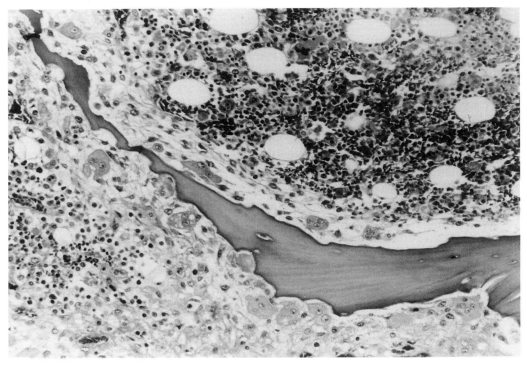

Fig. 6. Marked proliferation of osteoclasts along a bone trabecula. The edge of trabecula is serrated, displaying a saw-toothed appearance. (Figure courtesy of Dr. Takeya, the Second Department of Pathology, Kumamoto University School of Medicine.)

Skin Lesions

As stated previously, ATL cells infiltrate the skin, resulting in the various skin lesions, such as papules, erythema, and nodules that are frequently observed in ATL patients. ATL cells densely infiltrate the dermis and epidermis, forming Pautrier's microabscesses in the epidermis. In erythematous plaques and localized papules, ATL cells proliferate mainly in the epidermis, and proliferation of ATL cells can be seen throughout the entire skin as tumors or nodules. Some ATL patients manifest only skin lesions, which can be tumoral, erythematous, or papular. Although this subtype can be diagnosed as smoldering ATL according to recent criteria, it may also be the so-called cutaneous type of ATL.

Central Nervous System

CNS involvement occurs in about 9% of ATL patients, especially in acute type ATL *(our unpublished data)*. Although both leptomeningeal invasion and intracerebral masses are complications of ATL, leptomeningeal involvement is more common. In 1990, Teshima et al. found that CNS involvement developed in 10 of 99 ATL patients (10.1%), of whom nine had leptomeningeal involvement and two developed intracerebral invasion *(76)*.

Gastrointestinal Tract

ATL cells frequently infiltrate the gastrointestinal tract, and complaints such as diarrhea or abdominal pain suggest gastrointestinal involvement in ATL patients. It was reported that invasion of ATL cells into the gastrointestinal tract was detected in 59 of 139 autopsy cases (44%) *(77)*.

Involvement of Other Organs

Lytic bone lesions are rare complications in ATL patients, but the frequency of these lesions is higher in lymphoma type than in the other clinical types. Bone lesions include both lytic bone lesions and diffuse osteoresorption associated with hypercalcemia. Diffuse osteoresorption has been observed in patients with hypercalcemia.

Other Malignancies

ATL patients may also have complications due to other malignancies. B-cell lymphoma with the Epstein–Barr virus (EBV) genome has been reported in an ATL patient *(78)*, and Kaposi's sarcoma also has occurred with ATL *(79)*. EBV-positive lymphoma and Kaposi's sarcoma are well known to occur in AIDS patients, and impaired cell-mediated immunity in ATL, as in AIDS, is an important factor in these secondary malignancies.

TREATMENT OF ATL

ATL is generally treated with aggressive combination chemotherapy, but long-term success has been less than 10%. The acute form, with hypercalcemia, high LDH levels, and an elevated white blood cell count, shows a particularly poor prognosis. Sequential trials in Japan have resulted in an increase of the complete remission rate from 16% with a four-drug combination to 43% with eight drugs *(80)*. Unfortunately that advance did not translate into an improvement in overall survival. The median remains 8 mo, with death usually the result of severe respiratory infection or hypercalcemia, often associated with drug resistance. In contrast, smoldering ATL and some cases of chronic ATL may have a more indolent clinical course, which may be compromised by aggressive chemotherapy.

Regardless of the specific antileukemic therapy, the inevitable impairment of the T-cell function puts the patient at high risk of fungal, protozoal, and viral infections, against which prophylactic measures should be taken.

Deoxycoformycin, the nucleotide analog, was reported to induce long-term remission in a patient with ATL in 1985 *(81)*. Subsequently, Yamaguchi et al. *(82)* noted prolonged complete remissions in 2 out of 7 patients treated with deoxycoformycin. There was profound lymphopenia, but no neutropenia. Treatment with deoxycoformycin is not suitable for patients with highly aggressive disease activity. Interferon-α combined with azidothymidine was administrated to 19 patients with ATL, and major responses (complete plus partial remissions) were achieved in 58% of the patients (11 of 19), including complete remission in 26% (5 of 19) *(83)*. Other drugs, including arsenic trioxide, have been considered for treatment of ATL on the basis of in vitro data *(84)*. Successful allogeneic bone marrow transplantation for patients with ATL was reported *(85)*. We also performed bone marrow transplantation in a patient with acute ATL, who did not respond to combinational chemotherapy. The patient has been in complete remission for more than 24 mo.

PREVENTION OF HTLV-I INFECTION

Prevention of ATL by reducing transmission of HTLV-I is obviously a more attractive goal. To prevent infection with HTLV-I by blood transfusion, all donated blood in Japan was subjected to HTLV-I antibody testing beginning in November 1986. None of the subsequent recipients, even patients with hematologic disorders who received multiple transfusions, have seroconverted. An absolute decline of the carrier rate among young Japanese has been achieved through comprehensive blood donor screening and by persuading most carrier mothers to refrain from breast-feeding (86).

HTLV-I-RELATED DISORDERS

HTLV-I infection is a direct cause of ATL. In addition, infection with this virus has also been found to be an indirect cause of or a contributing factor in many other diseases, such as HAM/TSP (87,88), chronic lung diseases, opportunistic lung infections, strongyloidiasis (89), nonspecific intractable dermatomycosis (90), arthropathy (91), and uveitis (92). The association of HTLV-I infection with these diseases is considered to be due, to some extent, to the immunodeficiency induced by HTLV-I infection. High provirus load is reported in patients with HAM/TSP and HTLV-I uveitis (93,94), showing that HTLV-I-infected cells play an important role in the pathogenesis of those diseases, presumably by enhanced production of cytokines or activated phenotype with various adhesion molecules.

REFERENCES

1. Yodoi J, Takatsuki K, Masuda T. Two cases of T-cell chronic lymphocytic leukemia in Japan. N Engl J Med 1974; 290:572–573.
2. Uchiyama T, Yodoi J, Sagawa K, Takatsuki K, Uchino H. Adult T cell leukemia; clinical and hematological features of 16 cases. Blood 1977; 50:481–492.
3. Takatsuki K, Uchiyama T, Sagawa K, Yodoi J. Adult T cell leukemia in Japan. In: Seno S, Takaku F, Irino S. (eds). Topics in Hematology. Amsterdam: Excerpta Medica, 1977, pp. 73–77.
4. Poiesz BJ, Ruscetti FW, Gazder AF, Bunn PA, Minna JD, Gallo RC. Detection and isolation of type C retrovirus particles from fresh and cultured lymphocytes of patients with cutaneous T-cell lymphoma. Proc Natl Acad Sci USA 1980; 77:7415–7419.
5. Miyoshi I, Kubonishi I, Sumida M, Yoshimoto S, Hiraki S, Tsubota T, Kohashi H, Lai M, Tanaka T, Kimura I, Miyamoto K, Sato J. Characteristics of a leukemic T-cell line derived from adult T-cell leukemia. Jpn J Clin Oncol 1979; 9:485–494.
6. Hinuma Y, Nagata K, Hanaoka M, Nakai M, Maysumoto T, Kinoshita K, Shirakawa S, Miyoshi I. Adult T-cell leukemia: antigen in an adult T-cell leukemia cell line and detection of antibodies to the antigen in human sera. Proc Natl Acad Sci USA 1981; 78:6476–6480.
7. Seiki M, Hattori S, Hirayama Y, Yoshida M. Human adult T-cell leukemia virus: complete nucleotide sequence of the provirus genome integrated in leukemia cell DNA. Proc Natl Acad Sci USA 1983; 80:3618–3622.
8. Wong-Staal F, Gallo RC. Human T-lymphotropic retroviruses. Nature 1985; 317:395–403.
9. Yoshida M, Miyoshi I, Hinuma Y. Isolation and characterization of retrovirus from cell lines of human adult T-cell leukemia and its implication in the disease. Proc Natl Acad Sci USA 1982; 79:2031–2035.

10. Yoshida M, Suzuki T, Hirai H, Fujisawa J-I. Regulation of HTLV-I gene expression and its roles in ATL development. In: Takatsuki K (ed). Adult T-Cell Leukemia. Oxford: Oxford University Press, 1994, pp. 28–44.

11. Franchini G. Molecular mechanisms of human T-cell leukemia/lymphotropic virus type I infection. Blood 1995; 86:3619–3639.

12. Jeang KT, Widen SG, Semmes IV OJ, Wilson SH. HTLV-I trans-activator protein, Tax, is a transrepressor of the human b polymerase gene. Science 1990; 247:1082–1084.

13. Lemasson I, Robert-Hebmann V, Hamaia S, duc Dodon M, Gazzolo L, Devaux C. Transrepression of *lck* gene exression by human T-cell leukemia virus type 1-encoded p40tax. J Virol 1997; 71:1975–1983.

14. Suzuki T, Hirai H, Murakami T, Yoshida M. Tax protein of HTLV-I destabilizes the complexes of NF-κB and IκB-a and induces nuclear translocation of NF-κB for transcriptional activation. Oncogene 1995; 10:1199–1207.

15. Suzuki T, Kitano S, Matsushime H, Yoshida M. HTLV-I Tax protein interacts with cyclin-dependent kinase inhibitor p16INK4A and counteracts its inhibitory activity towards CDK4. EMBO J 1995; 7:1607–1614.

16. Jim DY, Spencer F, Jeang KT. Human T cell leukemia virus type 1 oncoprotein Tax targets the human mitotic checkpoint protein MAD1. Cell 1998; 93:81–91.

17. Cereseto A, Diella F, Mulloy JC, Cara A, Michieli P, Grassmann R, Franchini G, Klotman ME. p53 functional impairment and high p21waf1/cip1 expression in human T-cell lymphotropic/leukemia virus type I transformed T cells. Blood 1996; 88:1551–1560.

18. Pise-Masison CA, Radonovich M, Sakaguchi K, Appella E, Brady JN. Phosphorylation of p53: a novel pathway for p53 inactivation in human T-cell lymphotropic virus type 1-transformed cells. J Virol 1998; 72:6348–6355.

19. Etoh K-I, Tamiya S, Yamaguchi K, Okayama A, Tsubouchi H, Ideta T, Mueller N, Takatsuki K, Matsuoka M. Persistent clonal proliferation of human T-lymphotropic virus type I-infected cells in vivo. Cancer Res 1997; 57:4862–4867.

20. Cavrois M, Leclercq I, Gout O, Gessain A, Wain-Hobson S, Wattel E. Persistent oligoclonal expansion of human T-cell leukemia virus type 1-infected circulating cells in patients with tropical spastic paraparesis/HTLV-I associated myelopathy. Oncogene 1998; 17:77–82.

21. Tajima K, Tominaga S, Kuroishi T, Shimizu H, Suchi T. Geographical features and epidemiological approach to endemic T-cell leukemia/lymphoma in Japan. Jpn J Clin Oncol 1979; 9:495–504.

22. Blattner WA, Kalyanaraman VS, Robert-Guroff, Lister TA, Galton DA, Sarin PS, Crawford MH, Catovsky D, Greaves M, Gallo RC. The human type-C retrovirus, HTLV, in blacks from the Caribbean region, and relationship to adult T-cell leukemia/lymphoma. Int J Cancer 1982; 30:257–264.

23. Catovsky D, Greaves MF, Rose M, Galton DAG, Golden AWG, McCluskey DR, White JM, Lampert I, Bourikas G, Ireland R, Brownell AI, Bridges JM, Blattner WA, Gallo RC. Adult T-cell lymphoma-leukaemia in blacks from the West Indies. Lancet 1982; 1:639–643.

24. Fleming AF, Yamamoto N, Bhusnurmath SR, Maharajan R, Schneider J, Hunsmann G. Antibodies to ATLV (HTLV) in Nigerian blood donors and patients with chronic lymphatic leukaemia or lymphoma. Lancet 1983; 2:334–335.

25. Kazura JW, Saxinger WC, Wenger J, Forsyth K, Lederman MM, Gillespie JA, Carpenter CCJ, Alpers MA. Epidemiology of human T cell leukemia virus type I infection in East Sepik province, Papua New Guinea. J Infect Dis 1987; 155:1100–1107.

26. Yanagihara R, Ajdukiewicz AB, Garruto RM, Sharlow ER, Wu X-Y, Alemaena O, Sale H, Alexander SS, Gajudusek. Human T-lymphotropic virus type I infection in the Solomon Islands. Am J Trop Med Hyg 1991; 44:122–130.

27. Meytes D, Schochat B, Lee H. Serological and molecular survey for HTLV-I infection in a high-risk middle eastern group. Lancet 1990; 336:1533–1535.

28. Maeda Y, Fukuhara M, Takehara Y, Yoshimura K, Miyamoto K, Matsuura T, Morishima Y, Tajima K, Okochi K, Hinuma Y. Prevalence of possible adult T-cell leukemia virus carriers among volunteer blood donors in Japan: a nation-wide study, Int J Cancer 1984; 33:717–720.

29. Tajima K, Hinuma Y. Epidemiology of HTLV-I/II in Japan and the world. In: Takatsuki K, Hinuma Y, Yoshida M (eds). Advances in Adult T-Cell Leukemia and HTLV-I Research. Gann Monograph on Cancer Research, Vol. 39. Tokyo: Japan Scientific Societies Press, 1992, pp. 129–149.

30. Blattner WA, Gallo RC. Epidemiology of HTLV-I and HTLV-II infection. In: Takatsuki K (ed). Adult T-Cell Leukemia. Oxford: Oxford University Press, 1994, pp. 45–90.

31. Kinoshita K, Hino S, Amagasaki T, Ikeda S, Yamada Y, Suzumiya J, Momita S, Toriya K, Kamihira S, Ichimaru M. Demonstration of adult T-cell leukemia virus antigen in milk from three sero-positive mothers. Gann 1984; 75:103–105.

32. Tajima K, Inoue M, Takezaki T, Ito M, Ito S-I. Ethnoepidemiology of ATL in Japan with special reference to the Mongoloid dispersal. In: Takatsuki K (ed). Adult T-Cell Leukemia. Oxford: Oxford University Press, 1994, pp. 91–112.

33. Okochi K, Sato H, Hinuma Y. A retrospective study on transmission of adult T-cell leukemia virus by blood transfusion: seroconversion in recipients. Vox Sang 1984; 46:245–253.

34. Koyanagi Y, Itoyama Y, Nakamura N, Takamatsu K, Kira J, Iwamasa T, Goto I, Yamamoto N. In vivo infection of human T-cell leukemia virus type I in non-T cells. Virology 1993; 196:25–33.

35. Sagara Y, Ishida C, Inoue Y, Shiraki H, Maeda Y. 71-Kilodalton heat shock cognate protein acts as a cellular receptor for syncytium formation induced by human T-cell lymphotropic virus type 1. J Virol 1998; 72:535–541.

36. Richardson JH, Edwards AJ, Cruickshank JK, Dalgleish AG. In vivo cellular tropism of human T-cell leukemia viurs type 1. J Virol 1990; 64:5682–5687.

37. Etoh K-I, Yamaguchi K, Tokudome S, Watanabe T, Okayama A, Stuver S, Mueller N, Takatsuki K, Matsuoka M. Rapid quantification of HTLV-I provirus load: detection of monoclonal proliferation of HTLV-I-infected cells among blood donors. Int J Cancer 1999, 81:859–864.

38. Mueller N, Tachibana N, Stuver SO, Okayama A, Ishizaki J, Shishime E, Murai K, Shioiri S, Tsuda K. In: Blattner WA (ed). Epidemiologic Perspectives of HTLV-I in Human Retrovirology. New York: Raven Press, 1990, pp. 281–294.

39. Shinzato O, Ikeda S, Momita S, Nagata Y, Kamihira S, Nakayama E, Shiku H. Semiquantitative analysis of integrated genomes of human T-lymphotropic virus type I in asymptomatic virus carriers. Blood 1991; 78:2082–2088.

40. Wattel E, Mariotti M, Agis F, Gordien E, Ferrer Le Coeur F, Pin L, Rouger P, Chen ISY, Wain-Hobson S, Lefrere J-J. Quantification of HTLV-I proviral copy number in peripheral blood of symptomless carriers from the French West Indies. J Acquir Immune Defic Syndr 1992; 5:943–946.

41. Jacobson S, Shida H, McFarlin DE, Fauchi AS, Koenig S. Circulating CD8+ cytotoxic T lymphocytes specific for HTLV-I pX in patients with HTLV-I associated neurological disease. Nature 1990; 348:245–248.

42. Kannagi M, Harada S, Maruyama I, Inoko H, Igarashi H, Kuwashima G, Sato S, Morita M, Kidokoro M, Sugimoto M, Funahashi S, Osame M, Shida H. Predominant recognition of human T-cell leukemia virus type I (HTLV-I) pX against HTLV-I infected cells. Int Immunol 1991; 3:761–767.

43. Usuku K, Sonoda S, Osame M, Yashiki S, Takahashi K, Matsumoto M, Sawada T, Tsuji K, Tara M, Igata A. HLA haplotype-linked high immune responsiveness against HTLV-I in HTLV-I-associated myelopathy: comparison with adult T-cellleukemia/lymphoma. Ann Neurol 1988; 23:S143–150.

44. Sakashita A, Hattori T, Miller CW, Suzushima H, Asou N, Takatsuki K, Koeffler HP. Mutations of the *p53* gene in adult T cell leukemia. Blood 1992; 79:477–480.

45. Cesarman E, Chadburn A, Inghirami G, Gaidano G, Knowles DM. Structural and functional analysis of oncogenes and tumor suppressor genes in adult T-cell leukemia/lymphoma shows frequent p53 mutations. Blood 1992; 80:3205–3216.

46. Hatta Y, Hirama T, Miller CW, Yamada Y, Tomonaga M, Koeffler HP. Holozygous deletions of the *p15 (MTS2)* and *p16INK4A (CDKN2/MTS1)* genes in adult T-cell leukemia. Blood 1995; 85:2699–2704.

47. Uchida T, Kinoshita T, Watanabe T, Nagai H, Murate T, Saito H, Hotta T. The *CDKN2* gene alterations in various types of adult T-cell leukemia. Br J Haematol 1996; 94:665–670.

48. Tamiya S, Etoh K, Suzushima H, Takatsuki K, Matsuoka M. Mutation of *CD95 (Fas/Apo-1)* gene in adult T-cell leukemia cells. Blood 1998; 91:3935–3942.

49. Shimoyama M and members of The Lymphoma Study Group. Diagnostic criteria and classification of clinical subtypes of adult T-cell leukemia/lymphoma. Br J Hematol 1991; 79:428–439.

50. Kubota T, Ikezoe T, Hakoda E, Sawada T, Taguchi H, Miyoshi I. HTLV-I-seronegative, genome-positive adult T-cell leukemia: report of a case. Am J Hematol 1996; 53:133–136.

51. Luo SS, Tamura H, Yokose N, Ogata K, Dan K. Failure to detect anti-HTLV-1 antibody in a patient with adult T-cell leukemia. Br J Haematol 1998; 103:1207–1208.

52. Chosa T, Hattori T, Matsuoka M, Yamaguchi K, Yamamoto S, Takatsuki K. Analysis of anti-HTLV-I antibodies by strip radioimmunoassay—comparison with indirect immunofluorescence assay, enzyme-linked immunosorbent assay and membrane immunofluorescence assay. Leuk Res 1986; 10:605–610.

53. Hisada M, Okayama A, Shioiri S, Spiegelman DL, Stuver SO, Mueller NE. Risk factors for adult T-cell leukemia among carriers of human T-lymphotropic virus type I. Blood 1998; 92:3557–3561.

54. Yoshida M, Seiki M, Yamaguchi K, Takatsuki K. Monoclonal integration of human T-cell leukemia provirus in all primary tumors of adult T-cell leukemia suggests causative role of human T-cell leukemia virus in disease. Proc Natl Acad Sci USA 1984; 81:2534–2537.

55. Tamiya S, Matsuoka M, Etoh K, Watanabe T, Kamihira S, Yamaguchi K, Takatsuki K. Two types of defective human T-lymphotropic virus type I provirus in adult T-cell leukemia. Blood 1996; 88:3065–3073.

56. Hattori T, Uchiyama T, Tobinai T, Takatsuki K, Uchino H. Surface phenotype of Japanese adult T cell leukemia cells characterized by monoclonal antibodies. Blood 1981; 58:645–647.

57. Tsuda H, Takatsuki K. Specific decrease in T3 antigen density in adult T cell leukemia cells: I. Flow microfluorometric analysis. Br J Cancer 1984; 50:843–845.

58. Matsuoka M, Hattori T, Chosa T, Tsuda H, Kuwata S, Yoshida M, Uchiyama T, Takatsuki K. T3 surface molecules on adult T cell leukemia cells are modulated in vivo. Blood 1986; 67:1070–1076.

59. Kamihira S. Hemato-cytological aspects of adult T-cell leukemia. In: Takasuki K, Hinuma Y, Yoshida M (eds). Advances in Adult T-Cell Leukemia and HTLV-I Research. Gann Monograph on Cancer Research, vol. 39. Tokyo: Japan Scientific Societies Press, 1992, pp. 17–32.

60. Debatin KM, Goldman CK, Waldmann TA, Krammer PH. APO-1-induced apoptosis of leukemia cells from patients with adult T-cell leukemia. Blood 1993; 81:2972–2977.

61. Kamada N, Sakurai M, Miyamoto K, Sanada I, Sadamori N, Fukuhara S, Abe S, Shiraishi Y, Abe T, Kaneko Y, Shimoyama M. Chromosome abnormalities in adult T cell leukemia/lymphoma: a karyotype review committee report. Cancer Res 1992; 52:1481–1493.

62. Sanada I, Tanaka R, Kumagai E, Tsuka H, Nishimura H, Yamaguchi K, Kawano F, Fujiwara H, Takatsuki K. Chromosomal aberrations in adult T cell leukemia: relationship to the clinical severity. Blood 1985; 65:649–654.

63. Takatsuki K, Matsuoka M, Yamaguchi K. ATL and HTLV-I-related diseases. In: Takatsuki K (ed). Adult T-Cell Leukemia. Oxford: Oxford University Press, 1994, pp. 1–27.

64. Ogata M, Ogata Y, Kohno K, Uno N, Ohno E, Ohtsuka E, Saburi Y, Kamberi P, Nasu M, Kikuchi H. Eosinophilia associated with adult T-cell leukemia: role of interleukin 5 and granulocyte-macrophage colony-stimulating factor. Am J Hematol 1998; 59:242–245.

65. Tsuda H, Sawada T, Sakata K-M, Takatsuki K. Possible mechanisms for the elevation of serum b2-microglobulin levels in adult T-cell leukemia. Int J Hematol 1992; 55:179–187.

66. Yasuda N, Lai PK, Ip SH, Kung PC, Hinuma Y, Matsuoka M, Hattori T, Takatsuki K, Purtilo DT. Soluble interleukin 2 receptors in sera of Japanese patients with adult T-cell leukemia mark activity of disease. Blood 1988; 71:1021–1026.

67. Yamaguchi K, Nishimura Y, Kiyokawa T, Takatsuki K. Elevated serum levels of soluble interleukin-2 receptors in HTLV-I-associated myelopathy. J Lab Clin Med 1989; 114:407–410.

68. Yamaguchi K, Yul LS, Shimizu T, Nozawa F, Takeya M, Takahashi K, Takatsuki K. Concurrence of lymphoma type adult T-cell leukemia in three sisters. Cancer 1985; 56:1688–1690.

69. Yamaguchi K, Matutes E, Catovsky D, Galton DA, Nakada K, Takatsuki K. *Strongyloides stercoralis* as candidate co-factor for HTLV-I-induced leukaemogenesis. Lancet 1987; 2:94–95.

70. Gibbs WN, Lofters WS, Campbell M, Hanchard B, LaGrenade L, Clark J, Cranston B, Saxinger C, Gallo R, Blattner WA. Adult T-cell leukemia/lymphoma in Jamaica and its relationship to human T-cell leukemia/lymphoma virus type I-associated lymphoproliferative disease. In: Miwa M, Sugano H, Sugimura T. (eds). Retroviruses in Human Lymphoma/Leukemia. Tokyo: Japan Scientific Societies Press, 1985, pp. 77–90.

71. Kiyokawa T, Yamaguchi K, Takeya M, Takatsuki K. Hypercalcemia and osteoclast proliferation in adult T cell leukemia. Cancer 1987; 59:1187–1191.

72. Wano Y, Hattori T, Matsuoka M, Takatsuki K, Chua AO, Greene WC. Interleukin 1 gene expression in adult T cell leukemia. J Clin Invest 1987; 80:911–916.

73. Niitsu Y, Urushizaki Y, Koshida Y, Terui K, Mahara K, Kohgo Y, Urushizaki I. Expression of TGF-beta gene in adult T cell leukemia. Blood 1988; 17:263–266.

74. Suva LJ, Winslow GA, Wettenhall REH, Hammonds RG, Moseley JM, Diefenbach-Jagger H, Rodda CP, Kemp BE, Rodriguez H, Chen EY, Hudson PJ, Martin TJ, Wood WI. A parathyroid hormone related protein implicated in malignant hypercalcemia: cloning and expression. Science 1987; 237:893–896.

75. Watanabe T, Yamaguchi K, Takatsuki K, Osame M, Yoshida M. Constitutive expression of parathyroid hormone-related protein *(PTHrP)* gene in HTLV-I carriers and adult T cell leukemia patients which can be transcribed by HTLV-I *Tax* gene. J Exp Med 1990; 172:759–765.

76. Teshima T, Akashi K, Shibuya T, Taniguchi S, Okamura T, Harada M, Sumida I, Hanada M, Niho Y. Central nervous system involvement in adult T-cell leukemia/lymphoma. Cancer 1990; 65:327–332.

77. Utsunomiya A, Hanada S, Terada A, Kodama M, Uematsu T, Tsukasa S, Hashimoto S, Tokunaga M. Adult T-cell leukemia with leukemic cell infiltration into the gastrointestinal tract. Cancer 1988; 61:824–828.

78. Tobinai K, Ohtsu T, Hayashi M, Kinoshita T, Mastuno Y, Mukai K, Shimoyama M. Epstein–Barr virus (EBV) genome carrying monoclonal B-cell lymphoma in a patient with adult T cell leukemia and lymphoma. Leuk Res 1991; 15:837–846.

79. Greenberg SJ, Jaffe ES, Ehrlich GD, Korman NJ, Poiesz BJ, Waldmann TA. Kaposi's sarcoma in human T-cell leukemia virus type-I associated adult T cell leukemia. Blood 1990; 76:971–976.

80. Shimoyama M. Chemotherapy of ATL. In: Takatsuki K (ed). Adult T-Cell Leukemia. Oxford: Oxford University Press, 1994, pp. 221–237.

81. Daenen S, Rojer RA, Smit JW, Halie MR, Nieweg HO. Successful chemotherapy with deoxycoformycin in adult T-cell lymphoma-leukaemia. Br J Haematol 1984; 58:723–727.

82. Yamaguchi K, Yul LS, Oda T, Maeda Y, Ishii M, Fujita K, Kagiyama S, Nagai K, Suzuki H, Takatsuki K. Clinical consequences of 2'-deoxycorfomycin treatment in patients with refractory adult T-cell leukemia. Leuk Res 1986; 10:989–993.

83. Gill PS, Harrington W Jr, Kaplan MH, Ribeiro RC, Bennett JM, Liebman HA, Bernstein-Singer M, Espina BM, Cabral L, Allen S. Treatment of adult T-cell leukemia-lymphoma with a combination of interferon alpha and zidovudine. N Engl J Med 1995; 332:1744–1748.

84. Bazarbachi A, El-Sabban ME, Nasr R, Quignon F, Awaraji C, Kersual J, Dianoux L, Zermati Y, Haidar JH, Hermine O, de The H. Arsenic trioxide and interferon-alpha synergize to induce cell cycle arrest and apoptosis in human T-cell lymphotropic virus type I-transformed cells. Blood 1999; 93:278–283.

85. Borg A, Yin JA, Johnson PR, Tosswill J, Saunders M, Morris D. Successful treatment of HTLV-1-associated acute adult T-cell leukaemia lymphoma by allogeneic bone marrow transplantation. Br J Haematol 1996; 94:713–715.

86. Oguma S, Imamura Y, Kusumoto Y, Nishimura Y, Yamaguchi K, Takatsuki K, Tokudome S, Okuma M. Accelarated declining tendency of human T-cell leukemia virus type I carrier rates among younger blood donors in Kumamoto, Japan. Cancer Res 1992; 52:2620–2623.

87. Gessain A, Barin F, Vernant JC, Gout O, Maurs L Calender A, de The G. Antibodies to human T-lymphotropic virus type I in patients with tropical spastic paraparesis. Lancet 1985; 2:407–409.

88. Osame M, Usuku K, Izumo S, Ijichi N, Amitani H, Igata A, Matsumoto M, Tara M. HTLV-I associated myelopathy, a new clinical entity. Lancet 1986; 1:1031–1032.

89. Nakada K, Yamaguchi K, Furugen S, Nakasone T, Nakasone K, Oshiro Y, Kohakura M, Hinuma Y, Seiki M, Yoshida M, Matutes E, Catovsky D, Ishii T, Takatsuki K. Monoclonal integration proviral DNA in patients with strongyloidiasis. Int J Cancer 1987; 40:145–148.

90. LaGrenade L, Hanchard B, Fletcher V, Cranston B, Blattner W. Infective dermatitis of Jamaican children: a marker for HTLV-I infection. Lancet 1990; 336:1345–1347.

91. Nishioka K, Maruyama I, Sato K, Kitajima I, Osame M. Chronic inflammatory arthropathy associated with HTLV-I. Lancet 1989; I:441–442.

92. Mochizuki M, Watanabe T, Yamaguchi K, Takatsuki K, Yoshimura K, Shirao M, Nakashima S, Mori S, Araki S, Miyata N. HTLV-I uveitis: a distinct clinical entity caused by HTLV-I. Jpn J Cancer Res 1992; 83:236–239.

93. Yoshida M, Osame M, Kawai H, Toita M, Kuwasaki N, Nishida Y, Hiraki Y, Takahashi K, Nomura K, Sonoda S, Eiraku N, Ijichi S, Usuku K. Increased replication of HTLV-I in HTLV-I-associated myelopathy. Ann Neurol 1989; 26:331.

94. Ono A, Ikeda E, Mochizuki M, Matsuoka M, Yamaguchi K, Sawada T, Yamane S, Tokudome S, Watanabe T. Provirus load in patients with human T-cell leukemia virus type 1 uveitis correlates with precedent Graves' disease and disease activities. Jpn J Cancer Res 1998; 89:608–614.

13

Clonal HIV in the Pathogenesis of AIDS-Related Lymphoma

Sequential Pathogenesis

Michael S. McGrath, Bruce Shiramizu, and Brian G. Herndier

INTRODUCTION

Non-Hodgkin's lymphoma is one of the most common malignancies associated with human immunodeficiency virus (HIV) infection *(1–3)*. These lymphomas are predominantly of B-cell origin and a variety of studies have shown that abnormal B-cell immunologic differentiation occurs during the lymphomagenic process (*see also* Chapter 8) *(4–6)*. Current understanding regarding the pathogenesis of HIV-associated B-cell lymphoma involves evolution from a polyclonal antigen driven B-cell expansion into a polyclonal large cell lymphoma that can then become dominated by a single B-cell clone and at end stage appear as a monoclonal B-cell lymphoma *(4,6)*. Evidence for this polyclonal *(3,7,8)* to monoclonal evolution has been presented in detail; however, events critical to the pathogenesis of the polyclonal state of lymphoma have yet to be clearly defined.

Monoclonal HIV-associated lymphomas frequently have gene rearrangements at the c-*myc* locus *(1)*. This observation, particularly but not exclusively in the Burkitt's subtype, suggests that chromosomal translocations such as t(8;14) and/or infection with Epstein–Barr virus (EBV) are important in the pathogenesis of a subset of B-cell lymphomas. However, the presence of "fundamental" translocations in immunoglobulin gene loci such as t(14;18) [IgH—*bcl-2*] in follicular hyperphasias indicate that such translocations can precede and not be related to the formal advent of neoplasia (in this case follicular lymphoma) and ultimately not be sufficient to drive the pathogenesis of the lymphoma *(3)*. More likely, HIV lymphomas arise out of a setting of the gradual erosion of function and control of the immune system in the setting of chronic retroviral infection with the ultimately evolved B cell sometimes containing rearranged c-*myc* or *bcl-6*. A consensus is evolving that lymphomas in general are outgrowths of chronic antigen drive (mucosa-associated lymphoid tissue lymphomas ["maltomas"], follicular lymphomas), immunodeficiency, and EBV infection (post-transplant lymphoproliferative disease, congenital immunodeficiency lymphomas), and autoimmune disease (Sjögren's syndrome, angioimmunoblastic lymphadenopathy, etc.). HIV disease has many parallels with the above-mentioned examples of immune dysfunction and thus may be an important "model" for understanding lymphomagenesis. Chromosomal translocations and

From: *Infectious Causes of Cancer: Targets for Intervention*
Edited by: J. J. Goedert © Humana Press Inc., Totowa, NJ

infection with herpesviruses (such as EBV) likely play roles in the multistep evolution of lymphoma but do not explain all of HIV-associated lymphomagenesis.

HIV infection induces a state of profound immunodeficiency in individuals with end stage AIDS. The assumptions early in the AIDS epidemic were that AIDS lymphomas were expanded B-cell populations emerging in the face of profound immunosuppression similar to patients who receive allogeneic organ transplants *(3,9,10)*. This observation has been borne out in a few cases of AIDS-related lymphoma wherein the lymphomas are clearly expansions of EBV-positive B cells *(11,12)*, the clearest subset defining this class of lymphoma being the primary central nervous system lymphomas *(2)*. Other more recent studies have suggested the pathway for evolution of AIDS-related lymphoma is unique to HIV-infected individuals and represents a clear and stepwise evolution of an antigen-driven process *(4,5)*.

The current convention regarding lymphoma evolution relies on studies of B-cell immunoglobulin genes from monoclonal lymphomas in tracing their origin back to their polyclonal inception. Immunoglobulin heavy chain variable region genes *(V_H)* from AIDS lymphoma cells are highly modified, suggesting active macrophage and T-cell involvement in early stages of the abnormal B-cell maturation *(4,5,13,14)*. The fact that AIDS lymphoma B cells express highly mutated V_H region genes suggests this active immunologic cellular collaboration. The further finding that the mutations frequently are random also suggests a more fundamental problem in the antigen presentation and immune surveillance process. In the course of a normal immune response, B cells expressing randomly mutated variable region genes would have a negative selective pressure placed on them, and they would undergo programmed cell death (apoptosis). This process clearly has not occurred in the case of high-grade AIDS-related B-cell lymphoma.

The finding of abnormal B-cell maturation coupled with knowledge that HIV can infect a major antigen processing cell, the macrophage, suggests potential cooperation between the macrophage, T-cell, and B-cell compartments in the evolution of lymphoma *(3)*. Detailed studies on AIDS-associated B-cell V_H region gene modification suggest a stepwise process in which the B-cell compartment is either driven to proliferate and differentiate abnormally by the antigen presenting cells or is allowed to expand because of abnormal antigen presenting cell function *(4–6)*. This process may evolve into polyclonal and monoclonal lymphomas. When the first polyclonal lymphomas were described *(7)* and found to have molecular characteristics of a favorable long-term therapeutic outcome *(8,15)*, the concept was proposed that polyclonal lymphomas represented either a novel disease or a disease identified earlier in the pathogenesis of monoclonal lymphoma *(3)*. The major difference between other classes of lymphomas and the AIDS-associated lymphomas is of course the presence of HIV in the latter case.

HIV is a retrovirus and as such has the capability of integrating into infected host cell DNA. Retroviruses have the capability of integrating near and upregulating genes that in certain circumstances can trigger continued cellular proliferation. This is a process termed retroviral insertional mutagenesis *(16)*. Early studies of HIV in tumor B cells failed to find HIV integrated within the B-cell population *(17)*. However, macrophages are a major target for HIV infection and HIV-infected macrophage dysfunction has been implicated in driving lymphomagenesis. A central role for the macrophage in lymphomagenesis is suggested by its production of lymphostimulatory cytokines *(18)* and its chronic presentation of antigens (i.e., HIV) to an expanding B-cell population *(6,13)*.

A survey of AIDS lymphomas performed in the early 1990s identified a series of tumors wherein cells expressed high levels of HIV p24. One of these cases containing no clonal B cells was molecularly defined as a T-cell lymphoma, consisting of cells uniformly expressing high levels of HIV p24 antigen *(19)*. This was the first case identified wherein HIV appeared to be integrated in a clonally expanded cellular population. This observation was the first to suggest that HIV could in certain circumstances act as an insertional mutagenic agent not unlike those observed with Avian leukosis virus in B-cell lymphomas wherein an activated c-*myc* gene was implicated in lymphomagenesis *(20)*. The remainder of this chapter details studies performed to date on the role that HIV potentially plays as an insertional mutagen in vivo, those studies giving rise to the "sequential pathogenesis" hypothesis of AIDS-related lymphomagenesis.

FIRST CASE OF CLONAL HIV IN LYMPHOMAGENESIS

In 1992 Herndier et al. *(19)* described the first case of an AIDS-associated lymphoma containing a clonal form of HIV. This was a high-grade T-cell lymphoma that expressed CD4, CD5, and CD25, as well as high levels of HIV p24 antigen. The lymphoma was immunophenotypically T cell and contained a monoclonal T-cell receptor β-chain gene rearrangement. Although the immunophenotype (CD4+, CD25+) was consistent with that of a human T-cell leukemia virus type I (HTLV-I)-associated T-cell lymphoma, no evidence for HTLV-I infection was demonstrated. Southern blot analysis with an HIV probe, however, found a single form of HIV within this tumor. Parallel Southern blot analyses of lymph nodes that were not involved with tumor failed to find any dominant clonal HIV form. This was the first case wherein clonal HIV was implicated in the pathogenesis of an AIDS-related lymphoma.

EXPANDED STUDIES ON HIV P24 EXPRESSING TUMORS

To follow up the original case, lymphoma specimens obtained at San Francisco General Hospital during the period from 1985 through 1993 were screened with an anti-HIV p24 antibody. The original case was the only T-cell lymphoma in which all cells expressed HIV p24; however, many cases were identified in which tumor-associated macrophages were found to express high levels of HIV p24. In 1994, Shiramizu et al. *(21)* provided evidence for clonal HIV involvement in three more cases of AIDS-related lymphoma in addition to the first T-cell lymphoma described previously. The additional three cases were "ployclonal" or mixed immunophenotype and showed no evidence for a clonal B-cell or T-cell population of cells. This report evolved from the same type of Southern blot analysis performed in the original description of monoclonal HIV T cell lymphoma described previously. Figure 1 shows a Southern blot analysis of the original T-cell lymphoma and three polyclonal lymphomas reported in ref. *21*. This experiment shows that each of these lymphomas contained a single dominant form of HIV. Lane 1 contains an HIV in vitro infected lymphoma control, lanes 2 and 3 contain two different enzymatic digestions of DNA extracted from the original T-cell lymphoma, and lanes 4–6 contain DNA from three polyclonal lymphomas. Each of the three lymphomas in lanes 4–6 contained fewer than 5% clonal B cells as defined by immunoglobulin gene rearrangement studies, but immunohistochemical staining showed a high frequency of HIV-positive macrophages within these large-cell lymphoma specimens *(21)*.

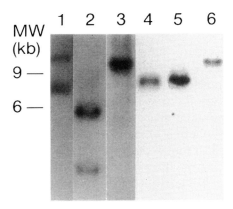

Fig. 1. Southern blot analysis with HIV probe. DNA was extracted from cell pellets and original tumor specimens and Southern blot analysis was performed as previously described *(19)*. *Lane 1*. DNA from HXB2 transfected T cell line. *Lanes 2, 3*. T-cell lymphoma specimen from *(19)* digested with *BAM-H1 (Lane 2)* and *Xba-1 (Lane 3)*. *Lanes 4–6*. *BAM-H1* digests of DNA from cases 2–4 (respectively) from ref. *21*.

The four cases shown in Fig. 1 were further studied and represent the analysis described in the Shiramizu paper in 1994. In this study the inverse polymerase chain reaction (IPCR) technique was performed on DNA extracted from all four tumors. IPCR utilizes primers within the HIV LTR facing away from each other followed by cutting with a restriction endonuclease and ligation into circular forms of DNA. This procedure allows identification of flanking sequence DNA and mapping of monoclonal HIV integration sites. In each of these four tumors the integration site was mapped to the region just upstream to the c-*fes* oncogene. The integrations all occurred within the 3′ exon (nontranslated) of the *fur* gene on chromosome 15, 1000–3000 basepairs upstream of the c-*fes* transcriptional initiation site. Southern blot analysis of IPCR products showed the presence of both LTR and *fur* gene sequence on each amplified IPCR product.

To prove that the IPCR-amplified products were related to the major HIV form within the tumor, a further Southern blot analysis was performed. Figure 2 shows the Southern blot analysis of a tumor associated IPCR product (lanes 1 and 2) as compared to tumor DNA (lane 3) cut with the same restriction enzyme. Lane 1 shows the ethidium bromide stained IPCR bands, which in lane 2 hybridized with a nonprimer HIV LTR probe (CW1B). Lane 3 shows the Southern blot results of a *Sau-3a*-digested tumor DNA probed with an exon-z *fur* gene probe. Note that all three lanes containing tumor and IPCR DNA have bands that co-migrate, a finding consistent with IPCR product sequencing results *(21)*. This is an important observation as it shows the IPCR products to be derived from the major integrated HIV form within the tumor.

As defined by Shiramizu et al. *(21)*, all four tumors had HIV integrated within the *fur* gene upstream of c-*fes*. Northern blot analysis was performed on RNA extracted from two of these tumors and from one follicular hyperplasia not involved with tumor. Figure 3 shows Northern blot analysis of these two tumors probed with a c-*fes* probe. Lane C is RNA extracted from a chronic myeloid leukemia cell line constituitively

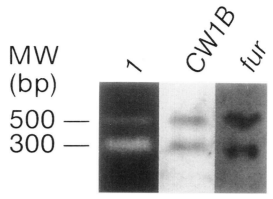

Fig. 2. IPCR and Southern blotting of HIV-LTR/*fur* junction region. DNA was extracted from the HIV T-cell lymphoma described in ref. *19* and *Sau3a* digested. IPCR *(lane 1)* was performed on 50 μg of DNA (1 μg of IPCR product) and 10 μg of digested tumor DNA were run on a gel and Southern blotted with an LTR probe (CW1B, ref.*21*) and *fur* probe *(lane 3, ref. 21)*. Sequence analysis confirmed the junction fragment as containing LTR and *fur* gene sequences.

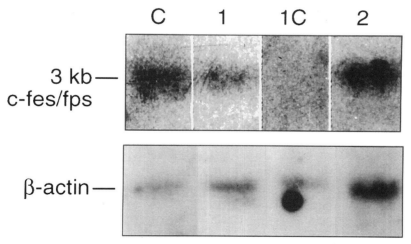

Fig. 3. Northern blot analysis of c-*fes* expression in HIV associated tumors. RNA was extracted from the HIV-associated T-cell lymphoma described in ref. *19 (lane 1)*, control hyperplastic lymph node *(lane 1C)*, polyclonal AIDS lymphoma (Case 3 in ref *21*) (lane 2) and compared with c-*fes* expressing TF-1 cell line (lane C). Northern blots with c-*fes* containing probe was performed as previously described *(26)*. A β-actin probe was used to control for level of RNA expression on original blot after washing.

expressing the normal 3-kb c-*fes* message. Lane 1 is the RNA extracted from the original T-cell lymphoma with lane 1C a follicular hyperplastic lymph node obtained from the same patient. The c-*fes* message was expressed only within the tumor and not a nontumor involved node. Lane 2 represents a Northern blot of RNA extracted from the mixed immunophenotype lymphoma described in Shiramizu et. al. (Case 3, ref. *21*) and shows the same 3-kb message hybridizing with a c-*fes* probe. All specimens contained similar levels of β-actin RNA.

To test whether the c-*fes* RNA expression coincided with expression of protein, monoclonal anti-*fes* antibody was used to stain a mixed immunophenotype lymphoma as compared to a follicular hyperplasia control (Case 2, ref. *21*). Figure 4A shows immunohistochemical staining of macrophages (not associated tumor cells) within the polyclonal lymphoma. Figure 4B shows that only a rare cell expressed *fes* protein within a follicular hyperplastic lymph node. These data taken together with data shown in Fig. 3 suggest that *fes* is expressed at both the RNA and protein level within these clonal HIV-containing tumors.

In an attempt to localize the clonal HIV, fluorescence activated cell sorting studies were performed in which CD14$^+$cells were sorted from CD3$^+$ and double-negative cells. Figure 5 shows the IPCR results of this experiment. Only sorted CD14$^+$ cells contained clonal forms of HIV. In conjuction with the immunohistochemical studies, these data are consistent with a clonal expansion of tumor associated macrophages (CD14 expressing cells) constitutively expressing c-fes protein. As described previously, c-*fes* encodes a 92-kD a protein tyrosine kinase that acts as an intracellular signal for such macrophage activating cytokines such as interleukin-3 (IL-3), GM-CSF, and M-CSF *(21)*. Constitutive expression of c-*fes* in macrophages may therefore contribute to clonal expansion of macrophages in this subset of tumors. Of interest is the observation that Reed–Sternberg cells of Hodgkin's disease also express c-*fes* RNA (*see also*, Chapter 7). The "sequential pathogenesis" model predicts that both the Reed–Sternberg cell in Hodgkin's disease and macrophages in AIDS lymphoma provide growth stimuli (factors) for the surrounding polyclonal cellular proliferations *(3,22)*.

SENSITIVITY OF IPCR

As shown in Fig. 5, input tumor material had only faint IPCR bands whereas the CD14$^+$ cell subset provided clear bands. This observation suggests a certain limitation in sensitivity of the IPCR procedure. In order to test the relative prevalence of clonal HIV within a tumor specimen, a sensitivity study was performed on the IPCR system employed thus far. Tumor DNA from the original T-cell lymphoma was serially diluted into DNA extracted from these same patients' follicular hyperplastic lymph nodes *(21)*. The results showed that the clonal IPCR bands began to disappear when the HIV containing DNA was in the 2–5% range (Fig. 6). Therefore the IPCR study shown in Fig. 5 and those shown previously *(21)* are capable of detecting clonal forms of HIV only if they represent 2–5% of the tumor DNA. This study confirms that IPCR is capable of identifying only a dominant clonal form of HIV within these tumors. This is important considering the recent report that different primer pairs (long terminal repeat [LTR] and GAG primers) apparently have a much higher sensitivity than that described in the studies cited earlier *(23)*.

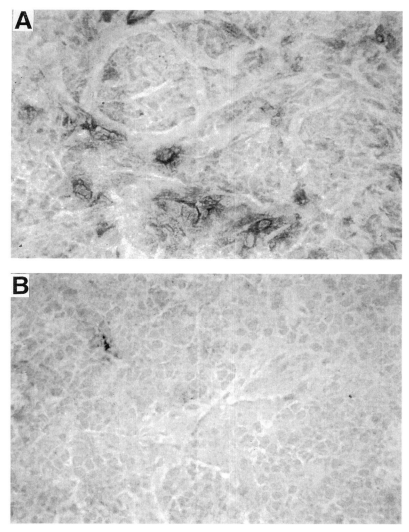

Fig. 4. C-*fes* expression in AIDS lymphoma vs hyperplastic lymph node tissue. Immunohistochemical staining was performed on tumor (Case 2 in ref. *21*) and on involved lymph node with mouse-anti-*fes* antibody (Oncogene Research Products, Cambridge, MA) as previously described *(19)*. **(A)** Tumor. **(B)** Lymph node (4× lower power than **A**). Monoclonal isotype matched control antibody staining was negative on both tissues.

MODEL FOR SEQUENTIAL PATHOGENESIS

The Shiramizu et al. article *(21)* and a follow-up study by McGrath et al. *(24)* identifying clonal IPCR products in an early form of Kaposi's sarcoma led to the proposal of the "sequential pathogenesis" model. In this model HIV randomly infects macrophages, however at a certain frequency that infection and subsequent integration can occur next to the c-*fes* oncogene. Fes is a 92-kDa tyrosine protein kinase associated

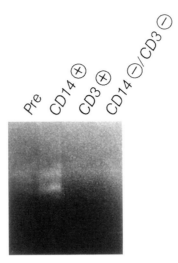

Fig. 5. HIV-IPCR on separated cells from AIDS lymphoma. HIV-IPCR was performed on cells as described in ref. *21* on tumor cells from Case 2 (ref. *21*), CD14+, CD3+, and CD14−/CD3− cells from Case 2.

with malignant transformation in animal tumor systems *(21)*. It is also an intracellular signal molecule communicating transmembrane signals in macrophages initiated by M-CSF, GM-CSF, and IL-3. The data presented earlier and in this review suggest that c-*fes* is constituitively expressed in macrophages containing clonal forms of HIV. Other studies have implicated macrophages as providing growth factors to support the expansion of lymphoma cells in vitro and in vivo. Growth factors implicated include IL-6 and IL-10 as well as other lymphostimulatory cytokines *(18)*. Constitutive expression of IL-10 by a macrophage clone would interfere predictably with activation of an anti-lymphoma T-cell response. The sequential pathogenesis model predicts that early stages in lymphomagenesis contain this clonal form of expanded macrophage that provides an environment that allows B-cell expansion into the experimentally observed polyclonal lymphoma process (reviewed in *3*). Over time these polyclonal lymphomas develop dominant clones and can then evolve into a monoclonal B-cell process. In this setting a preexistent B cell with c-*myc* locus translocation might have a considerable advantage and ultimately become the dominant clone. Similarly a *bcl-6* abnormality or herpesvirus infection could dominate tumor progression. The timing of such events is unclear—the possibility of superinfection with EBV of an already extant lymphoma process is intriguing—the EBV acting as a late hit in tumor progression. A schematic representation of this process is shown in Fig. 7.

This sequential pathogenesis process provides a new therapeutic intervention target for AIDS-related lymphoma. Conventional therapy, although capable of inducing remission in many patients with AIDS lymphoma is associated, with high rates of relapse or death from complications of chemotherapy associated immunosuppression. The identification of clonally expanded macrophages allows one to consider them as a new target for therapeutic intervention potentially earlier in the lymphomagenic process.

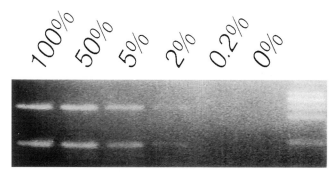

Fig. 6. Sensitivity of IPCR. DNA from a monoclonal tumor specimen containing a clonal HIV was diluted with increasing quantities of DNA from a hyperplastic node from Case 1 (ref. *21*) the same patient and subjected to IPCR. Agarose gel stained with ethidium bromide shows bands approx 200 and 450 basepairs.

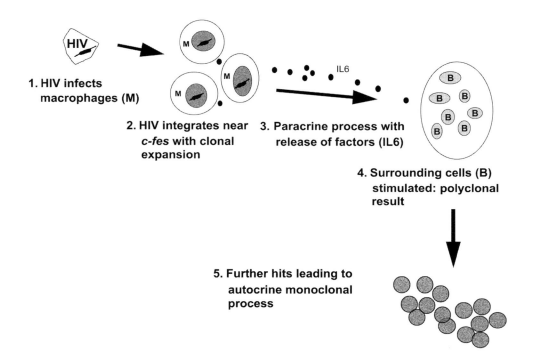

Fig. 7. Sequential pathogenesis of AIDS lymphoma schema.

Recent epidemiologic data suggest that macrophage dysfunction may be critical to the evolution of lymphomagenesis *(25)*. In a large recent case-control study of non-AIDS lymphoma, the two factors associated with a reduced risk of lymphoma are both related to inhibition of macrophage activation. The long-term use of nonsteroidal anti-inflammatory drugs, known to down regulate macrophage inflammatory mediator expression such as IL-1 and IL-6, was found to be protective for lymphoma development. The other major factor suggesting protection from lymphoma development was chronic use of cholesterol lowering agents such as cholestyramine. Fat ingestion by macrophages is known to induce activation and elaboration of inflammatory cytokines. Therefore both at the level of inflammatory cytokine production (nonsteroidal inflammatory drug [NSAID] use) and macrophage stimulation (cholestyramine use), drugs that reduce macrophage activation appear to decrease the risk for patients developing non-Hodgkin's lymphoma. Detailed follow-up studies on other subsets of AIDS and non-AIDS-associated lymphoma will be required to determine the generality of the "sequential pathogenesis" model of lymphomagenesis.

SUMMARY

The data described in this chapter suggest that HIV is capable of integrating within cells and allowing those cells to expand in a clonal manner. The first case involving clonal HIV integration was a monoclonal T-cell lymphoma, but three subsequent cases analyzed in detail have been expansions of HIV expressing macrophages involved in polyclonal lymphoproliferative processes representing early forms of lymphoma. Integration site mapping studies using IPCR, Southern blot, and DNA sequencing in each case identified the integration region within the *fur* gene upstream of c-*fes*. Studies on c-*fes* expression revealed normal c-*fes* message size and expression of c-*fes* protein within tumor tissue. Upon cell sorting, the clonal form of HIV was found exclusively in tumor associated macrophages within the polyclonal lymphomas. These observations gave rise to the "sequential pathogenesis" hypothesis wherein clonal forms of macrophage drive early events in lymphomagenesis. The recent epidemiologic data linking use of drugs that decrease macrophage inflammation with a decreased risk of lymphoma development are consistent with molecular studies implicating AIDS lymphoma B cells as outgrowths of antigen/mitogen driven processes. Studies currently underway include expanding investigations of the sequential pathogenesis model to other HIV-associated diseases wherein infected macrophages play a central role, such as in AIDS related dementia.

ACKNOWLEDGMENTS

This project was supported in part by NIH Grants U01 CA66529, P30MH59037 and R01CA87381, and by Bernie Sarafian with administrative assistance.

REFERENCES

1. Pelicci PG, Knowles DM, Zalmen AA, Wieczorek R, Luciw P, Dina D, Basilico C, Dalla-Favera R. Multiple monoclonal B cell expansions and c-*myc* oncogene rearrangements in acquired immune deficiency syndrome-related lymphoproliferative disorders. J Exp Med 1986; 164:2049–2076.
2. Meeker TC, Shiramizu BT, Kaplan L, Herndier BG, Sanchez H, Grimaldi JC, Baumgartner J, Rachlin J, Feigal E, Rosenblum M, McGrath MS. Evidence for molecular subtypes of HIV-1

associated lymphoma: division into peripheral monoclonal lymphoma, peripheral polyclonal lymphoma and central nervous system lymphoma. AIDS 1991; 5:669–674.

3. Herndier BG, Kaplan LD, McGrath MS. Pathogenesis of AIDS lymphomas. AIDS 1994; 8:1025–1049.

4. Ng VL, Hurt MH, Herndier BG, Fry KE, McGrath MS. V_H gene use by HIV type 1-associated lymphoproliferations. AIDS Res Hum Retrovir 1997; 13:135–149.

5. Przybylski GK, Goldman J, Ng VL, McGrath MS, Herndier BG, Schenkein DP, Monroe JG, Silberstein LE. Evidence for early B cell activation preceding the development of Epstein–Barr virus-negative acquired immunodeficiency syndrome-related lymphoma. Blood 1996; 88:4620–4629.

6. Ng VL, McGrath MS. The immunology of AIDS-associated lymphomas. Immunol Rev 1998; 162:293–298.

7. McGrath MS, Shiramizu BT, Meeker T, Kaplan L, Herndier BG. EBV negative polyclonal lymphoma: identification of a new HIV-associated disease process. J Acquir Immune Defic Syndr 1991; 4:408–415.

8. Shiramizu BT, Herndier BG, Meeker T, Kaplan L, McGrath MS. Molecular and immunophenotypic characterization of AIDS-associated Epstein–Barr virus-negative polyclonal lymphoma. J Clin Oncol 1992; 10:383–389.

9. Ziegler J, Beckstead J, Volberding P, Abrams DI, Levine AM, Lukes RJ, Gill PS, Burkes RL, Meyer PR, Metroka CE, Mouradian J, Moore A, Riggs SA, Butler JJ, Cabanillas FC, Hersh E, Newell GR, Laubenstein LJ, Knowles D, Odajnyk C, Raphael B, Koziner B, Urmacher C, Clarkson BD. Non-Hodgkin's lymphoma in 90 homosexual men: relation to generalized lymphadenopathy and the acquired immunodeficiency syndrome. N Engl J Med 1984; 311:565.

10. Knowles DM, Chamulak GA, Subar M, Burke JS, Dugan M, Wernz J, Slywotzky C, Pelicci G, Dalla-Favera R, Raphael B. Lymphoid neoplasia associated with the acquired immunodeficiency syndrome (AIDS): the New York University Medical Center experience with 105 patients (1981–1986). Ann Intern Med 1988; 108:744.

11. Shibata D, Weiss L, Hernandez A, Nathwani B, Bernstein L, Levine AM. Epstein–Barr virus-associated non-Hodgkin's lymphoma in patients infected with the human immunodeficiency virus. Blood 1993; 81:2102–2109.

12. Hamilton-Dutoit SJ, Pallesen G, Franzmann MB, Karkov J, Black F, Skinhoj P, Pedersen C. AIDS-related lymphoma: histopathology, immunophenotype, and association with Epstein–Barr virus as demonstrated by in situ nucleic acid hybridization. Am J Pathol 1991; 138:149.

13. Ng VL, Hurt MH, Fein CL, Khayam-Bashi F, Marsh J, Nunes WM, McPhaul LW, Feigal E, Nelson P, Herndier BG, Shiramizu B, Reyes GR, Fry KE, McGrath MS. IgMs produced by two acquired immune deficiency syndrome lymphoma cell lines: Ig binding specificity and V_H-gene putative somatic mutation analysis. Blood 1994; 83:1067–1078.

14. Riboldi P, Gaidano G, Schettino EW, Steger TG, Knowles DM, Dalla-Favera R, Casali P. Two acquired immunodeficiency syndrome-associated Burkitt's lymphomas produce specific anti-I IgM cold agglutinins using somatically mutated V_H 4–21 segments. Blood 1994; 83:2952–2961.

15. Kaplan LD, Shiramizu B, Herndier B, Kahn J, Meeker TC, Ng V, Volberding PA, McGrath MS. Influence of molecular characteristics on clinical outcome in HIV-associated non-Hodgkin's lymphoma: identification of a subgroup with favorable clinical outcome. Blood 1995; 85:1727–1735.

16. Kung HJ, Boerkoel C, Carter TH. Retroviral mutagenesis of cellular oncogenes: a review with insights into the mechanisms of insertional activation. Curr Top Micorbiol Immunol 1992; 171:1–25.

17. Gaidano G, Dalla-Favera R. Biologic aspects of human immunodeficiency virus-related lymphoma. Curr Opin Oncol 1992; 4:900–906.

18. Marsh JW, Herndier B, Tsuzuki A, Ng VL, Shiramizu B, Abbey N, McGrath MS. Cytokine expression in AIDS associated large cell lymphoma. J Interferon Cytokine Res 1995; 15:261–268.

19. Herndier BG, Shiramizu BT, Jewett NE, Aldape KD, Reyes GR, McGrath MS. Acquired immunodeficiency syndrome-associated T-cell lymphoma: evidence for human immunodeficiency virus type 1-associated T-cell transformation. Blood 1992; 79:1768–1774.

20. Hayward WS, Neel BG, Astrin SM. Activation of a cellular oncogene by promoter insertion in ALV-induced lymphoid leukosis. Nature (Lond.) 1981; 209:475–479.

21. Shiramizu B, Herndier BG, McGrath MS. Identification of a common clonal human immunodeficiency virus integration site in human immunodeficiency virus-associated lymphomas. Cancer Res 1994; 54:2069–2072.

22. Trumper LH, Brady G, Bagg A, Gray D, Loke SL, Griesser H, Wagman R, Braziel R, Gascoyne RD, Vicini S, Mak T. Single-cell analysis of Hodgkin and Reed-Sternberg cells: molecular heterogeneity of gene expression and *p53* mutations. Blood 1993; 81:3097–3115.

23. Finzi D, Hermankova M, Pierson T, Carruth LM, Buck C, Chaisson RE, Quinn TC, Chadwick K, Margolick J, Brookmeyer R, Gallant J, Markowitz M, Ho DD, Richman DD, Siliciano RF. Identification of a reservoir for HIV-1 in patients on highly active antiretroviral therapy. Science 1997; 278:1295.

24. McGrath MS, Shiramizu BT, Herndier BG. Identification of a clonal form of HIV in early Kaposi's sarcoma: evidence for a novel model of oncogenesis, "sequential neoplasia". J Acquir Immune Defic Syndr Hum Retrovirol 1995; 8:379–385.

25. Holly E, McGrath MS. A case control study of non-Hodgkin's lymphoma among heterosexual adults in the San Francisco Bay area. Am J Epidemiology 1999, 150:375–389.

26. Jücker M, Roebroek AJM, Mautner J, Koch K, Eick D, Dieehl V, Van de Ven WJM, Tesch H. Expression of truncated transcripts of the proto-oncogene c-*fps/fes* in human lymphoma and lymphoid leukemia cell lines. Oncogene 1992; 7:943–953.

IV
Papillomaviruses

14
Papillomaviruses in Human Cancers

Harald zur Hausen

Papillomas as benign tumors were the first proliferative condition for which the causation by a viral infection has been convincingly demonstrated. Tumor virology started with the cell-free transmission of oral dog warts by M'Fadyan and Hobday in 1898 *(1)*. These experiments preceded the frequently cited studies of a cell-free transmission of a chicken sarcoma by Peyton Rous *(2)* by 13 yr and those by Ellermann and Bang *(3)* on a viral origin of chicken leukemias by 10 yr. Also prior to these observations, in 1907 Ciuffo in Italy *(4)* showed the transmissibility of human warts in self-inoculation experiments. Thus, papillomas emerged as the first (though benign) tumors with a proven viral etiology.

The conversion of virus-caused papillomas into carcinomas was initially observed by Rous and Beard *(5)* and carefully analyzed by Rous and his associates in cottontail rabbits *(6–8)*. In these years, Rous analyzed synergistic effects of this virus infection with chemical carcinogens and formulated first ideas on tumor initiation. The frequent conversion of papillomas into carcinomas in the rabbit papillomavirus system has nevertheless for a long time been considered as a biological curiosity, particularly in view of the virtual absence of similar observations in humans. Only in the beginning of the 1950s a rare hereditary condition, epidermodysplasia verruciformis, a generalized verrucosis with frequent subsequent progression into squamous cell carcinomas of the skin, was recognized as a condition linked to wart virus infection *(9–11)*. Although in the following decade human papillomavirus particles were demonstrated electron microscopically and in the 1960s characterized as DNA viruses with a double-stranded circular genome, interest in this virus group remained at best marginal in this period of time. Besides the apparent clinical unimportance of warts, the inability to grow these viruses in tissue culture systems represented another contributing factor, discouraging most virologists.

The situation changed in the 1970s. Advances in molecular biology, the discovery of the heterogeneity of the human papillomavirus (HPV) group *(12–14)*, published speculations on a role of specific papillomaviruses in cancer of the cervix *(15–17)*, and the demonstration of a specific papillomavirus type in squamous cell carcinomas of patients with epidermodysplasia verruciformis *(18)* resulted in gradually increasing interest in this virus group. Since the early 1980s the situation changed more dramatically. The finding of novel HPV types in biopsies from cervical carcinomas *(19,20)* led

From: *Infectious Causes of Cancer: Targets for Intervention*
Edited by: J. J. Goedert © Humana Press Inc., Totowa, NJ

to a rapid increase in HPV studies and to a large number of attempts to prove their etiologic role in cervical as well as in other cancers.

GENERAL CHARACTERISTICS

The papillomavirus family emerges as the most complex family of human pathogenic viruses. Eighty-five different HPV types have been analyzed to date and the nucleotide sequence of most of them has been determined *(21,22* and de Villiers, *personal communication).* In addition, approx 120 putative novel genotypes were identified, based on more than 10% differences in their nucleotide sequence in a most conserved stretch of the major structural protein L1.

Structural properties of papillomavirus particles and the analysis of HPV DNA, as well as the mode of DNA replication, have been covered in previous reviews (e.g., *23).* In brief, the nonenveloped particle of approx 55 nm in diameter contains a double-stranded circular genome ranging in size between 7000 and 8000 basepairs. The structure renders these particles remarkably resistant against thermal inactivation. Genes are read in one direction only, and the genome contains two genes coding for late functions, the viral structural proteins, and six to eight early genes. Previous reviews covered the genomic structure of HPVs and animal papillomaviruses extensively (e.g., *23,24).* Three genes (E6, E7, and E5) possess growth-stimulating properties. In contrast to E5, however, E6 and E7 are able to transform a variety of human cells individually and to cooperate under conditions of simultaneous expression. E1 and E2 are engaged in viral DNA replication, E2 also in the transactivation of the viral long regulatory region. E3 and E8 genes have not been described in human anogenital HPV types. E4 is possibly a late nonstructural gene of these viruses, but its exact function remains to be elucidated.

As outlined previously, the papillomavirus group turned out to be extremely heterogeneous. The existing multitude of types can be subdivided into several individual subgroups: one of them covers anogenital HPV infections, the others contain HPV types infecting the skin. Depending on their relative risk to induce malignant transformation and on their ability to immortalize human cells in tissue culture, some anogenital HPV types are considered as "high-risk" infections, others as "low risk" *(25).* The following sections deal mainly with functions and control of E6 and E7 genes of high-risk infections and cover the host control of the virus.

NATURAL HISTORY OF HPV INFECTIONS

Infections with papillomaviruses require the availability of cells that are still able to replicate (reviewed in *24).* The outcome of an infectious event mainly depends on three factors: (1) the multiplicity of infection, (2) the interaction with chemical or physical carcinogens, and (3) immunologic responsiveness.

The role of the input multiplicity has been most carefully analyzed in cottontail rabbit papillomavirus (CRPV) infections *(26–28).* Infection of the rabbit skin with high doses of CRPV results in the emergence of papillomatous changes already 4–6 wk after inoculation. Low concentrations, however, result in papillomas only under conditions of treatment of the rabbit skin with chemical carcinogens *(7,8,26).* Without such treatment viral DNA can be demonstrated in normal tissue by the polymerase chain reaction (PCR). It appears that under these condition only the E1 gene is expressed which is required for the maintenance of the episomal state of the persisting viral DNA.

Immunosuppression of humans, either after receiving organ allografts or under conditions of an acquired immunodeficiency syndrome (AIDS), frequently results in extensive verrucosis *(29)*. Recent observations demonstrate the presence of papillomavirus DNA of a broad spectrum of genotypes in biopsies from normal skin and follicles of plucked hair *(30,31)*. This suggests that multiple infections with virus production are commonly taking place without any clinical symptoms. It is therefore highly likely that four modes of viral genome persistence exist: (1) latent infections (possibly only with *E1* gene expression), (2) inapparent infections (without clinical symptoms), (3) apparent infections (development of lesions), and (4) abortive infections (after integration of the viral genome into host cell DNA with the possible consequence of dysplasia and malignant progression).

Infections probably largely depend on the availability and the access to basal layer cells. These cells suppress viral functions efficiently, as long as this suppression is not overcome by a high input multiplicity. Only subsequent cell divisions and irreversible differentiation of the infected keratinocytes render these cells permissive for viral gene expression. The events are schematically shown in Fig. 1.

Low-input multiplicities in experimental settings lead to latent infections that can be reactivated by chemical or physical carcinogens or by severe immunosuppression. Particularly the activation of latent infections by chemical and physical carcinogens suggests the need for modifications in either host or viral DNA for the induction of proliferative changes. There exist no hints for modifications in the viral genome. In contrast, there is evidence for a tight host cell control in basal layer cells. This permits the following interesting speculation.

Papillomas in humans should then result mainly from HPV-infected cells acquiring specific modifications of the host cell genome in switching off the effective control of early viral gene expression. It is interesting to note that genital warts (condylomata acuminata) and CRPV-induced lesions of the rabbit skin reveal a remarkable degree of early viral gene transcription already in the proliferative zone *(27,32)*. Condylomata acuminata contain predominantly HPV-6 or -11 genomes. Similar to CRPV, a latent state of HPV-11 in the periphery of laryngeal papillomas has been reported *(33)*. It is therefore possible that the development of the respective lesions is the consequence of preexisting or induced genetic damage afflicting specific genes. The observed clonality of high-grade HPV lesions would also be in line with this speculation *(34,35)*. High-input multiplicities of the infecting agent that block intracellular inhibitory mechanisms by a gene-dosage effect could be an explanation for nonclonal development of papillomas.

In some contrast, early lesions induced by high-risk HPV types 16 and 18 frequently reveal very low, sometimes barely detectable, levels of viral oncogene expression *(36,37)*. One possible explanation would be a certain degree of leakiness for viral oncogene expression, specifically characterizing the high-risk HPV types, permitting in most instances the development of clinical symptoms and rarely or not at all resulting in a true state of latency. This point seems to require further investigation.

Viral DNA replication and particle formation in the stratum granulosum and stratum corneum may continue for long time intervals. The long-lasting release of infectious virus from cutaneous and mucosal surfaces accounts for the success of these infections. The frequent absence of an exposure to the immune system of the host is the most

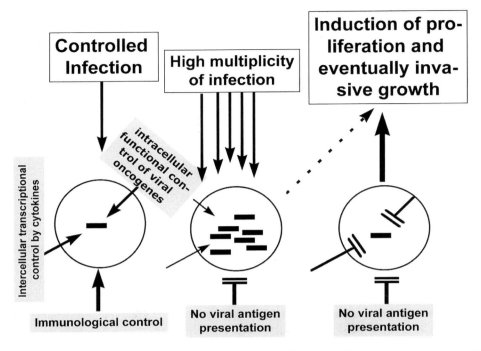

Fig. 1. Schematic model and outline of events following infection by human papillomaviruses. The *left part* symbolizes a cell harboring an HPV genome *(bar)*. The persisting viral genes are controlled by an intercellular control mechanism suppressing transcription, mediated by cytokines of surrounding cell compartments. In addition, an intracellular mechanism blocks the function of viral oncoproteins. Expressed viral genes moreover are subject to immunologic surveillance. High-input multiplicities seem to overcome the intracellular and intercellular control functions *(central part)*. Conversion toward malignant growth should still imply the nonrecognition of viral antigens by immunologic control mechanisms of the host. Conversion of cells containing low copy numbers of HPV DNA to malignant growth requires the modification of host cell genes regulating the inter- and intracellular (CIF-) cascades. In addition, nonrecognition by immunologic surveillance mechanisms seems to be a further requirement.

likely explanation for the development of this complex virus group. The evolution took place under minimal restraints from immunologic defense mechanisms.

CANCERS LINKED TO HPV INFECTIONS

Initial identifications of human papillomaviruses in human cancers were made in squamous cell carcinomas of the skin of patients with a rare hereditary disorder, epidermodysplasia verruciformis *(38)*. As early as 1972, Jablonska and co-workers considered this condition already as a model to study the role of papovaviruses in human cancers *(11)*.

A very common human cancer presently known to be caused by specific papillomavirus types is cancer of the cervix. The link of this cancer to HPV infections was proposed between 1974 and 1976 *(15,16)*. The first virus isolates from this tumor type, HPV-16 and HPV-18, were published in 1983 and 1984 *(19,20)*. Today > 95%

Table 1

Genotypes of HPV Detected in Benign and Neoplastic Lesions of the Cervix

Lesion	HPV genotypes[a]
Condyloma acuminata	**6, 11,** 42, 44, 51, 53, 83
Intraepithelial neoplasia	6, 11, **16,** 18, 26, 30, 31, 33, 34, 35, 39, 40, 42, 43, 45, 51, 52, 56, 57, 58, 59, 61, 62, 64, 67, 68, 69, 70, 71, 74, 79, 81, 82
Cervical and other anogenital cancers	6, 11, **16,** 18, 31, 33, 35, 39, 45, 51, 52, 54, 56, 58, 66, 68, 69

[a] Bold font indicates most common genotypes; small font indicates least common genotypes.

of cervical cancer biopsies contain HPV sequences. Although HPV-16 represents by far the most frequently identified virus, a number of additional genotypes has been identified in this tumor. Table 1 lists HPV genotypes found in cervical cancer biopsies.

Besides cervical cancer other anogenital cancers (anal, perianal, vulvar, penile, and vaginal) have been linked to the same infections (*see also* Chapter 15). Whereas anal and perianal cancers reveal a similar distribution of high-risk HPV infections, as found in cervical cancer, only about 50% of the other cancers turn out to contain high-risk HPV DNA. It is presently unknown whether the negative biopsies are indeed HPV-negative or contain other, possibly cutaneous, HPV types. In view of the scarcity of biopsies from such tumors no careful studies have been conducted to analyze the presence of cutaneous HPV in these conditions.

Besides anogenital cancers, approx 20% of oropharyngeal cancers have been found to contain anogenital high-risk HPV types *(39)*. Particularly frequent are HPV findings in cancers of the tonsils *(40,41)* and the tongue *(42)*. Occasional HPV positivity has also been reported for other cancers, such as cancer of the larynx *(43,44)*, hypopharynx *(45)*, nasal cavity *(46)*, palate, buccal mucosa, lips *(45)*, and even for a few lung cancer biopsies *(47)*. Since HPV-positive oral cancers, to the extent they have been investigated, express the viral oncoproteins E6 and E7 *(48,49)*, it is likely that the virus plays a causal role in these tumors (*see also* Chapter 16).

HPV infections have also been suspected to play a role in cancer of the esophagus *(50)*. The available data are not fully convincing, and the prevalence of HPV varies among laboratories and different geographic regions from zero to 67% (reviewed in *51*). A recent report finds a relatively high rate (34.9%) of HPV-positive biopsies in samples obtained from China and in 26.4% of samples obtained from cancer cases in South Africa *(52)*. Only a small fraction of the latter tumors contained anogenital HPVs; the others contained HPV types also found in cutaneous lesions. Three of the identified types represented putative novel HPV genomes.

Squamous cell carcinomas developing in patients with epidermodysplasia verruciformis (EV) were shown in 1979 to contain members of a specific subgroup of HPVs *(38)*. The development of broad-spectrum PCRs permitting the detection of a wide variety of HPV types resulted in the demonstration of a high percentage of squamous cell carcinomas in immunosuppressed as well as in immunocompetent individuals containing in part novel HPV sequences *(53–57)*. At present more than 80% of these tumors are HPV positive. A recent report describes a higher prevalence of some types in these lesions with HPVs 20, 23, 38 and two putative novel types accounting for 73% of the virus-positive biopsies *(58)*. The significance of these findings is difficult to assess. Problems arise from the high rate of HPV prevalence in plucked hair follicles and in biopsies from normal skin *(30,31)*, where up to 50% of the analyzed materials were found to be HPV-positive. In these materials a broad spectrum of different HPV genotypes has been detected, leading in addition to the identification of several putative novel genotypes *(see also* Chapter 16).

It is possible that, in contrast to high risk anogenital HPV infections, cutaneous HPV infections contribute by an indirect mode to squamous cell carcinoma development: their presence may protect against apoptosis after genetic damage due to solar exposure (Storey, *personal communication*), thus resulting in increased survival of the genetically modified cells. On the other hand, the development of papillomas in immunosuppressed patients specifically at sun-exposed sites points also to an involvement of genetic damage in wart development caused by these viruses. Further studies will have to clarify the picture.

PATHOGENIC MECHANISMS

Early observations analyzing HPV genomes and the viral transcription pattern in cervical carcinoma cell lines revealed frequent integration of viral DNA *(20)* and the consistent expression of the viral early genes E6 and E7 *(59,60)*. The same genes have subsequently been shown to be necessary for immortalization of various types of human cells (reviewed in *61)*. E6 as well as E7 genes can immortalize human cells independently *(62–64)*, although they cooperate efficiently in the immortalization of a wide spectrum of different human cells *(65,66)*.

E6 and E7 gene expression is also necessary for the proliferative phenotype of cultured cervical carcinoma cells *(67–69)*. Inducible E6/E7 antisense constructs or a hormone-inducible switch-off of HPV revealed that, in the cervical carcinoma cell lines tested, the expression of at least one of the viral oncogenes is necessary for the proliferative and the malignant phenotype.

The HPV16 E7 protein has been identified as a zinc binding phosphoprotein with two Cys-X-X-Cys domains composed of 98 amino acids. A similar zinc binding motif and two Cys-X-X-Cys motifs also occur in the E6 protein. This may point to an evolutionary relationship between the two proteins.

High-risk HPV E7 proteins complex with the retinoblastoma susceptibility protein pRB *(70)*. The binding affinity of high-risk HPVs' E7 for pRB is approx 10-fold higher than that of low-risk HPVs' E7 *(71)*. E7 is also able to cooperate with an activated *ras* gene in transformation of rodent and human cells *(72,73)*. pRB-binding, however, does not emerge as a general precondition for immortalization *(74,75)*, pointing to additional functions of the E7 protein. E7/pRB binding releases the transcription factor E2F from pRB complexes, thus activating transcription of genes regulating cell proliferation *(76)*.

Besides binding pRB high-risk HPV E7 proteins associate with related proteins, such as p107 and p130, and with the protein kinase p33cdk2 and with cyclin A *(77,78)*.

E7 expression in NIH3T3 cells results in a constitutive expression of cyclin E and cyclin A genes in the absence of external growth factors *(79)*.

High-risk E7 proteins, to a lesser extent than E6 proteins, can override DNA-damage p53-induced G_1 growth arrest *(80–83)*. This is considered as a potential mechanism for the reported E7 induction of chromosomal aberrations *(84)*.

A number of additional interactions of the E7 protein with host cell proteins have been revealed recently. E7 inactivates two cyclin-dependent kinase inhibitors, p21[CIP-1] and p27[KIP-1] *(85–87)*. It is possible that this inhibitory interaction is reciprocal and depends on the quantity of expressed E7 protein. In addition, a modulation of type M2 pyruvate kinase activity has been reported by the HPV16 E7 oncoprotein *(88)*, which seems to point to an important interference of viral oncoproteins with the carbohydrate metabolism of the infected cell.

The E6 protein binds p53 and abolishes its tumor-suppressive and transcriptional activation properties *(89)*. It promotes ubiquination of p53 and its subsequent proteolysis through interaction with the E6AP ubiquitin-protein ligase *(90,91)*. E6 and E7 are able to immortalize human keratinocytes independently, although both genes cooperate effectively in immortalization events. As observed for E7, E6 also targets other proteins: the focal adhesion protein paxillin *(92)* and the interferon regulatory factor 3 (IRF-3), blocking the induction of interferon-β mRNA after viral infection *(93)*. These data indicate the multifunctionality of viral oncoproteins, modifying a multitude of cellular functions.

The low efficiency of HPV immortalization, but even more so the recessive nature of immortalized cells, frequently complementing each other to senescence when cells of different clones are subjected to somatic cell hybridization *(94,95)*, strongly suggests that E6/E7 gene expression is necessary but not sufficient for immortalization. The same accounts for malignant conversion. As previously discussed, viral oncogene expression appears to be necessary for the malignant phenotype of HPV-positive cells. Yet, somatic cell hybridization of cells from different HPV-positive lines reveals three possible outcomes *(96)*: besides the failure to complement as seen for some lines (e.g., the HPV-18-positive HeLa and SW 756 cells), some complement each other for senescence (Rösl and zur Hausen, *unpublished data*), and still others complement each other for a nonmalignant phenotype (e.g., HeLa cells and the HPV 16-positive Caski line). Complementation to senescence on the one hand and complementation of malignant cells to immortalization on the other suggest that besides HPV gene expression at least two additional cellular signaling cascades need to be modified to permit malignant conversion.

HOST CELL FACTORS CONTROLLING HPV INFECTIONS: THE CIF CONCEPT

In most but not all cervical cancers viral DNA persists in an integrated state, whereas premalignant clinical lesions commonly contain exclusively episomal DNA *(97)*. Integration of the viral episome usually destroys its structural integrity, resulting in a partial dysregulation of viral oncogene transcription that results in part from upstream cellular enhancers, in part also from increased longevity of chimeric transcripts, encoding E6 and E7, but also flanking cellular sequences *(59,98)*. Integration seems to occur during the transition to high-grade lesions and seems to be partially responsible for the advanced dysplastic phenotype. Yet, it is clearly not sufficient, either for the immortalized or for the malignant phenotype of the cells. This can be judged from the analysis of somatic cell hybrids between different HPV-positive carcinoma cells or between different HPV-immortalized cells. In either instance these cells may complement each other to senescence, in spite of the exclusive presence of integrated viral DNA *(95)*. Some integration sites have been identified that correspond to fragile regions of the chromosomes *(99–103)*.

Mounting evidence points to specific chromosomal aberrations in either HPV-immortalized or malignantly transformed human cells. Although numerous aberrations have been demonstrated during the past 10 yr, some occur at higher frequency: they involve the chromosomal regions 3p14.2 and 3p21 *(104–106)*, 11p15 and 11q23 *(106–109)*, and 17p13.3 *(110)*. Besides these, additional apparently nonrandom modifications have been found in chromosomes 4p16, 4q21–35, 5p13–15, 6p21.3–22, and 18q12.2-22 *(107,111,112)*.

The chromosome region 3p14.2 harbors the Fragile Histidine Triad or *FHIT* gene *(113* and recently reviewed in *114)*. This exceptionally large locus is very frequently altered in common human cancers including cancer of the cervix. The gene seems to play a role as tumor suppressor gene, as replacement of *FHIT* expression in the respective cancer cells suppresses their tumorigenicity.

On a first glance the emergence of relatively specific chromosomal aberrations in a clearly virus-linked human cancer could be perplexing and may pose questions concerning the role of the persisting viral DNA. As previously pointed out, however, there exists ample evidence that viral oncogene expression is necessary for initiation and maintenance of the proliferative phenotype of HPV immortalized cells, and also for those HPV-positive cervical carcinomas cell lines that could be subjected to experimental analysis. As discussed previously, the viral oncoproteins are obviously necessary but not sufficient for the immortalized and malignant phenotypes of HPV-infected cells.

Early attempts to analyze a possible interaction between cellular functions and potential tumor viruses resulted in the postulation of a cellular interference factor (CIF), suppressing in normal cells transcription of viral oncogenes or their intracellular functions *(115,116)*. Data obtained later, revealed the existence of a network of CIFs adapted to the control of persisting high-risk HPV RNA transcription and the function of viral oncoproteins, resulting in a CIF-cascade concept *(24,117)*.

The transcriptional control is presently better understood than the functional control of persisting HPV oncogenes. Explantation of human HPV-immortalized cells into nude mice commonly results in small nodules without further progression and a very low rate of HPV E6/E7 RNA transcription in a limited number of cells *(118)*. This corresponds to observations made in proliferating layers of low-grade lesions of the cervix containing high-grade HPV *(36,37)*. Speculations that signals from the surrounding tissue mediate the suppression of HPV transcription led to experiments to expose HPV-immortalized and malignant cells to human macrophages under tissue culture conditions *(119–121)*. The data revealed that macrophages suppress selectively HPV transcription in immortalized, but not in malignant cells. Tumor necrosis factor-α (TNF-α) seems to play a prime role in the suppressing effect, as noted also in other systems *(122–124)*. Other cytokines, such as transforming growth factor-β

(TGF-β) *(125,126),* interleukin-1 *(123,127),* and interleukin-6 *(128)* had been shown previously to suppress preferentially HPV transcription in HPV immortalized cells. The proximal target of the TNF-α interaction appears to be the AP-1 complex in the HPV promoter, which upon TNF-α treatment of immortalized cells, but not malignant cells, changes its composition from preferential c-*jun*/c-*jun* homodimers to c-*jun*/Fra-1 heterodimers *(121).* In most malignant cells the AP-1 complex in the HPV promoter contains c-*jun*/c-*fos* heterodimers. Overexpression of c-*fos* in immortalized cells results in a single step to a malignant phenotype *(121).* The data point to the existence of a paracrine signaling pathway that blocks the transition of immortalized cells to a malignant phenotype (CIF-II cascade). This pathway is obviously interrupted in malignant cells.

Putative cellular genes engaged in transcriptional control are located on the short arm of chromosome 11, as deletion of this arm upregulates a regulatory component of protein phosphatase 2A (PP2A), resulting in lowered PP2A activity, and this again in an upregulation of persisting HPV DNA *(129).* Similar effects can be achieved with okadaic acid or SV40 small t-antigen, both known to interfere with PP2A function. How PP2A affects downstream targets and eventually may modify the composition of AP-1 dimers is still unknown.

The existence of a functional control of HPV oncoproteins (CIF-I cascade) can be deduced from several experimental approaches: in part from somatic cell hybridization studies revealing continued HPV oncogene transcription in senescent hybrid clones of different immortalized cells *(94),* in part also from observations revealing a switch-off of the p16^{ink4} cyclin-dependent kinase inhibitor in human keratinocytes immortalized by only the high-risk HPV E6 gene *(130,* Whitaker and zur Hausen, *unpublished data).* In E6- and E7-immortalized cells and in solely E7-immortalized cells, the situation is different. Here commonly an overexpression of p16 is observed, whereas two other cyclin-dependent kinase inhibitors become inactivated by E7, p21^{CIP1} and p27^{KIP1} *(85–87).* There is some probability that under conditions of low E7 expression p21 and p27 reciprocally interfere with functions of the viral oncoprotein, although this has not yet been proven directly. Thus, the cyclin-dependent kinase inhibitors may represent the most downstream targets for a functional inhibition of viral oncoproteins; their mode of regulation still needs to be clarified.

Thus, as summarized in Fig. 1, the available data point to the existence of an *intra* cellular control interfering with the function of viral oncoproteins (CIF-I cascade), whose interruption permits the transition of infected cells to an immortalized state and an *inter*cellular control (CIF-II cascade), triggered by different cell compartments, whose interruption as a second step mediates the conversion from immortalization to a malignant phenotype. Unlimited growth in tissue culture is achieved only after interruption of the CIF-I cascade. In the patient, modifications of these pathways may also occur in the reverse order. It is likely that the observed mutagenicity of high-risk E6 and E7 gene expression *(83)* even at a low level of expression contributes to modifications of the host cell genomes, thus permitting high-risk HPVs (by disregarding the factor time) a role as solitary carcinogens.

Today it becomes more and more evident that vertebrate hosts of evolutionary ancient viruses are adapted to subimmunologic control mechanisms that interfere intracellularly with functions of the viral genome.

CONTROL OF HPV INFECTIONS

The identification of papillomaviruses as cancer-inducing agents in humans permits the development of preventive strategies. The structural features of these viruses enabled the construction of virus-like particles consisting either of L1 and L2 or solely of L1 structural proteins *(131,132)*. The use of similar preparations in analogous systems in dogs *(133)*, cottontail rabbits *(134)*, and cattle *(135)* provides an excellent baseline for clinical trials in humans that have been started in recent years. Theoretically these vaccines could contribute to a measurable reduction of the cancer load, particularly in women, if applied globally. Besides attempts to develop preventive vaccines, efforts are also going on to construct therapeutic vaccines, based on modified E6 or E7 protein preparations or on chimeric particles expressing E7 antigenic epitopes within the L1 *(136)*. The latter preparations are anticipated to possess preventive and therapeutic properties.

The value of therapeutic interference based on these vaccination strategies is presently difficult to assess and will have to await the outcome of clinical trails. It will probably be difficult to treat cancer cases by using this regimen. On the other hand there seems to exist a reasonable possibility of therapeutically vaccinating against early lesions. It seems that after 20 yr of intensive research on anogenital papillomaviruses the efforts are finally beginning to pay off and hopefully will result in a global decrease of cervical cancer, which is still one of the most frequent cancers in women in major parts of this world.

REFERENCES

1. M'Fadyan J, Hobday F. Note on the experimental "transmission of warts in the dog." J Comp Pathol Ther 1898; 11:341–343.
2. Rous P. Transmission of a malignant new growth by means of a cell-free filtrate. Am J Med Assoc 1911; 56:198–211.
3. Ellermann V, Bang O. Experimentelle Leukämie bei Hühnern. Centralbl F Bakt Abt I (Orig) 1908; 46:595–609.
4. Ciuffo G. Innesto positivo con filtrado di verrucae volgare. G Ital Mal Venereol 1907; 48:12–17.
5. Rous P, Beard JW. Carcinomatous changes in virus-induced papillomas of the skin of the rabbit. Proc Soc Exp Biol Med 1934; 32:578–580.
6. Rous P, Beard JW. The progression to carcinoma of virus-induced rabbit papilloma (Shope). J Exp Med 1935; 62:523–548.
7. Rous P, Kidd JG. The carcinogenic effect of a papillomavirus on the tarred skin of rabbits. I. Description of the phenomenon. J Exp Med 1938; 67:399–422.
8. Rous P, Friedewald WF. The effect of chemical carcinogens on virus-induced rabbit papillomas. J Exp Med 1944; 79:511–537.
9. Lutz W. A propos de l'epidermodysplasie verruciforme. Dermatologica 1946; 92:30–43.
10. Jablonska S, Millewski B. Zur Kenntnis der Epidermodysplasia verruciformis Lewandowsky-Lutz. Dermatologica 1957; 115:1–22.
11. Jablonska S, Dabrowski J, Jakubowicz K. Epidermodysplasia verruciformis as a model in studies on the role of papovaviruses in oncogenesis. Cancer Res 1972; 32:583–589.
12. Gissmann L, zur Hausen H. Human papilloma viruses: physical mapping and genetic heterogeneity. Proc Natl Acad Sci USA 1976; 73:1310–1313.
13. Gissmann L, Pfister H, zur Hausen H. Human papilloma viruses (HPV): characterization of four different isolates. Virology 1977; 76:569–580.

14. Orth G, Favre M, Croissant O. Characterization of a new type of human papillomavirus that causes skin warts. J Virol 1977; 24:108–120.

15. zur Hausen H, Meinhof W, Scheiber W, Bornkamm GW. Attempts to detect virus-specific DNA sequences in human tumors: I. Nucleic acid hybridizations with complementary RNA of human wart virus. Int J Cancer 1974; 13:650–656.

16. zur Hausen H. Condylomata acuminata and human genital cancer. Cancer Res 1976; 36:530.

17. zur Hausen H. Human papillomaviruses and their possible role in squamous cell carcinomas. Curr Top Microbiol Immunol 1977; 78:1–30.

18. Orth G, Jablonska S, Favre M, Jarzabek-Chorzelska M, Rzesa G. Characterization of two new types of HPV from lesions of epidermodysplasia verruciformis. Proc Natl Acad Sci USA 1978; 75:1537–1541.

19. Dürst M, Gissmann L, Ikenberg H, zur Hausen H. A papillomavirus DNA from a cervical carcinoma and its prevalence in cancer biopsy samples from different geographic regions. Proc Natl Acad Sci USA 1983; 80:3812–3815.

20. Boshart M, Gissmann L, Ikenberg H, Kleinheinz A, Scheurlen W, zur Hausen H. A new type of papillomavirus DNA, its presence in genital cancer and in cell lines derived from genital cancer. EMBO J 1984; 3:1151–1157.

21. de Villiers E-M. Heterogeneity of the human papillomavirus group. J Virol 1989; 63:4898–4903.

22. de Villiers E-M. Human pathogenic papillomaviruses: an update. In: zur Hausen H (ed). Current Topics in Microbiology and Immunology, Vol. 86. Berlin–Heidelberg: Springer-Verlag, 1994, pp. 1–12.

23. Howley PM. Papillomavirinae: the viruses and their replication. In: Fields BN, Knipe DM, Howley PM (eds). Fields Virology Philadelphia: Lippincott-Raven, 1996, pp. 2045–2076.

24. zur Hausen H. Papillomavirus infections—a major cause of human cancers. Biochem Biophys Acta Rev Cancer 1996; 1288:F55–F78.

25. zur Hausen H. Genital papillomavirus infections. In: Rigby PWJ, Wilkie NM (eds). Viruses and Cancer. Cambridge: Cambridge University Press, 1986, pp. 83–90.

26. Amella CA, Lofgren LA, Ronn AM, Nouri M, Shikowitz MJ, Steinberg BM. Latent infection induced with cottontail rabbit papillomavirus. A model for human papillomavirus latency. Am J Pathol 1994; 144:1167–1171.

27. Schmitt A, Rochat A, Zeltner R, Borenstein L, Barrandon Y, Wetttstein FO, Iftner T. The primary target cells of the high risk cottontail rabbit papillomavirus colocalize with hair follicle stem cells. J Virol 1996; 70:1912–1922.

28. Breitburd F, Salmon J, Orth G. The rabbit viral skin papillomas and carcinomas: a model for the immunogenetics of HPV-associated carcinogenesis. Clin Dermatol 1997; 15:237–247.

29. Penn I. Post-transplant kidney cancers and skin cancers (including Kaposi's sarcoma). In: Schmähl D, Penn I (eds). Cancer in Organ Transplant Recipients. Heidelberg–Berlin: Springer-Verlag, 1991, pp. 946–953.

30. Boxman IL, Berkhout RJ, Mulder LH, Wolkers MC, Bouwes-Bavinck JN, Vermeer BJ, ter Schegget J. Detection of human papillomavirus DNA in plucked hairs from renal transplant recipients and healthy volunteers. J Invest Dermatol 1997; 108:712–715.

31. Astori G, Lavergne D, Benton C, Höckmayr B, Egawa K, Garbe K, de Villiers E-M. Human papillomaviruses are commonly found in normal skin of immunocompetent hosts. J Invest Dermatol 1998; 110:752–755.

32. Stoler MH, Wolinsky SM, Whitbeck A, Broker TR, Chow LT. Differentiation-linked human papillomavirus types 6 and 11 transcription in genital condylomata revealed by in situ hybridization with message-specific RNA probes. Virology 1989; 172:331–340.

33. Steinberg BM, Topp WC, Schneider PS, Abramson AL. Laryngeal papillomavirus infection during clinical remission. N Engl J Med 1983; 308:1261–1264.

34. Park TW, Richart RM, Sun XW, Wright TC Jr. Association between human papillomavirus type and clonal status of cervical squamous intraepithelial lesions. J Natl Cancer Inst 1996; 88:317–318.

35. Enomoto T, Haba T, Fujita M, Hamada T, Yoshino K, Nakashima R, Wada H, Kurachi H, Wakasa K, Sakurai M, Murata Y, Shroyer KR. Clonal analysis of high grade squamous intraepithelial lesions of the uterine cervix. Int J Cancer 1997; 73:339–344.

36. Dürst M, Glitz D, Schneider A, zur Hausen H. Human papillomavirus type 16 (HPV 16) gene expression and DNA replication in cervical neoplasia: analysis by in situ hybridization. Virology 1992; 189:132–140.

37. Stoler MH, Rhodes CR, Whitbeck A, Wolinsky SM, Chow LT, Broker TR. Human papillomavirus type 16 and 18 gene expression in cervical neoplasias. Hum Pathol 1992; 23:117–128.

38. Orth G, Jablonska S, Jarzabek-Chorzelska M, Rzesa G, Obalek S, Favre M, Croissant O. Characteristics of the lesions and risk of malignant conversion as related to the type of the human papillomavirus involved in epidermodysplasia verruciformis. Cancer Res 1979; 39:1074–1082.

39. IARC Monograph on the Evaluation of Carcinogenic Risks to Humans, Vol. 64. Human Papillomaviruses. IARC: Lyon, 1995.

40. Niedobitek G, Pitteroff S, Herbst H, Shepherd P, Finn T, Anagnostopoulos I, Stein H. Detection of human papillomavirus type 16 DNA in carcinomas of the palatine tonsil. J Clin Pathol 1990; 43:918–921.

41. Snijders PJ, Cromme FV, van den Brule AJ, Schrijnemakers HF, Snow GB, Meijer CJ, Walboomers JM. Prevalence and expression of human papillomavirus in tonsillar carcinomas, indicating a possible viral etiology. J Gen Virol 1992; 51:845–850.

42. de Villiers E-M, Weidauer H, Otto H, zur Hausen H. Papillomavirus DNA in human tongue carcinomas. Int J Cancer 1985; 36:575–578.

43. Kahn T, Schwarz E, zur Hausen H. Molecular cloning and characterization of the DNA of a new human papillomavirus (HPV 30) from a laryngeal carcinoma. Int J Cancer 1986; 37:61–65.

44. Scheurlen W, Stremlau A, Gissmann L, Höhn D, Zenner H-P, zur Hausen H. Rearranged HPV 16 molecules in an anal carcinoma and in a laryngeal carcinoma. Int J Cancer 1986; 38:671–676.

45. de Villiers E-M, Neumann C, Le JY, Weidauer H, zur Hausen H. Infection of the oral mucosa with defined types of human papillomaviruses. Med Microbiol Immunol 1986; 174:287–294.

46. Wu TC, Trujillo JM, Kashima HK, Mounts P. Association of human papillomavirus with nasal neoplasia. Lancet 1993; 341:522–524.

47. Stremlau A, Gissmann L, Ikenberg H, Stark E, zur Hausen H. Human papillomvirus type 16 DNA in an anaplastic carcinoma of the lung. Cancer 1985; 55:1737–1740.

48. Snijders PJ, Meijer CJ, van den Brule AJ, Schrijmemakers HF, Snow GB, Walboomers JM. Human papillomavirus (HPV) type 16 and 33 E6/E7 transcripts in tonsillar carcinomas can originate from integrated and episomal HPV DNA. J Gen Virol 1992; 73:2059–2066.

49. Snijders PJ, van den Brule AJ, Schrijnemakers HF, Raaphorst PM, Meijer CJ, Walboomers JM. Human papillomavirus type 33 in a tonsillar carcinoma generates its putative E7 mRNA via two E6* transcript species which are terminated at different early region poly(A)sites. J Virol 1992; 66:3172–3178.

50. Syrjänen KJ. Histological changes identical to those of condylomatous lesions found in esophageal squamous-cell carcinoma. Arch Geschwulstforsch 1982; 52:283–292.

51. Poljak M, Cerar A, Seme K. Human papillomavirus infection in esophageal carcinomas: a comparative study of 121 lesions using multiple broad-spectrum polymerase chain reactions and literature review. Hum Pathol 1998; 29:266–271.

52. Lavergne D, de Villiers E-M. Papillomavirus in esophageal papillomas and carcinomas. Int J Cancer 1999; 80:681–684.

53. Purdie KJ, Sexton CJ, Proby CM, Glover MT, Williams AT, Stables JN, et al. Malignant transformation of cutaneous lesions in renal allograft patients: a role for human papillomavirus. Cancer Res 1993; 53:5328–5333.

54. Shamanin V, Glover M, Rausch C, Proby C, Leigh I-M, zur Hausen H, de Villiers EM. Specific types of HPV found in benign proliferations and in carcinomas of the skin in immunosuppressed patients. Cancer Res 1994; 54:4610–4613.

55. Shamanin V, zur Hausen H, Lavergne D, Proby C, Leigh IM, Neumann C, Hamm H, Goos M, Haustein UF, Jung EG, Plewig G, Wolff H, de Villiers E-M. Human papillomavirus infections in non-melanoma skin cancers from renal transplant recipients and nonimmunosuppressed patients. J Natl Cancer Inst 1996; 88:802–811.

56. Berkhout RJ, Tieben LM, Smits HL, Bavinck JMN, Vermeer BJ, ter Schegget J. Nested PCR approach for detection and typing of epidermodysplasia verruciformis-associated human papillomavirus types in cutaneous cancers from renal transplant recipients. J Clin Microbiol 1995; 33:690–695.

57. Völter C, He Y, Delius H, Roy-Burman A, Greenspan JS, Greenspan D, de Villiers E-M. Novel HPV types present in oral papillomatous lesions from patients with HIV infections. Int J Cancer 1996; 66:453–456.

58. de Villiers E-M, Lavergne D, McLaren K, Benton EC. Prevailing papillomavirus types in non-melanoma carcinomas of the skin in renal allograft recipients. Int J Cancer 1997; 73:356–361.

59. Schwarz E, Freese UK, Gissmann L, Mayer W, Roggenbuck B, zur Hausen H. Structure and transcription of human papillomavirus type 18 and 16 sequences in cervical carcinoma cells. Nature 1985; 314:111–114.

60. Yee C, Krishnan-Hewlett Z, Baker CC, Schlegel R, Howley PM. Presence and expression of human papillomavirus sequences in human cervical carcinoma cell lines. Am J Pathol 1985; 119:361–366.

61. McDougall JK. Immortalization and transformation of human cells by human papillomavirus. Curr Top Microbiol Immunol 1994; 186:101–119.

62. Band V, Zaychowski D, Kulesa V, Sager R. Human papillomavirus DNAs immortalize normal human mammary epithelial cells and reduce their growth factor requirements. Proc Natl Acad Sci USA 1990; 87:463–467.

63. Band V, De Caprio JA, Delmolina L, Kulesa V, Sager R. Loss of p53 protein in human papillomavirus type 16 E6-immortalized human mammary epithelial cells. J Virol 1991; 65:6671–6676.

64. Halbert CL, Demers GW, Galloway DA. The E7 gene of human papillomavirus type 16 is sufficient for immortalization of human epithelial cells. J Virol 1991; 65:473–478.

65. Hawley-Nelson P, Vousden KH, Hubbert NL, Lowy DR, Schiller JT. HPV 16 E6 and E7 proteins cooperate to immortalize human foreskin keratinocytes. EMBO J 1989; 8:3905–3910.

66. Münger K, Phelps WC, Bubb V, Howley PM, Schlegel R. The E6 and E7 genes of human papillomavirus type 16 are necessary and sufficient for transformation of primary human keratinocytes. J Virol 1989; 63:4417–4423.

67. von Knebel Doeberitz M, Oltersdorf T, Schwarz E, Gissmann L. Correlation of modified human papillomavirus early gene expression with altered growth properties in C4-1 cervical carcinoma cells. Cancer Res 1988; 48:3780–3786.

68. von Knebel Doeberitz M, Rittmüller C, zur Hausen H, Dürst M. Inhibition of tumorigenicity of cervical cancer cells in nude mice by HPV E6-E7 antisense RNA. Int J Cancer 1992; 51:831–834.

69. von Knebel Doeberitz M, Rittmüller C, Aengeneyndt F, Jansen-Dürr P, Spitkovsky D. Reversible repression of papillomavirus oncogene expression in cervical carcinoma cells: consequences for the phenotype and E6–p53 and E7–pRB interactions. J Virol 1994; 68:2811–2821.

70. Dyson N, Howley PM, Münger K, Harlow E. The human papillomavirus-16 E7 oncoprotein is able to bind to the retinoblastoma gene product. Science 1989; 243:934–937.

71. Huibregtse JM, Scheffner M. Mechanisms of tumor suppressor protein inactivation by the human papillomavirus E6 and E7 oncoproteins. Semi Virol 1994; 5:357–367.

72. Matlashewski G, Schneider J, Banks L, Jones N, Murray A, Crawford L. Human papillomavirus type 16 DNA cooperates with activated *ras* in transforming primary cells. EMBO J 1987; 6:1741–1746.

73. Dürst M, Gallahan D, Jay G, Rhim JS Glucocorticoid-enhanced neoplastic transformation of human keratinocytes by human papillomavirus type 16 and an activated ras oncogene. Virology 1989; 173:767–771.

74. Banks L, Edmonds C, Vousden K. Ability of HPV16 E7 protein to bind RB and induce DNA synthesis is not sufficient for efficient transforming activity in NIH3T3 cells. Oncogene 1990; 5:1383–1389.

75. Jewers RJ, Hildebrandt P, Ludlow JW, Kell B, McCance DJ. Regions of human papillomavirus type 16 E7 oncoprotein required for immortalization of human keratinocytes. J Virol 1992; 66:1329–1335.

76. Bandara LR, Adamczewski JP, Hunt T, La Thangue NB. Cyclin A and the retinoblastoma gene product complex with a common transcription factor. Nature 1991; 352:249–251.

77. Dyson N, Guida P, Münger K, Harlow E. Homologous sequences in adenovirus E1A and human papillomavirus E7 proteins mediate interaction with the same set of cellular proteins. J Virol 1992; 66:6893–6902.

78. Tommasino M, Adamczewski JP, Carlotti F, Barth CF, Manetti R, Contorni M, Cavalieri F, Hunt T, Crawford L. HPV16 E7 protein associates with the protein kinase p33CDK2 and cyclin A. Oncogene 1993; 8:195–202.

79. Zerfass K, Schulze A, Spitkowsky D, Friedman V, Henglein B, Jansen-Dürr P. Sequential activation of cyclin E and cyclin A expression by human papillomavirus type 16 E7 through sequences necessary for transformation. J Virol 1995; 69:6389–6399.

80. Demers GW, Espling E, Harry JB, Etscheid BG, Galloway DA. Abrogation of growth arrest signals by human papillomavirus type 16 E7 is mediated by sequences required for transformation. J Virol 1996; 70:6862–6869.

81. Hickman ES, Bates S, Vousden KH. Perturbation of the p53 response by human papillomavirus type 16 E7. J Virol 1997; 71:3710–3718.

82. Slebos RJC, Lee MH, Plunkett BS, Kessis TD, Williams BO, Jacks T, Hedrick L, Kastan MB, Cho KR. p53-dependent G_1 arrest involves pRb-related proteins and is disrupted by the human papillomavirus 16 E7 oncoprotein. Proc Natl Acad Sci USA 1994; 91:5320–5324.

83. White AE, Livanos EM, Tlsty TD. Differential disruption of genomic integrity and cell cycle regulation in normal human fibroblasts by the HPV oncoproteins. Genes Dev 1994; 8:666–677.

84. Hashida T, Yasumoto S. Induction of chromosomal abnormalities in mouse and human epidermal keratinocytes by the human papillomavirus type 16 E7 oncogene. J Gen Virol 1991; 72:1569–1577.

85. Zerfass-Thome K, Zwerschke W, Mannhardt B, Tindle R, Botz JW, Jansen-Dürr P. Inactivation of the cdk inhibitor p27KIP1 by human papillomavirus type 16 E7 oncoprotein. Oncogene 1996; 13:2323–2330.

86. Jones DL, Alani RM, Münger K. The human papillomavirus E7 oncoprotein can uncouple cellular differentiation and proliferation in human keratinocytes by abrogating p21Cip1-mediated inhibition of cdk2. Genes Dev 1997; 11:2101–2111.

87. Funk JO, Waga S, Harry JB, Espling E, Stilman B, Galloway GA. Inhibition of CDK activity and PCNA-dependent DNA replication by p21 is blocked by interaction with the HPV–16 E7 protein. Genes Dev 1997; 11:2090–2100.

88. Zwerschke W, Mazurek S, Massimi P, Banks L, Eigenbrodt E, Jansen-Dürr P. Modulation of type M2 pyruvate kinase activity by the human papillomavirus type 16 E7 oncoprotein. Proc Natl Acad Sci USA 1999; 96:1291–1296.

89. Werness BA, Levine AJ, Howley PM. Association of human papillomavirus types 16 and 18 E6 proteins with p53. Science 1990; 248:76–79.

90. Scheffner M, Werness BA, Huibregtse JM, Levine JM, Howley PM. The E6 oncoprotein encoded by human papillomavirus types 16 and 18 promotes the degradation of p53. Cell 1990; 63:1129–1136.

91. Scheffner M, Huibregtse JM, Vierstra RD, Howley PM. The HPV 16 E6 and E6-AP complex functions as a ubiquitin-protein ligase in the ubiquination of p53. Cell 1993; 75:495–505.

92. Vande Pol SB, Brown MC, Turner CE. Association of bovine papillomavirus type 1 E6 oncoprotein with the focal adhesion protein paxillin through a conserved protein interaction motif. Oncogene 1998; 16:43–52.

93. Ronco L, Karpova AY, Vidal M, Howley PM. The human papillomavirus 16 E6 oncoprotein binds to interferon regulatory factor-3 and inhibits its transcriptional activity. Genes Dev 1998; 12:2061–2072.

94. Chen T-M, Pecoraro G, Defendi V. Genetic analysis of in vitro progression of human papillomavirus-transfected human cervical cells. Cancer Res 1993; 53:1167–1171.

95. Seagon S, Dürst M. Genetic analysis of an in vitro model system for human papillomavirus type 16-associated tumorigenesis. Cancer Res 1994; 54:5593–5598.

96. Harris H, Miller OJ, Klein G, Worst P, Tachibana T. Suppression of malignancy by cell fusion. Nature 1969; 223:363–368.

97. Cullen AP, Reid R, Campion M, Lorincz AT. Analysis of the physical state of different human papillomavirus DNAs in intraepithelial and invasive cervical neoplasm. J Virol 1991; 65:606–612.

98. Reuter S, Bartelmann M, Vogt M, Geisen C, Napierski I, Kahn T, Delius H, Lichter P, Weitz S, Korn B, Schwarz E. APM-1, a novel human gene, identified by aberrant co-transcription with papillomavirus oncogenes in a cervical carcinoma cell line, encodes a BTP/POZ-zinc finger protein with growth inhibitory activity. EMBO J 1998; 17:215–222.

99. Dürst M, Croce C, Gissmann L, Schwarz E, Huebner K. Papillomavirus sequences integrate near cellular oncogenes in some cervical carcinomas. Proc Natl Acad Sci USA 1987; 84:1070–1074.

100. Popescu NC, Zimonjic D, DiPaolo JA. Viral integration, fragile sites and proto-oncogenes in human neoplasia. Hum Genet 1990; 44:58–62.

101. Lazzo PA, Gallego MI, Ballester S, Feduchi E. Genetic alterations by human papillomaviruses in oncogenesis. FEBS Lett 1992; 300:109–113.

102. Zimonjic DB, Popescu NC, DiPaolo JA. Chromosomal organization of viral integration sites in human papillomavirus-immortalized human keratinocyte cell lines Cancer Genet Cytogenet 1994; 72:39–43.

103. Wilke CM, Hall BK, Hoge A, Paradee W, Smith DI, Glover TW. FRA3B extends over a broad region and contains a spontaneous HPV16 integration site: direct evidence for the coincidence of viral integration sites and fragile sites. Hum Mol Genet 1996; 5:187–195.

104. Yokota J, Tsukada Y, Nakajima T, Gotoh M, Shimosato Y, Mori N, Tsunokawa Y, Sugimura T, Terada M. Loss of heterozygosity on the short arm of chromosome 3 in carcinoma of the uterine cervix. Cancer Res 1989; 49:3598–3601.

105. Kohno T, Takayama H, Hamaguchi M, Takano H, Yamaguchi N, Tsuda H, Hirohashi S, Vissing H, Shimuzu M, Oshimura M, Yokota J. Deletion mapping of chromosome 3p in human uterine cervical cancer. Oncogene 1993; 8:1825–1832.

106. Kersemaekers AM, Kenter GG, Hermans J, Fleuren GJ, van de Vijver MJ. Allelic loss and prognosis in carcinoma of the uterine cervix. Int J Cancer 1998; 79:411–417.

107. Mitra AB, Murty V, Li RG, Pratap M, Luthra UK, Chaganbti RSK. Allelotype analysis of cervical carcinoma. Cancer Res 1994; 54:4481–4487.

108. Hampton GM, Penny LA, Baergen RN, Larson A, Brewer C, Liao S, Busby-Earle RMC, Williams AWR, Steel CM, Bird CC, Stanbridge EJ, Evans GA. Loss of heterozygosity in cervical carcinoma: subchromosomal localization of a putative tumor-suppressor gene to chromosome 11q22-q24. Proc Natl Acad Sci USA 1994; 91:6953–6957.

109. Mulklokandov MR, Kholodilov NG, Atkin NB, Burk RD, Johnson AB, Klinger HP. Genomic alterations in cervical carcinoma: losses of chromosome heterozygosity and human papillomavirus status. Cancer Res 1996; 56:197–205.

110. Fujita M, Inoue M, Tanizawa O, Iwamoto S, Enomoto T. Alterations of p53 gene in human primary cervical carcinoma with and without human papillomavirus infection. Cancer Res 1992; 52:5323–5328.

111. Hampton GM, Larson AA, Baergen RN, Sommers RL, Kren S, Cavenee WK. Simultaneous assessment of loss of heterozygosity at multiple microsatellite loci using semi-automated fluorescence based detection: subregional mapping of chromosome 4 in cervical carcinoma. Proc Natl Acad Sci USA 1996; 93:6704–6709.

112. Ku J-L, Kim W-H, Park H-S, Kang S-B, Park J-G. Establishment and characterization of 12 uterine cervical carcinoma cell lines: common sequence variation in the E7 gene of HPV-16 positive cell lines. Int J Cancer 1997; 72:313–320.

113. Le Beau MM. Chromosomal fragile sites and cancer-specific rearrangements. Blood 1986; 67:849–858.

114. Druck T, Berk L, Huebner K. *FHIT*ness and cancer. Oncology Res 1998; 10:341–345.

115. zur Hausen H. Cell-virus gene balance hypothesis of carcinogenesis. Behring Inst Mitt 1977; 61:23–30.

116. zur Hausen H. The role of viruses in human tumors. In: Klein G, Weinhouse S. (eds). Advances in Cancer Research, Vol. 33 1980; Academic Press, pp. 77–107.

117. zur Hausen H. Disrupted dichotomous intracellular control of human papillomavirus infection in cancer of the cervix. Lancet 1994; 343:955–957.

118. Dürst M, Bosch FX, Glitz D, Schneider A, zur Hausen H. Inverse relationship between human papillomvirus (HPV) type 16 early gene expression and cell differentiation in nude mouse epithelial cyysts and tumors induced by HPV positive human cell lines. J Virol 1991; 65:796–804.

119. Rösl F, Lengert M, Albrecht J, Kleine K, Zawatzky R, Schraven B, zur Hausen H. Differential regulation of the JE gene encoding the monocyte chemoattractant protein (MCP-1) in cervical carcinoma cells and derived hybrids. J Virol 1994; 68:2142–2150.

120. Rösl F, Das BC, Lengert M, Geletneky K, zur Hausen H. Antioxidant-induced changes in AP-1 composition result in a selective suppression of human papillomavirus transcription. J Virol 1997; 71:362–370.

121. Soto U, Das BC, Lengert M, Finzer P, zur Hausen H, Rösl F. Conversion of HPV 18 positive non-tumorigenic HeLa-fibroblast hybrids to invasive growth involves loss of TNF-α mediated repression of viral transcription and modification of the AP-1 transcription complex. Oncogene 1999; 18:3187–3198.

122. Villa LL, Vieira KB, Pei XF, Schlegel R. Differential effect of tumor necrosis factor on proliferation of primary human keratinocytes and cell lines containing human papillomavirus types 16 and 18. Mol Carcinogen 1992; 6:5–9.

123. Kyo S, Inoue M, Hayasaka N, Inoue T, Yutsudo M, Tanizawa O, Hakura A. Regulation of early gene expression of human papillomavirus type 16 by inflammatory cytokines. Virology 1994; 200:1330–1339.

124. Malejczyk J, Malejczyk M, Majewski S, Breifburd F, Luger TA, Jablonska S, Orth G. Increased tumorigenicity of human keratinocytes harboring human papillomavirus type 16 is associated

with resistance to endogenous tumor necrosis factor-alpha-mediated growth limitation. Int J Cancer 1994; 56:593–598.

125. Braun L, Dürst M, Mikumo R, Grupposo P. Differential response of nontumorigenic and tumorigenic human papillomavirus type 16-positive epithelial cells to transforming growth factor beta 1. Cancer Res 1990; 50:7324–7332.

126. Woodworth CD, Notario V, DiPaolo JA. Transforming growth factors beta 1 and 2 transcriptionally regulate human papillomavirus (HPV) type 16 early gene expression in HPV-immortalized human genital epithelial cells. J Virol 1990; 64:4767–4775.

127. Merrick DT, Winberg G, McDougall JK. Re-expression of interleukin 1 in human papillomavirus 18 immortalized keratinocytes inhibits their tumorigencity in nude mice. Cell Growth Different 1996; 7:1661–1669.

128. Kyo S, Inoue M, Nishio Y, Nakanishi K, Inoue H, Yutsudo M, Tanizawa O, Hakura A. NF-IL6 represses early gene expression of human papillomavirus type 16 through binding to the noncoding region. J Virol 1993; 67:1058–1066.

129. Smits PHM, Smits HL, Minnaar R, Hemmings BA, Mayer-Jaekel RE, Schuurman R, van der Noordaa J, ter Schegget J. The trans-activation of the HPV 16 long control region in human cells with a deletion in the short arm of chromosome 11 is mediated by the 55kDa regulatory subunit of protein phosphatase 2A. EMBO J 1992; 11:4601–4606.

130. Reznikoff CA, Yeager TR, Belair CD, Salevieva E, Puthenveettil JA, Stadler WM. Elevated p16 at senescence and loss of p16 at immortalization in human papillomavirus 16 E6, but not in E7, transformed human uroepithelial cells. Cancer Res 1996; 56:2886–2890.

131. Müller M, Zhou J, Reed TD, Rittmuller C, Burger A, Gabelsberger J, Braspenning J, Gissman L. Chimeric papillomavirus-like particles. Virology 1997; 234:93–111.

132. Wideroff L, Schiffman MH, Hoover R, Tarone RE, Nonnenmacher B, Hubbert N, Kirnbauer R, Greer CE, Lorincz AT, Manos MM, Glass AG, Scott DR, Sherman ME, Buckland J, Lowy DR Schiller JT. Epidemiologic determinants of seroreactivity to human papillomavirus (HPV) type 16 virus-like particles in cervical HPV-16 DNA-positive and -negative women. J Infect Dis 1996; 174:937–943.

133. Suzich JA, Ghim SJ, Palmer-Hill FJ, White WL, Tamura JK, Bell JA, Newsome JA, Jenson AB, Schlegel R. Systemic immunization with papillomavirus L1 protein completely prevents the development of viral mucosal papillomas. Proc Natl Acad Sci USA 1995; 92:11553–11557.

134. Breitburd F, Kirnbauer R, Hubbert NL, Nonnenmacher B, Trin-Dinh Desmarquet C, Orth G, Schiller JT, Lowy DR. Immunization with virus-like particles from cottontail rabbit papillomavirus (CRPV) can protect against experimental CRPV infection. J Virol 1995; 69:3959–3963.

135. Kirnbauer R, Chandrachud LM, O'Neil BW, Wagner ER, Grindlay GJ, Armstrong A, McGarvie GM, Schiller JT, Lowy DR, Campo MS. Virus-like particles of bovine papillomavirus type 4 in prophylactic and therapeutic vaccination. Virology 1996; 219:37–44.

136. Müller M, Zhou J, Reed TD, Rittmüller C, Burger A, Gabelsberger J, Braspenning J, Gissmann L. Chimeric papillomavirus-like particles. Virology 1997; 234:93–111.

15

Anogenital Squamous Cell Cancer and Its Precursors

Natural History, Diagnosis, and Treatment

Joel M. Palefsky

INTRODUCTION

Prior to the introduction of routine cervical cytology screening, the incidence of cervical cancer was 40–50/100,000. Currently the incidence of cervical cancer in the United States is approx 8/100,000 *(1)* and much of the reduction is attributed to the efficacy of cytology screening (Papanicolaou smears) to prevent cervical cancer. The corresponding decline in mortality from cervical cancer is seen vividly in the recently released atlas of US cancer mortality (http://www.nci.nih.gov/atlas). Despite the reduction, these data translate into the death of approx 4500 women each year in the United States of a disease that is preventable. Although some of the mortality can be attributed to failures in cervical cytology in the form of false-negative results, the majority of women diagnosed with cervical cancer in the United States were never screened at all. Thus, much of the mortality is concentrated in populations of women with inadequate access to health care, particularly minority populations such as Hispanic and African-American women. Consistent with this, the incidence of cervical cancer around the world is highest in those countries where there is no routine cervical cytology screening.

The incidence of anal cancer among human immunodeficiency virus (HIV)-negative men who have sex with men (MSM) is estimated to be as high as 35/100,000 *(2)* and may be twice that among HIV-positive MSM *(3)*. The incidence of anal cancer in these groups thus resembles that of cervical cancer prior to the introduction of cervical cytology screening, an observation that is not surprising, as there currently is no routine screening for anal cancer or its probable precursor, anal squamous intraepithelial lesion (anal SIL).

Screening and treatment of cervical squamous intraepithelial lesions (CSILs) to prevent cervical cancer is enormously expensive. Fortunately the etiologic association between cervical cancer and human papillomavirus (HPV) offers new approaches to the diagnosis of at-risk women to supplement cervical cytology. Other new approaches to improving diagnosis of SIL based on refinement of preparing cervical cytology smears and computer-assisted interpretation have recently become available as well. Prevention of cervical cancer may be achieved in the future through a prophylactic vaccine approach to prevent initial HPV infection. Finally, the traditional approach to

From: *Infectious Causes of Cancer: Targets for Intervention*
Edited by: J. J. Goedert © Humana Press Inc., Totowa, NJ

treating anogenital SIL, which is to physically remove the lesion, may yield to approaches that are more HPV-specific, including therapeutic vaccines designed to boost immunity against cells bearing HPV antigens.

NATURAL HISTORY OF CERVICAL HPV INFECTION AND CSIL

There are more than 100 anogenital HPV types and these are generally divided into oncogenic and nononcogenic types by virtue of the frequency of their association with invasive cervical cancer (*see* Chapter 14). Of the oncogenic types, HPV-16 is the most important because it is the most common type found in cervical cancer, followed by HPV types 18, 31, and 45. HPV 16 alone counts for about 50% of all cervical cancers worldwide *(4)*. HPV types 18, 31, and 45 are associated with an additional 20% of the cancers. HPV types 33, 52, 58, 35, 39, 56, 59, and 68 account for most of the remaining cancers, but many other HPV types are associated with small percentages of cervical cancers and these vary from country to country. There also exist a group of HPV types in the genital tract that are rarely if ever oncogenic; the most common of these are types 6, 11, 42, 43, and 44. The molecular mechanisms by which HPV contributes to the development of anogenital cancer are reviewed in Chapter 14.

For years there was debate about the modes of acquisition of anogenital HPV infection. There is now a consensus that the great majority of cervical HPV infections are acquired through sexual transmission *(5,6)*. HPV is one of the most common sexually transmitted agents, and estimates are that about 75% of the general population aged 15–49 yr acquires at least one genital HPV type during their lifetimes *(7)*.

Epidemiologic studies of cervical HPV infection suggest that the age-related prevalence of HPV infection, as determined by polymerase chain reaction (PCR), is highest among women in their late teens and early 20s *(8)*. These data suggest that most women acquire HPV infection relatively early after initiation of sexual activity. The age-related prevalence of cervical HPV infection declines thereafter, probably through development of immunity to HPV. HPV infection in these women has either been cleared or the level of infection may have been reduced to levels that are undetectable using current technology, perhaps with small foci of latent infection. In addition, low prevalence among older women may represent a cohort effect given changes in sexual behaviors that have occurred in the last few decades.

HPV infection is initially established in the basal layer of the anogenital epithelium. In the cervix, this is usually in the transformation zone (TZ), where the squamous epithelium of the exocervix meets the columnar epithelium of the endocervix. This squamocolumnar junction is a relatively thin, highly metabolically active area of epithelium. Most HPV infections occur here and most HPV-related lesions arise from this area, including invasive cancer. The significance of basal layer HPV infection is that this allows the virus to perpetuate itself and persist in the more differentiated cell layers of the epithelium. The basal and parabasal layers constitute the only dividing cell layers in the epithelium under normal circumstances. When the basal cells divide, the HPV genomes replicate as well and are passed to the daughter cells. This allows HPV to persist both in the cells that generate the remainder of the epithelium and in the progeny cells that are derived from the basal cells as they differentiate and rise through the epithelium. It is also possible that HPV may persist for long periods of time, perhaps indefinitely in latent form in the basal cell layers, where it can remain transcriptionally inactive and clinically silent. These clinically normal tissues may later develop into lesions if HPV reactivates. Consequently, treatment and removal of SIL rarely leads to "cure" of HPV infection.

Consistent with a role for HPV in the pathogenesis of anogenital SIL and invasive cancer, the epidemiology of these two diseases tracks closely with risk factors associated with sexual activity. These include a lower frequency of cervical cancer among nuns, higher risk among women whose husbands had more sexual partners, higher risk among second wives if the first wife had a diagnosis of cervical cancer, and higher risk among women whose husbands had penile cancer.

HPV infection of the basal layer may lead to a spectrum of histopathologic changes in the anogenital epithelium. Although HPV infection is established in the basal cell layer, the viral DNA replicates to a much higher level and becomes transcriptionally active in the more differentiated cell layers. Most viral protein expression therefore occurs in the more differentiated cell layers. At the more benign end of the spectrum of disease is condyloma and cervical intraepithelial neoplasia (CIN) grade 1, also known as mild dysplasia (Fig. 1). In the Bethesda system these have been combined into one diagnostic category, known as low-grade SIL (LSIL) for the purpose of grading cytology, and some pathologists combine these categories for histopathologic categorization as well. LSIL is characterized by relatively little basal cell proliferation and atypia, and in the case of condyloma, the presence of koilocytes (cells with an irregular, enlarged nucleus with a clear "halo") *(9)*. Koilocytosis may represent a direct cytopathic effect of HPV infection. Another diagnosis used in the Bethesda system is "atypical squamous cells of undetermined significance" (ASCUS), which describes cells that are neither clearly normal nor clearly dysplastic. In contrast to LSIL, high-grade SIL (HSIL) is characterized by increasingly severe cellular atypia, abnormal mitotic activity in the more superficial cell layers, and replacement of the normal epithelium with immature basaloid cells. In the Bethesda system HSIL includes CIN grades 2 and 3 (moderate and severe dysplasia, respectively) and carcinoma *in situ*.

Historically, precancerous lesions of the cervix were considered to be part of a continuum beginning with CIN 1, progressing to CIN 2, CIN 3, CIS, and ultimately invasive cancer. This was based in part on early studies of the natural history of CIN that showed that a high proportion of CIN 1 lesions progressed to higher grades of disease *(10)*. Subsequent studies failed to show a high progression rate, and it is now believed that the result of the Richart study reflected inclusion criteria (three consecutive cytology smears that showed CIN 1) biased toward women who were unlikely to regress spontaneously. Consequently, for most women, current thinking is that CIN 1 has relatively little potential to progress to invasive cancer. Moreover, the schema in which CIN 1 progresses to CIN 2 and CIN 3 has been questioned in light of studies showing not only that these grades of lesion can coexist in the same woman simultaneously, but also that some CIN 3 lesions may arise without going through a CIN 1 intermediate *(11)*. Moreover, CIN 2–3 lesions can develop early after infection with an oncogenic HPV type, with some lesions developing in one cohort study within 6 mo of HPV infection *(11)*. Consistent with the higher risk of progression to cancer from HSIL than LSIL, almost all HSIL lesions contain high- or medium-risk oncogenic HPV types whereas LSIL lesions may contain a wider range of types from low risk to high risk *(12)*.

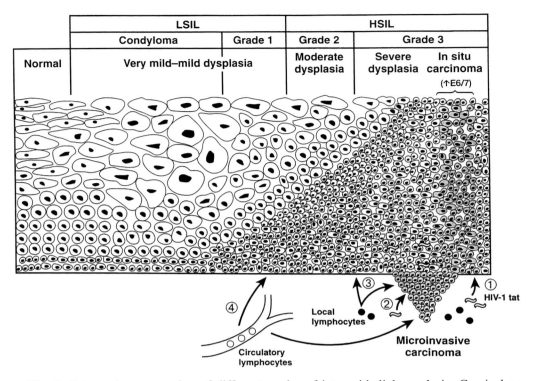

Fig. 1. Schematic presentation of different grades of intraepithelial neoplasia. Cervical or anal intraepithelial neoplasia grade 1 are characterized by 20–25% replacement of the epithelium with immature cells with high nucleus/cytoplasm ratios. Intraepithelial neoplasia grade 2 is characterized by approx 50% replacement with immature cells, and grade 3 by complete or nearly complete replacement. Microinvasion, shown at the bottom, occurs when the cells traverse the basement membrane. Although microinvasion can rarely occur in conjunction with intraepithelial neoplasia grade 1, it is likelier to occur in conjunction with intraepithelial neoplasia grade 3, as indicated schematically. Also depicted are hypothetical mechanisms by which HIV can potentiate development of neoplasia. (1) HIV-1 tat can be expressed by cells circulating in the stroma and be taken up by overlying HPV-infected keratinocytes resulting in upregulation of HPV E6 and E7 expression; (2) HIV-1 tat could potentiate migration of HPV-infected keratinocytes; (3) aberrant cytokine expression by locally circulating HIV-infected lymphocytes may modulate local immune response and may modulate HPV gene expression in overlying keratinocytes; and (4) systemic immune response to HPV-infected keratinocytes may be attenuated if HIV infection leads to loss of HPV-specific effector cells.

The incidence of carcinoma *in situ* among women aged 15–19 yr appears to have been rising in the last few decades compared to similarly aged women, perhaps due to changes in sexual activity during this time and earlier initiation of sexual intercourse *(13)*. The estimated incidence of carcinoma *in situ* among women aged 18–24 yr in Washington state was 196/100,000, which was similar to that of women aged 25–34 yr (212/100,000) *(14)*. Although the proportion of carcinoma *in situ* cases that progress to invasive cervical cancer remains unknown, some studies report progression in up to 71%. *(15)*. Thus, the clinical significance of distinguishing LSIL from HSIL is that most cases of LSIL will undergo spontaneous regression and do not require treatment to prevent cervical cancer. In contrast, HSIL requires therapy, as these may progress over time to invasive cancer. The time of progression of untreated HSIL to invasive cancer varies from individual to individual, and may take up to several decades. However, because a minority of cases of LSIL can progress to HSIL, women with LSIL require follow-up to ensure that the lesion has regressed. In addition, many clinicians recommend treatment of LSIL if it persists, because these lesions may be among those that progress to HSIL over time. Some clinicians also treat women with LSIL if compliance with follow-up is uncertain.

CHANGES IN CERVICAL CANCER INCIDENCE IN THE UNITED STATES

Cancer of the cervix is the third most common cancer of the female genital tract, following uterine cancer and ovarian cancer, respectively. From 1950 to 1991, data from the Surveillance, Epidemiology, and End Results (SEER) Program show that the incidence of cervical cancer declined nearly 77% among Caucasian women. However, a slight increase in cervical cancer was detected between 1986 and 1991 among women of all races, rising from 8.0/100,000 between 1981 and 1985 to 8.7/100,000 between 1986 and 1991. It is not clear if this represents a cohort effect reflecting a possible earlier initiation of sexual activity and more sexual partners among American women, or changes in cytology screening in at-risk populations. In 1995, there were 15,800 incident cases of cervical cancer in the United States and 4800 deaths from cervical cancer. For women diagnosed with cervical cancer between 1983 and 1989, the 5-yr survival rate was nearly 67%, and this rate has remained relatively stable since. The median age at diagnosis of cervical cancer is 48 yr *(16)*.

The incidence of cervical cancer is not distributed equally among racial groups. In 1992, the incidence of cervical cancer was approx 40% higher among African-American women than Caucasian women, and the greatest disparity was for women over the age of 50 yr. Mortality was also higher among African-American women. There may be several reasons for the differences between African-American and Caucasian women. African-American women have on average less adequate access to health care and are less likely to undergo routine cervical cytology screening. Consistent with this, women of lower socioeconomic status have higher rates of cervical cancer regardless of race *(17,18)*. Less adequate access to health care services may also explain the higher mortality rate among African-American women and women of lower socioeconomic status, as cervical cancers among African-American women are diagnosed on average at a later stage. Other factors may also play a role, as mortality among African-American women remains higher than among Caucasian women even after correction for stage of disease at the time of diagnosis.

RISK FACTORS FOR ANOGENITAL SIL AND CANCER OTHER THAN HPV INFECTION

Clearly HPV infection is one of the most important risk factors for anogenital SIL and cancer, and HPV infection is likely to be necessary for development of almost all of these lesions. Sexual risk factors such as number of sexual partners, age at first intercourse, and parity have long been associated with cervical cancer, but these likely reflect risk for acquisition of HPV infection. However, although the age-related prevalence of cervical LSIL parallels that of infection, only a small proportion of women who acquire HPV infection develop clinically detectable LSIL. An even smaller proportion of these women develop HSIL or invasive cervical cancer. This reflects the current understanding that HPV infection may be necessary but insufficient for development of CSIL and cervical cancer. The paradigm is that HPV infection contributes to carcinogenesis indirectly by stimulating cellular proliferation and rendering the epithelial cells susceptible to genetic damage through induction of chromosomal instability *(19,20)*. Consistent with this hypothesis, chromosomal mutations as shown by studies of loss of heterozygosity may be found in cervical cancer *(21–23)*. Other events that lead to genetic damage in the cells may play a more direct role in carcinogenesis.

Cigarette smoking has been shown to be associated with CSIL, and this was presumed to be mediated by exposure of tobacco-related carcinogens to HPV-infected epithelium and through attenuation of cervical epithelium Langerhans cell number and function. In more recent studies, however, in which the data were adjusted for HPV infection, cigarette smoking was not an independent risk factor *(24,25)*. The association between cervical cancer and oral contraceptive use is not clear, with some but not all studies showing an association. Dietary factors have been proposed and some studies suggest an association between folate deficiency and CSIL *(26,27)*. However, dietary supplements of folic acid appear to have little effect on the natural history of the disease *(28,29)*. In a study of women with CSIL compared to controls without CSIL, after adjusting for HPV infection and demographic factors there was an inverse correlation between plasma α-tocopherol and ascorbic acid levels and risk of CSIL *(30)*, a finding confirmed by a more recent study *(31)*. Further studies are needed to clarify these findings.

In vitro, several studies show that retinoic acid may stimulate cellular differentiation and inhibit proliferation of HPV-infected keratinocytes *(32–34)*. In clinical studies, however, CSIL was not associated with plasma retinol or β-carotene levels *(30)*; and in an earlier study, the association between increased risk of CSIL and retinol levels did not reach statistical significance *(35)*. Overall, the relationship between dietary factors and the incidence or natural history of CSIL remains unclear. In general, in vitro findings have not been matched by clear in vivo results, reflecting either a limited role for these factors in vivo or difficulties in precisely quantifying these factors in clinical studies.

Another risk factor of clear importance is that of immunodeficiency. The epidemiologic data described previously show that the prevalence of cervical HPV infection and CSIL decline with age. The presumed mechanism of this decline is a cell-mediated immune (CMI) response. Examples of loss of immune competence and its association with increased risk of anogenital and skin malignancies included women undergoing renal transplant who were iatrogenically immunosuppressed to prevent graft rejection *(36,37)*, as well as individuals with a rare immune disorder known as epidermodysplasia verruciformis.

More recently, HIV has emerged as the most common cause of immune suppression. There is a large body of literature that documents an increased risk of detection of HPV DNA in HIV-positive women, increased risk of CSIL, a slightly increased risk of cervical cancer, and greater difficulty treating the lesions. In a study from New York, the prevalence of HPV infection of any type was significantly greater in the 344 HIV-positive (60%) than the 325 HIV-negative (36%) women *(38)*. In addition, multiple types of HPV were present in 51% of the HIV-positive women compared to 26% of the HIV-negative women. These findings were confirmed in a more recent, larger study conducted at six Women's Interagency HIV Study (WIHS) sites around the United States, in which HPV infection was significantly more common among HIV-positive women than HIV-negative matched controls *(39)*. The strongest risk factors for HPV infection among HIV-positive women were indicators of more advanced HIV-related disease such as higher HIV viral load and lower CD4 levels. However, other factors that are commonly found in studies of HIV-negative women were important in HIV-positive women as well, including racial/ethnic background, current smoking, and age. Persistence of HPV infection may also be affected by HIV infection. In one study, persistent HPV infection with "high-risk" types was found in 20% of the HIV-positive women and 3% of the HIV-negative women *(40)*. The likelihood of persistent infection among the HIV-positive women was related to the level of immunosuppression. Women with CD4 counts < 200/mm^3 were more than twice as likely to have persistence as women with CD4 counts > 500/mm^3.

Cervical cytology is more often abnormal among HIV-positive women than in HIV-negative women *(41–43)*. In a study reported from San Francisco General Hospital (SFGH), CSIL was detected in 9 (20%) of 44 HIV-positive women compared to 2 (4%) of 52 HIV-negative women *(44)*. In the New York cohort, 20% of the HIV-positive women had CSIL compared to 4% of the HIV-negative women *(45)*. In a large recent study from the WIHS, cervical cytology was abnormal in 38% of HIV-infected women and 16% of HIV-negative women *(46)*. Among the risk factors for abnormal cytology in multivariate analysis in this study were HIV infection, lower CD4 cell count, higher HIV RNA level, HPV positivity, a prior history of abnormal cytology, and greater number of male sex partners within 6 mo of enrollment.

Many questions remain about the anti-HPV CMI response, including the nature of the effector cells, the HPV antigens to which they are directed, and whether the immune response leads to complete clearance of HPV infection or suppression of HPV to a level that is below the level of detection of current HPV DNA tests. The possibility of suppression, rather than clearance, is important because it implies that HPV could be reactivated at some point in the future by unknown factors, some of which may include loss of the CMI response that suppressed HPV.

Several lines of evidence point to the role of the CMI response in controlling cervical disease, but results have been somewhat conflicting. Earlier studies have shown that women with cervical lesions have decreased cellular proliferative responses to HPV type 16 E6 and E7 proteins compared to women without lesions *(47,48)*. In contrast both healthy women and women with CSIL produce T-cell responses to the HPV 16 L1 protein *(49–51)*, and responses to HPV 16 E7 peptides were linked to viral persistence and disease progression *(52)*. A study of cytotoxic T-cell response showed that fewer women with cervical lesions had responses to E6 and E7 than women without disease *(53)*. These results suggest the possibility that expression of E7 may induce T-cell tolerance, consistent with results in mouse models *(54–56)*. Again, conflicting results have been obtained in other studies *(57)*. Although the role of E7-specific CTL response in clearance of tumors in animal models has been demonstrated *(58,59)*, the role of these responses in vivo in prospective studies has not yet been determined. Host factors such as HLA haplotype have been shown to play a role as well, but these remain poorly defined *(60,61)*.

MECHANISMS OF INTERACTION BETWEEN HIV AND HPV

The increase in anogenital HPV infection and SIL in HIV-infected patients may be explained by several interactions between HIV and HPV, that are depicted schematically in Fig. 1. The observation of increased CSIL in patients who are iatrogenically immunocompromised or who have HIV infection underscores the role of the immune response to HPV infection. At the systemic level, it is speculated but not proven that HIV infection leads to generalized loss of memory T-cell subsets, among which may be HPV-specific clones. If true, loss of these cells would partially account for the increased prevalence of HPV infection and SIL in HIV-infected patients.

At the cellular level a direct interaction between HIV and HPV may occur, but this has not been proven to be active in vivo. Although HPV infects the epithelium, HIV may be found in Langerhans' cells, stromal cells, and infiltrating T cells. The HIV-1 tat protein has many potentially important biologic activities *(62,63)*. It has been shown to be secreted by HIV-infected cells and may be taken up by adjacent cells. In vitro it has been shown to transactivate E6 and E7, leading to increased expression of these onco-proteins *(64)*. Abnormal secretion of cytokines by HIV-infected lymphocytes that might activate HPV genes may also potentiate increased HPV-associated neoplasia. Thus, although HPV and HIV largely exist in two different cellular compartments— HPV in the epithelium and HIV in the stromal compartment beneath the basement membrane—there are multiple opportunities for HIV to modulate the expression of HPV and ultimately the natural history of CSIL.

DIAGNOSIS OF CERVICAL SIL

The goal of cervical cytology screening is to detect cervical cancer precursor lesions to allow them to be treated before they can progress to invasive cancer. Based on the data described previously, the primary focus of such as program should be detection of cervical HSIL. The current approach is to screen women repeatedly, often annually. The reason for this is the well-documented lack of sensitivity of a single cytology for the detection of HSIL. Studies show that the sensitivity of cervical cytology varies widely depending on the clinical setting, but in most studies it is between 50% and 70%. Thus, as a single screening test, cervical cytology smears perform poorly. Their strength is in their cumulative sensitivity, and the hope is that the progression rate of CSIL to invasive cancer is sufficiently slow that a cancer can still be prevented if the lesion is detected at one of the subsequent annual screenings.

The next step in the evaluation of a woman with abnormal cervical cytology is to visualize the source of the abnormal cells on the smear to allow for a biopsy. As described below, treatment of CSIL is based strictly on histopathology and not on cytology, as the grading of cervical smears is unreliable. To visualize the lesions, colposcopy is performed, in which a rolling microscope (colposcope) is brought to the opening of a vaginal speculum. This allows for the detailed inspection of the cervix and vagina under magnification.

For a colposcopic examination to be considered adequate, the clinician must visualize the squamocolumnar junction and the entire lesion. If part of the junction or lesion resides in the endocervical canal the examination is considered to be inadequate or unsatisfactory. Under these conditions, an endocervical curettage is necessary for completion of the evaluation. Unsatisfactory colposcopy occurs in 15–20% of women and increases in frequency with increasing age. Colposcopic criteria to distinguish low-grade lesions from high-grade lesions are well validated and are used to guide the clinician to biopsy the most severely abnormal-appearing areas *(65,66)*.

Other measures to improve sensitivity of the technique include application of 5% acetic acid, which leads an HPV-infected lesion to turn white compared to the nonlesional surrounding mucosa. A further measure that can be used to distinguish LSIL from HSIL includes application of Lugol's solution, in which lesional tissue excludes the iodine in the solution whereas normal tissue absorbs it and turns a deep brown color. Finally, a number of colposcopic criteria have been described to aid the clinician to distinguish LSIL from HSIL on the basis of the appearance of the lesion areas *(65,66)* and these include the topography of the lesion and the patterns of the blood vessels in the lesion. Unfortunately, colposcopy is expensive and can be uncomfortable for the patient.

Because grading on cervical cytology is not a reliable guide to determining the presence of HSIL, it is currently the practice to perform colposcopy on all women with HSIL on cytology and some with LSIL. In addition to its problem with sensitivity, cervical cytology suffers from low specificity and positive predictive value for detection of HSIL. Many women with LSIL undergo colposcopy unnecessarily. Some clinicians advocate repeating the cytology in 3 mo, performing colposcopy only if the cytology is repeatedly positive. This conundrum is even more pronounced for women with ASCUS on cytology, as the positive predictive value of ASCUS for the detection of cervical HSIL is even lower than that of LSIL.

EMERGING TECHNOLOGIES TO IMPROVE CERVICAL SIL DIAGNOSIS

Several technologies have emerged recently that are designed to improve the diagnostic sensitivity and positive predictive value of screening. These include cervical cell suspension methods that permit automated creation of single-cell monolayers such as the ThinPrep™ method; artifical intelligence methods to allow computerized screening of cervical smears such as PAPNET™ or AutoPap 300 QC™; and the use of HPV testing such as the Hybrid Capture™ test as an adjunct to cervical cytology.

The principal advantage of the monolayer cytology preparation methods such as ThinPrep™ is the consistently superior quality of the smears. Monolayer cytology methods rely on creation of cervical cell suspensions instead of smearing cervical cells on a glass slide for subsequent fixation. The cells are collected and suspended in 10 mL of a methanol-based solution. Specialized equipment is required to create the monolayers by using a vacuum to bring the cells onto a filter and then to blow the cells onto a glass slide. Interpreting a cellular monolayer is easier than a conventional smear because technical limitations such as cell clumping are largely eliminated. Studies have shown that they are equivalent to or better than routine smears in detecting HSIL or cancers *(67,68)*. Another advantage of this technology is that the creation of the monolayers typically uses only a small proportion of the total cellular sample. Several additional monolayer slides can therefore be made at any time, as the fixative in the suspension solution preserves the cells. The remaining sample may also be used for other purposes such as testing for HPV, as described later in this section. One of the major disadvantages of this technique is the higher cost of the sample collection apparatus and the cost of the machines used to make the monolayers, when compared to the cost of creating and interpreting conventional cervical cytology smears.

Another recent addition to the growing number of emerging technologies to improve detection methods for CSIL is the use of artificial intelligence methods to guide computerized screening of the smears. In one large recent study of more than 20,000 smears comparing PAPNET™ primary screening to manual primary screening, there was 89.8% agreement between the two methods (69). While the sensitivity of the two methods was similar for correctly identifying smears as abnormal, PAPNET™-assisted screening showed significantly better specificity (77%) than conventional screening (42%) for identification of negative smears. In one recent meta-analysis of studies evaluating PAPNET™ as a primary screening method, the PAPNET™ system detected approx 20% more positive smears than manual screening (70). When used to rescreen known false-negative slides, the system correctly identified on average only 33% of those slides as abnormal. Overall, the primary proposed use of this technique is to rescreen negative conventional cytology findings to reduce the false-negative rate.

The concept behind the addition of HPV testing to cervical cytology depends on the now accepted belief that most if not all cervical SIL and cancers are associated with HPV infection. Detection of oncogenic HPV types in a cervical specimen would therefore offer an alternative approach to identifying women at risk for high-grade SIL and cancer. At this time, the only Food and Drug Administration-approved test for detection of HPV in cervical smears or clinical purposes is the Hybrid Capture™ test (Digene Corporation, Beltsville, MD). This is not a PCR test but rather one that relies on signal amplification to achieve high sensitivity. The currently available version of the test does not indicate the presence of specific HPV types, but rather indicates the presence of one or more of the most common oncogenic genital HPV types using a probe mix. There is also a probe mix for the most common non-oncogenic genital HPV types.

Several studies indicate that the sensitivity of HPV testing alone for the detection of cervical HSIL is equivalent to or better than cervical cytology smears (71,72), and one recent study showed that detection of HPV 16 using hybrid capture at two different visits 6 mo apart had better sensitivity for detection of HSIL at colposcopy than repeated cytology screening (73). Nevertheless, most clinicians advocate using cytology and HPV testing together, and the clearest indication for the use of HPV testing currently is as an adjunctive test for women with ASCUS (74). Although many clinicians consider ASCUS to be low risk for concurrent or future cervical cancer, 39% of HSILs in a routine screening population were detected in the follow-up to an ASCUS diagnosis (75). Although a substantial number of HSIL cases would be detected upon follow-up of women with ASCUS, the positive predictive value of ASCUS for HSIL is low (5–10%). The clinical challenge is thus to identify those few individuals at high risk.

Three follow-up options have been proposed for women with ASCUS (76): immediate colposcopy; accelerated repeat cytology testing; and testing for the presence of HPV. Immediate colposcopy would theoretically detect all HSILs, but this is an expensive approach given the low positive predictive value. Repeat cytology also may not be cost-effective, because many women with ASCUS eventually require colposcopic evaluation owing to a high rate of repeat abnormal cytology *(77)*. Testing for HPV in specimens diagnosed as ASCUS has been proposed as an alternative approach, and the advent of the ThinPrep method provides a convenient way of performing HPV testing without requiring an additional patient visit. Thus if the laboratory diagnoses a specimen as ASCUS from a ThinPrep specimen, it can then perform HPV testing on the remaining portion of the specimen. In this algorithm, women with an oncogenic HPV type on Hybrid Capture™ would undergo colposcopy while women who test negative for one or more of these HPV types would be appropriately reassured and possibly undergo repeat cervical cytology testing. The largest study to date indicated that triage by HPV testing of women with ASCUS would provide more sensitive detection of HSIL with fewer colposcopy examinations and fewer follow-up visits than current management protocols *(74)*. This approach also has the advantage of improving the sensitivity of diagnosis of HSIL without increasing the costs of the cervical screening program.

Thus, future directions of cervical cytology screening include: (1) improvement of diagnostic sensitivity of cytology smears by incorporation of newer technologies such as monolayer smears and artificial intelligence-based computerized screening of smears; (2) using technologies such as HPV DNA testing to better rationalize who gets referred for colposcopy; and (3) development of less aggressive management approaches that lengthen screening intervals and minimize treatment of lesions such as LSIL that have little or no malignant potential.

TREATMENT OF CERVICAL SIL

As described previously, the first step in the workup of CSIL is performance of cervical cytology. If an abnormal cytology has been obtained, the two major decision points in the management algorithm for treatment of CSIL are (1) whether or not to perform colposcopy and (2) whether or not to treat a cervical lesion once it has been biopsied and the histopathology of the lesion has been established. A number of different organizations have published guidelines for cervical cytology screening in women. The American College of Obstetricians and Gynecologists and the American Cancer Society recommend that all women begin yearly Pap tests at age 18 or when they become sexually active, whichever occurs earlier. If a woman has had three consecutive negative annual cytology tests, testing may be performed less often at the judgment of a woman's health care provider.

Guidelines for management of women with abnormal cervical cytology have been established by the National Cancer Institute *(9)*. Currently women with ASCUS undergo repeat cytology every 4–6 mo for 2 yr until there have been three consecutive normal smears. If ASCUS is found in conjunction with an inflammatory process, then diagnostic measures to identify and treat concurrent vaginal infections should be initiated before the cytology is repeated. Most clinicians would perform colposcopy if a second ASCUS cytology is found within that 2-yr period. If LSIL is diagnosed on cytology, a similar follow-up plan may be initiated, but referral for colposcopy is recommended for women who may not return for follow-up. All women with HSIL on cytology should be referred for colposcopy.

Treatment of CSIL is based on the histology of biopsied lesions (CIN) and not on cytology (SIL), because of the inaccuracy of cervical cytology for grading lesions. Although treatment always is based on histology, the terms CIN and SIL often are used interchangeably. The purpose of performing biopsies is to determine if the lesions are low-grade or high-grade because the latter would mandate treatment, and to exclude the presence of invasive cancer, as this would invoke a different management algorithm. Several studies show that most biopsied lesions with mild (CIN 1) to moderate (CIN 2) dysplasia regress spontaneously with follow-up *(78–81)*. Thus, although treatment of all cases of CIN 2 may not be necessary, it likely does prevent some cases of cervical cancer particularly among women who may be less likely to return for regular follow-up. Therefore, CIN 2 usually is combined with CIN 3 for the purposes of initiating therapy. Until recently it was the practice to treat all cases of CIN, including CIN 1. However, as the majority of CIN 1 regress spontaneously, many clinicians opt to follow women with CIN 1 rather than treat automatically.

Once a decision to treat CIN is made and biopsies have excluded invasion, there are a number of therapeutic options. Because there currently is no specific therapy for HPV infection, analogous to the use of acyclovir for treatment of herpes simplex virus infection, current treatment methods rely on ablation or removal of the lesion. The simplest method is local excisional biopsy if the lesion is small enough, but this method is inadequate if the lesion extends into the endocervical canal. More often other methods are required such as cryotherapy or large loop excision of the T zone (LLETZ). This procedure is also known as loop electrosurgical excision procedure (LEEP) *(82–84)*. This procedure uses a fine wire to diathermically excise a cervical lesion or the entire transformation zone. The advantages of this procedure are that it preserves margins of the excised tissue for accurate pathologic assessment and is associated with less morbidity than other treatment methods *(85,86)*. Morbidity is related to the amount of tissue removed and may include bleeding during or after the procedure and, rarely, cervical stenosis or cervical incompetence, which can lead to preterm delivery and low birth weight *(87)*.

One of the disadvantages of LLETZ is that it is relatively expensive when compared to cryosurgery, which involves application of a liquid nitrogen cooled probe to the surface of the cervix *(88–90)*. The probe is typically applied twice for 2–3-min applications and leads to necrosis of the frozen areas. The advantages of this method are its low cost, easy applicability in many different clinical settings, low morbidity, and treatment of the entire exocervix. Although reepithelialization of the cervix occurs within 2–3 mo, one of the disadvantages is that scarring may reduce the value of subsequent cytology and colposcopy, especially if the procedure leads to the recession of the squamocolumnar junction into the endocervix. The procedure has a higher failure rate than LLETZ; and it cannot be used if a woman has an inadequate colposcopy, positive endocervical curettage, or especially large lesions. In this case, the treatment of choice is LLETZ.

Laser conization using a CO_2 laser is another treatment approach *(91,92)*. Performed under colposcopic guidance, it has the advantage of allowing the clinician to precisely determine the depth of the lesion excision and leads to minimal damage to surrounding tissues. The laser coagulates blood vessels, and thus there is a lower risk of bleeding than with some of the other therapies. Healing typically occurs without the scarring associated with cryosurgery, and thus there is usually little difficulty with follow-up cytology and colposcopy.

Cold-knife conization can be performed with patients in an ambulatory surgery setting and is usually effective if the margins are negative. It is typically performed only if the patient cannot be treated with LLETZ or laser conization. It is associated with a higher complication rate than the other procedures, including bleeding, stenosis, and scarring. Finally, hysterectomy can be performed if fertility is not a factor and if other gynecologic indications are present. Topical therapies such as retinoic acid and 5-fluorouracil have not been shown to be effective.

TREATMENT OF GENITAL WARTS

Like CIN 1, genital warts are low grade in histology, have low potential for progression to malignancy, and need not be treated to prevent development of cancer. They usually are associated with HPV-6 or -11. In contrast to cervical LSIL or HSIL, however, genital warts may be symptomatic and may lead to burning, itching, bleeding, and psychological discomfort for patients. Relief of these symptoms is an acceptable indication to treat genital warts, and the diagnosis and treatment of these lesions is well described in a recent American Medical Association position paper *(93,94)*.

Treatment of genital warts generally falls into two categories: patient-applied or provider-applied. Among the therapies now available for patients to use at home are purified podophyllotoxin (Condylox™) and imiquimod (Aldara™). These treatments have different mechanisms of action. Podophyllotoxin works by inhibiting microtubule formation and cell division; imiquimod is believed to work by stimulating local interferon production and possibly other cytokines as well. These therapies are approved for therapy of external genital warts and have roughly equivalent efficacy and safety profiles. Their advantage is that patients can apply the treatment themselves, but this also may prove to be a disadvantage if the lesions are too small to be seen by the patient. Therapy with these modalities may require several weeks of application.

Clinician-applied therapies include 80% trichloroacetic acid, liquid nitrogen, electrocautery, thermocoagulation, and laser. These are best reserved for patients whose lesions are too small to be treated by themselves or for lesions that are too large or widespread for home therapy. Most require more than one application of treatment. Each of these modalities, including patient-applied therapies, is associated with lesion recurrences. Patients therefore need to be followed closely after therapy and may require several treatment modalities before complete control is achieved. Counseling is also a critical part of the therapeutic approach to the patient.

DETECTION OF CSIL AND TREATMENT OF CIN IN HIV-POSITIVE WOMEN

HIV-positive women are advised to have a comprehensive gynecologic examination including a cervical cytology smear as part of their initial medical evaluation. If initial results are normal, at least one additional smear should be obtained in 6 mo to exclude a false-negative result on the initial cytology. If the second smear is normal, HIV-infected women should be advised to have an annual smear, similar to HIV-negative women. If the initial or follow-up cytology shows ASCUS or CSIL, the woman should be referred for a colposcopy. Although there was concern initially that cervical cytology may have an unusually high false-negative rate in HIV-positive women, this was not confirmed in subsequent studies. Thus, HIV infection alone does not constitute an indication for colposcopy.

Several studies suggest that HIV-positive women do not respond as well to standard therapy of CIN as HIV-negative women *(95,96)*. The natural history of CIN may be accelerated in HIV-positive women *(97)*. And, if cervical cancer does develop, treatment may be more difficult. Consequently, HIV-positive women with CIN should be followed very closely after therapy for recurrence and multiple treatment modalities may be needed *(98)*.

EMERGING APPROACHES TO PREVENTION AND TREATMENT OF HPV INFECTION

At this time, HPV infection cannot be prevented other than through sexual abstinence. There is no evidence to suggest that condoms effectively prevent HPV acquisition. This is because condoms probably do not completely cover all areas that may harbor HPV-associated lesions such as the base of the penis. However, efforts are now underway to prevent initial HPV infection through a vaccine-based approach, and it is assumed that induction of mucosal humoral immunity is the necessary protective effect. Most work on a prophylactic vaccine to date has focused on the use of recombinant L1 protein as a vaccine candidate. The L1 protein is the major capsid protein of the HPV virion. When expressed in vitro, it autoassembles into a structure that closely resembles native HPV virions *(99)*. These structures, termed "virus-like particles" (VLPs), have been shown to induce high titer neutralizing antibodies in animals *(100–102)* and in human Phase 1 trials *(103)* and to prevent lesion development in animal models *(104)*. Data thus far also indicate that the L1 vaccines are safe and well tolerated *(103)*. Trials to determine efficacy to prevent HPV infection are in progress. To date the data suggest that the antibodies raised against VLPs of specific viral types such as HPV-16 are relatively type-specific. Thus, it seems likely that a cocktail consisting of VLPs of several HPV types, for example, HPV-16,-18,-31, and -45, will be needed to prevent infection with the most common oncogenic HPV types. Efforts are also underway to determine if vaccine efficacy may be improved by genetically engineering early region HPV proteins such as E7 into the VLPs *(105)*.

In contrast to the attempt to use VLPs to induce prophylactic humoral immunity, it is assumed that a therapeutic response to a preexisting lesion requires induction of CMI response. Consequently, there is also an effort to develop therapeutic vaccines for individuals with high-grade CIN or cervical cancer as a primary mode of therapy or adjunctive to more standard therapeutic modalities. Unlike the VLPs which contain the L1 capsid protein, therapeutic vaccines typically target the E6 or E7 proteins, which are believed to be expressed continuously in high-grade lesions. In vitro animal data from several studies suggest that induction of a CMI response against these proteins may lead to resolution of tumors *(58,59)*. Phase 1 trials of recombinant vaccinia virus expressing E6 and E7 in patients with advanced cervical cancer demonstrated the safety of this approach, but relatively little immune response was seen *(106)*. Several other Phase 1 and Phase 1/2 studies are now underway using other preparations of E7 to determine their safety and efficacy against high-grade CIN.

ANAL CANCER AND ITS PRECURSORS

Anal cancer has traditionally been considered a rare disease, occurring in women at about one tenth the incidence of cervical cancer. However, unlike the declining incidence of cervical cancer, the incidence of anal cancer in women has been increasing at a rate of about 2% per year in the United States and also has been rising in European countries such as Denmark *(107)*. Anal cancer is more common in women than in men, but its incidence is highest among men who have practiced receptive anal intercourse, among whom the incidence of anal cancer was estimated to be as high at 35/100,000 *(2)*. Therefore, the incidence of anal cancer among these men is similar to that of cervical cancer among women prior to the introduction of routine cervical cytology screening. Moreover, because the data used to generate this estimate predated the onset of the HIV epidemic, they presumably reflect the incidence of anal cancer among HIV-negative men with a history of receptive anal intercourse (hereafter referred to as men who have sex with men, or MSM). The impact of the HIV epidemic on the incidence of anal cancer remains unclear. However, recent data suggest that the incidence of anal cancer among HIV-positive MSM may be about twice that of HIV-negative MSM *(2,3)*.

Biologically, cervical cancer resembles anal cancer in several ways, including similar histology. Both cervical and anal cancer frequently arise in the transformation zone *(107)*. In the cervix, this is where the columnar epithelium of the endocervix meets the squamous epithelium of the exocervix. In the anal canal, the transformation zone is located at the junction between the columnar epithelium of the rectum and the squamous epithelium of the anus. Cervical and anal cancer also share a strong association with HPV *(108–110)*. Finally, both cervical and anal and cancer are frequently associated with overlying HSIL. There are no published studies to date of the natural history of anal HSIL to demonstrate directly that anal HSIL progresses to invasive anal cancer. However, it seems likely that anal HSIL represents the true precursor lesion to anal cancer.

Unlike cervical HPV infection which declines substantially in prevalence after the age of 30, anal HPV infection is found in a large proportion (61%) of MSM well into their 30s and 40s *(111,112)*. Anal HPV infection is even more common in HIV-positive MSM, with nearly all such individuals having one or more HPV types. Infection with multiple HPV types is common, and the mean number of types increases with HIV positivity and lower CD4 levels.

Several studies have examined anal HPV infection in women *(44,113)*. Surprisingly, these studies demonstrate that anal HPV infection is found at a similar or higher rate as cervical HPV infection, and the spectrum of HPV types is similar in the anal canal and cervix. Notably, the same HPV types were found in the anus and cervix in only 50% of the women who were infected at both sites. The mode of acquisition of anal HPV infection was not clearly linked to receptive anal intercourse in these studies, but a more recent study of a larger number of women did show an association with receptive anal intercourse (JM Palefsky, *unpublished data*). However, insertion of inert objects or fingers exposed to other HPV-infected tissues of the individual or their sexual partner may also result in anal HPV infection.

The prevalence and natural history of anal SIL in HIV-positive and HIV-negative MSM have now been well characterized *(114–117)*. Consistent with the HPV infection data, the prevalence of anal SIL was higher in cross-sectional analysis among HIV-positive MSM than HIV-negative MSM, particularly among those with lower $CD4^+$ levels *(115)*. SIL was present in 36% (124/346) of HIV-positive men and 7% (19/262) of HIV-negative men, and the relative risk of SIL among HIV-positive men inversely correlated with CD4 count. In a study in Seattle of MSM who initially had no evidence of SIL, anal HSIL developed in 15% of HIV-positive and 8% of HIV-negative men after an average of 21 mo *(114)*. Risk factors for development of HSIL included infection with HPV 16 or 18, persistent detection of high levels of HPV DNA, and increased immunosuppression as reflected by a CD4 level < 500/mm^3. In a more recent study performed in San Francisco, HSIL developed in 49% of the HIV-positive men and 17% of the HIV-negative men over a 4-yr period *(117)*. The higher incidence in this study than the Seattle study likely reflects two factors: the longer follow-up time and the inclusion of subjects in the analysis who had LSIL or ASCUS at baseline as well as those with no signs of anal disease. Risk factors for progression to HSIL were similar among HIV-positive and HIV-negative men and included infection with multiple HPV types, persistent anal infection, and high level infection with oncogenic HPV types.

The incidence of anal cancer among HIV-positive women is not known. However, anal cytologic abnormalities are more common among HIV-positive women than among high-risk HIV-negative women *(44,113)*. Among the HIV-positive women, anal cytologic abnormalities were at least as common as cervical abnormalities although the severity of the anal lesions was less marked than those of the cervix. Fourteen percent of HIV-positive women had abnormal anal cytology; and, consistent with data obtained in studies of men, anal cytologic changes were associated with HIV infection and lower CD4 counts *(44)*. The natural history of anal SIL in HIV-positive women is not yet known. Anal cytologic abnormalities also have been detected in 4% of adolescent women. As in the HIV-positive women, anal HPV infection and receptive anal intercourse were independent risk factors *(118)*. Interestingly, history of CSIL was also an independent risk factor in this population, underscoring the concept of HPV infection as a "field" infection" of the entire anogenital region. Other risk factors for anal SIL in women include concurrent cervical HSIL or vulvar cancer and history of renal allograft *(119–121)*.

SCREENING AND TREATMENT ALGORITHMS FOR ANAL HSIL

The data presented here indicate a high prevalence of anal SIL among both HIV-positive and HIV-negative MSM, as well as a high incidence of HSIL and a high incidence of anal cancer among both HIV-positive and HIV-negative MSM. Given the similarity between cervical and anal cancer, it is possible that an anal cytology screening program in high-risk populations may reduce the incidence of anal cancer, similar to the reduction in cervical cancer associated with implementation of cervical cytology screening. As proposed, screening would be considered for the men and women at highest risk, that is, those with a history of receptive anal intercourse. Sexually active women, particularly those who are HIV-positive or who have a history of cervical HSIL or vulvar cancer, also appear to be at increased risk of anal HPV infection and anal SIL. Thus, other risk groups that could be considered for screening include all HIV-positive women, regardless of whether or not they have engaged in anal intercourse, and all women with high-grade cervical or vulvar lesions and cancer. However, few data exist at this time to support screening in the latter groups.

The elements of an anal screening program would likely closely resemble that of the cervix. Anal cytology and high-resolution anoscopy would be performed as described previously *(107)*. In the author's opinion, all patients with abnormal anal cytology, including those with ASCUS, should be referred for high-resolution anoscopy. Areas that appear suspicious for HSIL should be biopsied as described previously *(122)*. There is currently no accepted standard of care for treatment of anal SIL, and the medical literature is very limited on this subject. As with cervical lesions, only patients with HSIL should be routinely recommended for treatment, particularly those with the most advanced forms such as severe dysplasia. We do not routinely recommend treatment of low-grade lesions because of the high likelihood of pain associated with the treatment, high recurrence rate, and low risk of progression to cancer. However, many patients do opt for therapy to relieve symptoms associated with the lesions such as itching, burning, or psychological discomfort. The treatment of low-grade lesions is similar to that of high-grade lesions. For HIV-positive patients who have a reasonable life expectancy and good functional status, surgical excision or ablation is the primary form of treatment. Occasionally lesions may be small enough that they might respond to local application of 80% trichloroacetic acid in the office setting. Most lesions will require multiple applications over time for complete resolution, typically at intervals of 1–2 wk.

COST-EFFECTIVENESS OF ANAL CYTOLOGY SCREENING

To assess the clinical and cost-effectiveness of such an anal cytology screening program, Goldie and colleagues have been modeling anal cytology screening under a variety of conditions *(123)*. They used a combination of data from the literature and a range of assumptions in areas for which there are no data in the literature, such as the rate of progression from HSIL to invasive cancer and efficacy of treatment of HSIL to prevent anal cancer. The screening strategies considered included no screening, annual or semiannual anal cytology, and annual or semiannual anoscopies as screening tests. Overall, annual anal screening was found to be cost-effective for all HIV-positive MSM regardless of CD4 level *(123)*. Anal cytology was equivalent in cost-effectiveness to some of the most widely used practices in HIV-positive men, such as use of trimethoprim-sulfamethoxazole to prevent *Pneumocystis carinii* pneumonia. Using a similar model for HIV-negative MSM, anal cytology screening every 2–3 yr was found to be cost-effective (S. Goldie, submitted for publication).

SUMMARY

Cervical cancer remains one of the most common causes of mortality among young women worldwide. Associated with the sexually transmitted agent HPV, it is the most common source of cancer mortality due to viral infections. Cervical cancer is preceded by a series of precancerous changes known as SILs, and if these are detected through cytology screening and treated development of cancer is usually prevented. Thus, cervical cancer is also one of the most preventable cancers. Unfortunately routine cervical cytology screening is not available in many parts of the world where the incidence of cervical cancer remains high. Future efforts to reduce the incidence of cervical cancer are therefore largely being focused on development of vaccines to prevent initial infection with oncogenic HPV types. The advent of the HIV epidemic has also brought new challenges to clinicians treating SIL and cancer. CSIL is more common among HIV-positive women than among HIV-negative women and is more difficult to treat in this setting. Like cervical cancer, anal cancer is associated with HPV, and its current incidence among at-risk individuals, that is, those with a history of receptive anal intercourse, is similar to that of cervical cancer in the United States prior to the introduction of routine cervical cytology screening. Like CSIL, anal SIL is more common among HIV-positive MSM than among HIV-negative MSM, and recent data suggest that routine anal cytology screening of at-risk individuals may be cost-effective to prevent anal cancer. Women with a history of receptive anal intercourse may also be at increased risk of anal HPV infection, anal SIL, and anal cancer. Like vaccines to prevent initial infection with HPV, therapeutic vaccines targeted to HPV antigens are under development to treat anogenital SIL and, together with advances in diagnostic techniques for SIL, offer new promise in the control of HPV-associated lesions.

CONCLUSIONS

Prevention of cervical cancer through cervical cytology screening depends on identification and treatment of cervical HSIL before it progresses to cancer. Several methods such as monolayer cervical cytology, computerized screening of cervical smears, and adjunctive HPV testing will likely improve the diagnostic sensitivity and specificity of cervical cytology screening in a cost-effective manner. Advances in therapy for HPV-associated lesions have been slower in coming, but promising new HPV-specific approaches include therapeutic vaccines targeted at HPV antigens. Patients coinfected with HPV and HIV infection present a special challenge to the clinician owing to higher prevalence of CSIL and lower success rates with standard therapy. The HIV epidemic has also brought increased attention to the clinical problem of anal SIL and anal cancer. Although the risk of these lesions is highest among MSM, women are also at risk, particularly those with a history of receptive anal intercourse and HIV infection. As with the cervical cytology screening program, anal cytology screening program for those at risk is proposed and has been projected to be cost-effective.

Like herpes simplex virus, HPV may result in chronic infections at multiple anogenital sites, and may be difficult to treat. Although advances in diagnosis and therapy are encouraging, it is clear that the ultimate solution to the problems posed by HPV will be vaccine-based prevention of initial infection. Initial efforts in this direction appear to be very promising, and over the next few years studies examining the efficacy of this approach will be of great interest.

ACKNOWLEDGMENTS

This work was supported by Grants NCI R01CA54053 and R01CA 63933. Data in this chapter were derived in part from studies carried out in the General Clinical Research Center, University of California, San Francisco with funds provided by the Division of Research Resources 5 M01-RR-00079, U. S. Public Health Service.

REFERENCES

1. Qualters JR, Lee NC, Smith RA, Aubert RE. Breast and cervical cancer surveillance, United States, 1973–1987. Morbid Mortal Wkly Rep 1992; 41:1–15.

2. Daling JR, Weiss NS, Hislop TG, et al. Sexual practices, sexually transmitted diseases, and the incidence of anal cancer. N Engl J Med 1987; 317:973–977.

3. Goedert JJ, Cote TR, Virgo P, et al. Spectrum of AIDS-associated malignant disorders. Lancet 1998; 351:1833–1839.

4. Bosch FX, Manos MM, Munoz N, et al. Prevalence of human papillomavirus in cervical cancer: a worldwide perspective. International biological study on cervical cancer (IBSCC) Study Group. J Natl Cancer Inst 1995; 87:796–802.

5. Rylander E, Ruusuvaara L, Almströmer MW, Evander M, Wadell G. The absence of vaginal human papillomavirus 16 DNA in women who have not experienced sexual intercourse. Obstet Gynecol 1994; 83:735–737.

6. Burk RD, Ho GY, Beardsley L, Lempa M, Peters M, Bierman R. Sexual behavior and partner characteristics are the predominant risk factors for genital human papillomavirus infection in young women. J Infect Dis 1996; 174:679–689.

7. Koutsky L, Kiviat NB. Genital human papillomavirus. In: Holmes KK, Sparling PF, Mardh P-A, et al. (eds). Sexually Transmitted Diseases. New York: McGraw-Hill, 1998, pp. 347–359.

8. Schiffman MH. Recent progress in defining the epidemiology of human papillomavirus infection and cervical neoplasia. J Natl Cancer Inst 1992; 84:394–398.

9. Kurman RJ, Solomon D. The Bethesda system for reporting cervical/vaginal cytologic diagnoses:definitions, criteria and explanatory notes for terminology and specimen adequacy. New York: Springer-Verlag, 1994, p.81.

10. Richart RM, Barron BA. A follow-up study of patients with cervical dysplasia. Am J Obstet Gynecol 1969; 105:383–393.

11. Koutsky LA, Holmes KK, Critchlow CW, et al. A cohort study of the risk of cervical intraepithelial neoplasia grade 2 or 3 in relation to papillomavirus infection. N Engl J Med 1992; 327:1272–1278.

12. Lorincz AT, Reid R, Jenson AB, Greenberg MD, Lancaster W, Kurman RJ. Human papillomavirus infection of the cervix: relative risk associations of 15 common anogenital types. Obstet Gynecol 1992; 79:328–337.

13. Wiggins C. Cancer in Western Washington State 1974–1991. 1993.

14. Centers for Disease Control and Prevention. Special focus: behavioral risk factor surveillance—United States, 1991. Morbid Mortal Wkly Rep 1993; 42:1–23.

15. Spriggs AI, Boddington MM. Progression and regression of cervical lesions. Review of smears from women followed without initial biopsy or treatment. J Clin Pathol 1980; 33:517–522.

16. Krone MR, et al. The epidemiology of cervical neoplasms. In: Luesley D, et al. (eds). Intraepithelial Neoplasia of the Lower Genital Tract. New York: Churchill-Livingstone, 1995, p.49.

17. Miller BA, et al. (eds). SEER Cancer Statistics Review: 1973–1990. NIH Publication 93-2789, 1993.

18. Devesa SS. Descriptive epidemiology of cancer of the uterine cervix. Obstet Gynecol 1984; 63:605–612.

19. Livingstone LR, White A, Sprouse J, Livanos E, Jacks T, Tlsty TD. Altered cell cycle arrest and gene amplification potential accompany loss of wild-type *p53*. Cell 1992; 70:923–935.

20. Carder P, Wyllie AH, Purdie CA, et al. Stabilised *p53* facilitates aneuploid clonal divergence in colorectal cancer. Oncogene 1993; 8:1397–1401.

21. Magnusson PK, Wilander E, Gyllensten U. Analysis of loss of heterozygosity in microdissected tumor cells from cervical carcinoma using fluorescent dUTP labeling of PCR products. Biotechniques 1996; 21:844–847.

22. Rader JS, Kamarasova T, Huettner PC, Li L, Li Y, Gerhard DS. Allelotyping of all chromosomal arms in invasive cervical cancer. Oncogene 1996; 13:2737–2741.

23. Douc-Rasy S, Barrois M, Fogel S, et al. High incidence of loss of heterozygosity and abnormal imprinting of H19 and IGF2 genes in invasive cervical carcinomas. Uncoupling of H19 and IGF2 expression and biallelic hypomethylation of H19. Oncogene 1996; 12:423–430.

24. Bosch FX, Munoz N, de Sanjose S, et al. Risk factors for cervical cancer in Colombia and Spain. Int J Cancer 1992; 52:750–758.

25. Eluf-Neto J, Booth M, Munoz N, Bosch FX, Meijer CJLM, Walboomers JMM. Human papillomavirus and invasive cancer in Brazil. Br J Cancer 1994; 69:114–119.

26. Kwasniewska A, Tukendorf A, Semczuk M. Folate deficiency and cervical intraepithelial neoplasia. Eur J Gynaecol Oncol 1997; 18:526–530.

27. Butterworth CJ, Hatch KD, Macaluso M, et al. Folate deficiency and cervical dysplasia. JAMA 1992; 267:528–533.

28. Butterworth CJ, Hatch KD, Soong SJ, et al. Oral folic acid supplementation for cervical dysplasia: a clinical intervention trial. Am J Obstet Gynecol 1992; 166:803–809.

29. Childers JM, Chu J, Voigt LF, et al. Chemoprevention of cervical cancer with folic acid: a phase III Southwest Oncology Group Intergroup study. Cancer Epidemiol Biomarker Prev 1995; 4:155–159.

30. Ho GY, Palan PR, Basu J, et al. Viral characteristics of human papillomavirus infection and antioxidant levels as risk factors for cervical dysplasia. Int J Cancer 1998; 78:594–599.

31. Goodman MT, Kiviat N, McDuffie K, et al. The association of plasma micronutrients with the risk of cervical dysplasia in Hawaii. Cancer Epidemiol Biomarker Prev 1998; 7:537–544.

32. Behbakht K, DeGeest K, Turyk ME, Wilbanks GD. All-trans-retinoic acid inhibits the proliferation of cell lines derived from human cervical neoplasia. Gynecol Oncol 1996; 61:31–39.

33. Seewaldt VL, Dietze EC, Johnson BS, Collins SJ, Parker MB. Retinoic acid-mediated G1–S-phase arrest of normal human mammary epithelial cells is independent of the level of p53 protein expression. Cell Growth Different 1999; 10:49–59.

34. Hietanen S, Auvinen E, Syrjänen K, Syrjänen S. Anti-proliferative effect of retinoids and interferon-alpha-2a on vaginal cell lines derived from squamous intra-epithelial lesions. Int J Cancer 1998; 78:338–345.

35. Shimizu H, Nagata C, Komatsu S, et al. Decreased serum retinol levels in women with cervical dysplasia. Br J Cancer 1996; 73:1600–1604.

36. Sillman F, Stanek A, Sedlis A, et al. The relationship between human papillomavirus and lower genital intraepithelial neoplasia in immunosuppressed women. Am J Obstet Gynecol 1984; 150:300–308.

37. Penn I. Cancers of the anogenital regions in renal transplant recipients. Cancer 1986; 58:611–616.

38. Sun XW, Ellerbrock TV, Lungu O, Chiasson MA, Bush TJ, Wright TC Jr. Human papillomavirus infection in human immunodeficiency virus-seropositive women. Obstet Gynecol 1995; 85:680–686.

39. Palefsky JM, Minkoff H, Kalish LA, et al. Cervicovaginal human papillomavirus infection in human immunodeficiency virus-1 (HIV)-positive and high-risk HIV-negative women. J Natl Cancer Inst 1999; 91:226–236.

40. Sun XW, Kuhn L, Ellerbrock TV, Chiasson MA, Bush TJ, Wright TC Jr. Human papillomavirus infection in women infected with the human immunodeficiency virus. N Engl J Med 1997; 337:1343–1349.

41. Sillman FH, Sedlis A. Anogenital papillomavirus infection and neoplasia in immunodeficient women. Obstet Gynecol Clin North Am 1987; 14:537–558.

42. Maiman M, Fruchter RG, Serur E, Remy JC, Feuer G, Boyce J. Human immunodeficiency virus infection and cervical neoplasia. Gynecol Oncol 1990; 38:377–382.

43. Vermund SH, Kelley KF, Klein RS, et al. High risk of human papillomavirus infection and cervical squamous intraepithelial lesions among women with symptomatic human immunodeficiency virus infection. Am J Obstet Gynecol 1991; 165:392–400.

44. Williams AB, Darragh TM, Vranizan K, Ochia C, Moss AR, Palefsky JM. Anal and cervical human papillomavirus infection and risk of anal and cervical epithelial abnormalities in human immunodeficiency virus-infected women. Obstet Gynecol 1994; 83:205–211.

45. Wright TC Jr, Sun XW. Anogenital papillomavirus infection and neoplasia in immunodeficient women. Obstet Gynecol Clin North Am 1996; 23:861–893.

46. Massad LS, Riester KA, Anastos KM, et al. Prevalence and predictors of squamous cell abnormalities in Papanicolaou smears from women infected with HIV-1. Women's Intergency HIV Study Group. J Acquir Immun Defic Syndr 1999; 21:33–41.

47. Nakagawa M, Stites D, Farhat S, et al. T cell response to human papillomavirus type 16: relationship to cervical intraepithelial neoplasia. Clin Diagnost Lab Immunol 1996; 3:205–210.

48. Tsukui T, Hildesheim A, Schiffman MH, et al. Interleukin 2 production in vitro by peripheral lymphocytes in response to human papillomavirus-derived peptides: correlation with cervical pathology. Cancer Res 1996; 56:3967–3974.

49. Strang G, Hickling JK, McIndoe GA, et al. Human T cell responses to human papillomavirus type 16 L1 and E6 synthetic peptides: identification of T cell determinants, HLA-DR restriction and virus type specificity. J Gen Virol 1990; 71:423–431.

50. Shepherd PS, Rowe A, Cridland J, Chapman M, Luxton J, Rayfield L. An immunodominant region in HPV16.L1 identified by T-cell responses in patients with cervical dysplasias. In: Stanley MA (ed). Immunology of Human Papillomaviruses. New York: Plenum Press, 1994, pp. 169–174.

51. Shepherd PS, Rowe AJ, Cridland JC, Coletart T, Wilson P, Luxton JC. Proliferative T cell responses to human papillomavirus type 16 L1 peptides in patients with cervical dysplasia. J Gen Virol 1996; 77:593–602.

52. de Gruijl TD, Bontkes HJ, Walboomers JM, et al. Differential T helper cell responses to human papillomavirus type 16 E7 related to viral clearance or persistence in patients with cervical neoplasia: a longitudinal study. Cancer Res 1998; 58:1700–1706.

53. Nakagawa M, Stites DP, Farhat S, et al. Cytotoxic T lymphocyte responses to E6 and E7 proteins of human papillomavirus type 16: relationship to cervical intraepithelial neoplasia. J Infect Dis 1997; 175:927–931.

54. Frazer IH, Fernando GJ, Fowler N, et al. Split tolerance to a viral antigen expressed in thymic epithelium and keratinocytes. Eur J Immunol 1998; 28:2791–2800.

55. Doan T, Chambers M, Street M, et al. Mice expressing the E7 oncogene of HPV16 in epithelium show central tolerance, and evidence of peripheral anergising tolerance, to E7-encoded cytotoxic T-lymphocyte epitopes. Virology 1998; 244:352–364.

56. Doan T, Herd K, Street M, Bryson G, Fernando G, Lambert P, Tindle R. Human papillomavirus type 16 E7 oncoprotein expressed in peripheral epithelium tolerizes E7-directed cytotoxic T-lymphocyte precursors resticted through human (and mouse) major histocompatibility complex class I alleles. J Virol 1999; 73:6166–6170.

57. Nimako M, Fiander AN, Wilkinson GW, Borysiewicz LK, Man S. Human papillomavirus-specific cytotoxic T lymphocytes in patients with cervical intraepithelial neoplasia grade III. Cancer Res 1997; 57:4855–4861.

58. Feltkamp MC, Smits HL, Vierboom MP, et al. Vaccination with cytotoxic T lymphocyte epitope-containing peptide protects against a tumor induced by human papillomavirus type 16-transformed cells. Eur J Immunol 1993; 23:2242–2249.

59. Feltkamp MC, Vreugdenhil GR, Vierboom MP, et al. Cytotoxic T lymphocytes raised against a subdominant epitope offered as a synthetic peptide eradicate human papillomavirus type 16-induced tumors. Eur J Immunol 1995; 25:2638–2642.

60. Apple RJ, Erlich HA, Klitz W, Manos MM, Becker TM, Wheeler CM. HLA DR-DQ associations with cervical carcinoma show papillomavirus-type specificity. Nat Genet 1994; 6:157–162.

61. Helland A, Olsen AO, Gjøen K, et al. An increased risk of cervical intra-epithelial neoplasia grade II-III among human papillomavirus positive patients with the HLA-DQA1*0102-DQB1*0602 haplotype: a population-based case-control study of Norwegian women. Int J Cancer 1998; 76:19–24.

62. Barillari G, Gendelman R, Gallo RC, Ensoli B. The Tat protein of human immunodeficiency virus type 1, a growth factor for AIDS Kaposi sarcoma and cytokine-activated vascular cells, induces adhesion of the same cell types by using integrin receptors recognizing the RGD amino acid sequence. Proc Natl Acad Sci USA 1993; 90:7941–7945.

63. Buonaguro L, Barillari G, Chang HK, et al. Effects of the human immunodeficiency virus type 1 Tat protein on the expression of inflammatory cytokines. J Virol 1992; 66:7159–7167.

64. Vernon SD, Hart CE, Reeves WC, Icenogle JP. The HIV-1 tat protein enhances E2-dependent human papillomavirus 16 transcription. Virus Res 1993; 27:133–145.

65. Townsend DE, Ostergard DR, Mishell DR, Jr., Hirose FM. Abnormal Papanicolaou smears. Evaluation by colposcopy, biopsies, and endocervical curettage. Am J Obstet Gynecol 1970; 108:429–434.

66. Stafl A. Colposcopy in diagnosis of cervical neoplasia. Am J Obstet Gynecol 1973; 115:286–287.

67. Spitzer M. Cervical screening adjuncts: recent advances. Am J Obstet Gynecol 1998; 179:544–556.

68. Hutchinson ML, Zahniser DJ, Sherman ME, et al. Utility of liquid-based cytology for cervical carcinoma screening: results of a population-based study conducted in a region of Costa Rica with a high incidence of cervical carcinoma. Cancer 1999; 87:48–55.

69. Team PPM. Assessment of automated primary screening on PAPNET of cervical smears in the PRISMATIC trial. Lancet 1999; 353:1381–1385.

70. Abulafia O, Sherer DM. Automated cervical cytology: meta-analyses of the performance of the PAPNET system. Obstet Gynecol Surv 1999; 54:253–264.

71. Poljak M, Brencic A, Seme K, Vince A, Marin IJ. Comparative evaluation of first- and second-generation digene hybrid capture assays for detection of human papillomaviruses associated with high or intermediate risk for cervical cancer. J Clin Microbiol 1999; 37:796–797.

72. Clavel C, Masure M, Putaud I, et al. Hybrid capture II, a new sensitive test for human papillomavirus detection. Comparison with hybrid capture I and PCR results in cervical lesions. J Clin Pathol 1998; 51:737–740.

73. Nobbenhuis MAE, Walboomers JMM, Helmerhorst TJM, et al. Relation of human papillomavirus status to cervical lesions and consequences for cervical-cancer screening: a prospective study. Lancet 1999; 354:20–25.

74. Manos MM, Kinney WK, Hurley LB, et al. Identifying women with cervical neoplasia: using human papillomavirus DNA testing for equivocal Papanicolaou results. JAMA 1999; 281:1605–1610.

75. Kinney WK, Manos MM, Hurley LB, Ransley JE. Where's the high-grade cervical neoplasia? The importance of minimally abnormal Papanicolaou diagnoses. Obstet Gynecol 1998; 91:973–976.

76. Cox JT. Evaluating the role of HPV testing for women with equivocal Papanicolaou test findings. JAMA 1999; 281:1645–1647.

77. Ferris DG, Wright TC, Jr., Litaker MS, et al. Triage of women with ASCUS and LSIL on Pap smear reports: management by repeat Pap smear, HPV DNA testing, or colposcopy? J Fam Pract 1998; 46:125–134.

78. Kirby AJ, Spiegelhalter DJ, Day NE, et al. Conservative treatment of mild/moderate cervical dyskaryosis: long-term outcome. Lancet 1992; 339:828–831.

79. Fletcher A, Metaxas N, Grubb C, Chamberlain J. Four and a half year follow up of women with dyskaryotic cervical smears. Br Med J (Clin Res) 1990; 301:641–644.

80. Robertson JH, Woodend BE, Crozier EH, Hutchinson J. Risk of cervical cancer associated with mild dyskaryosis. Br Med J (Clin Res) 1988; 297:18–21.

81. Flannelly G, Anderson D, Kitchener HC, et al. Management of women with mild to moderate cervical dyskaryosis. Br Med J 1994; 308:1399–1403.

82. Prendiville W, Cullimore J, Norman S. Large loop excision of the transformation zone (LLETZ). A new method of management for women with cervical intraepithelial neoplasia. Br J Obstet Gynecol 1989; 96:1054–1060.

83. Wright TC, Jr., Gagnon S, Richart RM, Ferenczy A. Treatment of cervical intraepithelial neoplasia using the loop electrosurgical excision procedure. Obstet Gynecol 1992; 79:173–178.

84. Prendiville W. Large loop excision of the transformation zone. Baillieres Clin Obst Gynecol 1995; 9:189–220.

85. Bigrigg A, Haffenden DK, Sheehan AL, Codling BW, Read MD. Efficacy and safety of large-loop excision of the transformation zone. Lancet 1994; 343:32.

86. Ferenczy A, Choukroun D, Arseneau J. Loop electrosurgical excision procedure for squamous intraepithelial lesions of the cervix: advantages and potential pitfalls. Obst Gynecol 1996; 87:332–337.

87. Bloomfield PI, Buxton J, Dunn J, Luesley DM. Pregnancy outcome after large loop excision of the cervical transformation zone. Am J Obstet Gynecol 1993; 169:620–625.

88. Townsend DE, Ostergard DR. Cryocauterization for preinvasive cervical neoplasia. J Reprod Med 1971; 6:171–176.

89. Charles EH, Savage EW. Cryosurgical treatment of cervical intraepithelial neoplasia. Obstet Gynecol Surv 1980; 35:539–548.

90. Figge DC, Creasman WT. Cryotherapy in the treatment of cervical intraepithelial neoplasia. Obstet Gynecol 1983; 62:353–358.

91. Stein DS, Ulrich SA, Hasiuk AS. Laser vaporization in the treatment of cervical intraepithelial neoplasia. J Reprod Med 1985; 30:179–183.

92. Jordan JA, Woodman CB, Mylotte MJ, et al. The treatment of cervical intraepithelial neoplasia by laser vaporization. Br J Obstet Gynecol 1985; 92:394–398.

93. Beutner KR, Reitano MV, Richwald GA, Wiley DJ. External genital warts: report of the American Medical Association Consensus Conference. AMA Expert Panel on External Genital Warts. Clin Infect Dis 1998; 27:796–806.

94. Beutner KR, Wiley DJ, Douglas JM, et al. Genital warts and their treatment. Clin Infect Dis 1999; 28 (Suppl 1):S37–56.

95. Maiman M, Fruchter RG, Serur E, Levine PA, Arrastia CD, Sedlis A. Recurrent cervical intraepithelial neoplasia in human immunodeficiency virus-seropositive women. Obstet Gynecol 1993; 82:170–174.

96. Fruchter RG, Maiman M, Sedlis A, Bartley L, Camilien L, Arrastia CD. Multiple recurrences of cervical intraepithelial neoplasia in women with the human immunodeficiency virus. Obstet Gynecol 1996; 87:338–344.

97. Holcomb K, Maiman M, Dimaio T, Gates J. Rapid progression to invasive cervix cancer in a woman infected with the human immunodeficiency virus. Obstet Gynecol 1998; 91:848–850.

98. Maiman M. Management of cervical neoplasia in human immunodeficiency virus-infected women. J Natl Cancer Inst Monogr 1998; 68:43–49.

99. Schiller JT, Lowy DR. Papillomavirus-like particles and HPV vaccine development. Semin Cancer Biol 1996; 7:373–382.

100. Nardelli-Haefliger D, Roden RB, Benyacoub J, et al. Human papillomavirus type 16 virus-like particles expressed in attenuated *Salmonella typhimurium* elicit mucosal and systemic neutralizing antibodies in mice. Infect Immun 1997; 65:3328–3336.

101. Balmelli C, Roden R, Potts A, Schiller J, De Grandi P, Nardelli-Haefliger D. Nasal immunization of mice with human papillomavirus type 16 virus-like particles elicits neutralizing antibodies in mucosal secretions. J Virol 1998; 72:8220–8229.

102. Lowe RS, Brown DR, Bryan JT, et al. Human papillomavirus type 11 (HPV-11) neutralizing antibodies in the serum and genital mucosal secretions of African green monkeys immunized with HPV-11 virus-like particles expressed in yeast. J Infect Dis 1997; 176:1141–1145.

103. Schiller J, Lowy D. Papillomavirus-like particle vaccines for cervical cancer. Third National AIDS Malignancy Conference, Abstract S6, 1999.

104. Suzich JA, Ghim SJ, Palmer-Hill FJ, et al. Systemic immunization with papillomavirus L1 protein completely prevents the development of viral mucosal papillomas. Proc Natl Acad Sci USA 1995; 92:11553–11557.

105. Greenstone HL, Nieland JD, de Visser KE, et al. Chimeric papillomavirus virus-like particles elicit antitumor immunity against the E7 oncoprotein in an HPV 16 tumor model. Proc Natl Acad Sci USA 1998; 95:1800–1805.

106. Borysiewicz LK, Fiander A, Nimako M, et al. A recombinant vaccinia virus encoding human papillomavirus types 16 and 18, E6 and E7 proteins as immunotherapy for cervical cancer. Lancet 1996; 347:1523–1527.

107. Palefsky J. Anal cancer in HIV-positive individuals: an emerging problem. AIDS 1994: 283–295.

108. Zaki SR, Judd R, Coffield LM, Greer P, Rolston F, Evatt BL. Human papillomavirus infection and anal carcinoma. Retrospective analysis by in situ hybridization and the polymerase chain reaction. Am J Pathol 1992; 140:1345–1355.

109. Frisch M, Glimelius B, van den Brule AJ, et al. Sexually transmitted infection as a cause of anal cancer. N Engl J Med 1997; 337:1350–1358.

110. Frisch M, Fenger C, van den Brule AJ, et al. Variants of squamous cell carcinoma of the anal canal and perianal skin and their relation to human papillomaviruses. Cancer Res 1999; 59:753–757.

111. Critchlow CW, Holmes KK, Wood R, et al. Association of human immunodeficiency virus and anal human papillomavirus infection among homosexual men. Arch Intern Med 1992; 152:1673–1676.

112. Palefsky JM, Holly EA, Ralston ML, Jay N. Prevalence and risk factors for human papillomavirus infection of the anal canal in human immunodeficiency virus (HIV)-positive and HIV-negative homosexual men. J Infect Dis 1998; 177:361–367.

113. Melbye M, Smith E, Wohlfahrt J, et al. Anal and cervical abnormality in women—prediction by human papillomavirus tests. Int J Cancer 1996; 68:559–564.

114. Critchlow CW, Surawicz CM, Holmes KK, et al. Prospective study of high grade anal squamous intraepithelial neoplasia in a cohort of homosexual men: influence of HIV infection, immunosuppression and human papillomavirus infection. AIDS 1995; 9:1255–1262.

115. Palefsky JM, Holly EA, Ralston ML, et al. Anal squamous intraepithelial lesions in HIV-positive and HIV-negative homosexual and bisexual men: prevalence and risk factors. J Acquir Immune Defic Syndr 1998; 17:320–326.

116. Palefsky JM, Holly EA, Hogeboom CJ, et al. Virologic, immunologic, and clinical parameters in the incidence and progression of anal squamous intraepithelial lesions in HIV-positive and HIV-negative homosexual men. J Acquir Immune Defic Syndr 1998; 17:314–319.

117. Palefsky JM, Holly EA, Ralston ML, Jay N, Berry JM, Darragh TM. High incidence of anal high-grade squamous intra-epithelial lesions among HIV-positive and HIV-negative homosexual and bisexual men. AIDS 1998; 12:495–503.

118. Moscicki AB, Hills NK, Shiboski S, et al. Risk factors for abnormal anal cytology in young heterosexual women. Cancer Epidemiol Biomarker Prev 1999; 8:173–178.

119. Scholefield JH, Hickson WG, Smith JH, Rogers K, Sharp F. Anal intraepithelial neoplasia: part of a multifocal disease process. Lancet 1992; 340:1271–1273.

120. Ogunbiyi OA, Scholefield JH, Raftery AT, et al. Prevalence of anal human papillomavirus infection and intraepithelial neoplasia in renal allograft recipients. Br J Surg 1994; 81:365–367.

121. Ogunbiyi OA, Scholefield JH, Robertson G, Smith JH, Sharp F, Rogers K. Anal human papillomavirus infection and squamous neoplasia in patients with invasive vulvar cancer. Obstet Gynecol 1994; 83:212–216.
122. Jay N, Holly EA, Berry M, Hogeboom CJ, Darragh TM, Palefsky JM. Colposcopic correlates of anal squamous intraepithelial lesions. Dis Col Rectum 1997; 40:919–928.
123. Goldie SJ, Kuntz KM, Weinstein MW, Freedberg KA, Welton ML, Palefsky JM. The clinical-effectiveness and cost-effectiveness of screening for anal squamous intraepithelial lesions in homosexual and bisexual HIVpositive men. JAMA 1999; 281:1822–1829.

16
Human Papilloma Viruses and Cancers of the Skin and Oral Mucosa

Irene M. Leigh, Judy A. Breuer, John A. G. Buchanan,
Catherine A. Harwood, Sarah Jackson, Jane M. McGregor,
Charlotte M. Proby, and Alan Storey

INTRODUCTION

The major cellular component of skin and orogenital mucosa is the keratinocyte, which is characteristic of all stratified squamous epithelia. The keratinocyte is the target cell of the family of human papilloma viruses (HPVs), which may result in the development of benign "warts" (episomal infection) or the development of tumors (transformation of the tissue following viral integration). HPVs have an established role in anogenital carcinogenesis but their role in nonanogenital cancers of the skin (nonmelanoma skin cancer [NMSC]) or oral mucosa (oral squamous cell carcinomas [OSCC]) is less clear. Improving techniques for detection of HPV DNA have given rise to an increased understanding of the HPVs found in mucocutaneous sites and the viral–keratinocyte interactions. Thus we focus particularly on investigation of the expression and cellular functions of the subfamily of HPVs associated with epidermodysplasia verruciformis (EV HPVs).

KERATINOCYTE-DERIVED TUMORS: SKIN AND ORAL MUCOSA

Nonmelanoma skin cancers (NMSCs) are the most prevalent malignancies in fair-skinned populations worldwide (1). Epidemiologic and molecular data implicate ultraviolet (UV) radiation as an important etiologic factor, but other agents including the immune response, genetic predisposition, and viral infection may also be involved. A number of viruses have been proposed in the development of NMSC, but the most plausible evidence to date is that for HPV (2,3).

HPV is recognized increasingly as an important human carcinogen. In the established association with the so-called "high-risk" mucosal HPV types 16 and 18 with anogenital cancer, HPV is believed to act as a solitary carcinogen (3). HPV may also play a role in cutaneous malignancy, most prominently in the rare inherited condition epidermodysplasia verruciformis (EV) which is characterized by a predisposition to HPV infection and the development of cutaneous squamous cell carcinomas (SCCs) on sun-exposed sites (4). Tumor suppressor proteins p53 and pRb are important cellular

From: *Infectious Causes of Cancer: Targets for Intervention*
Edited by: J. J. Goedert © Humana Press Inc., Totowa, NJ

targets for the viral oncoproteins E6 and E7, respectively, in anogenital cancer, but the putative mechanisms of HPV in EV-associated skin malignancies are uncertain, with an almost invariable additional requirement for UV radiation *(4)*.

An association between HPV and skin cancer also has been proposed in renal transplant recipients *(5,6)*. Transplant patients have a 50–100-fold increased risk of NMSC, particularly squamous cell cancers, which occur predominantly on sun-exposed sites, often in close proximity to virus warts *(7,8)*. Histopathologic examination of squamous cell neoplasms in transplant recipients may show a spectrum of pathology, sometimes within single lesions, from benign wart, through increasing dysplasia, to frankly invasive squamous cell carcinoma *(9)*. HPV also is considered a possible cofactor in the development of sporadic skin cancers in the general population.

Oral squamous cell carcinoma (OSCC) accounts for in excess of 90% of all oral malignancies. In the United States some 30,000 new cases are diagnosed per year, with approx 8000 deaths *(10)*. The incidence may be increasing among black males in the United States in whom oral cancer is the fourth most common cancer *(11)*. Intraoral cancer has one of the lowest survival rates of any of the major cancer sites owing to late diagnosis *(12)*, with 5-yr survival rates of only 20–40% reported for nonlocalized oropharyngeal cancers *(13)*. A heterogeneous multifactorial, multistage etiology is envisaged. Suggested factors are included in Table 1 but in many cases the extent of their contribution to oral carcinogenesis is uncertain and varies among populations and from individual to individual. Together smoking and alcohol have been suggested to cause 75% of all OSCCs *(14)* and the two may act synergistically *(15,16)*. Strong evidence also links chewing tobacco in its various forms, particularly with lime and as betel quid or paan in the Asian subcontinent *(17–19)*, where OSCC accounts for in excess of 40% of all malignancies *(20–23)*. Only a relatively small proportion of people who use tobacco, alcohol, or betel quid develop OSCC *(24)*. There is an emerging population of patients with oral cancer who have not had obvious exposure to these agents *(25)*, and additional factors are likely to be involved. The integral role that HPV plays in anogenital carcinoma has suggested a possible role in oral carcinogenesis *(26)*.

HPVs: General Introduction (27)

Papillomaviruses, together with the polyomaviruses, are members of the papovavirus family. The family is characterized by its small (55 nm diameter in the case of papillomaviruses) nonenveloped virion, icosahedral capsid, and circular double-stranded DNA genome (of approx 8000 nucleotide bases in papillomaviruses). The general organization of the genome is the same for different HPV types and consists of three main regions: the early (E) region encoding viral regulatory, transforming, and replication proteins; the late (L) region encoding the structural capsid proteins L1 and L2; and the noncoding or upstream regulatory region. The HPV-encoded early genes appear to have multiple functions including (E1) ATPase and helicase activity necessary for initiating viral replication, (E2) regulation of viral transcription and replication, and (E4) proteins involved in maturation and release of viral particles. E5 has some transforming potential but this is not fully characterized, whereas E6 and E7 are the major transforming proteins of genital HPVs. HPV infects basal epithelial cells stimulating epithelial proliferation. In benign viral warts it is present as episomal DNA

Table 1
Etiologic Factors in OSCC

Tobacco smoking, e.g., pipes, cigars, cigarettes, bidis, reverse smoking; smokeless tobacco, e.g., chewing tobacco, tobacco sachets

Betel quid chewing

Alcohol, eg., spirits, wine, and beer

Nutritional deficiencies, e.g., iron deficiency as Plummer–Vinson syndrome; diets deficient in fruit, vitamins A and C

Chronic oral conditions, e.g., lichen planus, lupus erythematosus, submucous fibrosis

Mechanical irritation from dental factors, e.g., rough restorations

Ultraviolet light

Immunosuppression, e.g., in patients with organ transplants or possibly HIV infection

Chronic infections, e.g. candidosis, syphilis, herpes simplex virus, and human papilloma virus

with low level replication of viral episome within basal keratinocytes maintained by E1 and E2 expression. The full vegetative life cycle of HPV is tightly linked to keratinocyte differentiation, and other viral early genes are not switched on until the infected keratinocyte leaves the basal layer. Late gene expression with production of virus particles can take place only in highly differentiated keratinocytes.

The Relationship of EV-HPVs to a Phylogenetic Analysis of HPV

Improvements in HPV detection techniques have resulted from the advent of recombinant DNA technology. Distinguished originally by its restriction enzyme map, a papillomavirus isolate is now classified exclusively by characterization of its genome. A new type is one in which the nucleotide sequence of the most highly conserved part of the HPV genome, the L1 open reading frame (ORF), is shown to share < 90% identity to the homologous sequences of established prototypes *(28)*. Based upon this definition, 80 distinct HPV genotypes have now been described, and several groups have identified and partially characterized novel sequences predicting the existence of many more *(3)* (*see also*, Chapter 14).

Papillomaviruses show a marked host and epithelial cell specificity for infection and historically they have been grouped according to the location and clinical context from which they were initially isolated, hence the terminology cutaneous, mucosal, and EV types. Subsequent phylogenetic analyses based on sequence information have broadly justified this clinical classification *(29)*. Based on phylogenetic analysis of the L1 gene, four groups of EV-related HPV have been described: A to D. Viruses from all four groups appear to induce the characteristic EV macular lesions in sun-exposed skin and have been detected in NMSC occurring in EV patients or renal transplant recipients. The genomic diversity of the many different HPVs poses a considerable challenge to HPV detection and genotyping. Methods based upon DNA hybridization to specific HPV probes (Southern blot, slot blot, *in situ* hybridization) have now largely been superseded by polymerase chain reaction (PCR)-based techniques using degenerate and nested primers to increase sensitivity and specificity. This has revealed a diverse range of HPVs in skin and mucosal tissue including many HPV sequences that probably represent new, as yet uncharacterized EV-associated types *(27,30–33)*.

The complete genome sequence has been determined for more than 11 of the EV-related viruses *(34–38)*. Two features of the genome organization appear to be specific for this group. First the noncoding region (NCR) of the genome is much shorter than in all other HPVs (460 bp vs 1037 in HPV-1). Second, there is no equivalent of an ORF E5 in the 3′ part of the early region. The genome sizes of the EV-associated HPV fall into two classes, those of 7.7 kb (HPV-5,-8,-12,-14,-19,-20,-21,-24,-25,-47, and -50) and 7.4 kb (HPV-9,-15,-17,-22, and -23) *(38,39)*. The second class appears to have shorter NCRs *(40)* and E2 ORFs (100 and 200 bp, respectively). The small size of the EV-associated NCRs may explain why some of the replication control elements identified in prototypic viruses are located in the ORF L1 upstream or in the ORF E6 downstream. This contrasts with the situation in non-EV-associated HPVs.

EV-Related HPVs—Transcriptional Regulation

The EV-associated viruses appear to be transcriptionally active in both benign and malignant lesions from patients with EV. There appear to be at least two promoters in EV-associated HPVs, which generate both early and late region transcripts *(41)*. The late transcripts, L1 and L2, are detected only in terminally differentiated epithelial layers *(42)*. However, signals for the 5′ early region exon and the E4 exon are detectable throughout the epithelium. These differences underline the cell-differentiation-dependent nature of EV-associated HPV replication *(43)*.

Several of the mechanisms controlling the replication of EV-associated HPV are unique to this group. As in all HPVs, the main *cis*-acting responsive elements are located within the NCR of the genome. In addition to those regulatory elements common to all HPVs, EV types have been noted to encode certain unique elements within the NCR *(35,40,44)*. These are:

- four E2-binding palindromes P1–P4
- a cluster of sites between P2 and P3 that bind the NF1 protein
- a partially conserved motif of 33 nucleotides (M33 motif) followed by an AP1 binding site between P1 and P2.

Group A viruses (types 5, 8, 12, 36, 47, 14, 19, 20, 21, and 25) also share a conserved run of 29 nucleotides in their E6 proximal parts (M29), as well as a unique 50-base AT-rich region nearby and an E2 binding site in L1. These motifs are lacking in group B EV viruses, although two of them, HPV 9 and 17, contain an E2 palindrome in the E6 proximal part of the NCR, termed P5.

The regulation of transcription in the EV types has been most closely studied using HPV-8 as a prototype. HPV-8 has been described as having two promoters within the NCR, P175, which probably acts on E6 transcription, and P7535, which mediates expression of the L1 protein and E2 *(45)*. P7535 closely resembles other late gene promoters characterized in skin-specific HPVs. P7535 can also bind E2, suggesting a regulatory feedback circuit controlling its activity. Activation of the P2 E2-binding site appears to strongly repress the action of P7535, whereas the four distal E2 target sequences appear to transactivate the promoter.

EV NCRs also can act as transcriptional enhancers in C127 mouse fibroblasts *(46,47)*. In group A viruses this is dependent on E2 transactivation, whereas group B

EV viruses 9 and 17 appear to show constitutive activity in the same system. In this setting the major enhancing region within the HPV-8 NCR has been shown to be the M33 motif combined with the AP1 binding site *(48)*. Together with the AP1 complex and two other epithelial cell nuclear proteins these enhancer elements transcriptionally enhance the P7535 promoter. A 38-bp negative regulatory element located at the boundary of L1 ORF and the NCR and containing the E2 binding element P1 acts to downregulate P7535 *(49)*. It is possible therefore that the negative regulatory element can act as transcriptional enhancer or repressor depending on the level of E2. This may have important implications for the control of replication of EV-associated viruses.

Finally, the HPV-8 NCR, together with the proximal part of E6, encodes four sites that bind the negative cellular regulatory factor yin-yang 1 (YY1). These appear to mediate strong repression of both promoters P175 and P7535 *(50)*.

The State of Virus in EV-Associated Malignancies

In contrast to HPV-positive cervical cancers, integration of viral DNA into the cellular genome has been reported only with HPV-5 and -14 in two tumors occurring in EV patients *(51,52)*. Generally in EV patients, 100–300 copies per cell of episomal viral genome may be detected as well as variable numbers of oligomeric forms, or genomes with deletions *(51)* or duplications.

Does Human Papillomavirus Infection Play a Role in the Development of NMSC?

The study of HPV-associated skin carcinogenesis has been fraught with technical difficulties and, as a consequence, much of the literature in this area is inconsistent and confusing. The development of recombinant technology in the 1970s facilitated the detection, characterization, and examination of HPV in the skin, but until very recently even this was hampered by the diversity of HPV types now known to exist in keratinizing epithelia.

In early studies, detection of HPV DNA varied both in overall prevalence, from zero to 64%, and in the HPV types detected (reviewed in *[2]*). These discrepancies largely reflect the detection methods used; DNA-hybridization-based techniques were generally employed using a limited number of HPV probes that were not informative for the majority of HPV types. As a consequence, the true prevalence of HPV in cutaneous lesions was considerably underestimated. With PCR, which increased sensitivity, early studies used type-specific primers capable of detecting only a limited range of HPV *(53–55)*. This was frequently compounded by the use of paraffin-embedded material that yields suboptimal results compared with fresh frozen tissue *(56–58)*. Recently attempts have been made in several laboratories, including our own, to optimize conditions for HPV detection in the skin by employing frozen tissue and developing degenerate and nested PCR primers *(27,31–33,59)*. Using a combination of these primers, a comprehensive analysis of all known HPV types is now possible, including detection of mucosal, cutaneous, and EV types with high sensitivity and specificity *(60)*.

Detection of HPV DNA in NMSC in Organ Transplant Recipients

Risk factors for skin cancer in organ transplant recipients include fair skin (phototypes I–III), high cumulative sun exposure, older age, and longer duration of immunosuppression *(61)*. The role of HPV is unknown, but the high prevalence of HPV DNA detection in skin cancers from immunosuppressed individuals suggests it may be important. Early reports conflict, but recent studies from several independent laboratories have consistently found HPV DNA in approx 60–80% of premalignant keratotic lesions and of basal and squamous cell carcinomas from renal transplant patients *(32,33,60)*. There is some variation in HPV types reported by different groups, depending on the sensitivity and specificity of the primer combinations employed, but the overall consensus is that transplant-associated skin cancers contain a diverse range of HPV types, with no single HPV type predominating. In particular, HPV types 5 and 8, which are reported to be present in EV-associated skin cancers *(4)*, and HPV types 16 and 18, found in cervical and anogenital malignancies *(3)*, are not overrepresented here. In approx 80% of all lesions across several recent studies, EV-associated HPV types have been identified. In one study *(33)* just five HPV types (20, 23, 38, DL40, and DL267) were present in 73% of the cancers examined, but this is not the general experience. For example, in 82% of 40 transplant-associated SCCs we examined, a more diverse range of HPV types was found, including 24 different EV and EV-related HPV types (HPV-5, -14, -19, -20, -22, -23, -24, -25, -36, -37, -38, -49, -75, -RTRX1, -RTRX2, -RTRX5, RTRX32, -vs20-4, -vs42-1, -vs73-1,-vs92-1, Z95963). Seven cutaneous HPV types (10, 27, 2, 1, 3, 77, 28) and three mucosal types (HPV-11, -16, and -66) were also identified in several tumor specimens. Mixed infection with up to four different HPV types was found in approx 60% of lesions. We detected a similarly diverse range of HPVs in 75% of 24 basal cell carcinomas (BCCs) and in 88% of 17 carcinoma *in situ* (CIS). Whatever the minor discrepancies between groups, the majority of transplant-associated skin lesions in all recent studies has consistently shown a high prevalence of HPV DNA, usually mixed infection with EV, and cutaneous or, less commonly, EV and mucosal HPV types.

Detection of HPV DNA in NMSC in the General Population

Technical difficulties confused the literature on HPV and skin cancer in immunocompetent individuals for many years, just as in the transplant group. However, the use of a degenerate and nested PCR approach in the analysis of sporadic skin cancers has now, as for the transplant group, produced consistent results from several independent laboratories *(31,60)*. Detection rates are lower in all equivalent skin lesions in immunocompetent compared with immunosuppressed patients, with HPV DNA being found in approx 20–40% of actinic keratoses and basal and squamous cell carcinomas in the general population. Once again, no HPV type has been found to predominate, and HPV-5 and -8 are rarely detected. Instead all skin lesions contain diverse HPVs including EV-associated, cutaneous or, more rarely, "low-risk" mucosal types. Unlike transplant-associated skin lesions, however, skin cancers and premalignant lesions from immunocompetent individuals rarely show mixed infection. We found several differences in the prevalence of HPV DNA in skin cancers from immunocompetent patients compared with renal transplant recipients. The overall prevalence of HPV DNA was significantly lower for all lesions (SCC, BCC, and CIS: $p < .05$) in immunocompetent patients. The spectrum of types detected also differed. The HPV-positive lesions from immunocompetent patients most often had EV HPV types (19 of 23 [83%]), but these lesions infrequently had cutaneous HPV types (3 of 23 [13%]) or multiple HPV types (3 of 23 [13%]) compared with 39 of 66 (59%) of HPV-positive lesions from renal transplant recipients ($p < 0.001$).

Detection of HPV DNA in Normal Skin from Both Immunosuppressed and Immunocompetent Patients

The high prevalence of HPV DNA in premalignant and malignant skin lesions should be interpreted in the context of the HPV status of normal skin in a matched control population without skin cancer. The present technology is sensitive enough to detect HPV DNA in normal skin, presumably present as subclinical or latent infection, but few studies have addressed this. Preliminary data indicate that HPV DNA is present in normal skin of both immunocompetent and immunocompromised patients. Astori et al. *(62)* found EV-associated HPV types in 50% of six normal perilesional skin samples, adjacent to actinic keratoses, basal cell carcinomas, and benign nevi. Seven (35%) of 20 normal skin samples obtained during cosmetic surgery also were positive for HPV DNA in this study. We reported HPV DNA in 4 (33%) of 12 normal skin samples from patients who had undergone PUVA therapy for psoriasis *(63)* and have more recently found HPV DNA in approx 50% of 36 normal skin biopsies from 18 immunocompetent patients and 88% of 67 normal skin samples from 38 renal transplant recipients *(60)*. An earlier report from a separate group *(64)* found that plucked hair samples from 45% of 22 healthy volunteers and from 100% of 26 transplant patients were positive for EV-associated HPV DNA, indicating a very large potential reservoir of latent HPV in the population.

Is There a Role for HPVs in the Etiology of OSCC?

Our understanding of the natural history and biology of oral HPV infection is incomplete *(65,66)*. Acquisition may occur during birth from the mother's genital tract *(67)*, by autoinoculation from a genital or cutaneous site, or during orogenital contact between sexual partners *(68)*. The HPV genotypes commonly identified in oral mucosal lesions include types 2, 3, 6, 7, 11, 13, 16, 18, 31, 32, 33, 35, 55, 57, and 59. Types 1, 3, 10, 52, 69, 72, and 73 are more rarely isolated. A number of these types are associated with benign oral lesions such as squamous papilloma (mainly 6, 11, and 16), verruca vulgaris (2, 4, 6, 11, and 57), and focal epithelial hyperplasia (13 and 32). HPV may persist in the oral cavity in a latent form, perhaps acting as a reservoir for infection or activation subsequent to trauma or immunosuppression, and types 6, 7, 11, 16, 18, 31, and 33 have been detected on apparently healthy oral mucosa *(26, 65, 66)*. HPV types 16, 18, 31, and 33 have been classified as high risk in anogenital cancer *(69)*. Using PCR, a mean HPV infection prevalence of 25.4% of normal mucosa has been deduced *(26)*.

A role for high-risk HPV-16 and -18 in the development of OSCC is suggested by a number of studies demonstrating that these HPVs can immortalize oral keratinocytes in vitro *(70,71)* and molecular epidemiologic studies demonstrating an association of HPV with oral premalignant lesions and OSCC.

Detection of HPV DNA in OSCC

The reported HPV prevalence rates of OSCCs has varied from zero to 100% *(72)*, but studies need to be interpreted with caution. Many of these studies involved small, locally gathered samples, lacked unaffected controls, and were interpreted in the absence of information on contributory risk factors such as smoking and alcohol intake *(73)*. A large number of technical and biologic factors may also have contributed to the disparate findings including *(68,74)*:

1. The use of detection assays of differing sensitivity from the relatively low sensitivity *in situ* hybridization to the high-sensitivity PCR technique
2. The restriction of HPV to a limited subpopulation of cells at a low copy number in OSCC
3. Variable sampling techniques that may have excluded epithelial layers more likely to harbor HPV
4. Different methods of specimen storage studies (fresh or frozen has higher HPV DNA detection rates than does paraffin-embedded tissue)
5. The use of early gene primers in PCR which are two to three times more efficient than late gene primers at detecting HPV DNA in SCC *(26)*.

Interpretation of studies is thus difficult. However, HPV has been detected in up to 33% of premalignant lesions *(75)* and 42% of dysplastic lesions by various PCR techniques *(26)*. The mean rate of HPV detection in oral SCC by PCR has been reported as 36.6%, but when all methods are considered a mean prevalence of 26.2% has been reported *(26)*. High-risk HPV types 16 and 18 are found frequently in the HPV-positive specimens *(26)*. Recent reviews found that among specimens HPV positive by PCR, 40% contained HPV-16, 11.9% contained HPV-18, and 7.0% contained both HPV-16 and -18. It was found that 3.8% of OSCCs contained HPV-6, 7.4% contained HPV-11, and 10.9% contained HPV-6 and -11 *(74)*. There is some evidence for HPV-16 and -18 being associated with lesion aggressiveness: they are more likely to be detected in OSCC (up to 80%) as opposed to the less aggressive verrucous carcinomas (35.3%) *(26)*. In two studies, HPV infection with two high-risk types was associated with OSCC occurring 12.7 *(76)* and 9.6 yrs *(77)* earlier than carcinomas associated with one or no high-risk HPV types.

OSCC, in contrast to cervical carcinoma, seldom has HPV integrated into the host genome. Likewise, other high-risk HPV types 31, 33, and 39 *(68,69)* are rarely detected in OSCC, and the frequency of detection of HPV in OSCC is considerably less than that reported in cervical carcinoma (85–90%) *(3)*. These differences do not exclude a role for HPV in OSCC but may reflect the multifactorial etiology of oral SCC or a role in only a limited number of OSCCs. HPV types as yet undiscovered may be involved. The scattered distribution of HPV in OSCC evident in *in situ* PCR studies *(78)*, a higher frequency of HPV in younger OSCC patients *(79)*, and the loss of HPV-16 DNA sequences in OSCC cell lines during prolonged passage *(80)* have led to a hit-and-run hypothesis to explain the role of HPV in oral carcinogenesis *(68)*, with HPV's involvement being transitory, perhaps only during initiation. Interaction with other risk factors is suggested by the finding that oral keratinocytes immortalized by high-risk HPVs required exposure to tobacco-associated carcinogens prior to full malignant transformation *(81)*, by a case-control study suggesting HPV-16 involvement in a small number of OSCCs in combination with cigarette smoking *(82)*, and by reports of HPV-associated epithelial atypia in oral warts in HIV-positive patients *(83)*, although OSCC development in them has not been described so far.

FUNCTIONAL INTERACTIONS BETWEEN HPVs AND KERATINOCYTES

As previously described, HPVs are small DNA tumor viruses that display strict epitheliotropism by infecting stratified squamous epithelia at different body sites, as reviewed previously *(28,84)*. For stable viral maintenance to be achieved that would allow a productive viral infection to occur, the virus is presumed to infect cells of the basal layer. A candidate receptor for all HPV types, α-6 integrin, has been identified recently and is expressed on basal keratinocytes*(85)*. However, given the association between specific viral types at particular body sites, it would appear that other factors peculiar to the host cell at that site, in addition to its epithelial origin, must also be important.

Viral Gene Regulation

A clue to the viral tropism is suggested by analysis of the various viral DNA sequences, in particular the upstream regulatory region. This region of the viral genome, which can be up to about 1 kb in length, does not code for any structural proteins, but instead contains binding sites for cellular transcription factors that are important in directing expression of the viral genes in both basal and suprabasal differentiated cell layers. Indeed virus replication is intimately linked to and dependent upon keratinocyte differentiation. Portions of the upstream regulatory region critical for epithelial specific gene expression are termed the core enhancer, usually containing binding sites for transcription factors such as AP1 and TEF-1 *(86–92)*. It is most notable that divergent groups of HPVs have solved their individual requirements for host cell factors in different ways. Both the number and location of host transcription factor binding sites differ markedly among individual cutaneous or mucosal viruses, and individual viral types also may possess binding sites unique to that virus *(93–95)*. In those types that are commonly found in epidermodysplasia verruciformis (EV HPV types) such as HPV-5, the upstream regulatory region contains two specific DNA motifs, termed M29 and M33, that are found only in these HPV types. In contrast, in anogential viruses such as HPV-16, this region contains elements that enable the virus to respond to glucocorticoids and progesterones *(96,97)*. These are specific adaptations that may enable divergent viral types to survive in different epithelia.

Virally Encoded Oncogenes

Much of the recent work regarding the functions of virally encoded proteins has centered around anogenital HPV types most closely associated with the development of cervical carcinoma. In particular, much attention has focused on the E6 and E7 proteins of HPV-16 and -18 and the mechanisms by which they bring about cell transformation *(98–104)*. In contrast, comparatively little is known about the functions of the equivalent proteins of cutaneous HPVs. Dissection of the HPV-16 viral genome revealed that both E6 and E7 were powerful oncogenes able to transform cells in culture. Subsequent functional studies showed that the E6 and E7 proteins inactivate two important tumor suppressor proteins, p53 and the retinoblastoma gene product (pRb), respectively *(105–107)*. Studies on cutaneous HPV types have recapitulated these studies with differing results and have largely centered around HPV-5 and -8, which are associated with tumors in EV patients. Mutational studies revealed that the association of HPV-16 E7 with pRb hinged on the integrity of the LXCXE motif, and this motif also was required for the transforming activity of the protein *(108)*. Although the majority of E7 proteins of cutaneous viruses contain this motif, many associate with pRb weakly if at all and have a low transforming potential. This association with pRb is not, however, indicative of a transforming potential of the protein, as the HPV-1 E7 protein tightly associates with pRb but fails to transform cells in culture *(109)*. The HPV-10 E7 protein lacks this pRb binding motif entirely, suggesting that the virus uses other mechanisms to overcome this growth suppressive pathway. Furthermore, in contrast to the HPV-16 E7 protein, the E7 proteins of HPV types 8 and 47 fail to transform rodent cells *(110,111)*. Yet, in cooperation with activated Ha-*ras* the HPV-5 and -8 E7 genes are able to give rise to transformed colonies, and the HPV-1 E7 gene can fully transform mouse C127 cells *(112)*. The HPV-16 E7 protein has been shown to associate also with the p21 protein *(113,114)*, a cyclin-dependent kinase inhibitor, whose expression is induced by p53 in response to DNA damage and in a p53-independent manner in keratinocyte differentiation. Cells expressing the HPV-16 E7 protein show altered differentiation and an inhibition of PCNA and cyclin A/E-associated kinase activity *(113,114)*. There also is evidence that HPV-16 E6 and E7 proteins abrogate a mitotic spindle checkpoint through a p53-independent mechanism *(115)*. Whether cutaneous E6 and E7 proteins share this ability is worthy of future investigation. Close to the pRb binding domain in the HPV-16 E7 protein is a motif that is phosphorylated by casein kinase II (CKII). Phosphorylation of E7 at this site increases the affinity of the protein for TBP, a protein component of the basal gene transcription machinery *(116)*. Although most cutaneous virus E7 proteins lack this phosphorylation site, it appears to be conserved in HPV-77, a novel type isolated from warts and SCCs of immunocompromised individuals, suggesting a conservation of E7 function in this virus *(117)*. It appears then that the degree of morphologic transformation induced by cutaneous E7 proteins correlates poorly with the risk of malignant conversion in vivo. In difference to the combined immortalizing capacity of the HPV-16 E6/E7 genes in human keratinocytes, such immortalization studies using cutaneous HPVs have been unsuccessful to date.

In contrast to the E6 gene of anogenital viruses, the E6 gene of EV HPV types 5 and 8 appears to encode the major transforming activity. In rodent cell lines, EV E6 proteins are able to induce both morphologic transformation and anchorage-independent growth which, unlike the E7 gene, is reflective of their association with carcinomas. The association of the HPV-16 E6 protein with p53 leads to the rapid degradation of the protein. This is mediated by the binding of E6 to a cellular protein, E6-AP, leading to the ubiquitination of p53 followed by its rapid degradation by the ubiquitin-dependent proteolysis system*(118)*. Although this function of E6 is believed to be important in cellular transformation, E6 also has other p53-independent transforming activities *(119,120)*. This is highlighted by the cutaneous E6 proteins that function in transformation assays without associating with p53 or promoting its degradation *(121)*. These combined observations point toward as yet unidentified cellular targets of the cutaneous E6 and E7 proteins. Preliminary evidence also points toward a transforming activity encoded by the HPV-8 E2 protein *(110)*.

UV- and HPV-Associated Malignancy

In both EV and immunocompromised patients, HPV-containing tumors arise predominantly at body sites exposed to sunlight, indicating a fundamental role for UV as a cofactor in HPV-induced carcinogenesis, as well as its recognized role in skin cancer development in general *(122)*. UV leads to a strong induction of p53 in the skin *(123)*, playing an important role in protecting the integrity of the genome, either by inducing growth arrest allowing the repair of UV-induced DNA damage or by promoting apoptosis *(124)*. As noted previously, cutaneous E6 proteins fail to abrogate p53 function by degradation, yet their presence in lesions at UV-exposed sites implies that p53 responses to DNA damage have been overcome by other mechanisms. An anti-apoptotic activity of the E6 protein of anogenital HPV types has been noted *(125),* and such an activity encoded by cutaneous E6 may aid the survival of virally infected cells exposed to UV which in turn may facilitate the accumulation of UV-induced genetic changes.

Models of HPV Infection and Disease

The HPV viral life cycle in its natural host cell is intimately linked to and dependent upon the normal differentiation process. In basal layers, virus is maintained at low copy number in basal layers, which rises as vegetative viral DNA replication taking place in upper spinous layers. Concomitant with increased DNA replication, differential promoter usage coupled to the expression of viral genes has been detected in differentiating epidermis. The dependency of the virus upon host cell differentiation, coupled with the previous lack of an in vitro model of epidermal regeneration, has in the past proved a major obstacle in designing model systems to investigate HPV gene function under more physiologically relevant conditions. However, advances in keratinocyte biology coupled with the emergence of animal systems have gone a long way to fulfilling the necessary criteria. Much of the developmental work in the designing and testing of HPV model systems has been done using anogenital HPVs. The paucity of experimental data using cutaneous HPVs may stem from the lack of a keratinocyte immortalization assay.

Transformation of human skin was first demonstrated for HPV-11, a condyloma acuminata associated HPV type. HPV-11 viral particles were used to infect human skin that then was grafted beneath the renal capsule of athymic mice *(126,127)*. This resulted in production of viral particles and the development of condyloma similar to those seen in patients *(128)*. Such xenograft models were subsequently improved by the use of severe combined immunodeficiency (SCID) mice, producing larger xenografts that showed an increased rate of HPV-11 positivity *(129)*. This work was extended to include engraftment of HPV-16-infected foreskin keratinocytes onto the skin of SCID mice. The grafted skin expressed involucrin in differentiating keratinocytes and displayed features of HPV infection including koilocytosis and production of capsid antigen *(130)*. Direct grafting of HPV-6 or -11-containing lesions onto the skin of SCID mice also resulted in the formation of a macroscopic papillomata*(131)*. The first experimental system permitting the completion of the HPV-16 life cycle was achieved by grafting an immortal HPV-16 cell line isolated from a low-grade lesion onto a vascularized granulation bed on the flanks of nude mice *(132)*. Similar experiments using skin fragments from benign early premalignant EV lesions implanted under the kidney capsule of athymic mice led to the production of epidermal cysts displaying numerous mitoses and EV HPV DNA *(133,134)*.

Organotypic Cell Culture Systems and Drug Effects In Vitro

Although the mouse model xenograft systems have proved useful in studying HPV infected lesions, they are technically difficult and time consuming. Changes in HPV gene expression and induction of DNA replication can be induced by suspending keratinocytes harbouring episomal HPV DNA in semisolid medium *(135)*. Programmed differentiation of keratinocytes in vitro can be achieved by the use of organotypic cell cultures (rafts) *(136,137)*. In this system keratinocytes are seeded onto a dermal substitute and then raised to the air–liquid interface, allowing stratification and differentiation to occur. A variety of dermal substrates have been used, including collagen and deepidermalized human dermis. Grafting of HPV-16 immortalized keratinocytes in raft cultures leads to the reformation of epithelium; however, the epithelium exhibits parabasal crowding, enlarged nuclei in the upper layers, and features of a premalignant HPV-induced lesion *(138)*. These features included abnormal differentiation, mitotic figures, and abnormal mitoses in upper cell layers *(139,140)*. Biosynthesis of HPV-31 viral particles was first demonstrated by seeding onto collagen gels a cell line derived from a low-grade cervical intraepithelial neoplasia (CIN), that maintains episomal viral DNA *(141,142)*. Such organotypic systems are most useful in studying the effects of viral genes on epithelial proliferation and differentiation, and the relative contribution of transcription factor binding sites in the upstream regulatory region to altered HPV gene expression in stratified epithelia *(143)*. They also can be used to evaluate the effects of agents that may be important in modulating HPV gene function, such as tumor necrosis factor-α (TNF-α), interferon-γ (IFN-γ) *(144)*, UV, hormones, and retinoids. Although the lack of suitable cell lines harboring cutaneous HPVs has prevented similar studies from being undertaken to date, high-efficiency gene transfer into keratinocytes can be achieved using retroviruses. Recent advances in retroviral design now allow a high transduction efficiency coupled with a sustained expression of transgenes in regenerated epithelium *(145–147)*. The ability to use primary rather than immortalized cells for such assays has distinct advantages that will prove useful in studying HPV types with little or no inherent immortalizing potential.

Transgenic Animal Models

The use of transgenic mice is proving to be a powerful tool in studying tumor progression and dissecting the molecular events important in the multistage process of skin carcinogenesis. Although mouse skin has long been used to study tumor development and those changes important for the development of malignancy, the use of transgenic animals offers the ability to examine in greater detail the consequences of expression of specific viral genes (for reviews *see 148–150*). Transgenic animals expressing one or more wild type or mutated HPV genes allows the contribution of that gene to be evaluated for its contribution towards papilloma or tumour development. For example, crossing of HPV transgenics with mice knockouts for p21 or p53 would allow the contribution of the E6 and E7 genes to perturbation of differentiation and normal cell cycle control to be tested and compared to organotypic cultures *(113,151,152)*. HPV gene expression has been successfully targeted to the developing lens using the α-A crystallin promoter and to the epidermis using human keratin gene promoters such as K1 and K14 and bovine K10. K14-HPV-16 transgenic mice have been generated by a number of different groups *(148,150,153,154)*. The mice show progressive squamous epithelial neoplasias that can arise at many different anatomical sites including ears, skin, anus, cervix, and vagina, perhaps modulated by autocrine factors such as TGF-α or hormones such as progesterone acting through regulatory elements in the upstream regulatory region *(155–157)*. Mice transgenic for either E6 or E7 revealed the anti-apoptotic activity of the E6 protein in vivo and the proliferation-induced stimulation of apoptosis by E7 *(158,159)*. Mutations in the E7 gene revealed the importance of specific regions, including the pRb binding domain, in the induction of epidermal hyperplasia *(151)*. Karyotyping of primary tumors induced by bovine papillomavirus type 1 shows consistent changes on chromosomes 8 and 14 *(160)*. This suggests that papillomavirus transgenics may be useful to study the roles of cytogenetic changes in tumorigenesis and may also provide a model that will be helpful in evaluating potential anti-HPV agents *(161)*. This approach also will be useful in presenting viral antigens to the immune system in a way that can be modeled to the natural infection. Such immunologic studies on HPV-16 E6/E7 transgenic mice allow immunologic responses including antibody production, induction of cytotoxic T lymphocytes against viral proteins, and tolerance to be evaluated on different MCH genetic backgrounds.

THE ROLE OF HPV IN NMSC AND ORAL CANCER: CONCLUSIONS

The role of HPV in the development of skin cancer is still not clear. The viral epidemiology suggests that there is a large reservoir of latent HPV infection in the normal skin of the general population and in immunocompromised individuals. Preliminary evidence suggests that increased exposure, as in the transplant population, is associated with an increased risk of skin cancer but this needs to be confirmed in prospective studies. Malignant skin lesions in both immunocompetent and immunosuppressed patients frequently contain HPV DNA, and it is tempting to ascribe them a functional role. However, no particular HPV type predominates, and it remains a possibility that HPV is merely a "passenger," present but not active in the development of skin cancer. The technology is now in place to address this, to determine the molecular epidemiology of HPV infection in keratinizing epithelia, and to examine its role in skin carcinogenesis.

Similarly, because the association of HPV in oral squamous cell carcinoma is anecdotal at present, well designed, adequately controlled molecular epidemiologic studies are required to determine what if any role HPVs play. The epidemiologic association of HPV with OSCC and in vitro evidence of oral keratinocyte immortalization combined with growing knowledge of HPV oncogenes suggests a possible role for them in the etiology of OSCC. This putative role is not as clearcut as HPV's role appears to be in cervical carcinogenesis.

Functional studies of interactions between HPV oncogenes and keratinocytes do show that the EV HPVs' transforming activity does not lie in the association of EV-HPV E6 with p53. Elucidation of the cellular targets of EV-HPVs will further add to understanding the role of these viruses in keratinocyte-derived cancers, as well as potential strategies for their eradication or prevention.

REFERENCES

1. Ko CB, Walton S, Keczkes K, et al. The emerging epidemic of skin cancer. Br J Dermatol 1994; 130:269–272.
2. Proby C, Storey A, McGregor J, Leigh I. Does human papillomavirus infection play a role in non-melanoma skin cancer? Papillomavirus Rep 1996; 7:53–60.
3. zur Hausen H. Papillomavirus infections—a major cause of human cancers. Biochim Biophys Acta 1996; 1288:F55–78.

4. Majewski S, Jablonska S. Epidermodysplasia verruciformis as a model of human papillomavirus-induced genetic cancer of the skin. Arch Dermatol 1995; 131:1312–1318.

5. Walder BK, Robertson MR, Jeremy D. Skin cancer and immunosuppression Lancet 1971; ii:1282–1283.

6. Boyle J, McKie R, Briggs J, et al. Cancer, warts and sunshine in renal transplant recipients: a case control study. Lancet 1984; 1:702–705.

7. Glover MT, Proby CM, Leigh IM. Skin cancer in renal transplant patients. Cancer Bull 1993; 45:220–224.

8. McGregor JM, Proby CM. Skin cancer in transplant patients. Lancet 1996; 346:964–965.

9. Blessing K, McClaren KM, Benton EC, et al. Histopathology of skin lesions in renal allograft recipients: an assessment of viral features and dysplasia. Histopathology 1989; 14:129–139.

10. Boring CC, Squires TS, Tong T, Montgomery S. Cancer Statistics 1994. CA Cancer J Clin 1994; 44:7–26.

11. Harras A, Edwards BK, Blot WJ, Ries LA. Cancer rates and risks. Bethseda, MD: NIH, 1996, pp. 96–691.

12. Swango PA. Cancers of the oral cavity and pharynx in the United States: an epidemiologic overview. Pub Health Dent 1996; 56:309–318.

13. Horowitz AM, Goodman HS, Yellowitz JA, Nourjah PA. The need for health promotion in oral cancer prevention and early detection. J Pub Health Dent 1996; 56:319–330.

14. Blot WJ, McLaughlin JK, Winn DM, et al. Smoking and drinking in relation to oral and pharyngeal cancer. Cancer Res 1988; 48:3282–3287.

15. International Agency for Research on Cancer. Tobacco smoking. Lyons: IARC, 1986 (Monograph 38).

16. International Agency for Research on Cancer. Alcoholic beverages. Lyons: IARC, 1986 (Monograph 42).

17. International Agency for Research on Cancer. Tobacco Habits Other than Smoking: Betel-quid and Areca Nut; and Some Related Nitrosamines. Lyons: IARC, 1985 (Monograph 37).

18. Daftary DK, Murti PR, Bhonsole RB, et al. Risk factors and risk markers for oral cancer in high incidence areas of the world. In: Johnson NW (ed). Oral Cancer, Vol.2. Cambridge: Cambridge University Press 1991, pp. 29–63.

19. Binnie WH. Risk factors and risk markers for oral cncer in low incidence areas of the world. In: Johnson NW (ed). Oral Cancer, Vol.2. Cambridge: Cambridge University Press, 1991, pp.64–87.

20. Pindborg JJ. Control of oral cancer in developing countries. Bull WHO 1984; 62:817–824.

21. Parkin DM, Pisani P, Ferlay J. Estimates of the worldwide incidence of eighteen major cancers in 1985. Int J Cancer 1993; 54:594–606.

22. Boyle P, Macfarlane GJ, Maisonneuve P, et al. Epidemiology of mouth cancer in 1989: a review. JRSM 1990; 83:724–730.

23. Johnson NW. A global view of the epidemiology of oral cancer. In: Johnson NW (ed). Oral Cancer, Vol. 2. Cambridge: Cambridge University Press, 1991, pp. 3–26.

24. Sankaranarayanan R, Mohideen MN, Nair MK, et al. Aetiology of oral cancer in patients less than or equal to 30 years of age. Br J Cancer 1987; 59:439–440.

25. Wey PD, Lotz MJ, Triedman LJ. Oral cancer in women nonusers of tobacco and alcohol. Cancer 1987; 60:1644–1650.

26. Miller CS, White DK. Human papillomavirus expression in oral mucosa, premalignant conditions and squamous cell carcinoma. Oral Surg Oral Med Oral Pathol Oral Radiol Endod 1996; 82:57–68.

27. Berkhout RJM, Tieben LM, Smits HL, et al. Nested PCR approach to detection and typing of epidermodysplasia verruciformis-associated human papillomavirus types in cutaneous cancers from renal transplant recipients. J Clin Microbiol 1995; 33:690–695.

28. de Villiers EM. Human pathogenic papillomavirus types: an update. [Review] [83 refs]. Curr Top Microbiol Immunol 1994; 186:1–12.

29. Chan SY, Delius H, Halpern AL, Bernard HU. Analysis of genomic sequences of 95 papillomavirus types: uniting typing, phylogeny and taxonomy. J Virol 1995; 69:3074–3083.

30. Shamanin V, Glover M, Rausch C, et al. Specific types of human papillomavirus found in benign proliferations and carcinomas of the skin in immunosuppressed patients. Cancer Res 1994; 54:4610–4613.

31. Shamanin V, zur Hausen H, Lavergne D, et al. Human papillomavirus infections in nonmelanoma skin cancers from renal transplant recipients and non-immunosuppressed patients. J Natl Cancer Inst 1996; 88:802–811.

32. de Jong-Tieben LM, Berkhout RJ, Smits HL, et al. High frequency of detection of epidermodysplasia verruciformis-associated human papillomavirus DNA in biopsies from malignant and premalignant skin lesions from renal transplant recipients. J Invest Dermatol 1995; 105:367–371.

33. de Villiers E-M, Lavergne D, McLaren K, Benton EC. Prevailing papillomavirus types in nonmelanoma carcinomas of the skin in renal allograft recipients. Int J Cancer 1997; 73:356–361.

34. Fuchs PG, Iftner T, Weninger J, Pfister H. Epidermodysplasia verruciformis-associated human papillomavirus 8: genetic sequence and comparative analysis. J Virol 1986; 58:626–634.

35. Zachow KR, Ostrow RS, Faras AJ. Nucleotide sequence and genome organization of human papillomavirus type 5. Virology 1987; 158:251–254.

36. Kiyono T, Adachi A, Ishibashi M. Genome organization and taxonomic position of human papillomavirus type 47 inferred from its DNA sequence. Virology 1990; 177:401–405.

37. Pfister H, Fuchs PG. Papillomaviruses: particles, genome organization and proteins. In: Syrjanen KJ, Gissman L, Koss LG (eds). Papillomaviruses and Human Disease. Berlin: Springer-Verlag, 1987, pp. 1–18.

38. Delius H, Hofmann B. Primer-directed sequencing of human papillomavirus types. In: zur Hausen H (ed). Human Pathogenic Papillomaviruses. Berlin: Springer-Verlag, 1994, pp. 13–31.

39. de Villiers E. Heterogeneity of the human papillomavirus group. J Virol 1989; 63:4898–4903.

40. Ensser A, Pfister H. Epidermodysplasia verruciformis associated human papillomaviruses present a subgenus-specific organization of the regulatory genome region. Nucleic Acids Res 1990; 18:3919–3922.

41. Fuchs P, Pfister H. Papillomaviruses in epidermodysplasia verruciformis. Papillomavirus Rev 1999; 253–261.

42. Haller K, Stubenrauch F, Pfister H. Papilloma viruses in epidermodyslasia verruciformis. Int J Dermatol 1990, 32:806–810.

43. Hummel M, Lim HB, Laimins LA. Human papillomavirus type 31b late gene expression is regulated through protein kinase C-mediated changes in RNA processing. J Virol 1995; 69:3381–3388.

44. Krubke J, Kraus J, Delius H, et al. Genetic relationship among human papillomaviruses associated with benign and malignant tumours of patients with epidermodysplasia verruciformis. J Gen Virol 1987; 68:3091–3103.

45. Stubenrauch F, Malejczyk J, Fuchs PG, Pfister H. Late promoter of human papillomavirus type 8 and its regulation. J Virol 1992; 66:3485–3493.

46. Seeberger R, Haugen T, Turek L, Pfister H. An enhancer of human papillomavirus type 8 is trans-activated by the bovine papillomavirus type 1 E2 function. In: Steinberg BM, Brandsma JL, Taichman LB (eds). Papillomaviruses: Cancer Cells 5. Cold Spring Harbor, NY: Cold Spring Harbor Laboratory Press, 1987, pp. 33–38.

47. Reh H, Pfister H. Human papillomavirus 8 contains *cis*-active positive and negative transcriptional control sequences. J Gen Virol 1990; 71:2457–2462.

48. Horn S, Pfister H, Fuchs PG. Constitutive transcriptional activator of epidermodysplasia verruciformis-associated human papillomavirus 8. Virology 1993; 196:674–681.

49. May M, Grassmann K, Pfister H, Fuchs PG. Transcriptional silencer of the human papillomavirus type 8 late promoter interacts alternatively with the viral trans activator E2 or with a cellular factor. J Virol 1994; 68:3612–3619.

50. Pajunk HS, May C, Pfister H, Fuchs PG. Regulatory interactions of transcriptional factor YY1 with control sequences of the E6 promoter of human papillomavirus type 8. J Gen Virol 1997; 78:3287–3295.

51. Chan SWY, Reade PC. The role of ascorbic acid in oral carcinogenesis. Oral Dis 1998; 4:120–129.

52. Yabe Y, Tanimura Y, Sakai A, et al. Molecular characteristics and physical state of human papillomavirus DNA change with progressing malignancy: studies in a patient with epidermodysplasia veruciformis. Int J Cancer 1989; 43:1022–1028.

53. Soler C, Chardonnet Y, Allibert P, et al. Detection of mucosal human papillomavirus types 6/11 in cutaneous lesions from transplant recipients. J Invest Dermatol 1993; 101:286–291.

54. Stark LA, Arends MJ, McLaren KM, et al. Prevalence of human papillomavirus DNA in cutaneous neoplasms from renal allograft recipients supports a possible viral role in tumour promotion. Br J Cancer 1994; 69:222–229.

55. Arends MJ, Benton EC, McLaren KM, et al. Renal allograft recipients with high susceptibility to cutaneous malignancy have an increased prevalence of human papillomavirus DNA in skin tumours and a greater risk of anogenital malignancy. Br J Cancer 1997; 75:722–728.

56. Dyall-Smith D, Trowell H, Mark A, Dyall-Smith MA. Cutaneous squamous cell carcinoma and papillomaviruses in renal transplant recipients: a clinical and biological study. J Dermatol Sci 1991; 2:139–146.

57. Smith SE, Davis IC, Leshin B, et al. Absence of human papillomavirus in squamous cell carcinomas of nongenital skin from immunocompromised renal transplant patients. Arch Derm 1993; 129:1585–1588.

58. Ferrandiz C, Fuente MJ, Ariza A, et al. Detection and typing of human papillomavirus in skin lesions from renal transplant recipients and equivalent lesions from immunocompetent patients. Arch Dermatol 1997; 134:381–382.

59. Shamanin V, Delius H, de Villiers E-M. Development of a broad spectrum PCR assay for papillomaviruses and its application in screening lung cancer biopsies. J Gen Virol 1994a; 75:1149–1156.

60. Surentheran T, Harwood CA, Spink PJ, et al. Detection and typing of human papillomaviruses in mucosal and cutaneous biopsies from immunosuppressed and immunocompetent patients and patients with epidermodysplasia verruciformis: a unified diagnostic approach. J Clin Pathol 1998; 51:606–610.

61. Bouwes Bavincke JN. Epidemiological aspects of immunosuppression: roles of exposure to sunlight and human papillomavirus on the development of skin cancer. Hum Exp Toxicol 1994; 14:98–102.

62. Astori G et al. Human papillomaviruses are commonly found in normal skin of immunocompetent hosts. J Invest Dermatol 1998; 110:752–755.

63. Harwood CA, Spink PJ, Surentheran T, et al. Detection of human papillomavirus DNA in PUVA-associated non-melanoma skin cancers. J Invest Dermatol 1998; 111:123–127.

64. Boxman ILA, Berkhout RJM, Mulder LHC, et al. Detection of human papillomavirus DNA in plucked hairs from renal transplant recipients and healthy volunteers. J Invest Dermatol 1997; 108:712–715.

65. Chang F, Syrjanen S, Kellokoski J, Syrjanen K. Human papillomavirus (HPV) infections and their associations with oral disease. J Oral Pathol Med 1991; 20:305–317.

66. Praetorius F. HPV-associated diseases of oral mucosa. Clin Dermatol 1997; 15:399–413.

67. Puranen M, Yliskoski M, Saarikoski S, et al. Vertical transmission of human papillomavirus from infected mothers to their newborn babies and persistence of the virus in childhood. Am J Obstet Gynecol 1996; 174:694–699.

68. Sugerman PB, Shillitoe EJ. The high risk human papillomaviruses and oral cancer: evidence for and against a causal relationship. Oral Dis 1997; 3:130–147.

69. zur Hausen H. Human papilloma viruses in the pathogenesis of anogenital cancer. Virology 1991; 184:9–13.

70. Sexton CJ, Proby CM, Banks L, et al. Characterization of factors involved in human papillomavirus type-16 mediated immortalization of oral keratinocytes. J Gen Virol 1993; 74:755–761.

71. Oda D, Bigler L, Lee P, et al. HPV immortalization of human oral epithelial cells: a model for carcinogenesis. Exp Cell Res 1996; 226:164–169.

72. Yeudall WA, Paterson JC, Patel V, et al. Presence of human papillomavirus sequences in tumour-derived human oral keratinocytes expressing mutant p53. Eur J Cancer B Oral Oncol 1995; 31B:136–143.

73. Shah KV. Do Human papillomavirus infections cause oral cancer? J Natl Cancer Inst 1998; 90:1585–1586.

74. McKaig RG, Baric RS, Olshan AF. Human papillomavirus and head and neck cancer and molecular biology. Epidemiol Mol Biol 1998; 20:250–265.

75. Elamin F, Steigrimsdottir S, Wanakulasuriya S, et al. Prevalence of human papillomavirus infection in premalignant and malignant lesions of the oral cavity in UK subjects: a novel method of detection. Oral Oncol 1998; 34:191–197.

76. Woods KV, Shillitoe EJ, Spitz MR, et al. Analysis of human papillomavirus in oral squamous cell carcinomas. J Oral Pathol Med 1993; 22:101–108.

77. Miller CS, Zeuss MS, White DK. Detection of HPV DNA in oral carcinoma using polymerase chain reaction together with in situ hybridization. Oral Surg Oral Med Oral Pathol 1994; 77:776–777.

78. Milde K, Loning T. Detection of papillomavirus DNA in oral papillomas and carcinomas: application of insitu hybridization with biotinylated HPV 16 probes. J Oral Pathol Med 1985; 15:292–296.

79. Cruz IBF, Snijders PJF, Steenbergen RDM, et al. Age-dependence of human papillomavirus DNA presence in oral carcinomas. Eur J Cancer B Oral Oncol 1996; 32B:55–62.

80. Steenbergen RD, Hermsen AJ, Walboomers JM, et al. Integrated human papillomavirus type 16 and loss of heterozygosity at 11q22 and 18q21 in an oral carcinoma and its derivative cell line. Cancer Res 1995; 55:5465–5471.

81. Kim MS, Shin KH, Baek JH, et al. HPV 16, tobacco-specific *N*-nitrosamine and *N*-methyl-*N*-nitro-*N*-nitrosoguanidine in oral carcinogenesis. Cancer Res 1993; 53:4811–4816.

82. Schwartz SM, Daling JR, Doody DR, et al. Oral cancer risk in relation to sexual history and evidence of human papillomavirus infection. J Natl Cancer Inst 1998; 90:1626–1636.

83. Regezi JA, Greenspan D, Greenspan JS, et al. HPV-associated epithelial atypia in oral warts in HIV[+] patients. J Cutan Pathol 1994; 21:217–223.

84. zur Hausen H, de Villiers EM. Human papillomaviruses. Annu Rev Microbiol 1994; 48:427–447.

85. Evander M, Frazer IH, Payne E, et al. Identification of the alpha-6 integrin as a candidate receptor for papillomaviruses. J Virol 1997; 71:2449–2456.

86. Chan WK, Chong T, Bernard HU, Klock G. Transcription of the transforming genes of the oncogenic human papillomavirus-16 is stimulated by tumor promoters through AP1 binding sites. Nucleic Acids Res 1990; 18:763–769.

87. Chong T, Apt D, Gloss B, et al. The enhancer of human papillomavirus type 16: binding sites for the ubiquitous transcription factors oct-1, NFA, TEF-2, NF1, and AP-1 participate in epithelial cell-specific transcription. J Virol 1991; 65:5933–5943.

88. Chong T, Chan WK, Bernard HU. Transcriptional activation of human papillomavirus 16 by nuclear factor I, AP1, steroid receptors and a possibly novel transcription factor, PVF: a model for the composition of genital papillomavirus enhancers. Nucleic Acids Res 1990; 18:465–470.

89. Cripe TP, Haugen TH, Turk JP, et al. Transcriptional regulation of the human papillomavirus-16 E6-E7 promoter by a keratinocyte-dependent enhancer, and by viral E2 *trans*-activator and repressor gene products: implications for cervical carcinogenesis. Euro Mol Biol Org J 1987; 6:3745–3753.

90. Gius D, Grossman S, Bedell MA, Laimins LA. Inducible and constitutive enhancer domains in the noncoding region of human papillomavirus type 18. J Virol 1988; 62:665–672.

91. Ishiji T, Lace MJ, Pakkinen S, et al. Transcriptional enhancer factor (TEF)-1 and its cell-specific co-factor activate human papillomavirus-16 E6 and E7 oncogene transcription in keratinocytes and cervical carcinoma cells. EMBO J 1992; 11:2271–2281.

92. Thierry F, Spyrou G, Yaniv M, Howley P. Two AP1 sites binding JunB are essential for human papillomavirus type 18 transcription in keratinocytes. J Virol 1992; 66:3740–3748.

93. Apt D, Chong, T, Liu Y, Bernard HU. Nuclear factor I and epithelial cell-specific transcription of human papillomavirus type 16. J Virol 1993; 67:4455–4463.

94. Mack DH, Laimins LA. A keratinocyte-specific transcription factor, KRF-1, interacts with AP-1 to activate expression of human papillomavirus type 18 in squamous epithelial cells. Proc Natl Acad Sci USA 1991; 88:9102–9106.

95. Yukawa K, Butz K, Yasui T, et al. Regulation of human papillomavirus transcription by the differentiation-dependent epithelial factor Epoc-1/skn-1a. J Virol 1996; 70:10–16.

96. Gloss B, Bernard HU, Seedorf K, Klock G. The upstream regulatory region of the human papilloma virus-16 contains an E2 protein-independent enhancer which is specific for cervical carcinoma cells and regulated by glucocorticoid hormones. EMBO J 1987; 6:3735–3743.

97. Mittal R, Tsutsumi K, Pater A, Pater MM. Human papillomavirus type 16 expression in cervical keratinocytes: role of progesterone and glucocorticoid hormones. Obstet Gynecol 1993; 81:5–12.

98. Barbosa MS, Schlegel R. The E6 and E7 genes of HPV-18 are sufficient for inducing two-stage *in vitro* transformation of human keratinocytes. Oncogene 1989; 4:1529–1532.

99. Hawley-Nelson P, Vousden KH, Hubbert NL, et al. HPV 16 E6 and E7 proteins cooperate to immortalize human foreskin keratinocytes. EMBO J 1989; 8:3905–3910.

100. Münger K, Phelps WC, Bubb V, Howley PM. The E6 and E7 genes of the human papillomavirus type 16 together are necessary and sufficient for transformation of primary human keratinocytes. J Virol 1989; 63:4417–4421.

101. Münger K, Werness BA, Dyson N, et al. Complex formation between the human papillomavirus E7 protein with the retinoblastoma tumor suppressor gene product. EMBO J 1989; 8:4099–4105.

102. Phelps WC, Yee CL, Munger K, Howley PM. The human papillomavirus type 16 E7 gene encodes transactivation and transformation functions similar to those of adenovirus E1A. Cell 1988; 53:539–547.

103. Storey A, Banks L. Human papillomavirus type 16 E6 gene cooperated with EJ-*ras* to immortalize primary mouse cells. Oncogene 1993; 8:919–924.

104. Storey A, Pim D, Murray A, et al. Comparison of the *in vitro* transforming activities of human papillomavirus types. EMBO J 1988; 7:1815–1820.

105. Dyson N, Howley PM, Münger K, Harlow E. The human papillomavirus-16 E7 oncoprotein is able to bind to the retinoblastoma gene product. Science 1989; 243:934–936.

106. Scheffner M, Werness BA, Huibregste JM, et al. The E6 oncoprotein encoded by human papillomavirus types 16 and 18 promotes the degradation of p53. Cell 1990; 63:1129–1136.

107. Werness BA, Levine AJ, Howley PM. Association of human papillomavirus types 16 and 18 E6 proteins with p53. Science 1990; 248:76–79.

108. Edmonds C, Vousden KH. A point mutational analysis of human papillomavirus type 16 E7 protein. J Virol 1989; 63:2650–2656.

109. Ciccolini F, Di Pasquale G, Carlotti F, et al. Functional studies of E7 proteins from different HPV types. Oncogene 1994; 9:2633–2638.

110. Iftner T, Fuchs PG, Pfister H. Two independently transforming functions of HPV 8. Curr Topics Microbiol Immunol 1989; 144:167–173.

111. Kiyono T, Nagashima K, Ishibashi M. The primary structure of major viral RNA in a rat cell line transfected with type 47 human papillomavirus DNA and the transforming activity of its cDNA and E6 gene. Virology 1989; 173:551–565.

112. Schmitt A, Harry JB, Rapp B, et al. Comparison of the properties of the E6 and E7 genes of low-and high-risk cutaneous papillomaviruses reveals strongly transforming and high Rb-binding activity for the E7 protein of the low-risk human papillomavirus type I. J Virol 1994; 68:7051–7059.

113. Funk JO, Waga S, Harry JB, et al. Inhibition of CDK activity and PCNA-dependent DNA replication by p21 is blocked by interaction with the HPV-16 E7 oncoprotein. Genes Dev 1997; 11:2090–2100.

114. Jones DL, Thompson DA, Münger K. Destabilization of the RB tumor suppressor protein and stabilization of p53 contribute to HPV type 16 E7-induced apoptosis. Virology 1997; 239:97–107.

115. Thomas JT, Laimins LA. Human papillomavirus oncoproteins E6 and E7 independently abrogate the mitotic spindle checkpoint. J Virol 1998; 72:1131–1137.

116. Massimi P, Pim D, Storey A, Banks L. HPV16 E7 and adenovirus E1 a complex formation with TATA box binding protein is enhanced by casein kinase II phosphorylation. Oncogene 1996; 12:2325–2330.

117. Delius H, Saeling B, Bergmann K, et al. The genomes of three of four novel HPV types, defined by differences of their L1 genes, show high conservation of the E7 gene and the URR. Virology 1998; 240:359–365.

118. Huibregste JM, Scheffner M, Howley PM. A cellular protein mediates association of p53 with the E6 oncoprotein of human papillomavirus type 16 or 18. Eur Mol Biol Org J 1991; 10:4129–4135.

119. Iftner T, Bierfelder S, Csapo Z, Pfister H. Involvement of the human papillomavirus type 8 genes E6 and E7 in transformation and replication. J Virol 1988; 62:3655–3661.

120. Kiyono T, Hiraiwa A, Ishibashi M. Differences in transforming activity and coded amino acid sequence among E6 genes of several papillomaviruses associated with epidermodysplasia verruciformis. Virology 1992; 186:628–639.

121. Steger G, Pfister H. In vitro expressed HPV 8 E6 protein does not bind p53. Arch Virol 1992; 125:355–360.

122. Birkeland SA, Storm HH, Lamm LU, et al. Cancer risk after renal transplantation in the Nordic countries. Int J Can 1995; 60:183–189.

123. Hall PA, McKee PH, Menage HD, et al. High levels of p53 protein in UV-irradiated normal human skin. Oncogene 1993; 8:203–207.

124. Lane DP. p53, guardian of the genome. Nature 1992; 358:15–16.

125. Pan H, Griep AE. Altered cell cycle regulation in the lens of HPV-16 E6 or E7 transgenic mice: implications for tumor suppressor gene function in development. Genes Dev 1994; 8:1285–1299.

126. Kreider JW, Howett MK, Lill NL, et al. In vivo transformation of human skin with human papillomavirus type 11 from condylomata acuminata. J Virol 1986; 59:369–376.

127. Kreider JW, Howett MK, Wolfe SA, et al. Morphological transformation *in vivo* of human uterine cervix with papillomavirus from condylomata acuminata. Nature 1985; 317:639–641.

128. Kreider JW, Howett MK, Leure-Dupree AE, et al. Laboratory production in vivo of infectious human papillomavirus type 11. J Virol 1987; 61:590–593.

129. Bonnez W, Rose RC, Da Rin C, et al. Propagation of human papilloamvirus type 11 in human xenografts using the severe combined immunodeficiency (SCID) mouse and comparison to the nude mouse model. Virology 1993; 197:455–458.

130. Brandsma JL, Brownstein DG, Xiao W, Longley BJ. Papilloma formation in human foreskin xenografts after inoculation of human papillomavirus type 16 DNA. J Virol 1995; 69:2716–2721.

131. Sexton CJ, Williams AT, Topley P, et al. Development and characterisation of a novel xenograft model permissive for human papillomavirus DNA amplification and late gene expression. J Gen Virol 1995; 76:3107–3112.

132. Sterling J, Stanley M, Gatward G, Minson T. Production of human papillomavirus type 16 virions in a keratinocyte cell line. J Virol 1990; 64:6305–6307.

133. Adachi A, Kiyono T, Taguchi O, et al. Serial transplantation in SCID mice of epidermodysplasia verruciformis-associated squamous cell carcinoma without alteration of its histological and virological features. Virology 1996; 217:380–383.

134. Majewski S, Breitburd F, Skopinska M, et al. A mouse model for studying epidermodysplasia-verruciformis-associated carcinogenesis. Int J Cancer 1994; 56:727–730.

135. Ruesch MN, Laimins LA. Human papillomavirus oncoproteins alter differentiation-dependent cell cycle exit on suspension in semisolid medium. Virology 1998; 250:19–29.

136. Bell E, Sher S, Hull B, et al. The reconstitution of living skin. J Invest Dermatol 1983; 81:2s–10s.

137. Prunerias M, Regnier M, Woodley D. Methods of cultivation of keratinocytes at an air liquid interface. J Invest Dermatol 1983; 81:28–33.

138. McCance DJ, Kopan R, Fuchs E, Laimins LA. Human papillomavirus type 16 alters human epithelial cell differentiation *in vitro*. Proc Natl Acad Sci USA 1988; 85:7169–7173.

139. Blanton RA, Perez-Reyes N, Merrick DT, McDougall JK. Epithelial cells immortalised by human papillomavirus have premalignant characteristics in organotypic culture. Am J Pathol 1991; 138:673–685.

140. Merrick DT, Blanton RA, Gown AM, McDougall JK. Altered proliferation and differentiation markers in HPV16 and 18 immortalised epithelial cells grown in organotypic culture. Am J Pathol 1992; 140:167–178.

141. Frattini MG, Lim HB, Laimins LA. In vitro synthesis of oncogenic human papillomavirus requires episomal genomes for differentiation-dependent late expression. Proc Natl Acad Sci USA 1996; 93:3062–3067.

142. Meyers C, Frattini MG, Hudson JB, Laimins LA. Biosynthesis of human papillomavirus from a continuous cell line upon epithelial differentiation. Science 1992; 257:971–973.

143. Parker JN, Zhao W, Askins KJ, et al. Mutational analyses of differentiation-dependent human papillomavirus type 18 enhancer elements in epithelial raft cultures of neonatal foreskin keratinocytes. Cell Growth Different 1997; 8:751–762.

144. Delvenne P, al-Saleh W, Gilles C, et al. Inhibition of growth of normal and human papillomavirus-transfected keratinocytes in monolayer and prganotypic cultures by interferon-gamma and tumor necrosis factor-alpha. Am J Pathol 1995; 146:589–598.

145. Deng H, Choate KA, Lin Q, Khavari P. High-efficiency gene transfer and pharmacologic selection of genetically engineered human keratinocytes. Bio Techniques 1998; 25:274–279.

146. Deng H, Lin Q, Khavari P. Sustainable cutaneous gene delivery. Nature Biotech 1997; 15:1338–1391.

147. Krueger G, Jorgensen CM, Matsunami N, et al. Persistent transgene expression and normal differentiation of immortalized human keratinocytes *in vivo*. J Invest Dermatol 1999; 234:233–239.

148. Arbeit J M, Münger K, Howley PM, Hanahan D. Progressive squamous epithelial neoplasia in K14-human papillomavirus type 16 transgenic mice. J Virol 1994; 68:4358–4368.

149. Brown K, Balmain A. Transgenic mice and squamous multistage skin carcinogenesis. Cancer Metastas Rev 1995; 14:113–124.

150. Greenhalgh DA, Wang XJ, Dominey AM, et al. Development of transgenic mouse models of skin carcinogenesis: potential applications. Prog Clin Biol Res 1994; 387:75–94.

151. Gulliver GA, Herber RL, Liem A, Lambert PF. Both conserved region 1 (CR1) and CR2 of the human papillomavirus type 16 E7 oncogene are required for the induction of epidermal hyperplasia and tumor formation in transgenic mice. J Virol 1997; 71:5905–5914.

152. Jones DL, Alani RM, Münger K. The human papillomavirus E7 oncoprotein can uncouple cellular differentiation and proliferation in human keratinocytes by abrogating p21$^{CIP 1}$-mediated inhibition of cdk 2. Genes Dev 1997; 11:2101–2111.

153. Griep AE, Herber R, Jeon S, et al. Tumorigenicity by human papillomavirus type 16 E6 and E7 in transgenic mice correlates with alterations in epithelial cell growth and differentiation. J Virol 1993; 67:1373–1384.

154. Lambert PF, Pan H, Pitot HC, et al. Epidermal cancer associated with expression of human papillomavirus type 16 E6 and E7 oncogenes in the skin of transgenic mice. Proc Natl Acad Sci USA 1993; 90:5583–5587.

155. Arbeit JM, Olson DC, Hanahan D. Upregulation of fibroblast growth factors and their receptors during multi-stage eoidermal carcinogenesis in K14-HPV16 transgenic mice. Oncogene 1996; 13:1847–1857.

156. Auewarakul P, Gissmann L, Cid-Arregui A. Targeted expression of the E6 and E7 oncogenes of human papillomavirus type 16 in the epidermis of transgenic mice elicits generalized epidermal hyperplasia involving autoctine factors. Mol Cell Biol 1994; 14:8250–8258.

157. Michelin D, Gissmann L, Street D, et al. Regulation of human papillomavirus type 18 in vivo: effects of estrogen and progesterone in transgenic mice. Gynaecol Oncol 1997; 66:202–208.

158. Pan H, Griep AE. Temporally distinct patterns of p53-dependent and p53-independent apoptosis during mouse lens development. Genes Dev 1995; 9:2157–2169.

159. Song S, Gulliver GA, Lambert PF. Human papillomavirus type 16 E6 and E7 oncogenes abrogate radiation-induced DNA damage responses in vivo through p53-dependent and p53-independent pathways. Proc Natl Acad Sci USA 1998; 95:2290–2295.

160. Lindgren V, Sippola-Thiele M, Skowronski J, et al. Specific chromosomal abnormalities characterize fibrosacromas of bovine papillomavirus type 1 transgenic mice. Proc Natl Acad Sci USA 1989; 86:5025–5029.

161. Shindoh M, Sun Q, Pater A, Pater MM. Prevention of carcinoma in situ of human papillomavirus type 16-immortalized human endocervical cells by retinoic acid in organotypic raft culture. Obstet Gynaecol 1995; 85:721–728.

V
Hepatitis Viruses

17

Overview of Hepatitis B and C Viruses

Jia-Horng Kao and Ding-Shinn Chen

INTRODUCTION

Hepatocellular carcinoma (HCC) is one of the most common and devastating malignant tumors in the world, particularly in Asia and Africa *(1)*. With the estimated 1 million cases per year worldwide, HCC is the seventh most common cancer in men and the ninth most common in women. In high prevalence areas such as Southeast Asia, the Far East including Taiwan, and sub-Saharan Africa, the annual incidence of HCC reaches 30 cases per 100,000 population; this contrasts with an annual incidence of fewer than 2 cases per 100,000 population in low-risk areas such as the United States and most of Europe. Symptomatic HCCs usually run a rapidly progressive course with low rate of resectability and poor response to nonsurgical therapy and thus have a very poor prognosis *(2)*. The risk factors associated with the development of HCC include chronic infection with either hepatitis B virus (HBV) or hepatitis C virus (HCV), the presence of liver cirrhosis, carcinogen exposure especially aflatoxin B_1, alcohol abuse, genetic factors, male gender, cigaret smoking, and advanced age. Among these risk factors, chronic hepatitis virus infections, particularly those occurring in the presence of cirrhosis, show the strongest association with the development of HCC *(2,3)*. This chapter reviews the virologic characteristics, animal models, and molecular pathogenesis of both HBV and HCV.

HEPATITIS B VIRUS

Discovery

HBV is the first human hepatitis virus from which the proteins and genome could be identified and characterized. Before discovery of the viruses, two types of hepatitis (hepatitis A for infectious hepatitis and hepatitis B for serum hepatitis) were differentiated on the basis of transmission routes and other epidemiologic characteristics *(4)*. Hepatitis A virus (HAV) was transmitted by the fecal–oral route, whereas hepatitis B virus (HBV) was transmitted parenterally. In 1963, Blumberg et al. studied genetic polymorphisms of serum proteins, and discovered a previously unknown antigen in the blood of an Australian aborigine (Australia antigen) that formed a precipitin line with the serum of a multiply transfused hemophiliac*(5)*. The significance of Australia antigen was soon recognized by its specific association with hepatitis B. By using immune

From: *Infectious Causes of Cancer: Targets for Intervention*
Edited by: J. J. Goedert © Humana Press Inc., Totowa, NJ

electron microscopic methods, Dane and colleagues in 1970 first described the 42-nm particles that came to be known later as "Dane particles" *(6)* and are actually hepatitis B virions. The term Australia antigen was then replaced with hepatitis B surface antigen (HBsAg) to denote its association with the envelope of HBV. In 1973 the viral nature of Dane particles was confirmed by the detection of an endogenous DNA-dependent DNA polymerase within their core *(7)*. Subsequently, the HBV genome was found to be a small, circular DNA that was partially double-stranded *(8,9)*.

HBV Taxonomy

HBV is the prototype of a new family of closely related hepatotropic DNA viruses called hepadnavirus *(10)*. Included in this family are the woodchuck hepatitis virus (WHV), the ground squirrel hepatitis virus (GSHV), the duck hepatitis B virus (DHBV), as well as several other avian and mammalian variants. As in the situation of human HBV infection, chronic hepatitis and HCC are commonly observed in persistently infected woodchucks and less frequently in infected ground squirrels and ducks *(10)*. All the hepadnaviruses have similar hepatotropism and life cycles in their hosts. They all use the reverse transcription of viral RNA to form DNA within core particles as the initial step in replication. Thus the hepadnaviruses are also named pararetroviruses, in contrast to orthoretroviruses, which have an RNA genome (*see* Chapter 11).

Having only 3200 basepairs in its genome, HBV is the smallest known DNA virus *(9)*. The partially double-stranded circular DNA encodes four overlapping open reading frames *(10,11)*: *S* for the surface or envelope gene, *C* for the core gene, *P* for the polymerase gene, and *X* for the *X* gene (Fig. 1). The *S* and *C* genes also have upstream regions designated *pre-S* and *pre-C*. The whole virion, or Dane particle, is a 42-nm sphere that contains the nucleocapsid. The viral envelope encoded by the *S* gene contains three distinct components—large, middle, and major (or small) proteins—that are synthesized by beginning transcription with the *pre-S1, pre-S2,* or *S* gene alone, respectively (Fig. 1). Of interest, HBV can produce a large excess of surface antigens consisting of both small spheres and rods with an average diameter of 22 nm that can be found in the circulation. The pre-S1 and pre-S2 proteins are perhaps the more immunogenic components of HBsAg. Several specific antigenic determinants including the *a* determinant are common to all HBsAg, whereas the *d, y, w,* and *r* determinants are mainly of epidemiologic interest. Hepatitis B core antigen (HBcAg) is the nucleocapsid that encloses the viral DNA. When HBcAg-derived peptides are processed and expressed on the surface of liver cells, a cellular immune response can be induced for killing infected cells and clearing the virus. Hepatitis B e antigen (HBeAg) is a circulating peptide derived from the core gene, then modified and secreted from liver cells. It usually serves as a marker of active viral replication. HBeAg can act as a tolerogen to diminish host immune response against HBV because of its close resemblance to HBcAg, the putative target of the immune response. The long *P* gene encodes the DNA polymerase. However, because viral replication requires RNA intermediates, the polymerase also provides the reverse transcription function of HBV. The *X* gene encodes two proteins that have transactivation activities on HBV enhancer in aiding viral replication. These proteins can also transactivate other cellular genes that may play a role in hepatocarcinogenesis. In addition, several enhancers and promoters have been identified within the whole HBV genome.

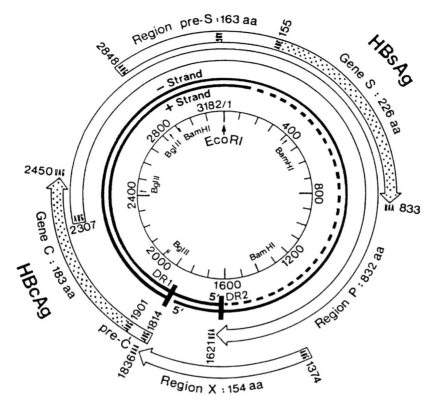

Fig. 1. Genetic organization of hepatitis B virus.

HBV Life Cycle and Viral Replication

The understanding of hepadnaviruses replication derives largely from animal models *(11–13)*. The process of HBV entry into the liver cell is not well understood because of the lack of susceptible cell lines for in vitro infection studies. However, cell membrane proteins may play a role in infection by association with the viral envelope binding to the cell surface and to facilitate viral penetration either by the fusion with the viral envelope or by receptor-mediated endocytosis. Following entry into the cell, the virus core is thought to be transported to the nucleus without processing, and the relaxed circular viral genome is repaired to form covalently closed circular DNA (cccDNA), which is thought to serve as the template for the transcription of both the pregenomic RNA, the precursor for replication, and mRNA from several promoters for viral protein synthesis. Integration of HBV DNA into the host genome does not occur during the normal course of replication, as it does with retroviruses. These mRNA encode the envelope, core, polymerase, and X proteins as previously mentioned. The 3.5-kb pregenomic RNA serves as a template for reverse transcription. Minus-strand DNA synthesis initiates at the 3′ DR1 with the terminal protein of the polymerase as a primer, and when synthesis progresses the RNA template is simultaneously degraded by RNaseH. Plus-strand DNA synthesis initiates at the 3′ end of DR2 and synthesis continues until the terminal protein at the 5′ end of the minus strand is passed. This produces an open circular DNA molecule similar to that of mature HBV. The mature core particles are then packed into the HBsAg/pre-S in the endoplasmic reticulum and released from the liver cell. A stable pool of cccDNA molecules is maintained in the nucleus by transporting the newly synthesized HBV DNA back into the nucleus. Because HBsAg can inhibit the formation of cccDNA, this may represent a negative feedback to HBV replication.

Animal Models of HBV

Although the chimpanzee has long served as a surrogate host for humans in modeling HBV infection *(14,15)*, the chronic liver disease in this model is less severe, and HCC has not been observed. Since the discovery of WHV in 1978, the virus and its host, the American eastern woodchuck, have been extensively studied and used as the most suitable model for human HBV infection *(13)*. WHV is closely related to the human HBV, having close similarities in morphology, genome structure and gene products, replication, epidemiology, the course of infection, and the development of illness including HCC. The woodchuck is thus used in the development of new vaccines, therapeutic vaccination, and antiviral agents. In addition, the woodchuck system is employed for testing viral inactivation procedures and for investigation of molecular mechanisms of the viral life cycle and the mechanisms of carcinogenesis and cell infection.

The molecular mechanism of WHV-related HCC in woodchuck has been reviewed recently *(16)*. Southern blot analysis of genomic DNA from a large number of woodchuck HCCs provides evidence of integrated WHV sequences in about 90%, including tumors from chronic carriers and from woodchucks that seroconverted and were not chronic carriers. Contrary to HBV, WHV seems to activate cellular protooncogenes by integration of viral sequences in the flanking host DNA. A high frequency (50%) of insertions of WHV DNA adjacent to c-*myc* and N-*myc* sequences has been reported *(17–19)*, and the N-*myc* mRNA was found to be overexpressed. The activation of N-*myc* expression in woodchuck HCC is similar to that caused by the murine leukemia virus (MuLV). In both cases, insertion of virus sequences occurs in the 3′ noncoding region of the N-*myc* locus in the same transcriptional orientation leading to chimeric RNA. These findings strongly suggest that WHV might act as an insertional mutagen to activate *myc* family genes (c-*myc* or N-*myc*) and then induce HCC in the animal.

Molecular Pathogenesis

HBV is a major public health problem worldwide. It is estimated that more than 350 million people are chronic HBV carriers *(10)*. Hepatitis B is the leading cause of chronic liver disease and HCC, accounting for 1 million deaths annually. Extensive prospective and retrospective studies in many parts of the world have provided a strong epidemiologic association between chronic HBV infection and HCC *(2,3)*. The increased risk of developing HCC has been estimated to be 100-fold for HBsAg carriers compared to uninfected populations, placing HBV in the first rank among known human carcinogens. Meantime, the existence of related animal viruses (such as WHV) that induce HCC in their hosts *(16)*, the weak oncogenicity of the viral X transcriptional transactivator, the long-term tumorigenic effect of surface glycoprotein, and the mutagenic action of viral integration into the host genome that may contribute to deregulate the normal cell growth control also support the connection between HBV and HCC *(20)*. The decrease of HCC in Taiwanese children after implementation of universal vaccination against HBV infection further strengthens the etiologic role of HBV in causing human HCC *(21)*.

Immunopathogenesis

The mechanisms of hepatocellular injury during HBV infection are predominantly immune-mediated *(22)*. The host immune attack against HBV is mainly mediated by a cellular response to small epitopes of HBV proteins, especially HBcAg, presented on the surface of liver cells. HLA class I-restricted $CD8^+$ cells recognize HBV peptide fragments derived from intracellular processing and presentation on the liver cell surface by class I molecules *(23)*. This process leads to direct cell killing by the $CD8^+$ cytotoxic T lymphocytes. However, progressive hepatic failure develops in certain patients, especially those with liver grafts but also occasionally in patients with renal or bone marrow transplants, due to a peculiar form of fibrosing cholestatic hepatitis *(24)*. Thus, high viral titers in serum and liver tissue may also have a direct cytopathic effect on liver cells in such immunosuppressed patients.

Hepatocarcinogenesis

The mechanisms of HBV-related HCC are not yet clear. Whether HBV acts through any recognized oncogenic mechanism, either directly or indirectly, represents an important but unsolved issue. However, it is generally believed that HBV has no direct oncogenic effect on the infected liver cell *(20)*. Malignant transformation of the liver cell occurs after a long period of chronic hepatitis, frequently associated with liver cirrhosis (Fig. 2). This fact also indicates that a multistep evolution involving many important and stagewise genetic changes is required for the development of HCC *(3,20)*, as in other human cancers. However, unlike the sequential genetic changes of colorectal cancers, most of those in hepatocarcinogenesis remain virtually unknown. On the other hand, the long latency of HCC development after the initial HBV infection may suggest an indirect action of the virus. The host immune response against the infected liver cells and/or a long-term toxic effect of viral proteins might cause continuous liver cell necrosis and consequent cellular regeneration, resulting in the accumulation of genetic changes. In addition, persistent HBV infection might potentiate the action of exogenous carcinogens such as aflatoxins and alcohol. Although integration of HBV DNA into the liver cell genome has been detected in most, but not all, patients with HBsAg-positive chronic hepatitis or HCC *(25,26)*, this may not contribute directly to hepatocarcinogenesis. Integration of viral DNA into the host genome may cause direct activation of cellular oncogenes or secondary chromosome instability. However, insertional activation of potential oncogenes has been described only in rare cases *(27,28)*, and the consequences of genetic instability resulting from viral integration have not been determined. In contrast, most of the woodchuck HCCs, like the human counterpart, contain integrated viral DNA with preferential integration sites that activate *myc* family genes (c-*myc* and N-*myc*) *(16)*. Whether these striking differences are related to viral determinants or to species-specific factors remains to be determined.

Many interesting relationships have been noted in cytogenetic and subsequent molecular genetic features of HCC in Taiwan. First, amplification and overexpression of known protooncogenes such as *cyclin D1* and c-*myc* in human HCC have been demon-

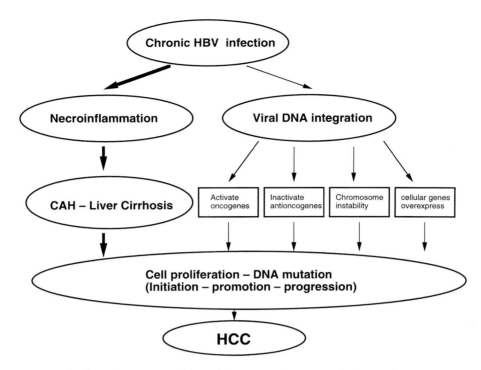

Fig. 2. Pathogenesis of hepatitis B-related hepatocellular carcinoma.

strated *(27,29),* and activation of c-*myc* occurs more frequently in young patients having elevated serum α-fetoprotein (AFP) levels or HBV infection.

Second, because cytogenetic analysis of HCC cell lines and primary HCC tissues show chromosome 1p to be the region most commonly affected, genetic abnormalities of chromosome 1p in HCC were explored by microsatellite polymorphism analysis *(30,31).* In half of the HCCs studied, aberrations of chromosome 1p were found *(32),* and the abnormalities could be classified into three groups: typical loss of heterozygosity, two- to threefold increase of allelic dosage, and novel microsatellite polymorphism. These abnormalities clustered at the telomeric (distal) part of chromosome 1p, with a common region mapped to 1p35–36, which is also the region with frequent loss of heterozygosity in neuroblastoma as well as colorectal and breast cancers. Using the same strategy, allelic loss on chromosomes 4q and 16q was also studied *(33).* The frequency of allelic loss on chromosome 16q was 70%, and the common region was mapped to 16q22–23. A similar high frequency (77%) was found on chromosome 4q with the common region mapped to 4q12–23. Of interest, the allelic loss of chromosome 4q in HCC was associated with elevated serum AFP levels, whereas the remaining portion (23%) without the 4q deletion had normal serum AFP *(33).* These findings suggest that further positional cloning may identify putative HCC-relevant tumor suppressor genes on chromosome 4q and 16q are promising, with one gene on chromosome 4q perhaps contributing to the AFP expression in HCC.

Third, the tumor-suppressor gene *p53* can transactivate the transcription of genes, with tumors developing when p53 protein is mutated or lost *(34).* The association between *p53* gene mutation and hepatocarcinogenesis has been extensively studied *(35–39)*. In Taiwan, 37% of HCC tissues had mutant p53 protein, 29% had mutations in the *p53* gene, and 13% had specific codon 249 mutations *(38)*. The p53 protein was overexpressed more frequently in HCC with elevated serum AFP level, in large HCC, and in invasive HCC *(37)*. Meanwhile, overexpression of p53 protein was closely correlated with p53 mRNA overexpression and *p53* gene mutation. Clinically, HCCs with p53 protein expression and those negative for both p53 protein and mRNA expression had an unfavorable outcome, while HCC with no p53 protein but with p53 mRNA overexpression had the best outcome; the 4-yr survival was 26.1%, 26.3%, and 62.5% in the three groups, respectively *(37)*. Thus, the p53 protein and mRNA expression patterns in HCC correlate with *p53* gene mutation and tumor behavior. This may serve as a molecular marker for prognosis. Although a specific hot-spot mutation at codon 249 of the *p53* gene has been frequently found in aflatoxin-related HCC, this specific mutation is much less frequently encountered in Taiwan, where contamination of food by aflatoxin has not been heavy in recent decades *(38,39)*. Mutations of the *p53* gene among Taiwanese HCC cases are widely distributed throughout exons 5–8; a new hot-spot for point mutations, T/A transversions with an amino acid change from serine to threonine, was identified in codon 166 of the *p53* gene *(35)*. In addition, alterations of the highly conserved consensus intervening sequences at the splice junctions may also lead to the inactivation of the *p53* gene *(36,40)*.

Therapy of HBV

The currently recommended therapy of chronic hepatitis B is a 4- to 6-mo course of interferon-α (IFN-α) in doses of 5–10 million units three times a week, a regimen that results in sustained clearance of HBV DNA and HBeAg from serum in approx 25–40% of patients, and a loss of HBsAg in 10% of Western patients *(41)*. Long-term follow-up of patients who respond to IFN-α treatment with clearance of HBeAg indicates that the majority ultimately clear HBsAg as well and have continued remission of liver disease. A recent report indicated that the clearance of HBeAg after treatment with IFN-α in patients with chronic hepatitis B is associated with improved clinical outcomes *(42)*. However, low levels of HBV DNA can still be detected in liver tissue and better therapies of hepatitis B are still needed. Recently, several oral "second-generation" nucleoside analogs such as lamivudine and famciclovir have been developed that have potent activity against HBV. The best studied is lamivudine (3-thiacytidine), which induced marked reduction of serum HBV DNA levels and improvement in serum aminotransferase activities and hepatic histology in the majority of patients *(43)*. When lamivudine was stopped, however, most patients relapsed. Of further concern, long-term therapy has led to viral resistance in up to 20% of patients within a year and even more with longer term therapy. Little is known regarding the clinical course of those HBsAg carriers whose HBV DNA has become resistant to this nucleoside analog. Future approaches to therapy for hepatitis B should focus on combinations with interferon, other antiviral nucleoside analogs, or therapeutic vaccines.

Prevention of HBV

The most practical and cost-effective way to prevent HBV-related HCC is vaccination against HBV. In Taiwan, we have already confirmed that universal vaccination is feasible and effective in reducing HBsAg carriers *(44)*. The carrier rate in children decreased dramatically from 10% to 1.3% 10 yr after the mass immunization *(45)*. Most importantly, a trend of declining incidence of childhood HCC was observed recently. The average annual incidence of HCC in children 6–14 yr of age declined from 0.70 per 100,000 children in 1981–1986 to 0.57 in 1986–1990, and further to 0.36 in 1990–1994 ($p < 0.01$) *(21)*. These data suggest the effect of HBV mass vaccination program in controlling HBV-related HCC is starting to be seen in the Taiwanese children, and a similar benefit likely will be seen in young adults within a few years. We anticipate seeing an 80–85% decrease of HCC in all adults within 3–4 decades of HBV vaccination *(44)*. The decrease of HCC in children after the implementation of universal vaccination against HBV represents a practical means of preventing a human cancer by vaccination for the first time in history.

HEPATITIS C VIRUS

Discovery

The term "non-A, non-B hepatitis" (NANBH) was introduced in the mid-1970s to describe inflammatory liver disease not attributable to infection with HAV or HBV *(4)*. In 1978, the NANBH agent was shown to be transmissible to chimpanzees, as evidenced by the development of liver pathology, including detection of characteristic cytoplasmic tubular structures by electron microscopy *(14)*. Filtration studies showed that the NANBH agent(s) was < 80 nm in size and thus likely to be a virus. Sensitivity to chloroform indicated that the NANBH virus is enveloped. In 1989, Choo et al. reported the molecular cloning of an NANBH agent from plasma collected from a well-characterized, chronically infected chimpanzee with a high infectious titer of NANBH agent *(46)*. The plasma was subjected to extensive ultracentrifugation to pellet small viruses, and total nucleic acid was extracted from the pellet. The nucleic acid was denatured and cDNA was synthesized by reverse transcription to obtain clones of any viral RNA present. The cDNA was cloned into λgt11, and one million clones were screened with human NANBH patient serum. A 155-bp clone called 5-1-1 was identified that did not hybridize to control human DNA or to DNA derived from two chimpanzees with NANBH. A larger, overlapping, 353-bp clone was then isolated that hybridized to liver and plasma RNA from the original chimpanzee but not the control chimpanzee. These data suggested that the clones were derived from an exogenous RNA molecule associated with NANBH infection. Ribonuclease and hybridization experiments showed that the clones were derived from a single-stranded, plus-sense RNA. This novel RNA virus was subsequently designated hepatitis C virus (HCV). With the subsequent development of antibody-based detection systems, HCV was found to be the major cause of chronic NANBH *(47–49)*.

Taxonomy

HCV has been classified as a separate genus, *Hepacivirus,* in the family *Flaviviridae* based on its similar hydrophobicity patterns and limited sequence homology to the other two genera, *Flavivirus* and *Pestivirus,* of the family *(50–53)*. The flaviviruses include a number of human viruses transmitted by arthropod vectors such as yellow fever virus, the dengue viruses, and Japanese encephalitis virus. Pestiviruses of animals

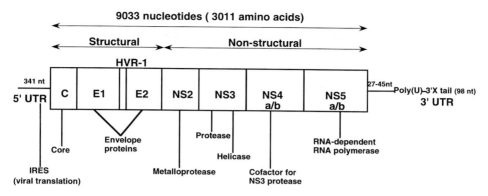

Fig. 3. Genetic organization of hepatitis C virus.

include bovine viral diarrhea virus, classical swine fever virus, and border disease virus of sheep. HCV also appears to be related to recently identified tamarin or human viruses known as GBV-A, GBV-B, and GBV-C or hepatitis G virus (HGV) *(54–56)*.

The RNA genome of HCV is approx 9500 nucleotides and contains highly conserved untranslated regions (UTRs) at both the 5′ and 3′ termini (5′ UTR and 3′ UTR), which flank a single, long open reading frame encoding a polyprotein of slightly more than 3000 amino acids *(50,51)*. The structural proteins are located in the N-terminal portion, and followed by the nonstructural (NS) proteins (Fig. 3). The HCV polyprotein is processed by a combination of host and virus-encoded proteases into at least 10 individual proteins. In order, from the N to C terminus of the polyprotein, these are C, E1, E2, p7, NS2, NS3, NS4a, NS4b, NS5a, and NS5b. Among these, C, E1, and E2 are thought to be structural components of the HCV virion. C is a positively charged protein presumed to form the core structure encapsidating the genomic RNA. E1 and E2 are glycoproteins likely to be integrated into the lipid envelope of the virion. The N-terminal end of the E2 protein contains two hypervariable regions (HVR-1 and HVR-2) that exhibit significant variation among HCV isolates. The nucleotide and amino acid sequences in this region vary over time within individuals, suggesting this variation in the envelope proteins may allow the virus to escape the neutralizing antibodies *(57,58)*. NS2–NS5 are putative nonstructural components that may participate in replication of the HCV genome.

HCV isolates cloned from different geographic areas show significant sequence divergence, classified into six major genotypes (types 1–6) based on phylogenetic tree analysis of subgenomic regions, with further divisions into subtypes (1a, 1b, 2a, 2b, etc.) *(59)*. Even within a single infected individual, HCV can exist as a population of viruses with closely related genomes, which are called quasispecies *(50,51,60)*. The increased diversity of HCV quasispecies has been linked to longer duration of HCV infection, older age, higher level of viremia, and HCV genotype 1 infection *(60,61)*.

HCV Life Cycle and Viral Replication

Electron microscopic analysis of HCV particles in serum, liver extracts, or human B- or T-cell lines infected with HCV in vitro has shown particles of 50–75 nm and smaller particles of 30–35 or 45–55 nm *(62,63)*. The smaller particles are observed after detergent treatment or in high-density sucrose fractions and are presumed to be the naked core structure, while the larger particles appear to be the intact virions *(51)*.

Because of the lack of an efficient culture cell system for HCV propagation, the mechanisms of intracellular replication of HCV remain largely speculative *(50)*. Based on analogy with flaviviruses, the replication strategy of HCV is thought to occur via a minus-strand intermediate. In brief, the HCV virion probably enters into the liver cell by receptor-mediated endocytosis. The incoming virus particle uncoats and releases the genomic plus strand, which is translated to produce a single long polyprotein that is probably processed co- and posttranslationally to produce individual structural and nonstructural proteins. The nonstructural proteins presumably form a replication complex that utilizes the viral RNA as a template for the synthesis of minus strands. The minus strands in turn serve as templates for synthesis of plus strands. The NS5b in the replication complex provides the RNA-dependent RNA polymerase for the elongation of the nascent minus-strand RNA, while the viral NS3 helicase provides the unwinding activity. The full-length plus-strand RNA genome is then assembled with the mature nucleocapsid to form the viral core, which is then encoated with the viral envelope to form the mature HCV virion. The core protein is then released to form the viral capsid, which in conjunction with the viral RNA forms the complete core of the viral particle. The envelope proteins subsequently mature to form the envelope that coats the viral core and virus assembly is complete. The HCV particles then bud out of the liver cell into the extracellular compartment.

Although HCV is essentially hepatotropic, several lines of evidence suggest that this virus can infect peripheral blood mononuclear cells (PBMCs) in most patients with chronic HCV infection *(53)*. Our recent study also showed that HCV indeed actively infects PBMC of patients with chronic hepatitis C. However, HCV infection of PBMC did not seem to correlate with the pathogenesis of liver cell damage, and PBMC tropism of HCV was not preferentially influenced by viral genotypes *(64)*. Nevertheless, more specific information is needed to clarify the mechanisms concerning the PBMC tropism of HCV.

Animal Models of HCV

At present, the chimpanzee is the only animal shown to be consistently infected with HCV *(65)*. Several features of human HCV infection are recapitulated in the chimpanzee model. Most importantly, the frequency of persistent infection is high in both species, and virus replication occurs despite evidence of cellular and humoral immune responses. A key difference is that necroinflammatory lesions in chronically infected chimpanzees are almost always mild, whereas in humans the disease spectrum is wide, ranging from mild to severe hepatitis and end-stage liver disease requiring liver transplantation. However, chimpanzees can indeed develop HCC after long-term HCV infection, suggesting that cofactors may not be needed for HCV-associated hepatocarcinogenesis. In addition, vertical transmission has not yet been identified in chimpanzees, and cross-challenge experiments have revealed only a limited degree of immunity after natural infection. Understanding the similarities and differences of chronic HCV infection in the two species is important for the development of preventive measures and effective therapy for HCV infection.

Molecular Pathogenesis of HCV

HCV, like HBV, is important globally. The World Health Organization (WHO) recently estimated that there are 170 million HCV carriers worldwide, and 80% of patients with acute HCV infection develop chronic hepatitis. Among them, up to 20% have been estimated to progress to liver cirrhosis, and 1–5% may develop HCC over a period of 20–30 yr *(49)*.

Immunopathogenesis

Despite advances in our knowledge of the epidemiology and molecular virology of HCV, the mechanisms of hepatocellular injury in HCV infection are not completely understood. Studies of the pathogenesis of chronic hepatitis C are difficult because of the lack of an animal or cell culture model. Indirect evidence suggests that HCV may be cytopathic at high levels, and this may lead to a unique pattern of rapidly progressive fibrosing cholestatic liver disease in a small proportion of immunosuppressed patients with very high levels of viremia, as in the situation of chronic HBV infection *(66)*. However, in most patients with chronic HCV infection, there is a growing body of evidence that the host immune response plays the major role in controlling HCV infection and causing hepatocellular damage *(67)*.

Hepatocarcinogenesis

So far, the mechanism of hepatocarcinogenesis of HCV remains unclear. Although replicative HCV intermediates, such as minus-strand HCV RNA, have been detected in HCC tissues *(68)*, HCV RNA does not integrate into the cellular genome as does HBV, and little is known about the biologic activities of HCV proteins. It is more likely that HCV-related HCC occurs against a background of repeated necroinflammation and regeneration, associated with liver injury due to chronic hepatitis, contributing to the complex multistep process of hepatocarcinogenesis *(20)*. Most, if not all, cases of HCV-related HCC occur in the presence of cirrhosis, suggesting that it is the underlying liver disease *per se* that is the risk factor for HCC rather than HCV infection (Fig. 4).

It is noteworthy, however, that patients with HCV-related HCC but without liver cirrhosis have been reported recently *(69)*. Although the absence of liver cirrhosis at the time of HCC presentation does not exclude the possible role of previous necroinflammation in the development of HCC, these cases may provide evidence for an association between HCV and HCC independent of liver cirrhosis. For example, the 5' half of the sequence encoding the HCV nonstructural protein NS3 has been shown to have oncogenic activity and can transform mouse fibroblast cells after transfection *(70)*. Recently, the transforming potential of the HCV core gene has been investigated by using primary rat embryo fibroblast (REF) cells that were transfected with or without cooperative oncogenes *(71)*. Integration of the HCV core gene resulted in expression of the viral protein in REF-stable transformants. REF cells cotransfected with HCV core and H-*ras* genes became transformed and exhibited rapid proliferation, anchor-independent growth, and tumor formation in athymic nude mice. These results suggest that the core protein plays an important role in the regulation of HCV-infected cell growth and in the transformation to tumorigenic phenotype. In addition, development of HCC in two independent lines of mice transgenic for the HCV core gene has been demonstrated. These mice had hepatic steatosis early in life, which is a histologic feature

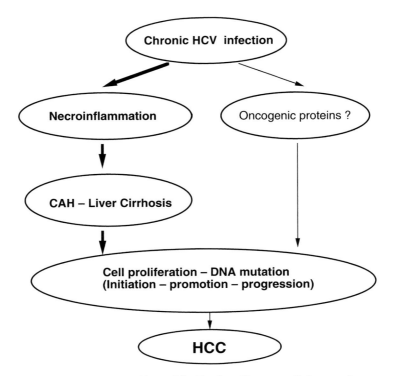

Fig. 4. Pathogenesis of hepatitis C-related hepatocellular carcinoma

associated with chronic hepatitis C *(72)*. After the age of 16 mo, mice of both lines developed hepatic tumors that first appeared as adenomas containing fat droplets in the cytoplasm. Subsequently, a more poorly differentiated HCC developed from within the adenomas, presenting in a "nodule-in-nodule" manner without cytoplasmic fat droplets. This closely resembles the histopathologic characteristics of the early stage of HCC in patients with chronic hepatitis C. Their results indicated that the HCV core protein may have a direct role in the development of HCC. Taken together, these findings suggest that HCV could be directly carcinogenic rather than acting simply through liver cirrhosis. On the other hand, *p53* gene mutations, consisting of a G to T transition in codon 249 and a G to T/A to T transversion, have been identified in patients with HCV-related HCC *(73)*. This suggests that HCV also may affect carcinogenesis via a *p53* mechanism. Nevertheless, a better understanding of the biology of HCV infection is needed to clarify its role in HCC development including promotion, induction, and malignant cell transformation.

Some reports have found that infection with HCV genotype 1b was associated with a higher incidence of liver cirrhosis and HCC compared to infection with other genotypes *(74–77)*. However, this needs to be confirmed in larger series and other populations.

Therapy

The currently recommended 12- to 18-mo course of IFN-α in doses of 3 million units three times a week for the therapy of chronic hepatitis C can clear HCV RNA and normalize serum aminotransferase levels as well as liver histology in approx 20% of patients *(41)*. Sustained responses have been associated with marked improvements in hepatic histology, and long-term studies indicate that the majority of patients remain free of virus in serum and liver, suggesting a "cure" of infection. New approaches to therapy for hepatitis C include combination therapy with IFN-α and ribavirin, for which the sustained response rate (40–50%) has been higher than that for interferon alone (10–20%) *(78–80)*.

It has been suggested that the progression of HCC can be halted or slowed down by treatment of the underlying HCV infection. A recent study from Japan indicated that patients with HCV-related liver cirrhosis have a significantly lower risk of HCC if treated with IFN-α than those who were not treated *(81)*. This decrease of HCC was noted not only in those who had a good response to interferon but also in those who did not. Nevertheless, these findings await further confirmation. Although combination therapy could induce a sustained response rate in 50% of patients, this is not adequate. Search for other antiviral compounds is in progress, and some new drugs may soon be available for HCV clinical trials. The current approaches include protease inhibitors, helicase inhibitors, and long-acting IFN (pegylated IFN). As was true in the search for the best therapy for human immunodeficiency virus infection, it will be a daunting challenge to develop the most effective yet least costly combination therapies for HCV infection. Ultimately, improvements in therapy against HCV infection will depend on the development of better in vitro cell culture and also on further elucidation of the molecular biology of HCV infection.

Prevention

The quasispecies nature and variation of amino acid sequences on the envelope proteins of the HCV virion may allow the virus to escape the neutralizing antibodies and then establish persistent infection *(57,58,61)*. As confirmed in chimpanzee experiments, antibody against E2 after vaccination was found either to confer only transient protection against HCV infection or to ameliorate the severity of clinical hepatitis, if animals were infected *(82)*. In addition, the lack of protective immunity against reinfection with heterotypic or homotypic HCV infection in an already infected host was documented in both chimpanzee experiments and human observations *(83–86)*. Taken together, these findings pose a major obstacle to the design of a preventive vaccine against HCV.

Until effective and safe immunoprophylaxis is available, interruption of transmission routes such as screening blood donors for anti-HCV, use of disposable medical instruments, especially needles and syringes, and avoidance of sharing personal tools remains the mainstay of prevention of HCV infection.

REFERENCES

1. Parkin DM, Stjernsward T, Muir CS. Estimates of the worldwide frequency of twelve major cancers. Bull World Health Org 1984; 62:163–182.
2. Colombo M. Hepatocellular carcinoma. J Hepatol 1992; 15:225–236.
3. Chen DS. From hepatitis to hepatoma: lessons from type B viral hepatitis. Science 1993; 262:369–370.
4. Purcell RH. The discovery of hepatitis viruses. Gastroenterology 1993; 104:955–963.

5. Blumberg BS, Alter HJ, Visnich S. A "new" antigen in leukemia sera. JAMA 1965; 191:541–546.

6. Dane DS, Cameron CH, Briggs M. Virus-like particles in serum of patients with Australia-antigen-associated hepatitis. Lancet 1970; 1:695–698.

7. Kaplan PM, Greenman RL, Gerin JL, Purcell RH, Robinson WS. DNA polymerase associated with human hepatitis B antigen. J Virol 1973; 12:995–1005.

8. Robinson WS, Greenman RL. DNA polymerase in the core of the human hepatitis B virus candidate. J Virol 1974; 13:1231–1236.

9. Robinson WS. The genome of hepatitis B virus. Annu Rev Microbiol 1977; 31:357–377.

10. Lee WM. Hepatitis B Virus Infection. N Engl J Med 1997; 337:1733–1745.

11. Lau JYN, Wright TL. Molecular virology and pathogenesis of hepatitis B. Lancet 1993; 342:1335–1344.

12. Nassal M, Schaller H. Hepatitis B virus replication. Trends Microbiol 1993; 1:221–228.

13. Roggendorf M, Tolle TK. The woodchuck: an animal model for hepatitis B virus infection in man. Intervirology 1995; 38:100–112.

14. Tabor E, Purcell RH, Gerety RJ. Primate animal model and titered inocula for the study of human hepatitis A, hepatitis B, and non-A, non-B hepatitis. J Med Primatol 1993; 12:305–318.

15. Thung SN, Gerber MA, Popper H, Hoyer BH, London WT, Ford EC, Bonino F, Purcell RH. Animal model of human disease: chimpanzee carriers of hepatitis B virus (chimpanzee hepatitis B carriers). Am J Pathol 1991; 3:328–332.

16. Buendia MA. Hepatitis B viruses and liver cancer: the woodchuck model. In: Mason A, Neil J, McCrea M (eds). Viruses and Cancer. Cambridge: Cambridge University Press, 1994, pp. 183–187.

17. Fourel G, Couturier J, Wei Y, Apiou F, Tiollais P, Buendia MA. Evidence for long-range oncogene activation by hepadnavirus insertion. EMBO J 1994; 13:2526–2534.

18. Fourel G, Trepo C, Bougueleret L, Henglein B, Ponzetto A, Tiollais P, Buendia MA. Frequent activation of N-*myc* genes by hepadnavirus insertion in woodchuck liver tumours. Nature 1990; 347:294–298.

19. Hsu T, Moroy T, Etiemble J, Louise A, Trepo C, Tiollais P, Buendia MA. Activation of c-*myc* by woodchuck hepatitis virus insertion in hepatocellular carcinoma. Cell 1988; 55:627–635.

20. Brechot C. Molecular mechanisms of hepatitis B and C viruses related to liver carcinogenesis. Hepatogastroenterology 1998; (Suppl 3): 1189–1196.

21. Chang MH, Chen CJ, Lai MS, Hsu HM, Wu TC, Kong MS, Liang DC, Shau WY, Chen DS, Taiwan Childhood Hepatoma Study Group. Universal hepatitis B vaccination in Taiwan and the incidence of hepatocellular carcinoma in children. N Engl J Med 1997; 336:1855–1859.

22. Chisari FV. Cytotoxic T cells and viral hepatitis. J Clin Invest 1997; 99:1472–1477.

23. Tsai SL, Chen MH, Yeh CT, Chu CM, Lin AN, Chiou FH, Chang TH, Liaw YF. Purification and characterization of a naturally processed hepatitis B virus peptide recognized by CD8+ cytotoxic T lymphocytes. J Clin Invest 1996; 97:577–584.

24. AI Faraidy K, Yoshida EM, Davis JE, Vartanian RK, Anderson FH, Steinbrecher UP. Alteration of the dismal natural history of fibrosing cholestatic hepatitis secondary to hepatitis B virus with the use of lamivudine. Transplantation 1997; 64:926–928.

25. Chen DS, Hoyer BH, Nelson J, Purcell RH, Gerin JL. Detection and properties of hepatitis B viral DNA in liver tissue from patients with hepatocellular carcinoma. Hepatology 1982; 2:42S–46S.

26. Lai MY, Chen DS, Chen PJ, Lee SC, Sheu JC, Huang GT, Wei TC, Lee CS, Yu SC, Hsu HC. Status of hepatitis B virus DNA in hepatocellular carcinoma: a study based on paired tumor and nontumor liver tissues. J Med Virol 1988; 25:249–258.

27. Peng SY, Lai PL, Hsu HC. Amplification of the c-*myc* gene in human hepatocellular carcinoma: biologic significance. J Formos Med Assoc 1993; 92:866–870.

28. Tabor E. Tumor suppressor genes, growth factor genes, and oncogenes in hepatitis B virus-associated hepatocellular carcinoma. J Med Virol 1994; 42:357–365.

29. Zhang YJ, Jiang W, Chen CJ, Lee CS, Kahn SM, Santella RM, Weinstein IB. Amplification and overexpression of cyclin D1 in human hepatocellular carcinoma. Biochem Biophys Res Commun 1993; 196:1010–1016.

30. Chen HL, Chen YC, Chen DS. Chromosome 1p aberrations are frequent in human primary hepatocellular carcinoma. Cancer Genet Cytogenet 1996; 86:102–106.

31. Chen HL, Chiu TS, Chen PJ, Chen DS. Cytogenetic studies on human liver cancer cell lines. Cancer Genet Cytogenet 1993; 65:161–166.

32. Yeh SH, Chen PJ, Chen HL, Lai MY, Wang CC, Chen DS. Frequent genetic alterations at the distal region of chromosome 1p in human hepatocellular carcinomas. Cancer Res 1994; 54:4188–4192.

33. Yeh SH, Chen PJ, Lai MY, Chen DS. Allelic loss on chromosomes 4q and 16q in hepatocellular carcinoma: association with elevated alpha-fetoprotein production. Gastroenterology 1996; 110:184–192.

34. Teramoto T, Satonaka K, Kitazawa S, Fujimori T, Hayashi K, Maeda S. *p53* gene abnormalities are closely related to hepatoviral infections and occur at a late stage of hepatocarcinogenesis. Cancer Res 1994; 54:231–235.

35. Diamantis ID, McGandy C, Chen TJ, Liaw YF, Gudat F, Bianchi L. A new mutational hot-spot in the *p53* gene in human hepatocellular carcinoma. J Hepatol 1994; 20:553–556.

36. Hsu HC, Huang AM, Lai PL, Chien WM, Peng SY, Lin SW. Genetic alterations at the splice junction of p53 gene in human hepatocellular carcinoma. Hepatology 1994; 19:122–128.

37. Hsu HC, Tseng HJ, Lai PL, Lee PH, Peng SY. Expression of *p53* gene in 184 unifocal hepatocellular carcinomas: association with tumor growth and invasiveness. Cancer Res 1993; 53:4691–4694.

38. Lunn RM, Zhang YJ, Wang LY, Chen CJ, Lee PH, Lee CS, Tsai WY, Santella RM. *p53* mutations, chronic hepatitis B virus infection, and aflatoxin exposure in hepatocellular carcinoma in Taiwan. Cancer Res 1997; 57:3471–3477.

39. Sheu JC, Huang GT, Lee PH, Chung JC, Chou HC, Lai MY, Wang JT, Lee HS, Shih LN, Yang PM, Wang TH, Chen DS. Mutation of *p53* gene in hepatocellular carcinoma in Taiwan. Cancer Res 1992; 52:6098–6100.

40. Lai MY, Chang HC, Li HP, Ku CK, Chen PJ, Sheu JC, Huang GT, Lee PH, Chen DS. Splicing mutations of the *p53* gene in human hepatocellular carcinoma. Cancer Res 1993; 53:1653–1656.

41. Hoofnagle JH, Di Bisceglie AM. The treatment of chronic viral hepatitis. N Engl J Med 1997; 336:347–356.

42. Niederau C, Heintges T, Lange S, Goldmann G, Niederau CM, Mohr L, Haussinger D. Long-term follow-up of HBeAg-positive patients treated with interferon alfa for chronic hepatitis B. N Engl J Med 1996; 334:1422–1427.

43. Lai CL, Chien RN, Leung NW, Chang TT, Guan R, Tai DI, Ng KY, Wu PC, Dent JC, Barber J, Stephenson SL, Gray DF. A one-year trial of lamivudine for chronic hepatitis B. Asia Hepatitis Lamivudine Study Group. N Engl J Med 1998; 339:61–68.

44. Chen DS, Hsu HM, Chang MH, Sung JL, and the Hepatitis Control Committee. Hepatitis B vaccines: status report on long-term efficacy. In: Rizzetto M, Purcell RH, Gerin JL, Verme G (eds). Viral Hepatitis and Liver Disease. Turin: Edizioni Minerva Medica, 1997, pp. 635–637.

45. Chen HL, Chang MH, Ni YH, Hsu HY, Lee PI, Lee CY, Chen DS. Seroepidemiology of hepatitis B virus infection in children: ten years of mass vaccination in Taiwan. JAMA 1996; 276:906–908.

46. Choo QL, Kuo G, Weiner AJ, Overby LR, Bradley DW, Houghton M. Isolation of a cDNA clone derived from a blood-borne non-A, non-B viral hepatitis genome. Science 1989; 244:359–362.

47. Kao JH, Tsai SL, Yang PM, Sheu JC, Lai MY, Hsu HC, Sung JL, Wang TH, Chen DS. A clinico-pathologic study of chronic non-A, non-B (type C) hepatitis in Taiwan: comparison between posttransfusion and sporadic patients. J Hepatol 1994; 21:244–249.

48. Kuo G, Choo QL, Alter HJ, Gitnick GI, Redeker AG, Purcell RH, Miyamura T, Dienstag JL, Alter MJ, Stevens CE, Tegtmeier GE, Overby LR, Bradley DW, Houghton M. An assay for circu-lating antibodies to a major etiologic virus of human non-A, non-B hepatitis. Science 1989; 244:362–364.

49. Sharara AL, Hunt CM, Hamilton JD. Hepatitis C. Ann Intern Med 1996; 125:658–668.

50. Fang JWS, Chow V, Lau JYN. Virology of hepatitis C virus. Clin Liver Dis 1997; 1:493–514.

51. Major ME, Feinstone SM. The molecular virology of hepatitis C. Hepatology 1997; 25:1527–1538.

52. Simmonds P. Virology of hepatitis C virus. Clin Ther 1996; 18 (Suppl B):9–36.

53. Trepo C, Vierling J, Zeytin FN, Gerlich WH. The first Flaviviridae symposium. Intervirology 1997; 40:279–288.

54. Linnen J, Wages J, Zhang-Keck ZY, Fry KE, Krawczynski KZ, Alter H, Koonin E, Gallagher M, Alter M, Hadziyannis S, Karayiannis P, Fung K, Nakatsuji Y, Shih JW, Young L, Piatak M, Hoover C, Fernandez J, Chen S, Zou JC, Morrris T, Hyams KC, Ismay S, Lifson JD, Hess G, Foung SKH, Thomas H, Bradley D, Margolis H, Kim JP. Molecular cloning and disease associa-tion of hepatitis G virus: a transfusion-transmissible agent. Science 1996; 271:505–508.

55. Simons JN, Leary TP, Dawson GJ, Pilot-Matias TJ, Muerhoff AS, Schlauder GG, Desai SM, Mushahwar IK. Isolation of novel virus-like sequences associated with human hepatitis. Nat Med 1995; 1:564–569.

56. Zuckerman AJ, Alphabet of hepatitis viruses. Lancet 1996; 347:558–559.

57. Farci P, Shimoda A, Wong D, Cabezon T, De Gioannis D, Strazzera A, Shimizu Y, Shapiro M, Alter HJ, Purcell RH. Prevention of hepatitis C virus infection in chimpanzees by hyperimmune serum against the hypervariable region 1 of the envelope 2 protein. Proc Natl Acad Sci USA 1996; 93:15394–15399.

58. Kato N, Sekiya H, Ootsuyama Y, Nakazawa T, Hijikata M, Ohkoshi S, Shimotohno K. Humoral immune response to hypervariable region 1 of the putative envelope glycoprotein (gp70) of hepatitis C virus. J Virol 1993; 67:3923–3930.

59. Simmonds P, Holmes EC, Cha TA, Chan SW, McOmish F, Irvine B, Beall E, Yap PL, Kolberg J, Urdea MS. Classification of hepatitis C virus into six major genotypes and a series of subtypes by phylogenetic analysis of the NS-5 region. J Gen Virol 1993; 74:2391–2399.

60. Kao JH, Chen PJ, Lai MY, Wang TH, Chen DS. Quasispecies of hepatitis C virus and genetic drift of the hypervariable region in chronic type C hepatitis. J Infect Dis 1995; 172:261–264.

61. Kato N, Ootsuyama Y, Sekiya H, Ohkoshi S, Nakazawa T, Hijikata M, Shimotohno K. Genetic drift in hypervariable region 1 of the viral genome in persistent hepatitis C virus infection. J Virol 1994; 68:4776–4784.

62. Kaito M, Watanabe S, Tsukiyama-Kohara K, Yamaguchi K, Kobayashi Y, Konishi M, Yokoi M, Ishida S, Suzuki S, Kohara M. Hepatitis C virus particle detected by immunoelectron micro-scopic study. J Gen Virol 1994; 75:1755–1760.

63. Takahashi K, Kishimoto S, Yoshizawa H, Okamoto H, Yoshikawa A, Mishiro S. p26 protein and 33-nm particle associated with nucleocapsid of hepatitis C virus recovered from the circulation of infected hosts. Virology 1992; 191:431–434.

64. Kao JH, Chen PJ, Lai MY, Wang TH, Chen DS. Positive and negative strand of hepatitis C virus RNA sequences in peripheral blood mononuclear cells in patients with chronic hepatitis C: no correlation with viral genotypes 1b, 2a, and 2b. J Med Virol 1997; 52:270–274.

65. Walker CM. Comparative features of hepatitis C virus infection in humans and chimpanzees. Springer Semin Immunopathol 1997; 19:85–98.

66. Toth CM, Pascual M, Chung RT, Graeme-Cook F, Dienstag JL, Bhan AK, Cosimi AB. Hepatitis C virus-associated fibrosing cholestatic hepatitis after renal transplantation: response to interferon-alpha therapy. Transplantation 1998; 66:1254–1258.

67. Nelson DR, Lau JYN. Pathogenesis of hepatocellular damage in chronic hepatitis C virus infection. Clin Liver Dis 1997; 1:515–527.

68. Gerber MA, Shieh CYS, Shim KS, Swan NT, Demetris AJ. Detection of replicative hepatitis C virus sequences in hepatocellular carcinoma. Am J Pathol 1992; 141:1271–1277.

69. De Mitri MS, Poussin K, Baccarini P, Pontisso P, D'Errico A, Simon N, Grigioni W, Alberti A, Beaugrand M, Pisi E. HCV-associated liver cancer without cirrhosis. Lancet 1995; 345:413–415.

70. Sakamuro D, Furukawa T, Takegami T. Hepatitis C virus nonstructural protein NS3 transforms NIH 3T3 cells. J Virol 1995; 69:3893–3896.

71. Ray RB, Lagging LM, Meyer K, Ray R. Hepatitis C virus core protein cooperates with *ras* and transforms primary rat embryo fibroblasts to tumorigenic phenotype. J Virol 1996; 70:4438–4443.

72. Moriya K, Fujie H, Shintani Y, Yotsuyanagi H, Tsutsumi T, Ishibashi K, Matsuura Y, Kimura S, Miyamura T, Koike K. The core protein of hepatitis C virus induces hepatocellular carcinoma in transgenic mice. Nat Med 1998; 4:1065–1067.

73. Puisieux A, Ozturk M. TP53 and hepatocellular carcinoma. Pathol Biol (Paris) 1997; 45:864–870.

74. Kao JH, Chen PJ, Lai MY, Yang PM, Sheu JC, Wang TH, Chen DS. Genotypes of hepatitis C virus in Taiwan and the progression of liver disease. J Clin Gastroenterol 1995; 21:233–237.

75. Kao JH, Lai MY, Chen PJ, Hwang LH, Chen DS. Serum hepatitis C virus titers in the progression of type C chronic liver disease. With special emphasis on patients with type 1b infection. J Clin Gastroenterol 1996; 23:280–283.

76. Kato N, Yokosuka O, Hosoda K, Ito Y, Ohto M, Omata M. Quantification of hepatitis C virus by competitive reverse transcription-polymerase chain reaction. Hepatology 1993; 18:16–20.

77. Mahaney K, Tedeschi V, Maertens G, Di Bisceglie AM, Vergalla J, Hoofnagle JH, Sallie R. Genotypic analyses of hepatitis C virus in American patients. Hepatology 1994; 20:1405–1411.

78. Davis GL, Esteban-Mur R, Rustgi V, Hoefs J, Gordon SC, Trepo C, Shiffman ML, Zeuzem S, Craxi A, Ling MH, Albrecht J. Interferon alpha-2b alone or in combination with ribavirin for the treatment of relapse of chronic hepatitis C. N Engl J Med 1998; 339:1493–1499.

79. Lai MY, Kao JH, Yang PM, Wang JT, Chen PJ, Chan KW, Chu JS, Chen DS. Long-term efficacy of ribavirin plus interferon alpha in the treatment of chronic hepatitis C. Gastroenterology 1996; 111:1307–1312.

80. Reichard O, Norkrans G, Fryden A, Braconier JH, Sonnerborg A, Weiland O. Randomized, double-blind, placebo-controlled trial of interferon alpha-2b and without ribavirin for chronic hepatitis C. Lancet 1998; 351:83–87.

81. Nishiguchi S, Kuroki T, Nakatani S, Morimoto H, Takeda T, Nakajima S, Shiomi S, Seki S, Kobayashi K, Otani S. Randomised trial of effects of interferon-α on incidence of hepatocellular carcinoma in chronic active hepatitis C with cirrhosis. Lancet 1995; 346:1051–1055.

82. Choo QL, Kuo G, Ralston R, Weiner A, Chien D, Van Nest G, Han J, Berger K, Thudium K, Kuo C, Houghton M. Vaccination of chimpanzees against infection by the hepatitis C virus. Proc Natl Acad Sci USA 1994; 91:1294–1298.

83. Farci P, Alter HJ, Govindarajan S, Wong DC, Engle Rpurcell RH. Lack of protective immunity against reinfection with hepatitis C virus. Science 1992; 258:135–140.

84. Kao JH, Chen PJ, Lai MY, Chen DS. Superinfection of heterologous hepatitis C virus in a patient with chronic type C hepatitis. Gastroenterology 1993; 105:583–587.

85. Kao JH, Chen PJ, Lai MY, Yang PM, Sheu JC, Wang TH, Chen DS. Mixed infections of hepatitis C virus as a factor in acute exacerbation of chronic type C hepatitis. J Infect Dis 1994; 170:1128–1133.

86. Kao JH, Chen PJ, Lai MY, Yang PM, Wang TH, Chen DS. Superinfection of homotypic virus in hepatitis C virus carriers: studies on patients with posttransfusion hepatitis. J Med Virol 1996; 50:303–308.

18
Hepatocellular Carcinoma

Michael C. Kew

INTRODUCTION

Hepatocellular carcinoma (HCC) is regarded as one of the major malignant diseases in the world today. There are a number of justifications for this view. Although uncommon or even rare in most countries, HCC is the most prevalent, or among the most prevalent, tumors in many parts of eastern and southeastern Asia and the western Pacific islands as well as throughout sub-Saharan Africa, regions that are among the most populous in the world (1,2). At least 310,000 new cases of the tumor are diagnosed each year, 140,000 in the People's Republic of China alone (1). Relative to other tumors, HCC ranks fifth in overall frequency, fourth in males and seventh in females, and it accounts for 4–5% of the global cancer burden (1,2). Its often rapid course, difficulty in diagnosis before the disease is advanced, small chance of resection when symptomatic, high recurrence rate after resection or liver transplantation, and failure to respond to chemotherapy and irradiation are responsible for a prognosis so grave that the annual mortality rate is virtually the same as the annual incidence (3). In developing countries in the Far East and Africa with the highest incidences of HCC, the tumor has far-reaching socioeconomic consequences, developing as it often does at a relatively young age (50% of Mozambican Shangaans are < 30 yr of age when they present with HCC [4]) and affecting men predominantly (3). For all these reasons, prevention of HCC is paramount.

Toward this end, a number of environmental risk factors for HCC have been identified during recent years, and primary prevention of the more important of these is already possible or should soon become possible. A start has also been made in unravelling the complex mechanisms of hepatocarcinogenesis, paving the way for strategies for secondary and tertiary prevention of the tumor to be developed and instituted, and contributing to our understanding of oncogenesis in general. HCC was one of the first human tumors to be linked causally with virus infection, and among the principal risk factors already recognized are two hepatotropic viruses, one of which, hepatitis B virus (HBV), is now considered to be, with tobacco, the most important environmental carcinogens to which humans are exposed.

Before reviewing what is known of the pathogenesis of virally induced HCC, some aspects of the diagnosis, pathology, and treatment of the tumor are briefly considered.

From: *Infectious Causes of Cancer: Targets for Intervention*
Edited by: J. J. Goedert © Humana Press Inc., Totowa, NJ

DIAGNOSIS

Clinical Recognition

Advanced HCC usually presents with symptoms and signs sufficiently characteristic to allow the diagnosis to be suspected, especially in populations in which this tumor is common or when a risk factor is known to be present *(3)*. In its early stages, however, HCC runs a silent course, making recognition difficult at the only time that the tumor is likely to be amenable to treatment.

Although HCC often coexists with cirrhosis *(5)*, the influence that the cirrhosis exerts on the diagnosis of the tumor differs between regions of high and low (or intermediate) incidence of HCC. In the latter (but also in Japan, a country with a high incidence), HCC commonly develops as a late complication of symptomatic cirrhosis resulting from chronic hepatitis C virus (HCV) infection or alcohol abuse, or both *(3,6)*. The patient has few, if any, symptoms attributable to the tumor. If, in addition, the tumor is small (as it often is in a cirrhotic liver in these regions) it is seldom obvious in the presence of advanced cirrhosis and is discovered only on hepatic imaging, during liver transplantation or other surgical intervention, or at necropsy. The onset of unexplained abdominal pain, weight loss, ascites, or liver enlargement in a patient known to have cirrhosis should alert the clinician to the possibility that HCC has supervened. In contrast, in ethnic Chinese and black African populations the associated cirrhosis either produces no symptoms or the symptoms are overshadowed by those ascribed to the tumor *(3,6)*. Consequently, the cirrhosis is uncovered only during the diagnostic workup or at necropsy. In addition, HCCs in these populations are typically appreciably larger than in those with low or intermediate incidences. Right hypochondrial or upper abdominal pain, weight loss, and weakness are the most common symptoms, and the patient may also be aware of a mass in the upper abdomen *(3,6)*. The liver is almost always enlarged, sometimes massively so, and tender with an irregular or smooth surface. An arterial bruit, or rarely a friction rub, may be heard over the tumorous liver. Overt jaundice is uncommon when the patient is first seen.

HCC may present in a number of atypical ways *(6)*. These include presentations with obstructive jaundice, hypoglycemia, hypercalcemia, acute hemoperitoneum, Budd–Chiari syndrome, inferior vena caval obstruction, superior mediastinal syndrome, bone pain, Virchow–Trossier node, fever of unknown origin, arterial hypertension, feminization, or skin rashes. Although none is common, an awareness of these presentations may prevent the diagnosis being delayed or even missed.

Tumor Markers

A sensitive and specific serum marker for HCC would greatly facilitate its diagnosis, and a large number of candidates have been advocated over the years *(7)*. None, however, is more useful than the one first described, α-fetoprotein (α-FP).

α-Fetoprotein

Serum concentrations of this glycoprotein are raised in most patients with HCC *(7)*. In countries with a high incidence of the tumor, levels are elevated in as many as 90% of patients and very high concentrations are often attained (the mean value is of the order of 70,000 ng/mL, normal < 20 ng/mL). Serum concentrations are less often raised in countries with a low or intermediate incidence of HCC and the level reached is generally lower (mean of the order of 8000 ng/mL). α-FP production by HCC is age related, younger patients being more likely to have raised levels and to attain very high concentrations *(8)*. The differences between countries may therefore be explained in part by the younger ages of many of the patients in high-risk black African and ethnic Chinese populations. No differences in α-FP concentrations exist between the sexes. Nor is there an obvious correlation between serum α-FP levels and any clinical or biochemical indices or with survival time of the patients. In countries with a low incidence of HCC, α-FP concentrations are generally higher when the tumor coexists with cirrhosis or in patients with current HBV infection, but this is not so in countries where the tumor is common. Although synthesis of α-FP in mice with chemically induced HCC correlates with the degree of differentiation of the tumor, the evidence in this regard in human HCC is conflicting.

As useful as α-FP undoubtedly is in the diagnosis of HCC, it falls short of being an ideal serum marker for the tumor. In addition to the false-negative results already mentioned, several diseases give false-positive results *(7)*. These include a variety of benign hepatic diseases, especially acute and chronic hepatitis and cirrhosis. Serum concentrations of α-FP are usually only slightly raised in these conditions, but moderately or even markedly elevated values are sometimes present. Raised levels also occur in approximately one-third of patients with undifferentiated teratocarcinoma or embryonal cell carcinoma of the ovary or testis, and in about 10% of patients with tumors of endodermal origin. If the threshold concentration of α-FP for the diagnosis of HCC is raised to 400 ng/mL (or 500 ng/mL in some laboratories), most false-positive results can be eliminated while still retaining a 70–75% positivity rate in high incidence countries. Inevitably, however, the positivity rate in low incidence regions falls below 50%.

α-FP is heterogeneous in structure. The microheterogeneity results from differences in the asparagine-linked biantenary oligosaccharide side chain of the molecule, and is the reason for the differential affinity of this glycoprotein for lectins. Reactivity with *Lens culinaris* agglutinin A is helpful in differentiating HCC from benign hepatic diseases, and, to a lesser extent, reactivity with concanavalin A in distinguishing between HCC and other α-FP-producing tumors *(7)*. Differential lectin reactivity is particularly useful in differentiating HCC from benign hepatic diseases when the serum α-FP level is only slightly raised. Small asymptomatic HCCs are usually associated with only modestly elevated α-FP levels, and a number of small benign hepatic masses may mimic HCC on hepatic imaging. Accordingly, reactivity with *Lens culinaris* agglutinin A can profitably be used in the surveillance of individuals at high risk of developing HCC. The drawback of the method is the cost, especially because the greatest numbers of patients with HCC occur in countries with the least resources.

Des-Γ-Carboxy Prothrombin

Des-Γ-carboxy prothrombin (also known as "protein induced by vitamin K absence or antagonism" [PIVKA-II]) is a precursor of vitamin K that has been used as a serum marker for HCC *(7)*. The explanation for the production of des-Γ-carboxy prothrombin by the tumor is uncertain. Among the suggested causes are a failure of HCC to express the prothrombin Γ-glutamyl carboxylase gene and abnormal uptake of vitamin K by malignant hepatocytes *(9)*. As a result, the precursor protein accumulates in the tumor and subsequently leaks into the bloodstream. In most populations des-Γ-carboxy pro-thrombin is less useful than α-FP as a serum marker of HCC, although the two markers can be used together to increase the sensitivity and specificity of diagnosis (7).

None of the many other candidate serum markers for HCC can match α-FP for sensitivity and specificity and accordingly they are not used in clinical practice.

Imaging

Hepatic imaging plays a central role in the diagnosis both of symptomatic HCCs and of small HCCs during surveillance programs aimed at the early detection of subclinical tumors in high-risk individuals. Nevertheless, with none of the imaging modalities now available is the picture obtained pathognomonic of HCC and definitive diagnosis still depends on histologic examination of the tissue.

Ultrasonography

Ultrasonography is commonly used to confirm the presence of hepatic masses in symptomatic patients (10). It is widely available, not invasive, relatively inexpensive, easy to perform, and detects almost all symptomatic and presymptomatic HCCs. Large tumors usually have a mixed echogenic/echolucent appearance and an ill-defined margin. Apart from delineating the number, size, and distribution of the lesions, ultrasonography is helpful in evaluating operability of the tumor because of its ability to detect invasion of the portal and hepatic venous systems and the biliary system. In the few symptomatic HCCs invisible on ultrasonography, computed tomography will almost always show the lesion.

Ultrasonography is also the modality of choice for screening the liver during long-term surveillance of individuals at high risk of HCC (10,11). In addition to the advantages already mentioned, ultrasonography can be used repeatedly and is highly sensitive, allowing tumors < 2 cm in diameter and even smaller (which have a better prognosis than larger lesions) to be detected by skilled operators. Moreover, the machine is portable. With very small tumor nodules the ultrasonographic pattern is usually hypoechoic, but about one-third are hyperechoic, reflecting the presence of fatty metamorphosis or clear cells. Some may be isoechoic. A mosaic pattern with septum formation, a peripheral halo, and posterior echo enhancement is a typical appearance.

Two recent refinements to ultrasonography have added new dimensions to its diagnostic capabilities. Dynamic contrast-enhanced ultrasonography with intraarterial infusion of CO_2 microbubbles provides information on the vascularity of small tumors that are undetectable angiographically, and can be used to differentiate HCC from adenomatous hyperplasia, small hemangiomas, metastases, and focal nodular hyperplasia (10). Color Doppler ultrasonography has advantages over pulsed Doppler ultrasonography and may be useful in differentiating a small HCC from focal nodular hyperplasia (10). A further refinement is intravenous contrast-enhanced color Doppler ultrasonography, which is expected to further improve the detection of subclinical HCCs and to aid in the choice of treatment of the tumor (10).

Computed Tomography and Hepatic Angiography

Computed tomography is used in visualizing both symptomatic and small HCCs when ultrasonography is unhelpful, as well as in evaluating operability of the tumor and in planning resection *(12)*. A difference of at least 10 Hounsfield numbers between normal and abnormal areas of the liver is generally needed for accurate detection of liver tumors. Intravenous contrast material infused in conjunction with computed tomography enhances normal liver tissue to a greater degree than most neoplastic tissues and may reveal the pattern of tumor perfusion. It also shows the course, caliber, and patency of blood vessels. Contrast computed tomography may thus facilitate characterization of the tumor. Spiral (helical) computed tomography has the advantage of rapid scanning and allows the peak hepatic enhancement (which occurs 70–120 s after intravenous injection) to be scanned. Tumor enhancement with this method approaches that achieved with arteriography *(12,13)*.

The use of hepatic arteriography in combination with computed tomography further increases the diagnostic capabilities of tomography *(12,13)*. Because HCCs obtain their blood supply from the hepatic artery, computed tomography/ arteriography produces a high attenuation blush of the tumor. In computed tomography/portography injection of contrast material into the superior mesenteric vein causes dense enhancement of portal venous blood and highlights the tumor as a negative image *(12,13)*. Because iodized poppy seed (Lipiodol) is concentrated and retained in tumor tissue, the injection of this material at the end of hepatic arteriography can be used to detect very small HCCs using computed tomography performed after a suitable delay *(12,13)*.

Magnetic Resonance Imaging

This form of imaging is seldom needed for the diagnosis of HCC. Contrast-enhanced magnetic resonance imaging with gadopenetate dimeglumine and fast images with gradient echo sequences or the use of the tissue-specific contrast medium superparamagnetic iron oxide is, however, one of the most accurate ways of differentiating between small HCCs and hemangiomas in the liver *(14)*.

PATHOLOGY

Advanced HCC is classified on visual inspection into expanding (massive), nodular, and diffuse types *(15,16)*. The expanding type consists of a large single tumor (although it may be accompanied by a few small satellite nodules); the nodular type of multiple nodules of different sizes, some of which may be confluent; and the diffuse type of multiple small, ill-defined tumors throughout the liver. The expanding type usually arises in an otherwise normal liver, whereas the diffuse type is typically found in the presence of cirrhosis. In Japan, in particular, the expanding type may be surrounded by a thick fibrous capsule. Early (small) HCCs are divided into distinct nodular and indistinct nodular varieties.

The majority of HCCs in all geographic regions arise in a cirrhotic liver. The morphologic features of HBV-induced cirrhosis differ from those of HCV-induced cirrhosis. In type B cirrhosis, the regenerative nodules are larger than those of type C cirrhosis, the fibrous septa are thin and regular, and active inflammation is infrequent. In type C cirrhosis the nodules are smaller, the fibrous septa are broad and irregular, and active inflammation is common. Cirrhosis resulting from alcohol abuse is typically micronodular, with features generally similar to those seen in type C cirrhosis but with additional specific findings such as pericellular fibrosis, giant mitochondria, and alcoholic hyaline.

HCC is classified according to histologic grade into well-differentiated, moderately differentiated, poorly differentiated, and undifferentiated tumors, and according to histologic pattern into trabecular, acinar (pseudoglandular), compact, scirrhous, and fibrolamellar varieties *(15,16)*. All grades and patterns are seen in advanced HCC, whereas early HCCs are usually well differentiated with a trabecular or acinar pattern. Pleomorphic, clear cell, oncocyte-like, and spindle cell variants may be seen on cytologic as well as histologic examination.

TREATMENT

The treatment of HCC is determined by the extent of the tumor burden, the presence or absence of cirrhosis, and the degree of hepatic dysfunction.

Surgical resection offers the best chance of cure *(17)*. A significant proportion of tumors uncovered during screening of high-risk individuals or populations are resectable, but symptomatic HCCs are seldom amenable to resection. Tumor recurrence, both intrahepatic and extrahepatic, is frequent *(18)*.

Liver transplantation may be performed for those tumors that are not resectable but have not spread beyond the liver *(17,19)*. Tumor recurrence is, however, common.

Alcohol injection may be used to eradicate small HCCs that are not suitable for resection because of their number or position, because liver function is poor, or because the patient refuses surgery *(20)*.

Embolization or chemoembolization has been used in selected patients to reduce the tumor bulk before surgery, but it has yet to be shown that the advantage gained offsets the disadvantages *(21)*.

Chemotherapy has never produced a predictable response rate of > 20% and is therefore used for palliation only *(22)*. Biologic response modifiers have not, to date, been proven to be of value, although the patients treated have always had advanced disease.

Because of the disappointing results of treating symptomatic HCC, much attention has been focussed on detecting the tumor at a presymptomatic stage when it is likely to be small and amenable to surgical or other invasive treatments. Detection of subclinical HCC has taken two forms: mass population screening and long-term surveillance of individuals at high risk of developing HCC *(11)*. Population screening can be contemplated only in those populations having the highest incidences of HCC, and even then the enormity of the task is daunting. The programs undertaken to date have been based solely on measuring serum α-FP concentrations. Because only about 45% of presymptomatic HCCs produce a diagnostic α-FP level, a substantial number of small tumors are overlooked in screening programs of this sort. Monitoring of high-risk individuals (mainly those with persistent HBV or HCV infection) is more feasible and is probably cost effective. It involves periodic imaging of the liver, using ultrasonography in the first instance, and measurement of serum α-FP concentrations.

VIRUS-INDUCED HEPATOCELLULAR CARCINOMA

HCC is multifactorial in etiology, and its pathogenesis, like that of other carcinomas, is a complex process that involves a number of sequential steps and evolves over several or many years. Among the causal associations now identified, two hepatitis viruses, HBV and HCV, predominate. There are some 360 million carriers of HBV in the world today and a further 170 million people are chronically infected with HCV, and all of these are at greatly increased risk for developing HCC. Between them, the two viruses contribute to the etiology of about 80% of global HCC. They do not act alone, however, but in conjunction with other environmental carcinogens and a variety of host factors. Of the other hepatotropic viruses, hepatitis A and E never produce long-term pathologic sequelae, and there is no compelling evidence that hepatitis D virus, which always occurs together with HBV, increases the oncogenic potential of that virus. Hepatitis G virus probably does not cause liver disease of any sort, including HCC, and no data are yet available on the carcinogenic effects of the most recently recognized transfusion-transmitted virus (TTV).

The cellular and molecular basis for virally induced HCC has yet to be fully elucidated. Nevertheless, evidence continues to accumulate that HBV and HCV contribute to hepatocarcinogenesis both indirectly, by causing chronic necroinflammatory hepatic disease, and directly.

HBV AS A HEPATOCARCINOGEN

HBV, a partially double-stranded DNA virus belonging to the Hepadnaviridae, is the single most important risk factor for HCC. Approximately 25% of chronic carriers of the virus develop the tumor *(23)*. In ethnic Chinese and black African populations, which have the highest incidences of HCC, the carrier rates may be as high as 15% *(23–25)*. In these populations HBV infection is acquired predominantly very early in life, as a result of either perinatal transmission from HBV e antigen-positive carrier mothers *(23)* or horizontal infection from recently infected and hence highly infectious young siblings or playmates *(26)*. About 90% of HBV infections contracted during the neonatal period or early in childhood become chronic, and it is these early-onset carriers that have a lifetime relative risk of developing HCC of > 100 *(27)*. HBV carriage has almost always been present for many years before HCC develops, an interval consistent with a cause-and-effect relationship. With increasing duration of infection the chance of tumor formation rises progressively *(23,28)*. In contrast, HBV infection acquired in adulthood seldom becomes chronic, and when it does it is rarely complicated by tumor formation *(29)*.

In those populations with a very high incidence of HBV carriage and HCC in which universal immunization of infants against the virus has been included in the Expanded Program of Immunization for a sufficient length of time, there has already been a decrease in the carrier rate of the virus and the incidence of HCC *(30)*, providing further proof, if any was needed, of the pivotal role of chronic HBV infection in the genesis of HCC in these populations.

Direct Carcinogenicity by Integration

Circumstantial evidence that HBV is directly carcinogenic comes from three sources. Although most HBV-related HCCs coexist with cirrhosis, supporting the belief that virally induced chronic necroinflammatory hepatic disease plays an important part in the pathogenesis of HCC *(31,32)*, the remaining tumors arise in an otherwise normal liver. Moreover, in populations with a high incidence of HBV-related HCC, markers of current infection with the virus are present as often in serum and liver and tumor tissue of HCC patients without cirrhosis as in those of those with cirrhosis *(33,34)*. The demonstration that HBV DNA is integrated into cellular DNA in the great majority of these tumors provides further support for a direct oncogenic effect of the virus *(35)*. Insertion of HBV DNA into chromosomal DNA precedes the development of HCC, and the presence of discrete hybridization bands in individual tumors indicates clonal expansion of cells with integrants. Nevertheless, integration of HBV DNA has not been proved to be indispensable to the pathogenesis of virally induced HCC. Additional circumstantial evidence comes from the observation that in animals chronically infected with certain Hepadnaviridae *(36)* and in transgenic mice into which the HBV *X* gene together with its regulatory sequences have been introduced *(37)*, HCC develops in the absence of chronic necroinflammatory hepatic disease.

A number of putative mechanisms for direct oncogenicity of HBV are supported by experimental evidence. The finding of HBV DNA integrants in chromosomal DNA in HCC is consistent with insertional mutagenesis, a mechanism of oncogenesis described with nonacutely transforming viruses. Viral DNA integration in HCC appears, however, to occur at random sites (although some chromosomes are affected more often than others) *(38)*, which argues against insertion in or near protooncogenes, growth regulatory genes, or tumor suppressor genes, or their regulatory elements, being a numerically important mechanism for initiating carcinogenesis. Indeed, in only a few human HCCs have integrants been detected in relation to a protooncogene or growth regulatory gene in or near a tumor suppressor gene *(39,40)*. In contrast, 41% of HCCs in woodchucks infected with woodchuck hepatitis virus (WHV) (another member of the Hepadnaviridae) contain rearrangements of N-*myc* loci secondary to viral integration that activate expression of the gene *(41)*. On the other hand, only 6% of ground squirrels infected with ground squirrel hepatitis virus (GSHV) have a rearranged N-*myc* allele, and gene amplification is responsible for overexpression of c-*myc (41)*. Moreover, transgenic mice develop HCC after wild-type woodchuck c-*myc* gene together with upstream WHV DNA has been incorporated into the germline *(42)*. Although c-*myc*, N-*ras*, and c-*fos* overexpression has been described in human HCC, expression of these genes is known to be increased during hepatic regeneration, and these findings may be the result rather than the cause of the increased cell proliferation in the tumors *(43)*. Loss or disruption (inversion, duplication, or translocation) of chromosomal DNA in the sequences flanking integrated HBV DNA is a frequent finding in human HCC *(38)*. These changes could promote genomic instability by deleting tumor suppressor genes, or, by altering the physical relation between protooncogenes or tumor suppressor genes and their regulatory elements, may perturb the expression of these genes.

Direct Carcinogenicity—HBV X, Other Viral and Host Genes

HBV DNA integrants may induce malignant transformation in another way. Integration of viral DNA at random sites in host DNA is compatible with activation of transcription in *trans*. The HBV genome is known to contain two *trans*-activators. The HBV *X* gene encodes a 17-kDa protein that is a potent *trans*-activator of a number of cellular promoters, including some that regulate cell proliferation and differentiation, and apoptosis *(44)*. Evidence for an oncogenic role for HBV *X* is mounting. This gene is highly conserved among different viral isolates and, because of its proximity to the preferred integration sites in the viral genome, is the region of HBV DNA most often included in integrants *(45,46)*. Integrated HBV *X,* even when truncated, frequently encodes functionally active *trans*-activator proteins and may overexpress X protein, which could perturb signal transduction pathways important for the regulation of cell growth during hepatocyte regeneration *(47)*. HB X protein transforms mouse fibroblasts in vitro and converts immortalized fetal hepatocytes into a fully malignant phenotype *(48)*. Furthermore, NIH 3T3 cells stably transfected with an HBV *X* expression plasmid are carcinogenic in nude mice *(49)*. Further evidence that X protein can induce malignant transformation is provided by the transgenic mouse model created with the HBV *X* gene together with its regulatory elements *(34)*. The progeny frequently develop HCC, and are also more susceptible to the hepatocarcinogenic effects of diethylnitrosamine *(49)*. Finally, other oncogenic hepadnaviruses, namely, WHV and GSHV, have a discrete *X* gene, whereas duck hepatitis B virus, which does not cause HCC, does not *(50)*.

One of the growth regulatory proteins whose function is affected by HB X protein is that expressed by the tumor suppressor gene, *p53*. This gene has pleiotropic functions including monitoring the integrity of the cellular genome, modulating DNA repair, and promoting cell senescence *(51,52)*. Among its actions are arrest of the cell cycle in G_1, regulation of the DNA damage-control response, and induction of apoptosis *(51,52)*. The nuclear protein encoded by *p53* modulates transcription of a number of genes by binding to specific DNA sequences and to other cellular factors such as MDM2, TBP, and WT-1. There is evidence that HB X protein complexes with the c-terminal end of p53 protein, preventing its DNA consensus binding and transcriptional *trans*-activator functions *(53–55)*. Binding takes place in the cytoplasm, and blocks entry of p53 protein into the nucleus. HB X protein also inhibits binding of XBP, a DNA repair protein, to p53 protein *(56)*. By preventing the p53-dependent checkpoint function of the cell cycle, surveillance of DNA damage, and apoptosis, HB X protein may allow the accumulation of cells with abnormal DNA from which clones with a survival advantage could be selected, thereby playing a role in the genesis of HCC.

HB X protein may interfere with DNA repair in at least two other ways. It complexes with XAP-1, which normally binds to damaged DNA in the first step in nucleotide excision-repair, thereby preventing the cell from efficiently repairing damaged DNA *(57)*. Cells that express HB X protein have been shown to be more susceptible to the lethal effects of low dose ultraviolet irradiation *(58)*. Moreover, this protein binds preferentially to ultraviolet-irradiated DNA through an association with nuclear proteins. HB X protein may thus interfere with cellular DNA repair by binding to damaged DNA. These two mechanisms would allow DNA mutations to accumulate, impairing genetic stability, and resulting eventually in cancer formation.

No obvious correlation has been shown between the presence of integrated HB *X* gene in HCCs and the inactivating guanine to thymine transversion at the third base of codon 249 of *p53* gene that results from heavy dietary exposure to the fungal toxin, aflatoxin B_1 *(45)*. Epidemiologic evidence from parts of Africa and the Far East indicates that repeated ingestion of aflatoxin B_1 is a major risk factor for HCC in these countries *(59)*. Because these populations also have high HBV carrier rates the two risk factors often occur together, although there is no clear evidence that integrated HBV DNA and the specific codon 249 mutation have a synergistic carcinogenic effect *(45)*.

Nevertheless, in these individuals the tumor suppressor effects of the p53 protein could be entirely or almost entirely abrogated, either by interaction between HB X protein and wild-type p53 protein or by an inactivating mutation of the *p53* gene induced by heavy dietary exposure to aflatoxin B_1.

Mutations of *p53* at various sites within the *p53* gene have been found in association with mutation of the retinoblastoma *(Rb)* tumor suppressor gene, and these together might contribute to malignant transformation of hepatocytes *(60)*. No correlation has been demonstrated between HBV DNA integration and these mutations in combination.

The HBV *pre-S2/S* gene, when 3' truncated, also has *trans*-activating properties *(61)*. This region of the genome is often included in HBV DNA integrants and 3' truncation is commonly present. Moreover, there is evidence that *pre-S2/S* cooperates with c-Ha-*ras* in cell transformation *(61)*.

Mutations in the HBV genome might also play a part in the pathogenesis of HCC, perhaps by increasing the likelihood of HBV persistence and integration. The basic core promoter region of the genome overlaps the *X* gene. In one study, nucleic acid and amino acid divergences in this region were shown to be more frequent in patients with HCC than in asymptomatic carriers of the virus. Paired 1762 adenine to thymine and 1764 guanine to adenine missense mutations were particularly common *(62)*. Deletions or insertions in this region were found in a second study *(63)*. Missense mutations of the bulge of the RNA encapsidation signal, a region that plays a pivotal role in HBV replication, have also been reported in patients with HCC *(64)*.

Transforming growth factor (TGF)-α, an autocrine regulator of cell growth and regeneration, can be detected in HCC and surrounding liver tissue *(65)*. In the latter, TGF-α has been shown to be overexpressed in hepatocytes in which hepatitis B surface antigen (HBsAg) is detected, and there is some evidence that it may also be overexpressed in malignant cells containing HBV DNA integrants *(66)*. These findings suggest that an interaction between HBV and TGF-α in regenerating liver tissue may play a role in hepatocarcinogenesis.

Indirect Carcinogenicity

The observations that the majority of HCCs coexist with cirrhosis *(5)* (a few coexist with chronic hepatitis) and that not all HBV-related HCCs contain viral integrants *(67,68)* support the hypothesis that this virus may also cause malignant transformation indirectly by inducing chronic necroinflammatory hepatic disease. Further support is provided by the findings in transgenic mice that are created with the HBV *pre-S/S* gene. These mice overproduce large envelope (pre-S1) protein that accumulates in the endoplasmic reticulum of hepatocytes, producing severe and persistent injury to these cells with inflammation, regenerative hyperplasia, and transcriptional deregulation, and progressing ultimately to neoplasia *(69)*. These findings imply that severe and prolonged hepatocyte injury *per se* may lead to unrestrained cell growth.

Malignant transformation developing in the presence of chronic necroinflammatory hepatic disease, whatever the cause of the latter, is probably related to continuous or recurring cycles of hepatocyte necrosis followed by regeneration *(31)*. The resulting accelerated cell turnover rate may act as a tumor promoter. It increases the probability of integration of HBV DNA, both because single-stranded DNA is more susceptible to viral insertion and because the increased intracellular topoisomerase I activity generated results in cleavage of viral DNA at specific motifs, linearizing the circular DNA, and promoting its integration *(70)*. In addition, the likelihood both of spontaneous mutation and of damage to DNA by exogenous mutagens is increased. The accelerated rate of cell division also allows less time for altered DNA to be repaired before the cell divides again, there "fixing" the abnormal DNA in the daughter cells. This facilitates the accumulation of a number of mutations, which are required for the multistep process of carcinogenesis. In addition, an increased hepatocyte turnover rate provides an opportunity for the selective growth advantage of initiated cells to be exercised.

Other mechanisms are also possible. Inflammation *per se* leads to the generation of oxygen reactive species in the affected tissue and these may be mutagenic *(71)*. N-nitroso compounds are produced endogenously in hepatitis virus-infected hepatocytes and cause the promutagenic and cytotoxic DNA lesion, O^6-alkylguanine *(72)*. Sequestration of the enzyme O^6-alkylguanine-DNA-alkyltransferase, which is responsible for the repair of O^6-alkylguanine, in the cytoplasm of these cells (and away from its site of action in the nucleus) in hepatitis B cirrhosis may impair DNA repair *(72)*. Because HB X modulates HBV replication *(73)*, its protein may contribute indirectly to hepatocarcinogenesis by maintaining the viral carrier state, thereby predisposing to the development of chronic hepatitis, cirrhosis, and ultimately HCC.

Hepatocarcinogenesis is a complex process that involves several or many cumulative genetic events. These could perturb the function of a variety of cellular genes including protooncogenes, growth factor genes, and tumor suppressor genes, altering growth regulatory pathways. Different events in HCC induction by viruses, direct or indirect, probably operate at different stages in the genesis of a particular tumor and in different ways in different tumors. Indeed, direct and indirect effects of the virus acting in concert are probably responsible for most HCCs caused by hepatitis viruses.

HCV AS A HEPATOCARCINOGEN

Evidence for a causal role for HCV, a single-stranded RNA virus related to the Flaviviridae, in HCC is more recent but almost equally compelling. In common with HBV infection, the importance of chronic HCV infection as a risk factor for the tumor differs between developed and developing countries *(74,75)*. In the former, whatever the incidence of HCC, HCV is a more important causal association of the tumor than is HBV, and in Japan, Italy, and Spain the virus accounts for as much as 80% of HCCs *(74,75)*. For patients in these countries who have been referred to a hepatology clinic with chronic HCV infection, the annual risk of developing HCC ranges from 1.0% to 8.9%, with the risk being greater both in countries with higher incidences of the tumor and in patients with cirrhosis than in those with chronic hepatitis. Persistent HCV infection and alcohol abuse often (and chronic HBV infection and alcohol abuse less often) coexist as causal associations of HCC in developed countries *(74,75)*. HCV plays a secondary role in the genesis of HCC in ethnic Chinese and black African populations, in which HBV is the dominant risk factor.

Patients with HCV-related HCC are generally older than those with HBV-induced tumors, especially in developing countries where the difference in mean age may be as much as 20 yr *(74,75)*. The interval between initial infection with the virus and the diagnosis of HCC is generally 25–30 yr, although a few patients present in as short a time as 5–10 yr. Controversy exists over whether HCV genotype 1b is more closely associated with HCC than the other genotypes and whether treatment of chronic hepatitis C infections with interferon-α lessens the risk of neoplastic supervention *(75)*.

Mechanisms of Carcinogenicity

Almost all HCV-related HCCs arise in cirrhotic livers and most of the remainder develop against a background of chronic hepatitis, an observation that strongly suggests that chronic necroinflammatory hepatic disease is an important contributor to the development of the tumor *(74,75)*. HCV replicative intermediates do not integrate into chromosomal DNA, but apart from this the mechanisms whereby an increased hepatocyte turnover rate may act as a tumor promoter already mentioned in respect to HBV would apply equally or to an even greater extent to HCV. An important pathogenetic role for chronic necroinflammatory hepatic disease offers one explanation for the frequent coexistence of HCV infection and alcohol abuse in patients with HCC, the two factors combining to induce more severe degrees of hepatocyte necrosis and regeneration.

The possibility that HCV could also be directly carcinogenic was initially suggested by the observation that a few HCV-related tumors arose in normal or near normal livers *(76)*. More convincing evidence was provided by the recent report that transgenic mice in which the core gene together with its regulatory sequences have been introduced develop HCC *(77)*. HCV would have to exert its direct carcinogenic effect from an extrachromosomal position, and possible mechanisms have been proposed. The deduced amino acid sequence of the HCV core protein shows it to be a basic protein that contains a putative DNA binding motif, as well as triplicate nuclear localization signals and several putative protein kinase A and C recognition sites *(78,79)*. These characteristics imply that the protein could function as a gene-regulatory protein. The nonstructural NS3 protein has both proteinase and helicase activity. NIH 3T3 cells transfected with the 5′ half of the HCV sequence encoding NS3 proliferated rapidly, lost contact inhibition, grew anchorage-independently in soft agar, and formed tumors in nude mice *(80)*. HCV replication may mediate the coexpression of TGF-α and insulin-like growth factor II, resulting in uncontrolled cell proliferation *(81)*.

A positive interaction between the carcinogenic effects of HBV and HCV has been demonstrated in the majority but not all populations that have been studied *(82)*. This interaction has usually taken the form of a synergistic effect. An interactive effect between excessive iron and persistent HCV infection has also been suggested. In the only study addressing this question, however, no correlation could be demonstrated between tissue iron and HCV (or HBV) infection *(83)*.

GENETIC ASPECTS

The geographic distribution of HCC, at both global and local levels, as well as time trends in its incidence and the effects of migration on its occurrence, imply a predominant role for environmental agents in the causation of this tumor. Evidence supporting an inherited component to the risk of HCC in humans is limited. Studies of histocompatibility antigens in patients with HCC have not shown a genetic predisposition to the tumor, although the published analyses have not included a full range of antigens *(84,85)*. HCC has been reported to have a familial occurrence, although in at least some of these studies the familial occurrence could be explained by several members of the family being infected with HBV. Nevertheless, in studies in Alaska and China a familial occurrence has remained even when chronic HBV infection has been excluded as a confounding factor *(86,87)*. Genetic factors may contribute indirectly to HBV-induced HCC because the immunologic basis for the development of persistent HBV infection may have an inherited component. The same may be true of HCV-induced HCC.

Further possible evidence for a role for genetic factors is suggested by the occurrence of HCC in a number of inherited metabolic diseases, including hereditary hemochromatosis, α_1-antitrypsin deficiency, hereditary tyrosinemia, glycogen storage disease (type I), and hypercitrullinemia *(88)*. Some of these conditions are complicated by the development of cirrhosis in addition to HCC, and chronic necroinflammatory hepatic disease may contribute to the neoplastic process. In others the genetic defect results in the accumulation of chemicals that are mutagenic. The latter is best illustrated by hereditary hemochromatosis, in which excessive amounts of iron accumulate in the tissues *(88)*. Excess hepatic iron is known to be mutagenic *(89)*.

Genetic variation may influence the carcinogenic potential of aflatoxin B_1. This mycotoxin is harmless before its metabolic activation in the phase I detoxification pathway in hepatocytes to aflatoxin 8,9-epoxide. The reactive epoxide is then rendered innocuous by phase II detoxification, in which glutathione-*S*-transferase M1 conjugates it to glutathione and epoxide hydrolase converts it into 1,2-dihydrodiol. If not detoxified, the epoxide can bind to DNA at the N^7 guanine residue. Mutant alleles of epoxide hydrolase have been shown to be overrepresented in Chinese and Ghanaian patients with HCC *(90)*. Furthermore, HBV carriers with high-risk genotypes are at an even greater risk of HCC than those with wild-type genotypes *(90)*.

REFERENCES

1. Parkin DM, Pisani P, Ferlay J. Estimates of the worldwide incidence of 18 major cancers in 1985. Int J Cancer 1993; 54:1–13.
2. Bosch FX. Global epidemiology of hepatocellular carcinoma. In: Okuda K, Tabor E (eds). Liver Cancer. New York: Churchill Livingstone, 1997, 13–28.
3. Kew MC. Hepatic tumors and cysts. In: Feldman M, Scharschmidt BF, Sleisenger MH (eds). Gastrointestinal and Liver Disease. Pathophysiology/Diagnosis/Management. Philadelphia: WB Saunders, 1998, pp. 1364–1387.
4. Prates MD, Torres FO. A cancer survey in Lourenco Marques, Portugese East Africa. J Natl Cancer Inst 1965; 35:729–757.
5. Kew MC, Popper. H. Relationship between hepatocellular carcinoma and cirrhosis. Semin Liver Dis 1984; 4:136–146.
6. Kew MC. Clinical manifestations and paraneoplastic syndromes of hepatocellular carcinoma. In: Okuda K, Ishak KG (eds). Neoplasms of the Liver. Tokyo: Springer-Verlag, 1987, pp. 199–214.
7. Kew MC. Tumor markers of hepatocellular carcinoma. J Gastroenterol Hepatol 1989; 4:373–384.
8. Kew MC, Macerollo P. Effect of age on the etiologic role of the hepatitis B virus in hepatocellular carcinoma in blacks. Gastroenterology 1988; 94:439–442.
9. Yamagata H, Nakanishi T, Furukawa M, Okuda H, Obata H. J Levels of vitamin K, immunoreactive prothrombin, des-Γ-carboxy prothrombin, and Γ-glutamyl carboxylase activity in hepatocellular carcinoma tissue. J Gastroenterol Hepatol 1995; 10:8–13.
10. Kudo M. Ultrasound. In: Okuda K, Tabor E, (eds). Liver Cancer. New York: Churchill Livingstone, 1997, pp. 315–330.

11. Kew MC. Detection and treatment of small hepatocellular carcinomas. In: Hollinger FB, Lemon SM, Margolis HS (eds). Viral Hepatitis and Liver Disease. Baltimore: Williams & Wilkins. 1991, pp. 535–540.

12. Choi BI. CT diagnosis of liver cancer. In: Okuda K, Tabor E (eds). Liver Cancer. New York: Churchill Livingstone, 1997, pp. 371–392.

13. Takayasu K. Hepatic angiography. In: Okuda K, Tabor E (eds). Liver Cancer. New York: Churchill Livingstone, 1997, pp. 347–360.

14. Ebara M. MRI diagnosis of liver cancer. In: Okuda K, Tabor E (eds). Liver Cancer. New York: Churchill Livingstone, 1997, pp. 361–370.

15. Nakashima T, Kojiro M. Hepatocellular carcinoma. An Atlas of Pathology. Tokyo: Springer-Verlag, 1987.

16. Craig JR, Peters RL, Edmondson HA. Tumors of the Liver and Intrahepatic Bile Ducts. Washington, DC: Armed Forces Institute of Pathology, 1989.

17. Ringe B, Pichlmayr R, Wittekind C, Tusch G. Surgical treatment of hepatocellular carcinoma: experience with liver resection and transplantation in 198 patients. World J Surg 1991; 15:270–285.

18. Terblanche J, Launois B. Liver resection. In: Terblanche J (ed). Hepatobiliary Malignancy. London: Arnold, 1994, pp. 505–506.

19. Werner ID, Williams R. Liver transplantation for malignancy: the current position. In: Terblanche J (ed). Hepatobiliary Malignancy. London: Arnold, 1994, pp. 595–620.

20. Livraghi T. Ethanol injection for the treatment of hepatocellular carcinoma. In: Okuda K, Tabor E (eds). Liver Cancer. New York: Churchill Livingstone, 1997, pp. 497–510.

21. Bronowicki J-P, Vetter D, Doffoel M. Chemoembolization for hepatocellular carcinoma. In: Okuda K, Tabor E (eds). Liver Cancer. New York: Churchill Livingstone, 1997, pp. 463–470.

22. Falkson G. Treatment of patients with hepatocellular carcinoma: state-of-the-art. Ann Oncol 1992; 3:336–337.

23. Beasley RP, Hwang LY. Hepatocellular carcinoma and the hepatitis B virus. Semin Liver Dis 1984; 4:113–121.

24. Chen PJ, Chen DS. Hepatitis B virus and hepatocellular carcinoma. In: Okuda K, Tabor E (eds). Liver Cancer. New York: Churchill Livingstone, 1997, pp. 29–37.

25. Kew MC. Chronic hepatitis B virus infection and hepatocellular carcinoma in Africa. S Afr J Sci 1992; 88:524–528.

26. Botha JF, Ritchie MJJ, Dusheiko GM, Mouton HWK, Kew MC. Hepatitis B virus carrier state in black children in Ovamboland: role of perinatal and horizontal infection. Lancet 1984; 2:1209–1212.

27. Beasley RP, Hwang L-Y, Lin CC, Chien CS. Hepatocellular carcinoma and HBV: a prospective study of 22,707 men in Taiwan. Lancet 1981; 2:1129–1133.

28. Szmuness W. Hepatocellular carcinoma and hepatitis B virus: evidence for a causal association. Prog Med Virol 1978; 24:40–69.

29. Seeff LB, Beebe GW, Hoofnagle JH, Norman JE, Buskell-Bakles Z, Waggoner JG, Kaplowitz N, et al. A serologic follow-up of the 1942 epidemic of post-vaccination hepatitis in the United States army. N Engl J Med 1987; 316:965–970.

30. Chang MH, Chen CJ, Lai MS, Hsu HM, Wu TC, Kong MS, et al. Universal hepatitis B vaccination in Taiwan and the incidence of hepatocellular carcinoma in children. N Engl J Med 1997; 336:1855–1859.

31. Kew MC. Role of cirrhosis on hepatocarcinogenesis. In: Bannasch P, Keppler D, Weber G (eds). Liver Cell Carcinoma. Dordrecht: Kluwer, 1989; pp. 37–46.

32. Kew MC. The hepatitis B virus and the genesis of hepatocellular carcinoma. GI Cancer 1996; 1:143–148.

33. Kew MC, Geddes EW, Macnab GM, Bersohn I. Hepatitis B and cirrhosis in Bantu patients with primary liver cancer. Cancer 1974; 34:539–541.

34. Prince AM, Szmuness W, Michon J, Demaille J, Diebolt G, Linhard J, Quenum C, et al. A case/control study of the association between primary liver cancer and hepatitis B infection in Senegal. Int J Cancer 1975; 16:376–383.

35. Matsubara K, Tokino T. Integration of hepatitis B virus DNA and its implications for hepatocarcinogenesis. Mol Med Biol 1990; 7:243–260.

36. Popper H, Roth L, Purcell RH, Tennant BC, Gerin JL. Hepatocarcinogenicity of the woodchuck hepatitis virus. Proc Natl Acad Sci USA 1987; 84:866–870.

37. Kim CM, Koike K, Saito I, Miyamura T, Jay G. HB *X* gene of hepatitis B virus induces liver cancer in transgenic mice. Nature 1991; 351:317–320.

38. Slagle BL, Lee TH, Butel JS. Hepatitis B virus and hepatocellular carcinoma. Prog Med Virol 1992; 39:167–203.

39. de The H, Marchio A, Tiollais P, DeJean A. A novel steroid thyroid hormone receptor-related gene inappropriately expressed in human hepatocellular carcinoma. Nature 1987; 330:667–670.

40. Wang J, Chenivesse X, Henglein B, Brechot C. Hepatitis B virus integration in a *cyclin A* gene in hepatocellular carcinoma. Nature 1990; 343:555–557.

41. Hansen LJ, Tennant BC, Seeger C, Ganem D. Differential activation of *myc* gene family members in hepatic carcinogenesis by closely related hepatitis B viruses. Mol Cell Biol 1993; 13:659–667.

42. Buendia MA, Etiemble J, Degott C, Babinet C, Tiollais P. Primary hepatocellular carcinoma in transgenic mice carrying a woodchuck c-*myc* gene activated by retroviral insertion. In: Cilberto B, Cortese R, Schibler U, Schutz G (eds). Gene Expression During Liver Differentiation and Disease. IRNBM, 1991, p. 187.

43. Arbuthnot P, Kew MC, Fitschen W. c-fos and c-myc oncoprotein expression in human hepoatocellular carcinomas. Anticancer Res 1991; 11:921–924.

44. Shirakata Y, Kawada M, Fujiki Y, Sana H, Oda M, Yaginuma K, Kobayashi M, et al. The *X* gene of hepatitis B virus induced growth stimulation and tumorigenic transformation of mouse NIH 3T3 cells. Jpn J Cancer Res 1989; 80:617–621.

45. Unsal H, Zakicier C, Marcais C, Kew MC, Volkmann M, Zentgraf H, Isselbacher K, et al. Genetic heterogeneity of hepatocellular carcinoma. Proc Natl Acad Sci USA 1994; 91:822–826.

46. Wang W, London WT, Feitelsohn MA. Hepatitis B X antigen in hepatitis B viris carriers with liver cancer. Cancer Res 1991; 51:4971–4977.

47. Paterlini P, Poussin K, Kew MC, Franco D, Brechot C. Selective accumulation of the X transcript of the hepatitis B virus in patients negative for hepatitis B surface antigen with hepatocellular carcinoma. Hepatology 1993; 21:313–321.

48. Henkler F, Koshy R. Hepatitis B virus transcriptional activators: mechanisms and possible role in oncogenesis. J Vir Hepatit 1996; 3:109–121.

49. Slagle BL, Lee TH, Medina D, Finegold MJ, Butel JS. Increased sensitivity to the hepatocarcinogen diethylnitrosamine in transgenic mice carrying the hepatitis B virus *X* gene. Mol Carcinogen 1996; 15:261–269.

50. Robinson WS. Hepadnaviruses and hepatocellular carcinoma. Cancer Det Prev 1989; 14:245–252.

51. Ullrich SJ, Anderson CW, Mercer WE, Appwella E. The p53 tumor suppressor protein, a modulator of cell proliferation. J Biol Chem 1992; 267:15259–15262.

52. Yonish-Rouach E, Grunwald D, Wilder S, Kimchi A, May E, Lawrence JJ, May P, et al. p53-mediated cell death: relationship to cell cycle control. Mol Cell Biol 1993; 13:1415–1423.

53. Wang XW, Forrester K, Yeh GH, Feitelsohn MA, Gu JR, Harris CC. Hepatitis B virus X protein inhibits p53 sequence-specific DNA binding, transcriptional activity, and association with transcription factor ERCC3. Proc Natl Acd Sci USA 1994; 91:2230–2234.

54. Truant R, Antunovic J, Greenblatt J, Prives C, Cromlish JA. Direct interaction of the hepatitis B virus HBX with p53 protein leads to the inhibition by HBX of p53 response element-directed transactivation. J Virol 1995; 69:1851–1859.

55. Ueda H, Ulrich SJ, Gangemi JD, Kappel CA, Ngol L, Feitelsohn MA, Jay G. Functional inactivation but not structural mutation of *p53* causes liver cancer. Nat Genet 1995; 9:41–47.

56. Wang XW, Yeh H, Schaeffer L, Roy R, Moncollin V, Egly JM, Wang Z, et al. *p53* modulation of TFIIH-associated nucleotide excision-repair activity. Nat Genet 1995; 10:188–195.

57. Becker SA, Lee TL, Butel JS Slagle BL. Hepatitis B virus X protein interferes with cellular DNA repair. J Virol 1998; 72:266–272.

58. Capovilla A, Carmona S, Arbuthnot P. Hepatitis B virus X protein binds to damaged DNA and sensitizes liver dells to ultraviolet irradiation. Biochem Biophys Res Commun 1997; 232:255–260.

59. Wogan GN. Aflatoxin exposure as a risk factor for hepatocellular carcinoma. In: Okuda K, Tabor E (eds). Liver Cancer. New York: Churchill Livingstone, 1993, pp. 51–58.

60. Murakami Y, Hayashi K, Hirohashi S, Sekiya T. Aberrations of the tumor suppressor *p53* and retinoblastoma genes in human hepatocellular carcinoma. Cancer Res 1993; 53:368–372.

61. Kekule AS, Lauer U, Meyer M, Caselmann WH, Hofschneider PH, Koshy R. The preS2/S region of integrated hepatitis B virus DNA encodes a transcriptional transactivator, Nature 1990; 343:63–64.

62. Baptista M, Kramvis A, Kew MC. High prevalence of 1762^T 1764^A mutations in the basic core promoter of hepatitis B virus isolated from black Africans with hepatocellular carcinoma compared with asymptomatic carriers. Hepatology, 1999; 29:946–953.

63. Laskus T, Radkowski M, Nowicki M, Wang LF, Vargas H, Rakela J. Association between hepatitis B virus core promoter rearrangements and hepatocellular carcinoma. Biochem Biophys Res Commun 1998; 244:812–814.

64. Kramvis A, Kew MC, Bukofzer S. Hepatitis B virus precore mutants in serum and liver of southern African blacks with hepatocellular carcinoma. J Hepatol 1998; 28:132–141.

65. Tabor E., Viral hepatitis and liver cancer. In: Goldin RD, Thomas HC, Gerber MA, (eds). Pathology of Viral Hepatitis. London: Arnold, 1998, pp. 161–177.

66. Tabor E, Farshid M, DiBisceglie A, Hsia CC. Increased expression of transforming growth factor α after transfection of a human hepatoblastoma cell line with hepatitis B virus. J Med Virol 1992; 37:271–273.

67. Brechot C, Hadchouel M, Scotto J, Fonck M, Potet F, Vyas GN, Tiollais P. State of hepatitis B virus DNA in hepatocytes of patients with hepatitis B surface antigen positive and negative liver diseases. Proc Natl Acad Sci USA 1981; 78:3906–3910.

68. Shafritz DA, Shouval D, Sherman HI, Kew MC. Integration of hepatitis B virus DNA into the genome of liver cells in chronic liver disease and hepatocellular carcinoma. N Engl J Med 1981; 305:1067–1073.

69. Chisari FV, Klopchin K, Moriyama T, Pasquinelli C, Dunsford HA, Sell S, Brinster RL, et al. Molecular pathogenesis of hepatocellular carcinoma in hepatitis B virus transgenic mice. Cell 1989; 4:1145–1156.

70. Wang JC. DNA topoisomerases. Ann Biochem 1985; 54:665–697.

71. Freeman BA, Crapo JD. Biology of disease: Free radicals and tissue injury. Lab Invest 1982; 47:412–456.

72. Lee SM, Portmann BC, Margison GP. Abnormal intracellular distribution of O^6-alkylguanine-DNA-alkyl transferase in hepatitis B cirrhotic human liver: a potential co-factor in the development of hepatocellular carcinoma. Hepatology 1996; 24:987–990.

73. Chen HS, Kaneko S, Girones R, Anderson RW, Hornbuckle WE, Tennant BC, Cote PJ, et al. The WHV *X* gene is important for establishment of virus infection in woodchucks. J Virol 1993; 67:1218–1226.

74. Kobayashi K, Purcell RH, Shimotohno K, Tabor E. Hepatitis C Virus and Its Involvement in the Development of Hepatocellular Carcinoma. Princeton: Princeton Scientific, 1995.

75. Kew MC. Hepatitis C virus and hepatocellular carcinoma in developing and developed countries. Vir Hepatit Rev 1998; 4:259–269.

76. De Mitri MS, Poussin K, Baccarini P, Pontisso P, D'Errico A, Simon N, Grigione W, et al. HCV-associated liver cancer without cirrhosis. Lancet 1995; 345:413–415.

77. Moriya K, Fujie H, Shintani Y, Yotsuyanagi H, Tsutsumi T, Ishibashi K, Matsura Y, et al. The core protein of hepatitis C virus produces hepatocellular carcinoma in transgenic mice. Nature Med 1998; 4:1065–1067.

78. Shih CM, Lo SJ, Miyamura T, Chen Sy, Lee YHW. Suppression of hepatitis B virus expression and replication by hepatitis C virus core protein in HUH-7 cells. J Virol 1993; 67:5823–5832.

79. Kin DW, Suzuki R, Harada T, Saito I, Miyamura T. Trans-suppression of gene expression by hepatitis C viral core protein. Jpn J Sci Biol 1994; 47:211–220.

80. Sakamura D, Fuukawa T, Takegami K. Hepatitis C virus non-structural protein NS3 transforms NIH 3T3 cells. J Virol 1995; 69:3893–3896.

81. Tanaka S, Takenaka K, Matsumata T, Mori R, Sugimachi K. Hepatitis C virus replication is associated with expression of transforming growth factor-α and insulin-like growth factor II in cirrhotic livers. Dig Dis Sci 1996; 41:208–215.

82. Kew MC, Yu MC, Kedda MA, Coppin A, Sarkin A, Hokinson J. The relative roles of hepatitis B and C viruses in the etiology of hepatocellular carcinoma in southern African blacks. Hepatology 1997; 112:184–187.

83. Mandishona E, MacPhail AP, Gordeuk VR, Kedda MA, Paterson AC, Roualt T, Kew MC. Dietary iron overload as a risk factor for hepatocellular carcinoma in black Africans. Hepatology 1998; 27:1563–1566.

84. Kew MC, Gear AJ, Baumgarten I, Dusheiko GM, Maier G. Histocompatibility antigens in patients with hepatocellular carcinoma and their relationship to chronic hepatitis B virus infection in these patients. Gastroenterology 1979; 77:537–539.

85. Gilmore IT, Harrison JM, Parkins RA. Clustering of hepatitis B virus infection and hepatocellular carcinoma in a family. J R Soc Med 1981; 74:843–845.

86. Shen FM, Lee MK, Gong HM, Cax XQ, King MC. Complex segregation analysis of hepatocellular carcinoma in Chinese families: interaction of inherited susceptibility and hepatitis B viral infection. Am J Hum Genet 1991; 49:88–93.

87. Alberts SR, Lanier AP, McMahon BJ, Harpster A, Bulkow LR, Hayward WL, Marray C. Clustering of hepatocellular carcinoma in Alaska Native families. Genet Epidemiol 1991; 8:127–139.

88. Hadchouel M. Metabolic liver diseases and hepatocellular carcinoma. In: Brechot C (ed). Primary Liver Cancer: Etiological and Progression Factors. Boca Raton, FL: CRC Press, 1994, pp. 79–88.

89. Loeb LA, James EA, Waltersdorph AM, Klebanoff SJ. Mutagenesis by the autoxidation of iron with isolated DNA. Proc Natl Acad Sci USA 1988; 85:3918–3922.

90. McGlynn KA, Rosvold EA, Lustbader ED, Hu Y, Clapper ML, Zhou T, Wild CP, et al. Susceptibility to hepatocellular carcinoma with genetic variation in the enzymatic detoxification of aflatoxin B_1. Proc Natl Acad Sci USA 1995; 92:2384–2387.

19

Hepatitis C Virus, B-Cell Disorders, and Non-Hodgkin's Lymphoma

Clodoveo Ferri, Stefano Pileri, and Anna Linda Zignego

HEPATITIS C VIRUS INFECTION

Since its identification in 1989 *(1,2)*, hepatitis C virus (HCV) has been recognized as the major causative agent of posttransfusion and sporadic parenterally transmitted non-A–non-B hepatitis *(3)*. HCV is a single-stranded, positive-sense RNA virus showing similarities of genomic organization with pestiviruses. The introduction of second- and third-generation enzyme-linked immunosorbent assay (ELISA) and recombinant immunoblot assay (RIBA) tests significantly improved the diagnostic procedures for the detection of HCV-related antibodies (anti-HCV). Unlike many other viral infections, the detection of serum IgG class antibodies often suggests active HCV infection. However, anti-HCV may persist long after viral clearance. Thus, detection of viral RNA sequences using polymerase chain reaction (PCR) or other amplification methods is required to demonstrate infectous HCV *(4)*. In patients with non-A, non-B hepatitis there is generally a good concordance between anti-HCV and PCR results. The detection of HCV RNA sequences in tissue specimens by *in situ* hybridization could be usefully employed mainly for etiopathogenetic investigations, although this still requires proper validation *(5)*.

HCV genotypes have been defined by means of nucleotide and amino acid sequence analyses. There is an increasing number of HCV types and subtypes; at least 6 major HCV genotypes with 11 subtypes have been demonstrated in patient populations from different geographic areas *(6)*. The presence of different HCV genotypes seems to be relevant for both pathogenetic and therapeutic implications, as suggested by the increased prevalence of genotype 1b in subjects with low response to interferon treatment and genotype 2a/c in lymphoproliferative disorders *(3–8)*. Although some HCV genotypes are prevalent in particular geographic areas, a large variety of types and subtypes appears in a given country. In addition, HCV shows marked genetic variability. The viral genome is a mixture of heterogeneous HCV RNA molecules, often designated as quasispecies *(9)*. The coexistence of multiple mutants provides an efficient and rapid mechanism for the virus to escape the immune response and therefore to persist in the host. The large majority of infected individuals develop chronic HCV infection *(3,10)*, with about 70% showing chronic hepatitis.

From: *Infectious Causes of Cancer: Targets for Intervention*
Edited by: J. J. Goedert © Humana Press Inc., Totowa, NJ

HCV infects not only liver cells, but also lymphoid tissues as suggested by the presence of active (minus-strand HCV RNA-positive) or "latent" viral replication (minus-strand HCV RNA only in mitogen-stimulated cells) in the peripheral lymphocytes of HCV seropositives *(11,12)*. The infection of the lymphoid tissues could represent an HCV reservoir that contributes significantly to viral persistence. On the whole, the hepato-and lymphotropism of HCV may explain the appearance of a constellation of both hepatic and extrahepatic disorders *(10,13)*, specifically chronic hepatitis, cirrhosis, autoimmune hepatitis, hepatocellular carcinoma, autoimmune thyroiditis, glomerulonephritis, porphyria cutanea tarda, lung fibrosis, mixed cryoglobulinemia, and B-cell lymphoma *(10,13)*.

MIXED CRYOGLOBULINEMIA

Mixed cryoglobulinemia (MC) is a multifaceted disease that represents an intersection of several autoimmune and lymphoproliferative disorders *(14,15)*. The term cryoglobulinemia refers to the presence in the serum of one or more immunoglobulins that precipitate reversibly at temperatures below 37° *(16)*. Circulating cryoglobulins are detectable in a wide number of infectious, immunologic, and hematologic disorders *(14,16,17)*.

According to Brouet et al. *(16)*, cryoglobulinemia is classified into three main subgroups. Type I is composed of one monoclonal immunoglobulin, generally an IgM. Type II (mixed) is composed of polyclonal IgG and monoclonal IgM, and type III (mixed) is composed of both polyclonal IgG and IgM components. The IgM is an autoantibody with rheumatoid factor (RF) activity. Moreover, IgG–IgM circulating immune complexes may include trace amounts of IgA, fibrinogen, complement, and antigens including viral particles.

Cryoglobulinemia type I is generally found in patients with lymphoproliferative disorders, such as Waldenstrom's macroglobulinemia or multiple myeloma. In contrast, MC (types II–III) can be detected in various chronic infectious or immune-mediated diseases *(14–17)*. Since its first description in 1966 *(17)*, so-called "essential" MC was considered to be a distinct entity when other systemic, infectious, or neoplastic disorders were excluded on the basis of a wide clinicoserologic workup. MC is characterized by a typical clinical triad—purpura, weakness, arthralgias—and by involvement of one or more organ systems manifesting as chronic hepatitis (70%), glomerulonephritis (30%), peripheral neuropathy (30–40%), skin ulcers (10–20%), diffuse vasculitis (15%), or less frequently lymphatic (10%) and hepatic (3%) malignancies *(13–17)*. Moreover, circulating mixed cryoglobulins with RF activity as well as reduced hemolytic complement activity with low C4 component are the typical serologic findings of the disease *(14–17)*. There are no differences between type II and type III MC in terms of clinical manifestations and prognosis *(15)*. It has been hypothesized, but never fully demonstrated, that polyclonal type III MC, often associated with chronic hepatitis, represents a precondition of the oligomonoclonal type II MC, occasionally complicated by B-cell non-Hodgin's lymphoma (NHL). The prevalence of MC is highly variable among different countries. It is more frequent in southern Europe than in northern Europe or North America *(14–18)*. On the whole, it is considered to be a relatively rare disorder, but it may be underestimated because of its heterogeneity.

Leukocytoclastic vasculitis is the histologic hallmark of cutaneous manifestations of MC *(14–17)*. Cryoglobulinemic vasculitis is secondary to the deposition of circulating immune complexes, mainly the cryoglobulins as well as complement, in the small blood vessels and, less frequently, in medium-sized arteries. Moreover, various organ involvement with diffuse or nodular lymphoid aggregates in the liver, bone marrow, and spleen is the expression of an underlying lymphoproliferative disorder *(14,15)*. Mono- or polyclonal B-lymphocyte expansion *(19)* is related to the production of immune complexes responsible for systemic vasculitis.

With chronic hepatitis in more than two-thirds of MC patients *(15–18)*, a possible role of hepatotropic viruses in the etiopathogenesis of the disease has long been suggested. Hepatitis B virus infection appears to be the etiologic factor of MC in only a few (<5%) patients *(15)*. On the contrary, HCV infection has been demonstrated in the large majority of cases *(20–24;* Table 1). Support for an etiopathogenetic role of HCV in this disease came from virologic studies demonstrating that HCV infects peripheral blood mononuclear cells, as well as lymphoid tissues in MC patients *(12,25,26)*. Chronic HCV infection is responsible for both the chronic hepatitis and the B-cell expansion that characterize the cryoglobulinemic syndrome *(3,12,19,25,26)*.

Circulating immune complexes and various autoantibodies, often associated with autoimmune manifestations, have been observed in many patients with B-cell neoplasias, including monoclonal gammopathies, chronic lymphocytic leukemia, and low-grade NHL *(14)*. In these lymphoproliferative disorders, serum monoclonal (IgMκ) RFs also have been detected. Like natural autoantibodies, monoclonal RFs share a major complementary determining region named Wa, and they invariably express a Vκ light chain derived from a single germinal gene, the human Kv 325 *(14,22)*. A large body of research indicates that autoimmune and B-cell lymphoproliferative disorders often are closely related *(14,15)*. MC, characterized by a large amount of circulating immune complexes, also can be regarded as a "benign" B-cell neoplasm. The presence in the serum of Wa RF *(14,22)*, and the clonal expansion of IgMκ-bearing B-cells *(19)*, together with lymphocyte and plasmacytoid cell infiltrates in the bone marrow, suggest that low-grade or *in situ* NHL is the underlying disorder of MC *(27)*. More interestingly, this lymphoproliferation can switch to frank, malignant B-cell NHL *(28,29)*, generally after a long follow-up period. These clinicoserologic and pathologic observations indicate that there is a continuum among some autoimmune disorders, MC, and B-cell neoplasias *(13–15)*. In this scenario, MC represents an interesting example of coexistence of autoimmune and lymphoproliferative disorders, for which HCV infection can be a common triggering factor.

EPIDEMIOLOGY OF HCV-ASSOCIATED LYMPHOMA

The etiology of NHL is poorly understood but of considerable interest because of the increasing incidence of these malignancies worldwide *(30)*. A possible causative link between hepatotropic viruses and malignant lymphomas has been hypothesized since 1971, when an autopsy study of 814 Belgian patients with neoplastic diseases reported a significant association between cirrhosis and lymphoproliferative disorders *(31)*. With the identification of HCV as a triggering factor of MC *(20–24)*, its potential role in NHL was suspected *(12)*. In 1994, HCV infection was first demonstrated in a significant percentage of Italian patients with unselected B-cell NHL,

Table 1
Hepatitis C Virus (HCV) Infection and Lymphoproliferative Disorders (LPDs)

Authors (ref. no.)	Prevalence of HCV infection in LPD[a]			
	Country	Diagnosis	No. of Patients	% HCV+
Ferri C et al., 1994 (32)	Italy	B-NHL	50	34[b]
Cavanna L et al., 1995 (33)	Italy	B-NHL	150	25[b]
Luppi M et al., 1996 (34)	Italy	B-NHL	69	42[b]
Silvestri F et al., 1996 (35)	Italy	B-NHL	311	9[b]
Luppi M et al., 1996 (43)	Italy	B-NHL MALT type	27	50[b]
Ferri C et al., 1996 (42)	Italy	B-NHL	100	25[b]
Mazzaro C et al., 1996 (36)	Italy	B-NHL	199	28[b]
Musto P et al., 1996 (46)	Italy	B-NHL	150	27[b]
Musolino C et al., (37)	Italy	B-NHL	24	21[b]
Hanley J et al., 1996 (47)	UK[c]	B-NHL	38	0
Brind AM et al., 1996 (48)	UK[c]	B-NHL	63	0
McColl MD et al., 1997 (49)	UK[c]	B-NHL	72	0
Izumi T et al., 1996 (52)	Japan	B-NHL	54	22[b]
Zignego AL et al., 1997 (38)	Italy	B-NHL	150	25[b]
Zuckerman E et al., 1997 (39)	USA[d]	B-NHL	120	22[b]
De Rosa G et al., 1997 (44)	Italy	B-NHL	91	23[b]
King PD et al., 1998 (50)	USA[e]	B-NHL	73	1.4
Ellenrieder V et al., 1998 (45)	Germany	B-NHL	69	4.3
Ohsawa M et al., 1998 (41)	Japan[f]	Primary hepatic B-NHL	9	100[b]
Ferri C et al., 1991 (20)	Italy	MC	42	90[b]
Disdier et al., 1991 (24)	France	MC	30	70[b]
Agnello et al., 1992 (23)	USA	MC	19	84[b]
Cavanna L et al., 1995 (33)	Italy	CLL	40	5
Mussini C et al., 1995 (51)	Italy	MGUS,MM,WM	70, 21, 12	14[b], 14[b], 8[b]
Ferri C et al., 1996 (42)	Italy	CLL	25	12[b]
Musto P et al., 1996 (46)	Italy	MM,MGUS, CLL,WM	90, 47, 41, 13	11[b], 13[b], 20[b], 23[b]
Silvestri F et al., 1996 (35)	Italy	MM	78	4
Hanley J et al., 1996 (47)	UK	MM,MGUS	24, 10	0, 0
McColl MD et al., 1997 (49)	UK	CLL	38	0
Izumi T et al., 1997 (52)	Japan	WM, MM	4, 21	25, 14[b]
De Rosa G et al., 1997 (44)	Italy	MM, MGUS, CLL, WM	56, 48, 48, 13	16[b], 23[b], 17[b], 61[b]

	Prevalence of LPD in patients with HCV infection			
				LPD (%)
Ferri C et al., 1995 (53)	Italy	HCV+	500	B-NHL (2.8)
Brind AM et al., 1996 (54)	UK	HCV+	25	B-NHL (4)
Sikuler E et al., 1997 (55)	Israel	HCV+	103	B-NHL (3.9)
Andreone P et al., 1998 (8)	Italy	HCV+	239	MC (10), MG (11)
Hausfater P et al., 1998 (57)	France	HCV+	1800	B-NHL, CLL,WM,MM, MALT (2.5)

[a] Presence of anti-HCV antibodies and/or HCV RNA.

[b] Significant association if compared to HCV infection in other hematologic malignancies and/or healthy controls.

[c] Studies from the same geographic area of Scotland.

[d] Studies from Southern California (78% Hispanic ethnicity).

[e] Studies from midwestern United States (Missouri).

[f] HCV detection by *in situ* hybridization technique.

CLL, chronic lymphocytic leukemia; MGUS, monoclonal gammopathies of uncertain significance; MM, multiple mieloma; WM, Waldenstrom's disease; MC, mixed cryoglobulinemia; MG, monoclonal gammopathies.

regardless of the grade of malignancy *(32)*. The prevalence of HCV-related markers (anti-HCV and HCV RNA) in 34% of NHL was particularly significant as compared to Hodgkin's lymphomas (3%) and healthy controls (1.5%). This association subsequently was confirmed in other series of B-cell NHL from Italy and other countries *(33–46;* Table 1). Apart from some important exceptions *(47–50)*, numerous clinicoepidemiologic studies reported an increased prevalence of HCV infection in B-cell NHL.

The association of HCV with B-cell NHL seems not to be fortuitous or artifactual, considering that no increased risk factors for HCV exposure were recorded in HCV-seropositive NHL compared to seronegatives and that the prevalence of HCV infection in B-cell NHL was statistically higher than in the general population and control groups of other hematologic malignancies *(32–46)*. A surprisingly high prevalence of HCV infection has been detected in two series of mucosa-associated lymphoid tissue (MALT) type and primary hepatic NHL, from Italy and Japan, respectively *(41,43;* Table 1). A significant association with HCV also has been observed, though to a lesser extent, for other benign and malignant B-cell neoplasias, including Waldenstrom's macroglobulinemia, monoclonal gammopathies of uncertain significance, chronic lymphocytic leukemia, and multiple myeloma *(33,35,42,44,46,51,52;* Table 1). Moreover, the above findings were mirrored by the increased incidence of lymphoproliferative disorders, including B-cell NHL, in large series of unselected patients with chronic HCV infection *(8,53–57;* Table 1).

A decisive contribution for direct involvement of HCV in lymphomagenesis came from investigations showing the presence of HCV-related proteins and/or HCV replication intermediates in peripheral lymphocytes and tissue biopsy specimens of NHL patients by means of immunohistochemistry, reverse transcriptase-polymerase chain reaction (RT-PCR), or *in situ* hybridization studies *(53,58–60)*. Although limited by the use of controversial methods *(5)*, HCV-related antigens and HCV RNA have been demonstrated in neoplastic infiltrates of bone marrow, lymph nodes, salivary glands, and liver in HCV-associated B-cell NHL patients with or without MC *(26,53,58–61)*.

Epidemiologic studies suggest geographic and racial heterogeneity in the involvement of HCV in B-cell lymphomas (Table 1). There seems to be a gradient from northern to southern Europe—strongest in Italy *(32–38,44,46)*, but weak in France *(57)*, and United Kingdom, particularly in Scotland *(47–49,54)*. Studies from the United States suggest a similar discrepancy. Among patients with NHL in Southern California, many of whom were Hispanic, the prevalence of HCV infection (22%) was significantly higher as compared to patients with hematologic malignancies other than B-cell NHL (4.5%) or with benign hematologic disorders (5%) *(39)*. This association was not confirmed in NHL patients from the midwestern United States *(50)*. As the prevalence of HCV infection is quite homogeneous among Western countries, the variable distribution of HCV-associated NHL suggests that HCV *per se* is not sufficient, but that genetic and/or environmental cofactors are necessary for the full expression of malignancy. A confounding factor, which does vary geographically, is the distribution of HCV genotypes among different patient populations. Genotype 2a/c is found more frequently in subjects with MC and other benign or malignant lymphoproliferative disorders complicating type C hepatitis *(7,8,53)*.

Other epidemiologic evaluations indirectly support the possible role of HCV in NHL together with the multifactorial origin of the lymphomagenesis. First, a significantly increased risk of developing NHL has been reported, but not uniformly confirmed, in population-based studies of individuals with a history of previous transfusion *(62)*. Interestingly, in a Swedish survey this risk was lower for subjects who received leukocyte-depleted transfusions *(63)*. This finding can speculatively be correlated with the observation that HCV RNA may be detectable more frequently in peripheral blood mononuclear cells than in sera of infected individuals *(12)*. Moreover, NHL is one of the most commonly diagnosed malignancies worldwide, and its incidence has increased markedly in recent decades *(30)*. Concomitantly, HCV is emerging as a common and insidiously progressive disease *(10)*. In this scenario, HCV could be regarded as one of the most important exogenous triggering agents potentially involved in lymphomagenesis.

Finally, the oncogenic potential of HCV could be supported indirectly by the results of an epidemiologic study of 592 Japanese NHL patients, among whom an increased risk of developing hepatocellular carcinoma was noticed. Interestingly, HCV seropositivity was detectable in the majority (88%) of patients with complicating liver cancer *(64)*. Chronic hepatitis and/or cirrhosis was found in about 80% of patients with NHL following type II MC *(28)*, whereas in HCV-associated NHL without cryoglobulinemic syndrome the prevalence of liver involvement ranged from 16% to 50% *(32–46)*. It is likely that the prevalence of liver involvement in HCV-associated NHL is underestimated owing to both the insidious, often subclinical course of type C hepatitis, and the lack of thorough histologic evaluation in the published studies. Similarly, the incidence of hepatocellular carcinoma in HCV-associated NHL has not been adequately investigated, although in MC patients the incidence of liver cancer is probably lower than that observed in the general population of HCV-infected individuals.

PATHOLOGIC FEATURES OF HCV-ASSOCIATED LYMPHOMA

On diagnostic grounds, clonal lymphoid proliferations in HCV-positive patients can be divided into two main groups, monotypic lymphoproliferative disorders of undetermined significance (MLDUS) and overt lymphomas *(27,28,32,65)*. The former cannot be recognized without clinical data, as their histopathologic picture is basically indistinguishable from that of some lymphoid tumors, which are indolent but nevertheless invariably fatal. In this section, we use the concepts and terminology of the Revised European–American–Lymphoma (REAL) Classification *(66)*, which recently has been validated in a study sponsored by the National Cancer Institute (NCI) of the United States *(67)* and has been adopted as operational guidelines by the World Health Organization *(68)*. MLDUS occur in HCV-positive patients, who often show the clinical and laboratory pattern of type II MC *(21,22,27,65,69)*. Histologically (Fig. 1), they have lymphoid infiltrates in the bone marrow and liver that resemble peripheral B-cell lymphomas of the small cell/B-chronic lymphocytic leukemia (CLL) type or, more rarely, immunocytoma/lymphoplasmacytic lymphoma (Ic). The main morphologic, phenotypic, and genotypic findings are summarized in Table 2.

Some groups have reported that MLDUS show immunocytic morphology *(35,36,46,51,70,72,73)*. This does not correspond to our experience, perhaps owing to differences in terminology between the Updated Kiel Classification (UKC) *(73)* and

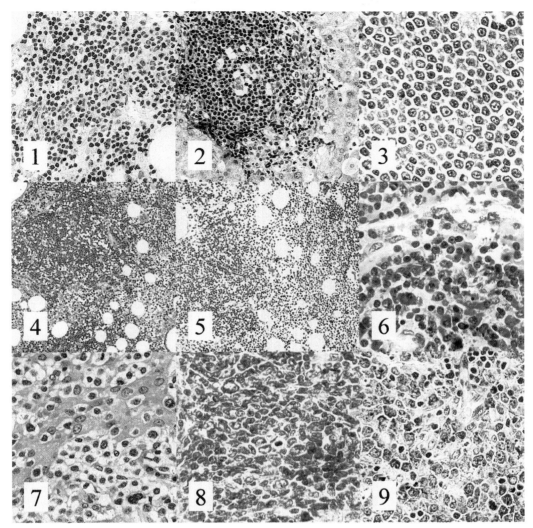

Fig. 1. Main histopathologic patterns of HCV-related MLDUS and overt lymphomas. **1:** B-CLL-like MLDUS: nodular infiltrate in the bone marrow showing vaguely defined borders and consisting of small lymphocytes, prolymphocytes, and paraimmunoblasts (Giemsa, ×250). **2:** B-CLL-like MLDUS: liver portal tract infiltrated by the same lymphoid population as in **1**; note the mild activity of the infiltrate (Giemsa, ×200). **3:** B-CLL-like MLDUS; cytological details of the infiltrate at higher magnification. Medium-sized prolymphocytes and large paraimmunoblasts are easily seen (Giemsa, ×600). **4:** B-CLL-like MLDUS: positivity at the determination of κ Ig-light chain (Immunohistochemistry, APAAP technique, specific polyclonal antibody, provided by Dako, Denmark, Gill's hematoxylin nuclear counterstain; ×150). **5:** B-CLL-like MLDUS: negativity at the determination of λ Ig-light chain (Immunohistochemistry, APAAP technique, specific polyclonal antibody, purchased by Dako, Denmark, Gill's hematoxylin nuclear counterstain; ×150). **6:** Ic-like MLDUS: the lymphoid infiltrate consists of small lymphocytes, lymphoplasmacytoid elements and mature plasma cells (Giemsa, ×600). **7:** MZL: neoplastic cells show centrocyte-like morphology; some of them infiltrate a gastric gland producing a lymphoepithelial lesion (Giemsa, ×600). **8:** FCL: the lymphoid population within a neoplastic follicle consists of centrocytes and a few centroblasts (Giemsa, ×600). **9:** DLBCL: the neoplastic population consists of variably shaped large elements (Giemsa, ×600).

Table 2
Histopathology of HCV-Related MLDUS and Overt Lymphomas according to the REAL Classification

MLDUS

B-chronic lymphocytic leukemia (B-CLL)-like

Morphology: In liver and bone marrow, lymphoid infiltrates consist of a mixture of small lymphocytes, prolymphocytes, and paraimmunoblasts; the latter two cell types can form pseudofollicles with numerous mitoses; bone marrow infiltrates are nodular or paratrabecular; liver infiltrates are in portal tracts and show minimal/mild activity.

Phenotype: Lymphoid elements carry B-cell markers (CD19, CD20, CD22, CD79a), CD5, CD23, and monotypic surface Ig (IgM/κ), as typically observed in B-CLL; *bcl-2* expression is rather strong; Ki-67 marking is low; numerous T cells are comprised within liver infiltrates.

Genotype: Preliminary studies by microdissection-PCR show the presence of oligoclonality in portal lymphoid infiltrates; thus, the monotypic pattern seen by immunohisto-chemistry appears to reflect more than one clone.

Immunocytoma (Ic)-like

Morphology: In liver and bone marrow, infiltrates consist of small lymphocytes, lympho-plasmacytoid elements, and plasma cells, with occasional blasts; neither prolympho-cytes nor pseudofollicles are seen; the infiltrates show the same location as in B-CLL-like MLDUS.

Phenotype: Lymphoid elements carry B-cell markers (CD19, CD20, CD22, CD79a) and monotypic surface and cytoplasmic Ig (IgM/κ), but are negative for CD5 and CD23; *bcl-2* expression is moderate; Ki-67 marking is low.

Genotype: There are no extensive reports on the topic.

Overt lymphomas

B-CLL

Morphology: Cytology corresponds to the one described in MLDUS; the lymph node struc-ture is diffusely effaced with infiltration of the capsule and obliteration of the sinuses; in the spleen, there is involvement of both the white and red pulp.

Phenotype: *See* B-CLL MLDUS.

Genotype: Molecular studies regularly show clonal rearrangements of Ig encoding genes.

Ic

Morphology: Cytology is the same as in Ic-like MLDUS; the lymph node structure is dif-fusely effaced with preservation and partial dilatation of the sinuses; in the spleen, there is involvement of the white pulp.

Phenotype: *See* Ic-like MLDUS; cases with A or G heavy-chain Ig expression are seen.

Genotype: Molecular studies regularly show clonal rearrangements of Ig encoding genes.

(continues)

Table 2 (continued)

Marginal zone lymphoma (MZL)

Morphology: Neoplastic cells of small size show centrocyte-like or monocytoid profile and variable degrees of plasmacellular differentiation; when aggregates of 10–15 blasts are seen, possible transformation into a more aggressive form should be suspected; marginal zone derivation of blastic tumors can be accepted only in the presence of a small-cell component.

MALT-derived MZL shows: (1) multifocal distribution within the organ of origin, (2) tendency to colonize preexisting follicles, (3) infiltration of epithelial mucosal structures with formation of lymphoepithelial lesions, and (4) tendency to infiltrate the sinuses and marginal zone of regional lymph nodes.

Primary nodal MZL: The tumor infiltrates the sinuses and marginal zone.

Primary splenic MZL: The neoplasm diffuses through sinuses and infiltrates the marginal zone of Malpighi's corpuscles producing progressive obliteration.

Phenotype: Neoplastic cells express B-cell markers (CD19, CD20, CD22, CD79a), surface and cytoplasmic monotypic Ig (IgM$^+$/IgD$^-$, IgM$^+$/IgD$^+$ only for the splenic type) and—variably—CD43, CD68, DBA.44, and Ki-B3/CD45R; CD5, PRAD1, and CD10 are negative; *bcl-2* is weakly expressed; Ki-67 marking is low.

Genotype: Molecular studies have mainly focused on gastric MALT lymphoma, because of its frequency and response to *H. pylori:* eradication; HCV may be the equivalent for extragastric MZLs; in particular, a chronic inflammatory stimulus might facilitate the onset of clones incapable of DNA repair (i.e., with RER phenotype); some of these clones carrying abnormalities such as t(11;18) might take advantage over the others, producing an early lymphoma, that still needs the microbial stimulus and T-cell cooperation; further genomic aberrations, such as t(1;14) or +3, might make the growth independent of the microenvironment; finally, p53 point mutations or loss of homozygosity, *p16* deletion or c-*myc* rearrangements might produce the switch of the growth from low-grade to high-grade histology.

Follicle center lymphoma (FCL)

Morphology: Neoplastic cells resemble centrocytes and centroblasts of normal germinal centers and show a follicular growth pattern in most cases; three cytological grades are distinguished: 1 (centroblasts cover <25% of follicular areas), 2 (centroblasts cover from 25% to 50% of follicular areas), and 3 (centroblasts cover more than 50% of follicular areas).

Phenotype: Lymphomatous elements express B-cell markers (CD19, CD20, CD22, and more weakly CD79a), CD10 and the *bcl-6* gene product, but are negative for CD5; monotypic Ig are often detected on the cell surface and more rarely in the cytoplasm; *bcl-2* is overexpressed in >95% of cases; Ki-67 marking is variable: it usually parallels the content of centroblasts; antibodies against CD21, CD23, and CD35 show a more or less tight meshwork of follicular dendritic cells.

Genotype: In a randomly selected population, about 70% of cases show a translocation [t(14;18), t(2;18) or t(18;22)], which causes *bcl-2* gene rearrangement and overexpression of its product, which is a potent antiapoptotic agent; clonal rearrangements of the Ig encoding genes are regularly encountered.

(continues)

Table 2 (continued)

Diffuse large B-cell lymphoma (DLBCL)

    Morphology: Neoplastic cells of large size display variably shaped nuclei, numerous distinct nucleoli, and a rim of basophilic cytoplasm; tumors with homogeneous cytology (centroblastic, immunoblastic, multilobated, or anaplastic) can be seen; mitotic figures are numerous; the content of apoptotic bodies varies from case to case; T-cell-rich B-cell lymphoma represents a peculiar variant of the tumor, characterized by a high content of T-lymphocytes: immunohistochemistry is mandatory for its diagnosis, as it can easily be misdiagnosed as peripheral T-cell lymphoma or mixed cellularity Hodgkin's disease on morphology alone.

    Phenotype: Lymphomatous elements express CD19, CD20, CD22, and—more variably—CD79a and CD10; CD30 is regularly found in the anaplastic subtype; detection of surface and cytoplasmic Ig is inconstant; a proportion of cases is positive for *bcl-2* and *bcl-6:* however, the expression of these molecules is not indicative of specific gene rearrangements; Ki-67 marking is high.

    Genotype: In a randomly selected population, about 40% of DLBCLs carry rearrangements of the *bcl-6* gene (located at 3q27): this finding seems to be associated with a very good response to chemotherapy; about 30% of DLBCLs display *bcl-2* gene rearrangements: this might indicate their derivation from a preexisting FCL and heralds a poor clinical course; clonal rearrangements of Ig encoding genes are regularly encountered.

Multiple myeloma

    Morphology: In HCV-positive patients, the tumor more often shows low-grade cytology, interstitial infiltration, and pathological stage 1.

    Phenotype: Neoplastic cells express monotypic Ig, EMA, and in half the cases CD79a, while they are negative for both CD45 and most B-cell markers; occasional dot-like positivity for cytokeratin 8 can be seen in the Golgi area.

    Genotype: clonal rearrangements of Ig encoding genes are regularly found.

the REAL Classification *(66)*. With a critical review of the literature, most of the immunocytoma-like proliferation described by others does not satisfy the criteria of the REAL Classification *(66)*. In subtypes of MLDUS, repeated biopsies usually do not show expansion of monotypic B-cell infiltrates in the bone marrow *(65)*. In the liver these can even undergo histologic regression, in the course of cirrhotic evolution as reported by Monteverde et al. in 14 patients with MLDUS and type II MC *(69)*. Interestingly enough, in a few patients with MLDUS who received repeated bone marrow biopsies before and after interferon administration, regression of the lymphoid infiltrates was observed in conjunction with the clearance of HCV *(74,75)*.

    Monoclonal gammopathy of undetermined significance (MGUS) was diagnosed in many (11%) HCV-positive patients without cryoglobulinemia *(8)*. These cases were characterized by discrete interstitial infiltrates of the bone marrow by typical plasma cells, which did not always show clear-cut monotypia by immunohistochemistry. It is likely that the clone responsible for the M-spike in the serum was too small to modify the normal 2:1 or 3:1 ratio between κ- and λ-producing plasma cells. In a few cases, the monoclonal component reflected an overt myeloma. These MGUS cases in HCV-positive patients differ from MLDUS by histologic pattern, the frequent absence of cryoglobulinemia, and the type of M-component in the serum.

Most overt malignant lymphomas do not develop in patients with a previous history of MLDUS. This finding strengthens the concept that NHL does not necessarily stem from a preexisting HCV-associated "benign" lymphoproliferation, but rather that the virus might be indirectly involved in the pathogenesis of these malignancies *(32,34,72,76–79)*. Both small lymphocytic lymphoma/B-CLL and immunocytoma (Ic) can be encountered in HCV-positive patients (Fig. 1, panel 7), although in our files and those of other groups they do not represent the most common histologies *(78)*.

Malignant lymphomas can arise from the marginal zone of lymphoid follicles both in the nodes and at extranodal sites. In our experience, all three varieties of marginal zone lymphoma (MALT-derived, nodal, and splenic) can be observed in HCV-positive patients. Marginal zone lymphoma (Fig. 1) is one of the most common types of lymphoid tumor observed in HCV-positive patients. It has been suggested that in cases occurring in lymph nodes or at extranodal sites other than the stomach, HCV might play the same pathogenetic role as *Helicobacter pylori* in the development of gastric marginal zone (MALT) lymphoma *(see* Chapter 22) *(43,61,78)*. The two agents, however, do not seem to be mutually exclusive as some cases have been infected with both HCV and *Helicobacter pylori (43)*.

Follicular center lymphoma (Fig. 1, panel 8) is the most common variety of malignant lymphoma encountered in HCV-positive patients *(78)*. In the same patient population, diffuse large B-cell lymphoma (DLBCL) also has been reported rather frequently *(78)*. Recently, in Japan *(40)* and the United States *(80)*, a new clinicopathologic variant of DLBCL has been described, which primarily presents in the liver and sometimes the spleen and is associated in 71% of cases with HCV infection (Fig. 1, panel 9).

Finally, in a number of HCV-positive patients, the M-component actually reflected multiple myeloma *(8)*. In our experience, these are usually low-grade, pathologic stage 1 tumors with prevalent interstitial infiltration *(81)*. As the amount of neoplastic plasma cells can be modest, immunohistochemical tests in paraffin sections are useful to assess the monotypic nature of the infiltrate and its differentiation from florid reactive plasma-cytosis, which is polytypic by the determination of Ig light chains *(81)*.

HCV AND LYMPHOMAGENESIS

A causative role of viral agents in malignant lymphomas has been established for at least two viruses, namely, Epstein–Barr virus (EBV) and human T-cell leukemia/lymphoma virus I (HTLV-I). EBV is involved in lymphomas complicating immunocompromised patients and in 30% of non-African Burkitt's lymphoma, while HTLV-I is responsible for the adult T-cell leukemia/lymphoma syndrome in some geographic areas *(13)* *(see* Chapters 5 and 12, respectively). Since EBV has been ubiquitous for years and the role of HTLV-I is limited to particular patient populations, they cannot explain the increasing incidence of NHL in all parts of the world *(30)*. HCV-associated lymphomas may represent a new model for virus-induced cancer in humans.

In asymptomatic or symptomatic HCV chronically infected individuals, the intimate mechanism(s) responsible for the appearance of malignancy remains largely obscure. A variable combination of co-factors in the development of hepatic and/or lymphatic disorders in HCV-positive individuals should be considered. The presence of specific

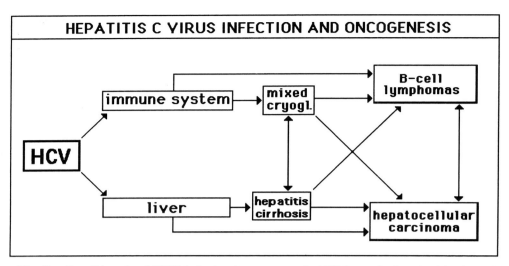

Fig. 2. Possible role of HCV infection in oncogenesis: HCV may be involved in the pathogeneis of hepatocellular carcinoma and/or B-cell lymphomas directly *(13,32–39,82)* or through liver and/or immune system disorders; namely, chronic hepatitis (±cirrhosis) and mixed cryoglobulinemia *(3,13,28,29,53,55–57)*. Both hepatocellular carcinoma and B-cell lymphoma may develop during the natural course of HCV chronic infection *(64)*. (Modified from ref. *13*.)

HCV mutants, possibly with higher oncogenic potential, other infectious or environmental agents, and genetically driven host reactivity may affect the clinical expression of HCV infection, including chronic hepatitis, systemic autoimmune disorders, and cancer *(10,13,15,21,22)*. HCV infection may lead to hepatocellular carcinoma and B-cell neoplasia through a network of events (Fig. 2). On the basis of clinico-epidemiological observations, cancer may develop directly with chronic HCV infection *(13,32–39,82)* or through intermediate steps of "benign" disorders *(13,28,29)*. The observation in the same subject of autoimmune and neoplastic diseases, concomitantly or sequentially, indicates that HCV-related disorders could be the result of a multifactorial and multistep process. In this respect, the example of MC described earlier, a condition with a mixture of different clinical features characterized by a generally benign clinical course, is particularly illuminating *(15–17,21,27)*.

Chronic HCV infection is the most frequent condition predisposing to hepatocellular carcinoma, regardless of cirrhosis, alcohol abuse, age, gender, or hepatitis B virus coinfection *(3,13,82)*. NHL may develop in patients with both immune suppression and immune stimulation conditions, such as acquired immunodeficiency syndrome (AIDS) or Sjögren's syndrome and rheumatoid arthritis, respectively *(13)*. Lymphotropism is a well recognized biologic characteristic of HCV *(11,12,25,26)*, and the mono- or polyclonal B-lymphocyte proliferation observed in chronically infected individuals may play an important pathogenetic role in HCV-associated disorders *(10,13)*. HCV is a positive, single-stranded RNA virus without a DNA intermediate in its replicative cycle, so that viral nucleic acid sequences cannot be integrated into the host genome. Thus, HCV-related NHL may be the product of complex oncogenic mechanisms for which this virus could be only a triggering factor. First, HCV might reactivate a latent infection of lymphocytes by a DNA virus, such as EBV or other human herpesviruses (HHV-6, HHV-7, HHV-8), which have been correlated with lymphomagenesis *(13,83)*. However, a preliminary observation on a small patient series indicates that coinfection with lymphotropic viruses is uncommon in HCV-associated NHL patients *(84)*. Possible cooperation between HCV and other RNA hepatitis viruses, such as hepatitis G virus (HGV), has been investigated in HCV-related MC *(85,86)*, but the possible contribution of HGV or other RNA viruses to lymphoproliferation remains unknown. Finally, a potential association between chronic HCV infection and the development of AIDS-related lymphoma seems to be excluded by recent clinicoepidemiologic observations *(see* Chapter 8) *(87)*.

The quasispecies nature of HCV *(9)* permits it to escape immune surveillance and favors the persistence of infection in the host. During long-lasting, asymptomatic HCV infection, viral antigens and/or HCV-induced autoantigens may exert a chronic stimulus to the immune system with consequent abnormally active lymphocyte proliferation. This condition per se could predispose to further cell alterations. Moreover, a mechanism of molecular mimicry between epitopes of virus and host may play an important pathogenetic role, as suggested by the frequent detection of anti-GOR antibodies in HCV seropositives *(13,88)*. These antibodies are specific for both HCV core and a host nuclear antigen termed GOR, which is detected only in the nuclei of cancer cells, in which it is probably overexpressed. On this basis, it has been hypothesized that *GOR* gene may be an oncogene *(88)*. Although not definitely demonstrated, such an immune-mediated process could be involved in the first steps of HCV-related oncogenesis.

In a single patient with type II MC, a monoclonal B-cell expansion has been correlated with genetic aberrations involving, in sequence, *bcl-2* and c-*myc* oncogenes *(89)*. An increased expression of bcl-2 protein has been observed in liver and bone marrow sections in patients with type II MC *(65)*. More interestingly, *bcl-2* recombination [t(14;18)] has been documented in the peripheral blood lymphocytes of HCV-infected individuals, with or without MC or B-cell lymphoma *(90)*. T (14;18) translocation is frequently involved in NHL *(91)*. The *bcl-2* protooncogene codes for the bcl-2 protein that is able to inhibit apoptosis *(92)*. Dysfunction of *bcl-2* leads to extended cell survival that allows other genetic aberrations, such as translocation of the *myc* oncogene, perhaps inducing more malignant characteristics, as observed in high-grade lymphomas *(93)*.

A beneficial effect of antiviral treatment by α-interferon in MC patients, including regression of low-grade lymphomatous infiltrates in the bone marrow *(75)*, has been observed *(94)*. This may indirectly support the hypothesis that viral factors can be involved in lymphoproliferation and probably in its maintenance, at least during the early stages of the disease. Another model of infectious antigen-driven lymphoma has been proposed in patients with *Helicobacter pylori* gastric infection, among whom a MALT type B-cell lymphoma may evolve from gastritis to frank lymphoma through a reactive lymphoid hyperplasia *(95) (see also* Chapter 22). Gene rearrangement studies suggested that multiple genetic aberrations, in a stepwise fashion, are involved in the clonal B-cell expansion preceding the overt lymphoma. This lymphoma may be responsive to *Helicobacter pylori* eradication *(96)*. There are clear analogies between *Helicobacter pylori* and HCV-associated lymphomagenesis, in particular MLDUS. The monotypic/oligoclonal lymphoproliferation observed in HCV-positive patients might arise within the context of an inflammatory process that fosters some clones over others through genetic alterations. As postulated to explain the sensitivity of gastric MALT lymphoma to *Helicobacter pylori*-eradicating therapy *(96)*, maintenance of these selected clones might require the persistence of the microbial stimulus and T-cell cooperation. Thus, eradication of the microbe might produce regression of the lymphoid clone. Further molecular studies are needed to test this hypothesis and to understand whether the frank lymphomas developing in about 10% of patients with MLDUS are clonally related to the preexisting lymphoproliferation *(79)*. At this time, there is no definitive proof that this relationship does indeed exist. Finally, the study of NHL patients with *Helicobacter pylori* and HCV coinfection might give us new interesting pathogenetic insights *(43)*.

Among numerous agents so far proposed, HCV infection could represent a novel etiologic factor of B-cell NHL. These are a heterogeneous group of malignancies with regard to their etiopathogenesis and clinicoepidemiologic characteristics. Therefore, it is not surprising that the role of HCV varies greatly among patient populations from different geographical areas *(13)*. Larger studies, with intensive molecular biology and virology, are needed to clarify the clinical relevance and the pathogenesis of HCV-associated lymphomas.

TREATMENT OF HCV-ASSOCIATED LYMPHOMA

The treatment of HCV-associated lymphomas does not differ substantially from that of "idiopathic" B-cell NHL *(97)*. However, the occurrence in the same subject of chronic viral infection and cancer and, in some cases, of other HCV-related disorders may be a conditioning factor for an optimal therapeutic strategy (Fig. 3). In all patients with B-cell NHL, the detection of HCV-related markers (anti-HCV and HCV RNA) is obviously mandatory, together with histologic classification and staging of the disease. Before the treatment and during the patient's clinical follow-up, HCV-positive NHL patients should be carefully evaluated for chronic hepatitis, cirrhosis, hepatocellular carcinoma, mixed cryoglobulinemia syndrome, and other HCV-related disorders, such as thyroiditis and glomerulonephritis. To date, there is not sufficient information on specific complications of cancer chemotherapy in HCV-positive NHL. In a series of patients with lymphoplasmacytoid lymphoma/immunocytoma, the presence or absence of HCV infection did not affect overall survival, although the quality of life was significantly worse in HCV-positive individuals regardless the therapeutic interventions *(72,78)*. These differences were mainly related to one or more manifestations of HCV infection, such as chronic hepatitis, glomerulonephritis, or cryoglobulinemic vasculitis.

For isolated B-cell NHL, a standard treatment can be followed according to clinical and pathologic assessment of the disease *(97)*. In the presence of severe liver and/or renal impairment, some precautions should be followed to tailor the treatment for the individual patient. In patients with MC complicated by B-cell NHL, but without severe visceral organ involvement, chemotherapy is usually well tolerated and improvement of the cryoglobulinemic syndrome may be observed. In MC with low-grade NHL, cycles of single-agent (cyclophosphamide) therapy are often sufficient for a complete remission. In HCV-infected individuals, with or without MC, a low-grade NHL can be observed at bone marrow biopsy examination. This is often a clin-

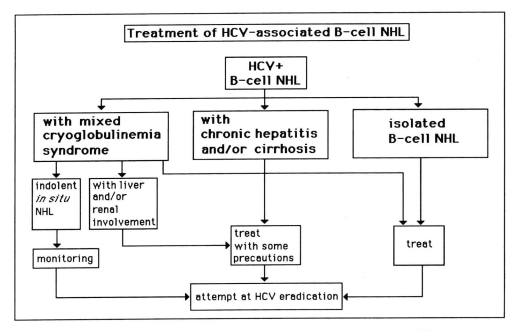

Fig. 3. Therapeutic strategies in HCV-associated B-cell NHL.

ically asymptomatic, nonprogressive lymphoma that may not require any specific treatment (Fig. 3).

Following the positive results observed in HCV-related chronic hepatitis *(98),* an attempt for HCV eradication with combined α-interferon and ribavirin treatment might also be tried in HCV-associated NHL, particularly with low-grade lymphomas (Fig. 3).

With the rapid growth of molecular biology we can hopefully try new and more efficient therapeutic strategies. The recent identification of the interaction between HCV envelope protein E2 and CD81 on both hepatocytes and lymphocytes *(99)* suggests the possibility of interfering with HCV binding to target cells. A vaccine-based therapy with recombinant HCV proteins may be able to prevent the evolution from viral infection to life-threatening clinical complications.

REFERENCES

1. Choo GL, Kuo G, Weiner AJ, Overby LR, Bradley DW, Houghton M. Isolation of a cDNA clone derived from a blood-borne non-A non-B viral hepatitis genome. Science 1989; 244:359–361.
2. Kuo G, Choo QL, Alter HJ. An assay for circulating antibodies to a major etiologic virus of human NANBH hepatitis. Science 1989; 362–364.
3. Hollinger FB. NANBH viruses. In: Hollinger FB, Robinson WS, Purcell RH, Garin JL, Ticehurst J (eds). Viral Hepatitis, Biological and Clinical Features, Specific Diagnosis and Prophylaxis. New York: Raven Press, 1991, pp. 139–173.
4. Garson JA, Tedder RS, Briggs M. Detection of HCV sequences in blood donations by "nested" PCR and prediction of infectivity. Lancet 1990; 335:1419–1422.
5. Lau JY, Krawczynski K, Negro F, Gonzalez-Peralta RP. In situ detection of hepatitis C virus—a critical appraisal. J Hepatol 1996; 24 (2 Suppl):43–51.

6. Simmonds P, Holmes EC, Cha TA, Chan SW, McOmish F, Irvine B, et al. Classification of hepatitis C virus into six major genotypesand a series of subtypes by phylogenetic analysis of the NS-5 region. J Gen Virol 1993; 74:2391–2399.

7. Zignego AL, Ferri C, Giannini C, Monti M, La Civita L, Careccia G, et al. Hepatitis C virus genotype analysis in patients with type II mixed cryoglobulinemia. Ann Intern Med 1996; 124:31–34.

8. Andreone P, Zignego AL, Cursaro C, Gramenzi A, Gherlinzoni F, Fiorino S, et al. Prevalence of monoclonal gammopathies in patients with hepatitis C virus infection. Ann Inter Med 1998; 129:294–298.

9. Martell M, Esteban JI, Quer J. Hepatitis C virus (HCV) circulates as a population of different but closely related genomes: quasispecies nature of HCV genome distribution. J Virol 1992; 66:3225–3229.

10. Gumber S, Chopra S. Hepatitis C: a multifaceted disease. Review of extrahepatic manifestations. Ann Intern Med 1995; 123:615–620.

11. Zignego AL, Macchia D, Monti M, Thiers V, Mazzetti M, Foschi M, et al. Infection of peripheral mononuclear blood cells by hepatitis C virus. J Hepatol 1992; 15:382–386.

12. Ferri C, Monti M, La Civita L, Longombardo G, Greco F, Pasero G, et al. Infection of peripheral blood mononuclear cells by hepatitis C virus in mixed cryoglobulinemia. Blood 1993; 82:3701–3704.

13. Ferri C, La Civita L, Zignego AL, Pasero G, Viruses and cancer: possible role of hepatitis C virus [review]. Eur J Clin Invest 1997; 27:711–718.

14. Gorevic PD, Frangione B: Mixed cryoglobulinemia cross-reactive idiotypes: implication for relationship of mixed cryoglobulinemia to rheumatic and lymphoproliferative diseases. Semin Hematol 1991; 28:79–94.

15. Ferri C, La Civita L, Longombardo G, Zignego AL, Pasero G. Mixed cryoglobulinemia: a crossroad between autoimmune and lymphoproliferative disorders [review]. Lupus 1998; 7:275–279.

16. Brouet JC, Clouvel JP, Danon F, Klein M, Seligmann M. Biologic and clinical significance of cryoglobulins. Am J Med 1974; 57:775–788.

17. Meltzer M, Franklin EC, Elias K, McCluskey RT, Cooper N. Cryoglobulinemia. A clinical and laboratory study. II. Cryoglobulins with rheumatoid factor activity. Am J Med 1966; 40:837–856.

18. Monti G, Galli M, Invernizzi F, Pioltelli P, Saccardo F, Monteverde A, et al. Cryoglobulinaemias: a multi-centre study of the early clinical and laboratory manifestations of primary and secondary disease GISC. Italian Group for the Study of Cryoglobulinaemias. Q J Med 1995; 88:115–126.

19. Perl A, Gorevic PD, Ryan DH, Condemi JJ, Ruszkowski RJ, Abraham GN. Clonal B cell expansion in patients with essential mixed cryoglobulinemia. Clin Exp Immunol 1989; 76:54–60.

20. Ferri C, Greco F, Longombardo G, Palla P, Moretti A, Marzo E, et al. Association between hepatitis C virus and mixed cryoglobulinaemia. Clin Exp Rheumatol 1991; 9:621–624.

21. Ferri C, La Civita L, Longombardo G, Greco F, Bombardieri S. Hepatitis C virus and mixed cryoglobulinemia [review]. Eur J Clin Invest 1993; 23:399–405.

22. Abel G, Zhang Q-X, Agnello V. Hepatitis C virus infection in type II mixed cryoglobulinemia [review]. Arthritis Rheum 1993; 36:1341–1349.

23. Agnello V, Chung RT, Kaplan L.M. A role for hepatitis C virus infection in type II cryoglubulinemia. N Engl J Med 1992; 327:1490–1495.

24. Disdier P, Harlé JR, Weiller PJ: Cryoglobulinemia and hepatitic infection [letter]. Lancet 1991; 338:1151–1152.

25. Gabrielli A, Manzin A, Candela M, Caniglia ML, Paolucci S, Danieli MG. Active hepatitis C virus infection in bone marrow and peripheral blood mononuclear cells from patients with mixed cryoglobulinemia. Clin Exp Immunol 1994; 97:87–93.

26. Sansonno D, De Vita S, Cornacchiulo V, Carbone A, Baiocchi M, Dammacco F. Detection and distribution of hepatitis C-related proteins in lymph nodes of patients with type II cryoglobulinemia and neoplastic or non-neoplastic lymphoproliferation. Blood 1996; 88:4638–4645.

27. Monteverde A, Rivano MT, Allegra GC, Monteverde Al, Zigrossi P, Baglioni P, et al. Essential mixed cryoglobulinemia, type II: a manifestation of low malignant lymphoma? Clinical-morphological study of 12 cases with special reference to immunohistochemical findings in liver frozen sections. Acta Haematol 1988; 79:20–25.

28. Ferri C, Monti M, La Civita L, Careccia G, Mazzaro C, Longombardo G. et al. Hepatitis C virus infection in non-Hodgkin's B-cell lymphoma complicating mixed cryoglobulinaemia. Eur J Clin Invest 1994; 24:781–784.

29. Pozzato G, Mazzaro C, Crovatto M, Modolo ML, Ceselli S, Mazzi G, Sulfaro S, Franzin F, Tulissi P, Moretti M, Santini GF.: Low-grade malignant lymphoma, hepatitis C virus infection, and mixed cryoglobulinemia. Blood 1994; 84:3047–3053.

30. Devesa SS, Fears T. Non-Hodgkin's lymphomas time trends. United States and international data. Cancer Res 1992; 52/S5432–40.

31. Heimann R, Lespagnard L, Dargent JL, Desmet VJ: Is there a link between viral hepatitis and lymphoproliferative disorders? From the autopsy room to the PCR thermal cycler [review]. Curr Diagn Pathol 1996; 3:177–181.

32. Ferri C, Caracciolo F, Zignego AL, La Civita L, Monti M, Longobardo G, et al. Hepatitis C virus infection in patients with non-Hodgkin's lymphoma. Br J Haematol 1994; 88:392–394.

33. Cavanna L, Sbolli G, Tanzi E, Romanò L, Civardi G, Buscarini E, et al. High prevalence of antibodies to hepatitis C virus in patients with lymphoproliferative disorders [letter]. Haematologica 1995; 80:486–487.

34. Luppi M, Grazia FM, Bonaccorsi G, Longo G, Narni F, Barozzi P, et al. Hepatitis C virus infection in a subset of neoplastic lymphoproliferations not associated with cryoglobulinemia. Leukemia 1996; 10:351–355.

35. Silvestri F, Pipan C, Barillari G, Zaja F, Fanin R, Infanti L, et al. Prevalence of hepatitis C virus infection in patients with lymphoproliferative disorders. Blood 1996; 87:4296–4301.

36. Mazzaro C, Zagonel V, Monfardini S, Tulissi P, Pussini E, Fanni M, et al. Hepatitis C virus and non-Hodgkin#alOs lymphomas. Br J Haematol 1996; 94:544–550.

37. Musolino C, Campo S, Pollicino T, Squadrito G, Spatari G, Raimondo G. Evaluation of hepatitis B and C virus infections in patients with non-Hodgkin's lymphoma and without liver disease. Haematologica 1996; 81:162–164.

38. Zignego AL, Ferri C, Innocenti F, Giannini C, Monti M, Bellesi G, et al. Lack of preferential localization of tumoral mass in B-cell non-Hodgkin's lymphoma associated with hepatitis C virus infection [letter]. Blood 1997; 89:3066–3068.

39. Zuckerman E, Zuckerman T, Levine AM, Douer D, Gutekunst K, Mizokami M, et al. Hepatitis C virus infection in patients with B-cell non-Hodgkin's lymphoma. Ann Intern Med 1997; 127:423–428.

40. Izumi T, Sasaki R, Miura Y, Okamoto H: Primary hepato-splenic lymphoma: association with hepatitis C virus infection [letter]. Blood 1996; 87:5380–5381.

41. Ohsawa M, Tomita Y, Hashimoto M, Kanno H, Aozasa K. Hepatitis C viral genome in a subset of primary hepatic lymphomas. Mod Pathol 1998; 11:471–478.

42. Ferri C, La Civita L, Caracciolo F, Bellesi G, Zignego AL. Hepatitis C virus and lymphoproliferative disorders [letter]. Blood 1996; 88:4730–4731.

43. Luppi M, Longo G, Ferrari MG, Ferrara L, Marasca R, Barozzi P, et al. Additional neoplasms and HCV infection in low-grade lymphoma of MALT type. Br J Haematol 1996; 94:373–375.

44. De Rosa G, Gobbo ML, De Renzo A, Notaro R, Garofalo S, Grimaldi M, et al. High prevalence of hepatitis C virus infection in patients with B-cell lymphoproliferative disorders in Italy. Am J Hematol 1997; 55:77–82.

45. Ellenrieder V, Weidenbach H, Frickhofen N, Michel D, Prummer O, Klatt S, et al. HCV and HGV in B-cell non-Hodgkin's lymphoma. J Hepatol 1998; 28:34–39.

46. Musto P, Dell'Olio M, Carotenuto M, Mangia A, Andriulli A. Hepatitis C virus infection: a new bridge between hematologists and gastroenterologists? [letter]. Blood 1996; 88:752–753.

47. Hanley J, Jarvis L, Simmonds P, Parker A, Ludlam C. HCV and non-Hodgkin lymphoma [letter]. Lancet 1996; 347:1339.

48. Brind AM, Watson JP, Burt A, Kestevan P, Proctor SJ, et al. Non-Hodgkin's lymphoma and hepatitis C virus infection. Leukemia Lymphoma 1996; 21:127–130.

49. McColl MD, Singer IO, Tait RC, McNeil IR, Cumming RL, Hogg RB. The role of hepatitis C virus in the aetiology of non-Hodgkin's lymphoma—a regional association? [letter]. Leukemia Lymphoma 1997; 26:127–130.

50. King PD, Wilkes JD, Diaz-Arias AA. Hepatitis C virus infection in non-Hodgkin's lymphoma. Clin Lab Haematol 1998; 20:107–110.

51. Mussini C, Ghini M, Mascia MT, Giovanardi P, Zanni G, Lattuada l, et al. Monoclonal gammopathies and hepatitis C virus infection [letter]. Blood 1995; 85:1144–1145.

52. Izumi T, Sasaki R, Tsunoda S, Akutsu M, Okamoto H, Miura MT. B-cell malignancy and hepatitis C virus infection. Leukemia 1997; 11:516–518.

53. Ferri C, La Civita L, Monti M, Longombardo G, Greco F, Pasero G, et al. Can type C hepatitis be complicated by B-cell malignant lymphoma? [letter]. Lancet 1995; 346:1426–1427.

54. Brind AM, Watson JP, James OF, Bassendine MF. Hepatitis C virus infection in the elderly. Q J Med 1996; 89:291–296.

55. Sikuler E, Shnaider A, Zilberman D, Hilzenrat N, Shemer-Avni Y, Neumann L, et al. Hepatitis C virus infection and extrahepatic malignacies. J Clin Gastroenterol 1997; 24:87–89.

56. Andreone P, Gramenzi A, Cursaro C, Bernardi M, Zignego AL. Monoclonal gammopathy in patients with chronic hepatitis C virus infection. [letter]. Blood 1996; 88:1122.

57. Hausfater P, Cacoub P, Bernard N, Loustaud-Ratti V, Le Lostec Z, Laurichesse H, et al. Hepatitis C virus infection and malignant lymphoproliferative disease: French national study. Arthritis Rheum 1998; 41 (9 Suppl): Abstr 1648.

58. Sansonno D, Iacobelli AR, Cornacchiulo V, Iodice G, Dammacco F. Detection of hepatitis C virus (HCV) proteins by immunofluorescence and HCV RNA genomic sequences by non-isotopic in situ hybridization in bone marrow and peripheral blood mononuclear cells of chronically HCV-infected patients. Clin Exp Immunol 1996; 103:414–421.

59. Agnello V, Abel G. Localization of hepatitis C virus in cutaneous vasculitic lesions in patients with type II cryoglobulinemia. Arthritis Rheum 1997; 40:2007–2015.

60. Manzin A, CAndela M, Paolucci S, Caniglia ML, Gabrielli A, Clementi M. Presence of hepatitis C virus (HCV) genomic intermediates in bone marrow and peripheral blood mononuclear cells from HCV-infected patients. Clin Diagn Lab Immunol 1994; 1:160–163.

61. De Vita S, Sansonno D, Dolcetti R, Ferraccioli GF, Carbone A, Cornacchiulo V, et al. Hepatitis C virus within malignant lymphoma lesion in the course of type II mixed cryoglobulinemia. Blood 1995; 86:1887–1892.

62. Alexander FE. Blood transfusion and risk of non-Hodgkin lymphoma. Lancet 1997; 350:1414–1415.

63. Blumberg N, Moller T, Olsson JI, Anderson H, Mollet T. Cancer morbidity in blood recipients—result of a cohort study. Eur J Cancer 1993; 29A:2101–2105.

64. Tanaka H, Tsukuma H, Teshima H, Ajiki W, Koyama Y, Kinoshita N, et al. Second primary cancers following non-Hodgkin's lymphoma in Japan: increased risk of hepatocellular carcinoma. Jpn J Cancer Res 1997; 88:537–542.

65. Monteverde A, Sabattini E, Poggi S, Ballarè M, Bertoncelli MC, de Vivo A. Bone marrow findings further support the hypothesis that essential mixed cryoglobulinemia type II is characterized by a monoclonal B-cell proliferation. Leukemia Lymphoma 1995; 20:119–124.

66. Harris N, Jaffe E, Stein H, Banks P, Chan J, Cleary M. A revised European-American Classification of lymphoid neoplasms: a proposal from the International Lymphoma Study Group. Blood 1994; 84:1361–1392.
67. The non-Hodgkin's lymphoma classification project. A clinical evaluation of the International Lymphoma Study Group Classification of non-Hodgkin's lymphoma. Blood 1997; 89:3909–3918.
68. Pileri S A, Milani M, Fraternali Orcioni G, Sabattini E. From the R.E.A.L. Classification to the upcoming WHO scheme: a step forward to a universal categorizing of lymphoma entities? Ann Oncol 1998; 9:607–612.
69. Monteverde A, Ballarè M, Pileri S. Hepatic lymphoid aggregates in chronic hepatitis C and mixed cryoglobulinemia. Springer Semin Imunopathol 1997; 19:99–110.
70. Mangia A, Clemente R, Musto P, Casciavilla I, La Foresta P, Sanpaolo G. Hepatitis C virus infection and monoclonal gammopathies not associated with cryoglobulinemia. Leukemia 1996; 10:1209–1213.
71. Santini GF, Crovatto M, Modolo ML, Martelli P, Silvia C, Mazzi G. Waldenstrom's macroglobulinemia: a role of HCV infection? [letter]. Blood 1993; 82:2932.
72. Silvestri F, Barillari G, Fanin R, Salmaso F, Pipan E, Puglisi F, et al. Impact of hepatitis C virus infection on clinical features, quality of life and survival with lymphoplasmacytoid lymphoma/immunocytoma. Ann Oncol 1998; 9:499–504.
73. Lennert K, Feller AC. Histopathology of non-Hodgkin's lymphomas (based on the Updated Kiel Classification). Berlin: Spinger-Verlag, 1992.
74. Lai R, Weiss LM. Hepatitis C virus and non-Hodgkin's lymphoma. Am J Clin Pathol 1998; 109:508–510.
75. Mazzaro C, Franzin F, Tulissi P, Pussini E, Crovatto M, Carniello GS, et al. Regression of monoclonal B-cell expansion in patients affected by mixed cryoglobulinemia responsive to α-interferon therapy. Cancer 1996; 77:2604–2613.
76. Ascoli V, Lo Coco F, Artini M, Levrero M, Martelli M, Negro F. Extranodal lymphomas associated with hepatitis C virus infection. Am J Clin Pathol 1998; 109:600–609.
77. De Vita S, Sacco C, Sansonno D, Gioghini A, Dammacco F, Crovatto M, et al. Characterization of overt B-cell lymphomas in patients with hepatitis C virus infection. Blood 1997; 90:776–782.
78. Luppi M, Longo G, Ferrari MG, Barozzi P, Marasca R, Morselli M, et al. Clinico-pathological characterization of hepatitis C virus-related B-cell non-Hodgkin's lymphomas without symptomatic cryoglobulinemia. Ann Oncol 1998; 9:495–498.
79. Magalini AR, Facchetti F, Salvi L, Fontana M, Puoti M, Scarpa A. Clonality of B-cells in portal lymphoid infiltrates of HCV-infected livers. J Pathol 1998; 185:86–90.
80. Page RD, Romaguera J, Osborne B, Cabanillas F. Primary hepatic lymphoma and association with hepatitis C viral infection [letter]. Blood 1996; 88 (Suppl. l):223.
81. Pileri S, Poggi S, Baglioni P, Montanari M, Sabattini E, Galieni P, et al. Histology and immunohistology of bone marrow biopsy in multiple myeloma. Eur J Haematol 1989; (Suppl. 51) 43:52–59.
82. De Mitri MS, Poussin K, Baccarini P, Pontisso P, D'Errico A, Simon N, et al. HCV-associated liver cancer without cirrhosis. Lancet 1995; 345:413–415.
83. Luppi M, Torelli G. The new lymphotropic herpesviruses (HHV-6, HHV-7, HHV-8) and hepatitis C virus (HCV) in human lymphoproliferative diseases: an overview. Haematologica 1996; 81:265–281.
84. Ferri C, Lo Jacono F, Monti M, Caracciolo F, La Civita L, Barsanti LA et al. Lymphotropic virus infection of peripheral blood mononuclear cells in B-cell non-Hodgkin's lymphoma. Acta Haematol 1997; 98:89–94.
85. Zignego AL, Giannini C, Gentilini P, Bellesi G, Hadziyannis S, Ferri C. Could HGV infection be implicated in lymphomagenesis? [letter] Br J Haematol 1997; 98:778–779.

86. Tepper JL, Feinman SV, D'Costa L, Sooknannan R, Pruzanski W. Hepatitis G and hepatitis C RNA viruses coexisting in cryoglobulinemia. J Rheumatol 1998; 25:925–928.

87. Levine AM, Nelson R, Zuckerman E, Zuckerman T, Govindarajan S, Valinluck, et al. Lack of association between hepatitis C infection and development of AIDS-related lymphoma. J Acquir Defic Syndr Hum Retrovirol 1999; 20:255–258.

88. Mishiro S, Takeda K, Hoshi Y, Yoshikawa A, Gotanda T, Itoh Y. An autoantibody crossreactive to hepatitis C virus core and a host nuclear antigen. Autoimmunity 1991; 10:269–273.

89. Ellis M, Rathaus M, Amiel A, Manor Y, Klein A, Lishner M. Monoclonal lymphocyte proliferation and *bcl-2* rearrangement in essential mixed cryoglobulinaemia. Eur J Clin Invest 1995; 25:833–837.

90. Zignego AL, Giannelli F, Marrocchi, Giannini C, Gentilini P, Innocenti F, et al. Frequency of *bcl-2* rearrangement in patients with mixed cryoglobulinemia and HCV-positive liver diseases [letter]. Clin Exp Rheumatol 1997; 15:711–712.

91. Ngan BY, Chen LZ, Weiss LM, Warnike RA, Cleary ML. Expression in non-Hodgkin's lymphoma of the bcl-2 protein associated with the t(14 : 18) translocation. N Engl J Med 1988; 318:1638–1644.

92. Korsmeyer SJ. *Bcl-2:* a repressor of lymphocyte death. Immunol Today 1992; 13:285–287.

93. Strasser A, Harris AW, Bath ML, Cory S. Novel primitive lymphoid tumors induced in trangenic mice by cooperation between *myc* and *bcl-2*. Nature 1990; 348:331–334.

94. Ferri C, Marzo E, Longombardo G, Lombardini F, La Civita L, Vanacore R, et al.: Alpha-Interferon in mixed cryoglobulinemia patients: a randomized crossover controlled trial. Blood 1993; 81:1132–1136.

95. Stolte M. *Helicobacter pylori* gastritis and gastric MALT-lymphoma. Lancet 1992; 339:745–746.

96. Carlson SJ, Yokoo H, Vanagunas A. Progression of gastritis to monoclonal B-cell lymphoma with resolution and recurrence following eradication of *Helicobacter pylori.* JAMA 1996; 275:937–939.

97. Wintrobe's Clinical Hematology, 10th edit. Lee GR, Foerster J, Lukens J, Paraskevas F, Greer JP, Rodgers GM (eds). Baltimore: Williams & Wilkins, 1998, pp. 2076–2101.

98. McHutchison JG, Gordon SC, Schiff ER, Shiffman ML, Lee WM, Rustgi VK, et al. Interferon alpha-2b alone or in combination with ribavirin as initial treatment for chronic hepatitis C. Hepatitis Interventional Therapy Group. N Engl J Med 1998; 339:1485–1492.

99. Pileri P, Uematsu Y, Campagnoli S, Galli G, Falugi F, Petracca R, et al. Binding of hepatitis C virus to CD81. Science 1998; 282:938–941.

VI
Bacterial and Helminthic Oncology

20

Overview of *Helicobacter pylori*

James G. Fox and Timothy C. Wang

DISCOVERY AND TAXONOMY

Discovery

Although diseases such as peptic ulcer disease and gastric cancer have been recognized for centuries, an infectious cause was not actively pursued until the latter part of the 20th century. Prior to 1982, peptic ulcer disease was attributed to excessive acid or stress, while gastric cancer was linked to a number of dietary factors suggested by extensive epidemiologic surveys. Both were known to be associated with chronic inflammation (gastritis) of the stomach, but this association remained unexplained. Nevertheless, the existence of gastric bacteria and a possible association with ulcer disease had been reported by investigators dating as far back as the 19th century. For example, in 1875, Bottcher and Letulle were able to demonstrate the presence of bacteria within the floor and margins of ulcers *(1)*, and Jaworski in 1889 described the presence of spiral organisms in the sediment of gastric washings. In 1924, Luck detected the presence of urease activity within the gastric mucosa. His work on gastric urease was confirmed by Conway and Fitzgerald, who also concluded that urease was endogenously produced by gastric epithelial cells and probably functioned as a mucosal protective agent to neutralize gastric acid *(2)*.

In 1938, Doenges studied 242 human gastric autopsy specimens, and found "spirochaetes" in 43% of these specimens, but was unable to reach any conclusions because of the presence of significant autolysis *(3)*. However, this observation led to a study in 1941 by Freedburg and Barron of 35 partial gastrectomy specimens, in which they detected "spirochaetes" in 37% of the samples analyzed *(4)*. Even with the aid of silver staining methodologies, these investigators found the organism extremely difficult to detect; nevertheless, they noted that the bacteria were more often associated with ulcers, both benign and malignant. Finally, in the early 1950s, Palmer conducted an extensive survey of 1140 gastric biopsy specimens that were examined histologically (although without silver stains); not surprisingly, without the aid of silver stains, he reported the finding that "no structure which could reasonably be considered to be of a spirochaetal nature" *(5)*. Consequently, the previous reports of spiral bacteria were interpreted as oral contaminants that multiplied in the postmortem setting. In the

From: *Infectious Causes of Cancer: Targets for Intervention*
Edited by: J. J. Goedert © Humana Press Inc., Totowa, NJ

1950s, the principle was established that because of its low pH the stomach was for the most part sterile and bacteria could not survive.

In the 1970s, upper endoscopy became established at many centers, leading to more frequent mucosal sampling of the gastric epithelium through endoscopic biopsy. In 1975, Steer and Colin-Jones reported the finding of bacteria closely related to the gastric mucosa in association with biopsy specimens showing gastritis but not in biopsies from normal stomachs *(6,7).* The bacteria in their samples appeared to be under the mucous layer and in close contact with surface mucous cells. They observed the presence of flagellae—"at least one filum projecting from one end of the bacterium"—and their ultrastructural studies actually revealed that the bacteria were spiral, although this was not highlighted in their reports. They hypothesized that the polymorphonuclear leukocytes present in the mucosa may have migrated in response to the presence of these bacteria, and believed that they were not contaminants. Steer attempted to isolate and culture the organisms, but was able to grow only *Pseudomonas aeruginosa* which was almost certainly a contaminant *(8).*

However, the observation that spiral bacteria were present in the gastric mucosa was concurrently pursued in Western Australia by a pathologist, Dr. J. Robin Warren, at the Royal Perth Hospital. Warren had observed for many years the presence of bacteria in the stomachs of gastritis patients, and in 1980 began compiling a series of cases in which he carried out both H&E and silver staining. In 1982, he was joined in his studies by a gastroenterology fellow, Barry Marshall. In 1983, Warren reported that "unidentified curved bacilli" were present in about half of all routine gastric biopsies and were strongly associated with the presence of "active, chronic gastritis" *(9).* He stated his belief that "these organisms should be recognized and their significance investigated." In an accompanying letter in the same issue of *The Lancet,* Marshall reported that he was able (after 34 previous failures) to culture the organisms on chocolate agar using *Campylobacter* isolation techniques and that he identified spiral bacteria about 2.5 μm in length with up to five sheathed flagellae that bore some resemblance to *Campylobacter* species *(10).* Although his initial studies did not address the possible pathogenic role of these bacteria, he concluded that "…they may have a part to play in other poorly understood, gastritis associated diseases (i.e., peptic ulcer and gastric cancer)."

Marshall and Warren, in 1984, published a subsequent paper in which they tested (through Warthin-Starry silver stains) for the presence of bacteria in 100 consecutive patients undergoing gastroscopy *(11).* In this prospective study, they found spiral or curved bacteria in 58 of 100 patients, and they cultured bacteria from 11 of these patients. They characterized the bacteria more definitively as Gram-negative, flagellate, microaerophilic, and named the bacteria *Campylobacter pyloridis.* They found the bacteria in "…almost all patients with active chronic gastritis, duodenal ulcer, or gastric ulcer," suggesting a possible etiologic role in these diseases. Over the next several years, the bacteria were isolated and cultured in a number of different countries (United Kingdom, Holland, Germany, the United States, Canada, Japan, and Peru), and the bacteria were characterized in much greater detail.

To demonstrate more convincingly that *C. pyloridis* could directly produce gastritis and/or symptoms (and thus fulfill Koch's postulates), Marshall orally ingested an isolate obtained from a 66-yr-old man with nonulcer dyspepsia *(12).* Prior to self-inoculation, he underwent upper endoscopy with biopsy which revealed no ulceration or gastritis or evidence of infection. After premedication with cimetidine, Marshall swallowed ~10^9 colony-forming units (cfu). Over the next several weeks, he developed a mild illness, characterized by symptoms of indigestion, bloating, nausea, vomiting, headache, irritability, and breath that was "putrid." At 10 d post-inoculation, gastroscopy revealed active gastritis. Surprisingly, at 14 d post-inoculation, symptoms resolved, and gastroscopy showed resolution of gastritis. This experiment was repeated by another investigator, Arthur Morris, in New Zealand. Morris ingested a different isolate (3×10^5 cfu) obtained from a 69-yr-old woman with dyspepsia and chronic gastritis; following which he developed moderate to severe attacks of epigastric pain, acute achlorhydria, and evidence of histologic gastritis *(13)*. Morris' symptoms evolved into a chronic dyspepsia that persisted through three courses of antibiotics, but they eventually resolved 3 yr later after a course of triple therapy with bismuth, metronidazole, and tetracycline *(14)*.

Taxonomy

The organism identified by Marshall and Warren initially was named *Campylobacter pyloridis,* and at first glance the organism appeared to be quite similar to other *Campylobacter* species. The gastric organisms were observed to be microaerophilic, Gram-negative, spiral shaped bacteria that morphologically closely resembled bacteria of the *Campylobacter* genus. Given this similarity, these "campylobacter-like organisms" achieved official recognition in 1985 as *Campylobacter pyloridis (15),* and in 1987 the name was officially changed to *Campylobacter pylori.* From the beginning, however, it was recognized that the organisms had a flagellar morphology that was distinct from organisms belonging to the *Campylobacter* genus *(11)*. Whereas members of the *Campylobacter* genus possessed a single unsheathed flagellum, the organism isolated by Marshall and Warren was characterized by four sheathed flagella at one end. In addition, the DNA base composition and the cell wall components of Marshall's bacterium differed substantially from those of other species of the *Campylobacter* genus. Finally, antibodies to Marshall's gastric bacterium showed little cross-reactivity with *C. jejuni* and other pathogenic *Campylobacter* species, indicating significant antigenic diversity. Thus, in 1989, Marshall's bacterium was recognized as belonging to a separate genus, and the organism was renamed *Helicobacter pylori (16)*.

Part of the decision to rename the Marshall's organism was related to the discovery of a second species that appeared to belong to the same genus. This second species, *Helicobacter mustelae,* was a small, rod-shaped bacterium that colonized primarily the antrum of ferrets and was first cultured by Fox et al. *(17)*. Over the last 10 yr, many additional members of the *Helicobacter* genus have been identified, which have included both gastric and nongastric *Helicobacter* species. All together, more than 18 distinct organisms have been identified and assigned to the *Helicobacter* genus, mainly on the basis of 16S ribosomal RNA sequencing data. There are an additional 30 species of novel *Helicobacter* spp. that have not been formally named. *(18,19)*. Ribosomal RNA codes for proteins that facilitate protein synthesis, and these sequences have been highly conserved over the course of bacterial evolution. The degree of 16S ribosomal RNA sequence similarity is thought to correlate closely with the ancestry of bacterial species, and bacteria with sequences that are >90% homologous to *H. pylori* have been assigned to the genus *Helicobacter.*

Helicobacter species have been found to colonize commonly the gastrointestinal tracts of mammals and birds, and some may be responsible for several types of gastrointestinal disease. In terms of gastric helicobacters, *Helicobacter felis,* the third species in the genus isolated, was found to be a spiral bacterium that naturally colonizes the gastric mucosa of both cats and dogs *(20). Gastrospirillum hominis,* which has been renamed *Helicobacter heilmannii,* has been observed to have a wide distribution and can be found in a large number of different hosts, including cats, dogs, pigs, cheetahs, nonhuman primates, and humans. *H. heilmannii* has been observed in association with mild gastric inflammation in humans, and thus is the only other helicobacter (except for isolated case reports of *H. felis*) that may be associated with stomach diseases in human patients *(18,21,22).* Several other gastric helicobacters—*H. nemenstrinae* and *H. acinonyx*—isolated from the stomachs of nonhuman primates and cheetahs, respectively, appear to be the most similar morphologically to *H. pylori (18,21).*

In addition to gastric helicobacters, a large number of bacteria have been identified that can be classified as nongastric helicobacters *(18). Helicobacter muridarum* was isolated initially from the ileum of rats and mice. It naturally colonizes both the small and large bowel of rodents, but also was found to be able to colonize the stomachs of mice, particularly elderly mice. Other lower bowel helicobacters were isolated and included *H. cinaedi, H. fennelliae, H. canis, H. hepaticus, H. pametensis, H. pullorum, H. rappini,* and *H. bilis.* Although most of the organisms appear to colonize primarily the intestine of the host, a number of these organisms also have been found in the hepatobiliary tract. For example, *H. hepaticus* was observed to be an efficient colonizer of the intestinal tract but also elicited a persistent hepatitis in some strains of mice. In A/JCr mice, *H. hepaticus* is associated with hepatoma and hepatocellular cancer *(23).* More recently, a number of *Helicobacter* species have been detected in the gallbladders of Chilean patients with chronic cholecystitis. Using polymerase chain reaction (PCR) analysis, Fox and colleagues were able to detect *H. bilis, H. rappini,* and *H. pullorum,* and suggested a possible relationship between these bile-resistant *Helicobacter* species with gallbladder disease *(24).*

Epidemiology of H. pylori

Soon after its discovery by Marshall and Warren, several serologic tests were developed and proved useful for studies of the epidemiology of *H. pylori.* Studies from around the world verified the association of *H. pylori* infection with peptic ulcer disease, and follow-up studies demonstrated unequivocally that triple antibiotic treatment of *H. pylori* resulted in decreased recurrences of peptic ulcer disease, as well as cure of ulcer disease when the infection was eradicated *(25–28).* Moreover, although epidemiologic investigation confirmed that *H. pylori* infection was more common in ulcer disease, these studies also revealed that infection was quite common even in asymptomatic individuals. *H. pylori* antibodies were found in 30–40% of asymptomatic individuals in the United States and in 70% or more of asymptomatic individuals in developing countries. In developed countries such as the United States, the seroprevalence of *H. pylori* appeared to have declined markedly over the last 50 yr, but this was not the case in developing nations. Overall, it has been estimated that possibly half the world's population is infected with *H. pylori (29),* making it the world's most common bacterial infection.

The association of *H. pylori* with chronic superficial gastritis was followed later by studies indicating that *H. pylori* gastritis can progress over several decades to chronic atrophic (type B) gastritis, a histopathologic condition that is a precursor of gastric carcinoma and that is characterized by a loss of specialized glandular tissue, including both parietal and chief cells *(30)*. The association with this preneoplastic lesion, and the epidemiologic parallel between *H. pylori* infection rates and gastric cancer incidence, suggested a possible role for *H. pylori* in the pathogenesis of gastric cancer. Gastric cancer was known to be very common in regions of the world (such as Peru, Mexico, Columbia, and parts of Asia) where virtually all adults were infected with *H. pylori* and where infection frequently occurred in early in childhood. Three prospective, case-control studies using stored sera obtained 6–14 yr prior to cancer diagnosis showed clearly that *H. pylori* infection was significantly more common in gastric cancer patients compared to controls with an odds ratio of approx 4.0 *(31–33)*. Studies by Forman et al. showed that the odds ratio increased to approx 9.0 when cancer cases were limited to those diagnosed more than 15 yr after testing positive for *H. pylori (34)*. Based on this epidemiologic evidence, a Working Group of the International Agency for Research on Cancer (IARC) concluded that infection increased the risk of cancer, and classified *H. pylori* infection as representing a group I carcinogenic exposure (*see also* Chapter 21) *(35)*.

In addition, *H. pylori* was strongly linked to other stomach diseases, including gastric mucosa-associated lymphoid tissue (MALT) lymphoma, a rare disorder in which there is transformation of a clonal B-cell population within the gastric mucosa (*see also* Chapter 22) *(36)*. Finally, *H. pylori* was associated strongly with Menetrier's hypertrophic gastropathy *(37)* and hyperplastic gastric polyps *(38)*, but only weakly (if at all) with nonulcer dyspepsia *(39,40)*.

The recognition that *H. pylori* represented a significant risk factor for gastric cancer raised the possibility that antibiotic treatment might reduce the overall risk of gastric cancer. Decision analysis studies indicated that, if *H. pylori* eradication could reduce gastric cancer risk by 30% or more, a strategy of screening and treating patients for *H. pylori* infection could in theory be cost effective *(41)*. However, the critical question continues to be whether *H. pylori* eradication can reduce gastric cancer risk, and at what stage the histopathologic progression is reversible. Initial studies from Japan involving *H. pylori* eradication in patients who had undergone partial gastrectomy for early gastric cancer suggested a reduction in risk of recurrent gastric cancer *(42)*. However, complete resolution of this question will require large randomized controlled trials with long-term follow-up, most likely carried out in countries where gastric cancer rates are high. Such trials are currently underway.

More recently, the approach of widespread eradication of *H. pylori* for the purpose of reducing gastric cancer risk has been complicated by speculation that *H. pylori* may actually be protective against gastroesophageal (GE) junction tumors *(43,44)*. The prevalence of *H. pylori* has clearly been declining in most developed countries such as the United States, in concert with declining rates of well-differentiated, intestinal-type adenocarcinomas. However, the rates of cancers involving the esophagus or gastric cardia, the so-called GE junction cancers, have been increasing rapidly over the last decade. Eradication of *H. pylori* was shown in some studies to result in increased rates of gastroesophageal reflux, a known factor in the pathogenesis of Barrett's esophagus and esophageal cancer *(45,46)*. In addition, reports from one group indicated that infection with *H. pylori*, particularly cagA strains, was inversely associated with GE junction cancers, suggesting that it may be protective *(47)*. Thus, many questions remain with respect to the role of *H. pylori* in specific gastric diseases and the precise recommendations regarding diagnosis and treatment of *H. pylori* in asymptomatic patients.

LIFE CYCLE, SPECIFICITY, AND VIRULENCE DETERMINANTS

Transmission of H. pylori

H. pylori is most likely spread via human-to-human transmission. Humans appear to be the only natural host for the organism, and no clear animal reservoir of infection has been identified. Early reports suggested that gastric *Helicobacter*-like organisms (GHLOs) colonized the gastric mucosa of pigs *(48)*. However, others have failed to identify or isolate *H. pylori* in abattoir pigs from Brazil and Germany using serology and culture techniques *(49,50)*. Studies to identify the pig as a natural reservoir for *H. pylori* have been complicated by the florid gastric microbiota because of the pig's copraphagic habits, making GHLO isolation attempts difficult. *"H. suis,"* closely related to *H. heilmannii* type 1, has been identified in pigs *(51–53)*. Thus, detailed molecular analysis of *Helicobacter*-like organisms isolated from pigs continues to be required for identity. At present, however, there is no convincing evidence that pigs are a reservoir for *H. pylori*. Recent data have shown that cats from one commercial source were found to be infected with *H. pylori (54)*. However, most domestic cats do not appear to represent a significant vector for transmission of the infection. *Helicobacter pylori* and *H. heilmannii* are the most common species reported in monkeys. *H. pylori* has been recovered from two species of old world macaques, rhesus *(M. mulatta)* and cynomolgus macaques *(Macaca fascicularis) (55–58)*. Rhesus macaques and Japanese macaques *(M. fuscata)* have been experimentally infected with human strains of *H. pylori (59–61)*. Based on biochemical, phenotypic and molecular analysis (and in limited studies using molecular techniques), it is believed that *H. pylori* isolated from macaques is highly related or identical to isolates from humans. Their limited numbers and minimal direct contact with humans render them an unlikely source of human infection.

It has been difficult to demonstrate the presence of *H. pylori* in the environment, in contrast to most other enteric bacteria. The possibility has been raised that a contaminated water supply could serve as a source of *H. pylori* infection, and *H. pylori* DNA has been detected in water samples from Lima, Peru using PCR techniques *(62)*. The municipal water supply (vs well water) was implicated as an important source of *H. pylori* infection, irrespective of whether the families were of high or low socioeconomic status *(62)*. These water sources, however, were linked within the neighborhood of residence. In addition, variables including population density, family age distribution, household density, and frequency of drinking untreated water were not considered *(62)*. Interestingly, recent epidemiologic data collected on 684 children residing in the southern Colombian Andes indicated that there was a strong association of infection with swimming in rivers or streams a few times a year *(63)*. In another cross-sectional study, *H. pylori* infection was best predicted by childhood living conditions such as lack of fixed hot water supply *(64)*. Studies in southern China showed no correlation between fecal contamination (using fecal coliform counts) of the water supply and the prevalence of *H. pylori* infection. However, it was determined that most subjects boiled their drinking water, irrespective of origin, and stored the water in vacuum flasks, prior to ingestion. Based on these results, the authors concluded that water was not an important source of transmission of *H. pylori* in this region of China *(65)*.

A large epidemiologic study in 1815 young adult Chileans under 35 yr old showed an association of ingestion of uncooked vegetables to increased *H. pylori* infection *(66)*. They speculated that contamination of vegetables by raw sewage could have played a role in *H. pylori* transmission. Confounding factors such as measuring socioeconomic status on a dichotomized scale without taking into consideration that 3 of the 14 items—water supply, sewage disposal, and indicators of residential crowding—are directly related to disease transmission *(66)*. In the Colombian study, children who frequently consumed raw vegetables in general and lettuce in particular were more likely to be infected with *H. pylori (63)*. Children eating lettuce several times a week had a higher risk of infection *(63)*.

There has been a great deal of speculation regarding whether the coccoid form of *H. pylori* may play a role in the organism's survival outside its host *(67–70)*. Experimental data indicate *H. pylori* coccoid forms can survive for more than 1 yr in river water and *H. pylori* could be cultured at 10 d from river water at 40°C *(71,72)*. *H. pylori* also can survive in milk for several days *(71)*, implying that milk contaminated with feces containing *H. pylori* could potentially be infectious to humans. To definitively test the relevance of the coccoid forms, in vivo experiments must be performed. That is, coccoid (unculturable) forms should be inoculated into a suitable animal model to ascertain whether indeed they are infectious. Until this is accomplished the importance of coccoidal forms in transmission of the organism from host to host will be unknown.

The natural acquisition of *H. pylori* infection occurs, for the most part, in childhood, and is associated with a low socioeconomic status early in life *(73)*. For example, *H. pylori* transmission is strongly linked to conditions associated with household crowding during childhood and supports the hypothesis of person-to-person transmission *(64)*. Using molecular techniques, others have found similar strains among siblings and parents, although some family members also have unique strains *(74)*.

Although *H. pylori* DNA has been detected by PCR in dental plaque, there are few reports of viable organisms within the oral cavity. Thus, an oral source of transmission remains speculative. *H. pylori* has been detected in the feces of children and dyspeptic adults *(75,76)*, and studies in ferrets colonized with *H. mustelae* have supported the notion of fecal–oral transmission, particular during the acute achlorhydric stage *(77,78)*. Because early childhood (<3 yr) appears to be the most frequent age of acquisition of infection, and because diarrhea is particularly frequent in this age group, a fecal–oral route seems plausible. Nevertheless, definitive evidence for fecal–oral transmission is lacking, and many questions remain regarding the mechanisms involved in acquisition of *H. pylori* infection *(79)*.

Bacterial Factors Responsible for Cell Specificity and Virulence

Helicobacter pylori is highly adapted to survive in the highly acidic environment of the stomach. In addition, the organism has specific tropism for gastric epithelial cells. Thus, in addition to being able to colonize the stomach, the organism is infrequently found in areas of gastric metaplasia that occur in the duodenum, esophagus *(80)*, jejunum and in isolated gastric metaplasia of the rectum *(29,81)*. The organism is actively motile and free-living, existing within or beneath the mucous layer of the stomach overlaying the gastric epithelial cells. Motility is essential for colonization of the stomach. Colonization of the gastric mileau is achieved through its spiral shape and the flagella that allow movement through and below the viscous, mucous layer of the stomach. A small percentage of organisms adhere to gastric epithelial cells, and rare organisms may be found intracellularly, suggesting actual invasion

(82). Adherence of *H. pylori* to the gastric epithelium most likely involves a number of surface receptors, possibly including the recently described the Lewis B-binding adhesin, BabA *(83)*. Most bacteria are however, nonadherent, and colonize the extracellular, mucous environment, which may account for lack of host in immune clearance or failures in antibiotic eradication. In addition, *H. pylori* has been found to adhere preferentially, to epithelial cells of the gastric pits. Organisms generally do not adhere to mucous neck, parietal, or chief cells *(84)*. However, *H. pylori* can invade deeply within the gastric glands, particularly within the non-acid-secreting mucosa of the gastric antrum *(85)*.

The bacterial factors that enable for persistence of *H. pylori* within the gastric lumen are still being investigated, but several critical factors have been determined. Some of this information derives from animal models and the creation of *H. pylori* isogenic mutants. A critical factor for *H. pylori* survival is the abundant production of urease, enabling hydrolysis of urea to ammonia and carbon dioxide. *H. pylori* synthesizes extremely high quantities of urease *(86)*. The generation of urease, assists in neutralizing gastric acidity and enables the organism to survive in the low pH of the stomach. *H. pylori* is an acid-tolerant neutrophile *(87)*, and isogenic mutants of *H. pylori* that are deficient in urease are unable to colonize the gastric mucosa of the gnotobiotic piglet *(88)*. Motility is achieved by means of multiple polar flagella. Two protein subunits that are components of the flagella have been identified, and the genes encoding these flagellins have been cloned. Nonmotile mutants, otherwise isogenic with wildtype *H. pylori*, have been constructed by allelic exchange. Detailed in vitro analysis of a *flaA*, a *flaB*, and a *flaA flaB* double mutant, all isogenic with the N6 strain of *H. pylori*, revealed that both flagellin subunits are necessary for full motility *(89)*. Although *flaA flaB* double mutants are completely nonmotile and are devoid of flagella, *flaA* mutants retain residual motility of the parent strain and have flagella that appear similar to those of the wild type. In gnotobiotic piglets, the *flaA* mutant and the *flaB* mutant were impaired in their ability to colonize with respect to the wild type parental strain, but only the double mutant failed to colonize *(90)*. *H. pylori* also produces enzymes involved in the breakdown of the surfactant layer overlying the gastric epithelium, such as phospholipase A2. Isogenic mutants of the gene *pldA*, which encodes for an outer member phospholipase, is unable to colonize mouse models.

Virulence determinants that have received the greatest amount of study are the *cag* locus and the *vacA* gene, which encodes for the vacuolating cytotoxin. The vacuolating cytotoxin first described by Leunk et al. induces a vacuolating effect in several cell lines including gastric cell lines *(91)*. The vacuolating toxin of *H. pylori* has been identified and characterized as a secreted protein; isogenic mutants lacking the toxin (Tox⁻) do not induce a vacuolating effect on cell lines *(92,93)*. Similarly, Tox⁻ *H. pylori* strains may not induce gastric cell damage in vivo, whereas some Tox⁺ *H. pylori* strains cause gastric damage in mouse models *(94, 94a)*. Nevertheless, it is important to remember that about 50% of *H. pylori* strains are Tox⁻ but are still capable of inducing gastritis in humans *(95)*. Also a vac A isogenic mutant of *H. pylori* can still conlonize gnotobiotic pigs and cause gastritis and vacuolation of epithelial cells *(95a)*.

The cytotoxin associated *(cagA)* gene initially was considered essential for vacuolating toxin activity because of the high degree of correlation between presence of *cagA* and ability of *H. pylori* to express the toxin *(96)*. However, subsequent publications indicated that isogenic mutants of *cagA* still were able to produce the toxin *(97–99)*.

The *cagA* is now known to be part of the *cag* locus, considered an important virulence determinant. This 40-kb DNA fragment, consisting of a cluster of more than 25 genes, known as the *cag* pathogenicity island, is more commonly found in *H. pylori* strains isolated from patients with peptic ulcer and gastric cancer *(100)*.

Strains of *H. pylori* with the *cag* pathogenicity island (PAI) *(101)*, the so-called *H. pylori* type I vs type II strains that lack the *cag* island *(99)*, are capable of inducing interleukin-8 (IL-8) expression and tyrosine phosphorylation of a 145-kDa protein from gastric epithelial cells *(102,103)*. Furthermore, isogenic mutants lacking numerous genes of the *cag* PAI abolish these in vitro effects *(100,103,104, 105)*. Importantly, however, these *H. pylori* isogenic mutants lacking either *cagA, cagF,* or *cag N* failed to abolish IL-8 production *(105)*.Recent studies show that multiple genes in the left half of the *cag* PAI are essential for the transcription of the IL-8 gene in gastric epithelial cells and that this depends on protein tyrosine activation *(105a)*.

The recent sequencing of the entire genome of two strains of *H. pylori* will allow investigators to more fully explore virulence factors already described as well as to determine the presence of others *(106,107)*.

Natural History and Stages of Infection

The initial stages of *H. pylori* infection occur soon after initial ingestion of the organism. Again, *H. pylori* is generally acquired in early childhood (<5 yr), even in highly developed, industrialized countries such as the United States and Western Europe *(108–111)*. The precise dose of organisms needed to establish infection in humans is not clear, given that the only experience reported to date is derived from ingestion by two human volunteers. Based on the reports of Marshall *(12)* and Morris *(13,14)*, a dose of 3×10^5 cfu is clearly sufficient to establish permanent infection, but the minimum required dose is likely much smaller, based on reports of endoscopic transmission of the disease *(112,113)*. Shortly after ingestion, there is a period of intense bacterial proliferation as *H. pylori* colonizes predominantly the antrum of the stomach; during this initial stage of colonization, the infection moves from gland to gland in a proximal direction, and along the way initiates a significant acute inflammatory response characterized by neutrophilic infiltration of the mucosa. Antral inflammation leads to downregulation of somatostatin secretion, resulting in increased circulating levels of gastrin. During the initial few weeks after infection, upper digestive symptoms may be present, including nausea, vomiting, belching, and anorexia. Based on reports of outbreaks of *H. pylori* infection secondary to endoscopic transmission, achlorhydria may be seen often during acute infection that in most cases resolves spontaneously *(112,113)*. Based on the ferret model of *H. mustalae* infection *(77,78)*, it is likely that this acute achlorhydria increases fecal shedding of the organism and facilitates transmission to other hosts, particularly in children. Within several weeks after infection, humoral immune responses as measured by IgG and IgM *H. pylori*-specific antibodies can be observed, but these immune responses are not effective in eliminating the infection. However, epidemiologic studies in children have suggested that spontaneous elimination of the infection does occur, especially in young children and the elderly. Thus, studies from Peru indicate that *H. pylori* infection is present in 71% of children at 6 mo of age but in only 48% of children at 18 mo of age, suggesting that the infection is cleared in some children in this early age group (114).

Once H. pylori has become firmly entrenched within the gastric mucosa, however, it generally persists in most infected individuals for decades. Moreover, it appears to coexist comfortably with its host, resulting in minimal signs or symptoms. However, although a benign relationship between organism and host is the most likely end result, there are a number of possible outcomes consequent to gastric Helicobacter infection (115). In a significant proportion of individuals, the infection and inflammation remains severe but still confined to the gastric antrum, and these individuals are at increased risk for duodenal ulcer disease. Approximately 15–20% of patients manifest evidence of peptic ulcer disease at some time, with duodenal ulcer disease being more common than gastric ulcer. Another possible outcome from infection is the development of uncontrolled B-cell proliferation within the gastric mucosa, resulting in MALT lymphoma (see Chapter 22).

However, in a greater number of infected individuals, the inflammation progresses and spreads to involve not only the antrum but also the body and fundus of the stomach. In these individuals, the infection and inflammation leads to destruction of glandular structures and loss of parietal and chief cell populations, resulting in atrophic gastritis and achlorhydria. Several clinical studies have suggested that treatment of patients with high doses of proton pump inhibitors, which worsens both achlorhydria and hypergastrinemia, may accelerate this progression to atrophy (30,116). Studies in mice have supported the notion that acid suppression can alter the distribution of organisms within the murine stomach (117). With the loss of acid secretion, serum gastrin levels gradually rise even further. During this process, both apoptosis and proliferation rates within the gastric mucosa are markedly elevated, and may lead to increased rates of mutagenesis in stem cell populations. The development of atrophic gastritis and its associated intestinal metaplasia may take 30 or more years to develop, and the appearance of metaplasia is often accompanied by the loss of active H. pylori infection (118,119). Atrophic gastritis is now recognized as the major precursor of gastric cancer, and is an established premalignant lesion. Overall, it has been estimated that, after many decades of chronic, asymptomatic infection, up to 0.5–1.0% of patients will develop gastric cancer.

Recent studies have raised the possibility that the pathways to acid hypersecretion and duodenal ulcer disease may be distinct from the pathway to acid hyposecretion and gastric cancer. Epidemiologic studies have shown that the risk of developing gastric cancer is much lower in patients with a history of duodenal ulcer disease, and much greater in patients with a history of gastric ulcer disease (120). Patients with duodenal ulcer disease are generally acid hypersecretors, whereas patients with gastric ulcer disease often show atrophic gastritis and acid hyposecretion. However, it is unclear if these two H. pylori-related disorders—duodenal ulcer disease and gastric cancer—really represent separate pathophysiologic pathways, or simply different stages in the same disease process. The decreased gastric cancer risk was shown for an average follow-up period of 9 yr, but multifocal atrophic gastritis often can develop in duodenal ulcer patients several decades after the onset of ulcer disease (120).

ANIMAL MODELS FOR HELICOBACTER-INDUCED GASTRIC CANCER

Although administration of N-nitro chemicals with and without salt in animals addressed the possible roles and mechanisms of promoters and nitrosamine induced gastric cancer, it now is clear that *H. pylori* is an important factor in gastric tumorigenesis. Furthermore, despite the presence of high nitrites in drinking waters and possible mutagenicity of nitrosated foods, the inconsistency of epidemiologic data suggests that high levels of dietary nitrites/nitrates and high-salt diets alone are not sufficient to produce overt gastric cancer in humans. Therefore animal models are being developed to study the role of *Helicobacter* species in gastric cancer, particularly in combination with other agents. During the last decade, several animal models have been described for *Helicobacter*-induced gastric disease. Of the animal models recently reviewed *(121)*, gastric adenocarcinoma occurred only with *H. mustelae (122)*. Recently, the gerbil has been shown to have particular relevant features that can be used to address whether *H. pylori* can induce gastric cancer. Gerbils, animals sparingly used for biomedical research, were first reported as a model for experimental *H. pylori* infection in 1991 *(123)*. The interest in using gerbils to study gastric cancer increased when Japanese investigators noted intestinal metaplasia, atrophy, and gastric ulcer in gerbils experimentally infected with *H. pylori* *(124,125)*. In one study, acute gastritis with erosions of the gastric mucosa occurred shortly after infection, whereas gastric ulcers, cystica profunda, and atrophy with intestinal metaplasia were observed 3–6 mo post infection *(125)*. Following these findings two separate research groups have noted that gerbils infected with *H. pylori* from periods ranging from 15 to 18 mo develop gastric adenocarcinoma *(126,127)*.

In the Watanabe study, gerbils were observed for up to 62 wk, and 37% were found to develop adenocarcinoma in the pyloric region *(127)*. The gastric cancers were clearly documented histologically. Vascular invasion and metastases were not observed, although it is possible that they may develop with longer periods of observation. It is also important to note that Honda et al., who reported *H. pylori* adenocarcinoma 15 mo post-inoculation, also did not record metastases or vascular invasion *(126)*.

Interestingly, the development of cancer is preceded by invagination of atypical glands (cystica profunda) into the submucosa considered by some to be a premalignant lesion. The histological progression in the gerbil closely resembled that observed in humans, including early appearance of intestinal metaplasia, well-differentiated histologic patterns of the gastric malignancy, and antral location of the gastric cancers. The association with gastric ulcers in this model is also of interest, given recent clinical studies in human patients indicating a link between gastric ulcer disease and gastric cancer *(120)*. The development of metaplasia with production of predominantly acid sialomucins was associated with tumor development. Although the long-standing question whether the cancers arose directly from these metaplastic cells has not been answered, the tumors clearly originated deep in the gastric glands, in close proximity to these metaplastic cells. Despite the lack of labeling studies to illustrate the point, the proliferative zone in these chronically infected animals most likely extended to the base of the glands.

Although most of the tumors in this *H. pylori* gerbil model originated in the pyloric region of the stomach, significant changes in the oxyntic mucosa consistent with chronic atrophic gastritis were seen. Glandular tissue in the gastric body and fundus were atrophied and replaced by hyperplastic epithelium of the pseudopyloric type. The differences between this lesion and gastric atrophy in human patients is that the gerbil corpus is not "thinner" consequent to the pseudopyloric hyperplasia *(127)*. A similar type of gastric atrophy (loss of oxyntic glands and neck cell hyperplasia) has been reported in *H. felis*-infected C57B1 mice *(128)*. Thus, the diagnosis of atrophy has less to do with the thickness of the mucosa and more to do with the loss of oxyntic (parietal and chief) cell populations within the gastric glands. Growing evidence suggests that the parietal cell may regulate key differentiation decisions within the gastric glands. For example, ablation of parietal cells using transgenic technology *(129)* or *H. felis* infection leads to altered glandular differentiation and neck cell proliferation as well as changes in gastric acid and gastrin physiology.

The expansion of an aberrant neck cell ("regenerative hyperplasia" or "pseudopyloric hyperplasia") in the gerbils is similar to that observed in the *H. felis* mouse model. This lineage of cells has been shown to be spasmolytic polypeptide (SP)-positive *(128),* and this SP-positive lineage also develops in *H. pylori*-associated gastric cancers in humans *(130).* The loss of oxyntic glandular tissue in response to *H. pylori* infection suggests that the gerbil becomes achlorhydric before the development of gastric cancer. The gerbil appears to be uniquely susceptible to *Helicobacter*-induced gastric neoplasia, and further characterization of the gerbil model may provide some clues to gastric cancer progression and host–bacteria interaction. The unusual susceptibility of this animal species to gastric cancer using a fairly standard *H. pylori* strain underscores once again the overriding importance of host factors in determining the outcome from *Helicobacter* infection *(131).* Finally, a possible role for altered gastrin physiology in the pathogenesis of gastric cancer has been rasied by several recent studies. In Mongolian gerbils, *H. pylori* leads to marked elevation of serum gastrin levels withic coincide temporally with increases in gastric mucosal proliferation rates *(132).* Further, inbred (FVB/N) mice that are rendered moderately hypergastrinemic through an insulin-gastrin (INS-GAS) transgene develop increased mucosal proliferation and progressive atrophy (parietal cell loss), and spontaneous gastric carcinomas after prolonged (20 mo) observation periods *(133).* In addition, infection of these hypergastrinemic mice with *H. felis* leads to accelerated tumorigenesis, with the majority (85%) of infected mice under 8 mo of age showing gastric cancer. These data support the notion that elevations in circulating gastrin-17, a common finding in *H. pylori*-infected patients, can contribute to the development of both atrophy and gastric cancer.

REFERENCES

1. Bottcher I. Dorpater Medicinische Zeitschrift 1874; 5:148.
2. Modlin IM, Sachs G. *Helicobacter pylori.* In: Acid Related Diseases: Biology and Treatment. 1998. Schnetztor-Verlag Gmb H Konstanz (eds.). Germany p. 315–364.
3. Doenges JL. Spirochetes in the gastric glands of *Macaca rhesus* and of man without related disease. Arch Pathol 1939; 27:469–477.
4. Freedburg AS, Barron LE. The presence of spirochetes in human gastric mucosa. Am J Dig Dis 1940; 7:443–445.
5. Palmer ED. Investigation of the gastric spirochetes of the human. Gastroenterology 1954; 27:218–220.
6. Steer HW. Ultrastructure of cell migration through the gastric epithelium and its relationship to bacteria. J Clin Pathol 1975; 28:639–646.
7. Steer HW, Colin-Jones DG. Mucosal changes in gastric ulceration and their response to carbenoxolone sodium. Gut 1975; 16:590–597.
8. Steer HW. Surface morphology of the gastroduodenal mucosa in duodenal ulceration. Gut 1984; 25:1203–1210.

9. Warren JD, Marshall BJ. Unidentified curved bacilli on gastric epithelium in active chronic gastritis. Lancet 1983; 1:1273–1275.

10. Marshall BJ, Warren JR. Unidentified curved bacillus on gastric epithelium in active chronic gastritis. Lancet 1983; i:1273–1275.

11. Marshall BJ, Warren JR. Unidentified curved bacilli in the stomach of patients with gastritis and peptic ulceration. Lancet 1984; i:1311.

12. Marshall BJ, Armstrong JA, McGechie B, Glancy RJ. Attempt to fulfill Koch's postulates for pyloric *Campylobacter.* Med J Aust 1985; 142:436–439.

13. Morris A, Nicholson G. Ingestion of *Campylopyloridis* causes gastritis and raised fasting gastric pH. Am J Gastroenterol 1987; 82:192–199.

14. Morris AJ, Nicholson GI, Perez-Perez GI, Blaser MJ. Long term follow up of voluntary ingestion of *Helicobacter pylori.* Ann Intern Med 1991; 114:662–663.

15. Anonymous. Validation of publication of new names and new combinations previously effectively published outside the IJSB. Int J Syst Bacteriol 1985; 85:223–225.

16. Goodwin CS, Armstrong JA, Chilvers T, et al. Transfer of *Campylobacter pylori* and *Campylobacter mustelae* to *Helicobacter pylori* gen. nov. and *Helicobacter mustelae* comb. nov., respectively. Int J Syst Bacteriol 1989; 39:397–405.

17. Fox JG, Edrise BM, Cabot E, Beaucage C, Murphy JC, Prostak KS. Campylobacter-like organisms isolated from gastric mucosa of ferrets. Am J Vet Res 1986; 47:236–239.

18. Fox JG. The expanding genus of *Helicobacter:* pathogenic and zoonotic potential. In: MH Sleisenger and JS Fordtram (eds). Seminars in Gastrointestinal Diseases, Vol. 8. Philadelphia: W B Saunders, 1997, pp. 124–141.

19. Fox JG, Wang TC. Helicobacter and liver disease (editorial). Ital J Gastroenterol 1997; 29:5–10.

20. Lee A, Hazell SL, O'Rourke J. Isolation of a spiral-shaped bacterium from the cat stomach. Infect Immun 1988; 56:2843–2850.

21. Lee A, Fox JG, Hazell S. Pathogenicity of *Helicobacter pylori:* a perspective. Infect Immun 1993; 61:1601–1610.

22. Lee A, O'Rourke J. Gastric bacteria other than *Helicobacter pylori.* Gastroenterol Clin North Am 1993; 22:21–42.

23. Ward JM, Fox JG, Anver MR, et al. Chronic active hepatitis and associated liver tumors in mice caused by a persistent bacterial infection with a novel *Helicobacter* species. J Natl Cancer Inst 1994; 86:1222–1227.

24. Fox JG, Dewhirst FE, Shen Z, et al. Hepatic *Helicobacter* species identified in bile and gallbladder tissue from Chileans with chronic cholecystitis. Gastroenterology 1998; 14:755–763.

25. Graham DY, Lew GM, Klein PD, et al. Effect of treatment of *Helicobacter pylori* infection on the long-term recurrence of gastric or duodenal ulcer: a randomized controlled study. Ann Intern Med 1992; 116:705–708.

26. Hentschel E, Brandstatter G, Dargosics B, et al. Effect of ranitidine and amoxicillin plus metronidazole on the eradication of *Helicobacter pylori* and the recurrence of duodenal ulcer. N Engl J Med 1993; 328:308–312.

27. Sung JJ, Chung SC, Lin TK, et al. Antibacterial treatment of gastric ulcers associated with *Helicobacter pylori.* N Engl J Med 1995; 332:139–142.

28. van der Hulst RW, Rauws EA, Koycu B, et al. Prevention of ulcer recurrence after eradication of *Helicobacter pylori:* a prospective long term follow up study. Gastroenterology 1997; 113:1082–1086.

29. Hunt RH. The role of *Helicobacter pylori* in pathogenesis: the spectrum of clinical outcomes. Scand J Gastroenterol 1996; 220:3–9.

30. Kuipers EJ, Uyterlinde AM, Pena AS, et al. Long-term sequelae of *Helicobacter pylori* gastritis. Lancet 1995; 345:1525–1528.

31. Forman D, Newell DG, Fullerton F, et al. Association between infection with *Helicobacter pylori* and risk of gastric cancer: evidence from a prospective investigation. Br Med J 1991; 302:1302–1305.

32. Nomura A, Stemmerman GN, Chyou PH, Kato I, Perez-Perez GI, Blaser MJ. *Helicobacter pylori* infection and gastric carcinoma among Japanese Americans in Hawaii. N Engl J Med 1991; 325:1132–1136.

33. Parsonnet J, Friedman GD, Vandersteen DP, et al. *Helicobacter pylori* infection and the risk of gastric carcinoma. N Engl J Med 1991; 325:1127–1131.

34. Forman D. *Helicobacter pylori* and gastric cancer. Scand J Gastroenterol 1996; 220:23–26.

35. IARC working group on the evaluation of carcinogenic risks to humans. Schistosomes, liver flukes and *Helicobacter pylori* Lyon, France: International Agency for Research on Cancer, 1994, pp. 177–240.

36. Parsonnet J, Hanson S, Rodriguez L, et al. *Helicobacter pylori* infection and gastric MALT lymphoma. N Engl J Med 1994; 330:1267–1271.

37. Bayerdorffer E, Ritter MM, Hatz R, Brooks W, Ruckdeschel G, Stolte M. Healing of protein losing hypertrophic gastropathy by eradication of *Helicobacter pylori*—is *Helicobacter pylori* a pathogenic factor in Menetrier's disease? Gut 1994; 35:701–704.

38. Ohkusa T, Takashimizu I, Fujiki K, et al. Disappearance of hyperplastic polyps in the stomach after eradication of *Helicobacter pylori*. A randomized clinical trial. Ann Intern Med 1998; 129:712–715.

39. Blum AL, Talley NJ, O'Morain C, et al. Lack of effect of treating *Helicobacter pylori* infection in patients with nonulcer dyspepsia. Omeprazole plus clarithromycin and amoxicillin effect one year after treatment (OCAY) study group. N Engl J Med 1998; 339:1875–1881.

40. McColl K, Murray L, El-Omar E, et al. Symptomatic benefit from eradicating *Helicobacter pylori* infection in patients with nonulcer dyspepsia. N Engl J Med 1998; 339:1869–1874.

41. Parsonnet J, Harris RA, Hack HM, Owens DK. Modeling cost effectiveness of *H. pylori* screening to prevent gastric cancer: a mandate for clinical trials. Lancet 1996; 348:150–154.

42. Uemura N, Mukai T, Okamoto S, et al. Effect of *Helicobacter pylori* eradication on subsequent development of cancer after endoscopic resection of early gastric cancer. Cancer Epidemiol Biomarkers Prev 1997; 6:639–642.

43. Blaser MJ. Hypothesis: the changing relationships of *Helicobacter pylori* and humans: implications for health and disease. J Infect Dis 1999; 179:1523–1530.

44. Blaser MJ. In a world of black and white, *Helicobacter pylori* is gray. Ann Intern Med 1999; 130:695–697.

45. Labenz J, Blum AL, Bayerdorffer E, Meining A, Stolte M, Borsch G. Curing *Helicobacter pylori* infection in patients with duodenal ulcer may provoke reflux esophagitis. Gastroenterology 1997; 112:1442–1447.

46. Vicari JJ, Peek RM, Falk GW, et al. The seroprevalence of cagA-positive *Helicobacter pylori* strains in the spectrum of gastroesophageal reflux disease. Gastroenterology 1998; 115:50–57.

47. Chow WH, Blaser MJ, Blot WJ, et al. An inverse relation between cagA+ strains of *Helicobacter pylori* infection and risk of esophageal and gastric cardia adenocarcinoma. Cancer Res 1998; 58:588–590.

48. Ho SA, Hoyle JA, Lewis FA, et al. Direct polymerase chain reaction test for detection of *Helicobacter pylori* in humans and animals. J Clin Microbiol 1991; 29:2543–2549.

49. Rocha GA, Queiroz DM, Mendes EN, Oliveira AM, Moura SB, Silva RJ. Source of *Helicobacter pylori* infection: studies in abbatoir workers and pigs [letter]. Am J Gastroenterol 1992; 87:1525.

50. Korber-Golze B, Scupin E. *Helicobacter pylori:* studies in domestic swine. Dtw Deutsche Tierarztliche Wochenschr 1993; 100:465–468.

51. Queiroz DM, Rocha GA, Mendes E, Lage AP, Carvalho AC, Barbosa AJ. A spiral microorganism in the stomach of pigs. Vet Microbiol 1990; 24:199–204.

52. Solnick JV, O'Rourke J, Lee A, Paster BJ, Dewhirst FE, Tompkins LS. An uncultured gastric spiral organism is a newly identified Helicobacter in humans. J Infect Dis 1993; 168:379–385.

53. Mendes EN, Queiroz DMM, Dewhirst FE, Paster BJ, Rocha GA, Fox JG. Are pigs a reservoir host for human Helicobacter infection? (Abstr 45). Am J Gastroenterol 1994; 89:1296.

54. Handt LK, Fox JG, Dewhirst FE, et al. *Helicobacter pylori* isolated from the domestic cat: public health implications. Infect Immun 1994; 62:2367–2374.

55. Baskerville A, Newell DG. Naturally occurring chronic gastritis and *C. pylori* infection in the Rhesus monkey: a potential model for gastritis in man. Gut 1988; 29:465–472.

56. Bronsdon MA, Schoenknecht FD. *Campylobacter pylori* isolated from the stomach of the monkey, *Macaca nemistrina.* J Clin Microbiol 1988; 26:1725–1728.

57. Dubois A, Fiala N, Heman-Ackah LM, et al. Natural gastric infection with *Helicobacter pylori* in monkeys: a model for spiral bacteria infection in humans. Gastroenterology 1994; 106:1405–1417.

58. Reindel JF, Fitzgerald AL, Breider MA, et al. An epizootic of lymphoplasmacytic gastritis attributed to *Helicobacter pylori* infection in cynomolgus monkeys *(Macaca fascicularis)* Vet Pathol 1999; 36:1–13.

59. Fukuda Y, Yamamoto I, Tonokatsu Y. Inoculation of rhesus monkeys with human *Helicobacter pylori:* a long-term investigation on gastric mucosa by endoscopy. Dig Endosc 1992; 4:19–30.

60. Fujioka T, Shuto R, Kodama R. Experimental model for chronic gastritis with *Helicobacter pylori:* long term follow up study in *H. pylori*-infected Japanese macaques. Eur J Gastroenterol Hepatol 1993; S1:S73–77.

61. Shuto R, Fujioka T, Kubota I, Nasu M. Experimental gastritis induced by *Helicobacter pylori* in Japanese monkeys. Infect Immun 1993; 61:933–939.

62. Hulten K, Han SW, Enroth H, et al. *Helicobacter pylori* in the drinking water in Peru. Gastroenterology 1996; 110:1031–1035.

63. Goodman KJ, Correa P, Tengana Aux HJ, et al. *Helicobacter pylori* infection in the Colombian Andes: a population-based study of transmission pathways. Am J Epidemiol 1996; 144:290–299.

64. Mendall MA, Goggin PM, Molineaux N, et al. Childhood living conditions and *Helicobacter pylori* seropositivity in adult life. Lancet 1992; 339:896–897.

65. Mitchell HM, Li YY, Hu PJ, et al. Epidemiology of *Helicobacter pylori* in Southern China: identification of early childhood as the critical period for acquisition. Infect Dis 1992; 166:149–153.

66. Hopkins RJ, Vial PA, Ferreccio C, et al. Seroprevalence of *Helicobacter pylori* in Chile: vegetables may serve as one route of transmission [note]. J Infect Dis 1993; 168:222–226.

67. Jones DM, Curry A. The genesis of coccal forms of *Helicobacter pylori.* In: Malfertheiner P, Ditschuneit H (eds). *Helicobacter pylori,* Gastritis and Peptic Ulcer. Berlin: Springer-Verlag, 1990, pp. 29–37.

68. Mai UEH, Schahamat M, Colwell RR. Survival of *Helicobacter pylori* in the aquatic environment. In: Menge H, Gregor M, Tytgat GNJ, Marshall BJ, McNulty CAM (eds). *Helicobacter pylori.* Berlin: Springer-Verlag, 1991, pp. 91–94.

69. Bode G, Mauch F, Ditschuneit H, Malfertheiner P. Identification of structures containing polyphosphate in *Helicobacter pylori.* J Gen Microbiol 1993; 139:3029–3033.

70. Bode G, Mauch F, Malfertheiner P. Coccoid forms of *Helicobacter pylori:* criteria for their viability. Epidemiol Infect 1993; 111:483–490.

71. Karim QN, Maxwell RH. Survival of *Campylobacter pylori* in artificially contaminated milk (letter). J Clin Pathol 1989; 42:778.

72. West AP, Miller MR, Tompkins DS. Survival of *Helicobacter pylori* in water and saline (letter). J Clin Pathol 1990; 43:609.

73. Xia HH, Talley NJ. Natural acquisition and spontaneous elimination of *Helicobacter pylori* infection: clinical implications. Am J Gastroenterol 1997; 92:1780–1787.

74. Mitchell HM, Hazell SL, Kolesnikow R, Mitchell J, Frommer D. Antigen recognition during progression from acute to chronic infection with a *cagA*-positive strain of *Helicobacter pylori*. Infect Immun 1996; 64:1166–1172.

75. Thomas JE, Gibson GR, Darboe MK, Dale A, Weaver LT. Isolation of *Helicobacter pylori* from human feces. Lancet 1992; 340:1194–1195.

76. Kelly SM, Pitcher MCL, Farmery SM, Gibson GR. Isolation of *Helicobacter pylori* from feces of patients with dyspepsia in the United Kingdom. Gastroenterology 1994; 107:1671–1674.

77. Fox JG, Paster BJ, Dewhirst FE, et al. *Helicobacter mustelae* isolation from feces of ferrets: evidence to support fecal–oral transmission of a gastric Helicobacter. *Infect Immun* 1992; 60:606–611.

78. Fox JG, Blanco M, Yan L, et al. Role of gastric pH in isolation of *Helicobacter mustelae* from the feces of ferrets. Gastroenterology 1993; 104:86–92.

79. Cave DR. How is *Helicobacter pylori* transmitted? Gastroenterology 1997; 113:S9–14.

80. Borhan-Manesh F, Farnum JB. Study of *Helicobacter pylori* colonization of patches of heterotopic gastric mucosa (HGM) at the upper esophagus. Dig Dis Sci 1993; 38:142–146.

81. Hill P, Rode J. *Helicobacter pylori* in ectopic gastric mucosa in Meckel's diverticulum. Pathology 1998; 30:7–9.

82. Wilkinson SM, Uhl JR, Kline BC, Cockerill FR. Assessment of invasion frequencies of cultured HEp-2 cells by clinical isolates of *Helicobacter pylori* using an acridine orange assay. J Clin Pathol 1998; 51:127–133.

83. Ilver D, Arnqvist A, Ogren J, et al. *Helicobacter pylori* adhesin binding fucosylated histoblood antigens revealed by retagging. Science 1998; 279:373–377.

84. Falk P, Roth KA, Boren T, Westblom TU, Gordon JI, Normark S. An in vitro adherence assay reveals that *Helicobacter pylori* exhibits lineage-specific tropism in the human gastric epithelium. Proc Natl Acad Sci USA 1993; 90:2035–2039.

85. Thomsen LL, Gavin JB, Tasman-Jones C. Relation of *Helicobacter pylori* to the human gastric mucosa in chronic gastritis of the antrum. Gut 1990; 31:1230–1236.

86. Mobley HLT. *Helicobacter pylori* factors associated with disease development. Gastroenterology 1997; 113:S21–S28.

87. Rektorschek M, Weeks D, Sachs G, Melchers K. Influence of pH on metabolism and urease activity of *Helicobacter pylori*. Gastroenterology 1998; 115:628–641.

88. Eaton KA, Brooks CL, Morgan DR, Krakowka S. Essential role of urease in pathogenesis of gastritis induced by *Helicobacter pylori* in gnotobiotic piglets. Infect Immun 1991; 59:2470–2475.

89. Josenhans C, Labigne A and Suerbaum S. Comparative ultrastructural and functional studies of *Helicobacter pylori* and *Helicobacter mustelae* flagellin mutants: both flagellin subunits, FlaA and FlaB, are necessary for full motility in *Helicobacter* species. *J Bacteriol* 1995; 177:3010–3020.

90. Eaton K, Suerbaum S, Josenhans C, Krakowka S. Colonization of gnotobiotic piglets by *H. pylori* deficient in two flagellin genes. Infect Immun 1996; 64:2445–2448.

91. Leunk RD, Johnson PT, David BC, Kraft WG, Morgan DR. Cytotoxic activity in broth-culture filtrates of *Campylobacter pylori*. J Med Microbiol 1988; 26:93–99.

92. Harris PR, Cover TL, Crowe DR, et al. *Helicobacter pylori* cytotoxin induces vacuolation of primary human mucosal epithelial cells. Infect Immun 1996; 64:4867–4871.

93. Smoot DT, Resau JH, Earlington MH, Simpson M, Cover TL. Effects of *Helicobacter pylori* vacuolating cytotoxin on primary cultures of human gastric epithelial cells. Gut 1996; 39:795–799.

94. Marchetti M, Arico B, Burroni D, Figura N, Rappuoli R, Ghiara P. Development of a mouse model of *Helicobacter pylori* infection that mimics human disease. Science 1995; 267:1655–1658.

94a. Lee A, O'Rourke J, DeUngria MC, Robertson B, Daskslopoulos G, Dixon MF. A standardized mouse model of *Helicobacter pylori* infection: introducing the Sydney strain. Gastroenterology 1997; 112:1386–1397.

95. Cover TL. The vacuolating cytotoxin of *Helicobacter pylori*. Mol Microbiol 1996; 20:241–246.

95a. Eaton KA, Cover TL, Tummuru, MKR, Blaser MJ, Krakowka S. Role of vacuolating cytotoxin in gastritis due to *Helicobacter pylori* in gnotobiotic piglets. *Infect Immun* 1997; 65:3462–3464.

96. Tummuru MK, Cover TL, Blaser MJ. Cloning and expression of a high molecular-mass major antigen of *Helicobacter pylori:* evidence of linkage to cytotoxicity. Infect Immun 1993; 61:1799–1809.

97. Tummuru MK, Cover TL, Blaser MJ. Mutation of the cytotoxin-associated *cagA* gene does not affect vacuolating cytotoxin activity of *Helicobacter pylori.* Infect Immun 1994; 62:2609–2613.

98. Crabtree JE, Xiang Z, Lindley IJ, Tompkins DS, Rappuoli R. Induction of interleukin-8 secretion from gastric epithelial cells by cagA isolgenic mutant of *Helicobacter pylori.* J Clin Pathol 1995; 48:967–969.

99. Xiang Z, Censini S, Bayeli PF, et al. Analysis of expression of CagA and VacA virulence factors in 43 strains of *Helicobacter pylori* reveals that clinical isolates can be divided into two major types and that CagA is not necessary for expression of the vacuolating cytotoxin. Infect Immun 1995; 63:94–98.

100. Censini S, Lange C, Xiang Z, et al. Cag, a pathogenicity island of *Helicobacter pylori,* encodes type I-specific and disease-associated virulence factors. Proc Natl Acad Sci USA 1996; 93:14648–14653.

101. Covacci A, Censini S, Bugnoli M, et al. Molecular characterization of the 128-kDa immunodominant antigen of *Helicobacter pylori* associated with cytotoxicity and duodenal ulcer. Proc Natl Acad Sci USA 1993; 90:5791–5795.

102. Crabtree JE, Farmery SM, Lindley IJD, Figura N, Peichl P, Tompkins DS. CagA/cytotoxic strains of *Helicobacter pylori* and interleukin-8 in gastric epithelial cell lines. J Clin Pathol 1994; 47:945–950.

103. Segal ED, Lange C, Covacci A, Tompkins LS, Falkow S. Induction of host signal transduction pathways by *Helicobacter pylori.* Proc Natl Acad Sci USA 1997; 94:7595–7599.

104. Tummuru MKR, Sharma SA, Blaser MJ. *Helicobacter pylori picB,* a homologue of the *Bordatella pertussis* toxin secretion protein, is required for induction of IL-8 in gastric epithelial cells. Mol Microbiol 1995; 18:867–876.

105. McGee DJ, Mobley HLT. Mechanisms of *Helicobacter pylori* infection: bacterial factors. In: Westblom TU, Czinn SJ, Nedrud JG (eds). Gastroduodenal Disease and *Helicobacter pylori.* New York: Springer-Verlag, 1999, pp. 155–180.

105a. Li SD, Kersulyte D, Lindley IJD, Neelam B, Berg DE, Crabtree JE. Multiple genes in the left half of the cag pathogenicity island of *Helicobacter pylori* are required for tyrosine kinase-dependent transcription of interleukin-8 in gastric epithelial cells. Infect Immun 1999; 67:3893–3899.

106. Tomb JF, White O, Kerlavage AR, et al. The complete genome sequence of the gastric pathogen *Helicobacter pylori.* Nature 1997; 388:539–547.

107. Alm RA, Ling LS, Moir DT, et al. Genomic sequence comparison of two unrelated isolates of the human gastric pathogen *Helicobacter pylori.* Nature 1999; 397:176–180.

108. Klein PD, Gilman RH, Leon-Barua R, Diaz F, Smith EO, Graham DY. The epidemiology of *Helicobacter pylori* in Peruvian children between 6 and 30 months of age. Am J Gastroenterol 1994; 89:2196–2200.

109. Lindkvist P, Asrat D, Nilsson I, et al. Age at acquisition of *Helicobacter pylori* infection: comparison of a high and a low prevalence country. Scand J Gastroenterol 1996; 28:181–184.

110. Jones NL, Sherman PM. *Helicobacter pylori* infection in children. Curr Opin Pediatr 1998; 10:19–23.

111. Ma JL, You WC, Gail MH, et al. *Helicobacter pylori* infection and mode of transmission in a population at high risk of stomach cancer. Int J Epidemiol 1998; 27:570–573.

112. Ramsey EJ, Carey KV, Peterson WL, et al. Epidemic gastritis with hypochlorhydria. Gastroenterology 1979; 76:1449–1457.

113. Graham DY, Alpert LC, Smith JL, Yoshimura HH. Iatrogenic *Campylobacter pylori* infection is a cause of epidemic achlorhydria. Am J Gastroenterol 1988; 83:974–980.

114. Granstrom M, Tindberg Y, Blennow M. Seroepidemiology of *Helicobacter pylori* infection in a cohort of children monitored from 6 months to 11 years of age. J Clin Microbiol 1997; 35:468–470.

115. Parsonnet J. *Helicobacter pylori* in the stomach-a paradox unmasked. N Engl J Med 1996; 335:278–280.

116. Eissele R, Brunner G, Simon B, Solcia E, Arnold R. Gastric mucosa during treatment with lansoprazole: *Helicobacter pylori* is a risk for argyrophil hyperplasia. Gastroenterology 1997; 112:707–717.

117. Danon J, O'Rourke JL, Moss ND, Lee A. The importance of local acid production !in the distribution of *Helicobacter felis* in the mouse stomach. Gastroenterology 1995; 108:1386–1395.

118. Karnes WE, Jr, Samloff IM, Siurala M, et al. Positive serum antibody and negative tissue staining for *Helicobacter pylori* in subjects with atrophic body gastritis. Gastroenterology 1991; 101:167–174.

119. Genta RM, Graham DY. Intestinal metaplasia, not atrophy or achlorhydria, creates a hostile environment for *Helicobacter pylori*. Scand J Gastroenterol 1993; 28:924–928.

120. Hansson LE, Nyren O, Hsing AW, et al. The risk of stomach cancer in patients with gastric or duodenal ulcer disease. N Engl J Med 1996; 335:242–249.

121. Fox JG, Lee A. The role of *Helicobacter* species in newly recognized gastrointestinal tract diseases of animals. Lab Anim Sci 1997; 47:222–255.

122. Fox JG, Dangler CA, Sager W, Borkowski R, Gliatto JM. *Helicobacter mustelae* associated gastric adenocarcinoma in ferrets *(Mustela putorius furo)*. Vet Pathol 1997; 34:225–229.

123. Yokota K, Kurebayashi Y, Takayama Y, et al. Colonization of *Helicobacter pylori* in the gastric mucosa of Mongolian gerbils. Microbiol Immunol 1991; 35:475–480.

124. Hirayama F, Takagi S, Kusuhara H, Iwao E, Yokoyama Y. Induction of gastric ulcer and intestinal metaplasia in Mongolian gerbils infected with *Helicobacter pylori*. J Gastroenterol 1996; 31:755–757.

125. Honda S, Fujioka T, Tokeida M, Gotoh T, Nishizono A, Nasu M. Gastric ulcer, atrophic gastritis, and intestinal metaplasia caused by *Helicobacter pylori* infection in Mongolian gerbils. Scand J Gastroenterol 1998; 33:454–460.

126. Honda S, Fujioka T, Tokieda M, Satoh R, Nishizono A, Nasu M. Development of *Helicobacter pylori*-induced gastric carcinoma in Mongolian gerbils. Cancer Res 1998; 58:4255–4259.

127. Watanabe T, Tada M, Nagai H, Sasaki S, Nakao M. *Helicobacter pylori* infection induces gastric cancer in Monglian gerbils. Gastroenterology 1998; 115:642–648.

128. Wang TC, Goldenring JR, Ito S, et al. Mice lacking secretory phospholipase A2 show altered apoptosis and differentiation with *Helicobacter felis* infection. Gastroenterology 1998; 114:675–689.

129. Li Q, Karam SM, Gordon JI. Diptheria toxin-mediated ablation of parietal cells in the stomach of transgenic mice. J Biol Chem 1996; 271:3671–3676.

130. Schmidt PH, Lee JR, Goldenring JR, Wright NA, Poulsom R. Association of an aberrant spasmolytic polypeptide-expressing cell lineage with gastric adenocarcinoma in humans. Gastroenterology 1998; 114:G2781.

131. Wang TC, Fox JG. *Helicobacter pylori* and gastric cancer: Koch's postulates fulfilled (editorial). Gastroenterology 1998; 115:780–783.

132. Peek RM, Wirth HP, Moss SF, Yang M, Abdalla AM, Tham KT, Zhang T, Tang LH, Modlin IM, Blaser MH. *Helicobacter pylori* alters gastric epithelial cell cycle events and gastrin secretion in Mongolian gerblis. Gastroenterology 2000; 118 (in press).

133. Wang TC, Dangler CA, Chen D, Goldenring JR, Koh TJ, Raychowdhury R, Coffey RJ, Ito S, Varro A, Dockray GJ, Fox JG. Synergistic interaction between hypergastrinemia and Helicobacter infection in a mouse model of gastric cancer. Gastroenterology 2000; 118:1–14.

21
Gastric Adenocarcinoma

Catherine Ley and Julie Parsonnet

Gastric cancer is the second most frequent cancer worldwide, representing almost 10% of all new cancers and surpassed only by lung cancer *(1)*. It is also the 14th most common cause of death and the second most common cause of cancer death *(2)*. Since the beginning of the century, however, gastric cancer incidence has been declining at a rate of 20–50% per decade *(3)*. In the United States, for example, it has gone from, in 1940, the leading cause of cancer death to, in 1998, the ninth and tenth leading cause of cancer death in men and women, respectively (Fig. 1). Today, the incidence of gastric cancer in the United States is on the order of eight per 100,000 persons, although rates are higher among men than women and vary substantially across various racial and ethnic groups *(4)*.

Gastric adenocarcinoma includes cancers of the noncardia, the cardia, and the gastroesophageal junction. Noncardia cancers, which are the most common, are defined as cancers of the antrum, corpus, and fundus *(5–7)*; it is the incidence of these cancers that is declining around the world. Noncardia tumors have been directly associated with *Helicobacter pylori* and are the focus of the current chapter. Cancers of the cardia and gastroesophageal junction, which are less common, appear to be on the increase, currently constituting up to 50% of stomach cancers in some areas *(7)*.

Several histologic systems exist to classify gastric cancers. The Lauren system classifies gastric adenocarcinoma into two types: intestinal and diffuse *(8)*. The intestinal type, which predominates around the world, is decreasing rapidly in frequency *(9,10)*. It commonly arises in the gastric antrum and is characterized by cohesive cells that form discrete glands. Such intestinal tumors are preceded by a series of precancerous lesions, starting with chronic atrophic gastritis, progressing to intestinal metaplasia, dysplasia, and finally to cancer; this sequence occurs over several decades *(9)* (Fig. 2). Diffuse-type carcinomas are declining in incidence at a slower rate. They are more common in developed countries, generally involve the fundus and cardia, and are less differentiated, characterized by cells without gland formation and with occasional ring cells and mucin. Precursor conditions for diffuse type adenocarcinomas are not defined.

The prognosis of gastric adenocarcinoma relates to the extent of the disease. In Japan, where gastric cancer is extremely common, persons undergoing routine screen-

From: *Infectious Causes of Cancer: Targets for Intervention*
Edited by: J. J. Goedert © Humana Press Inc., Totowa, NJ

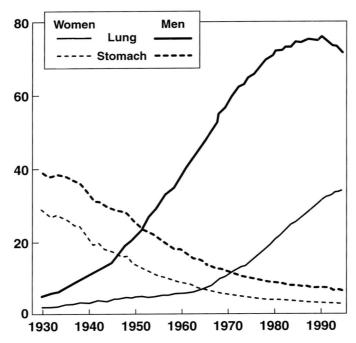

Fig. 1. Age-adjusted gastric and lung cancer death rates, by gender, US, 1930–1994. Rates are per 100,000 population and are age-adjusted to the 1970 US standard population. (Adapted with permission from the American Cancer Society, Cancer Facts and Figures)

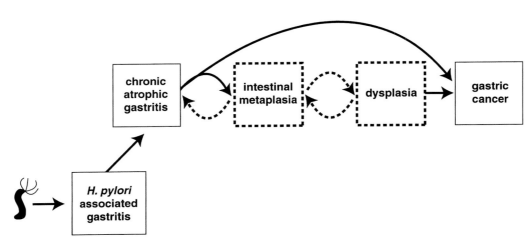

Fig. 2. Model of progression of precancerous lesions. Over time, chronic atrophic gastritis can lead to gastric cancer, potentially through intestinal metaplasia and dysplasia. Each lesion type has the potential to advance to, or regress from, the next type. *Dotted lines* indicate associations that are less well substantiated. *H. pylori* infection causes gastritis, a precursor to chronic atrophic gastritis.

ing for early gastric cancer have a 50% lower risk of dying from gastric malignancy than those who are not screened *(11)*. In most of the rest of the world, however, screening is not standard practice. In the United States, patients are rarely diagnosed with early gastric cancer, and survival rates at 1 and 5 yr are fairly low (46% and 21%, respectively) *(4)*. Survival rates in Europe are similarly poor *(12)*.

Although a large number of risk factors predisposing to gastric cancer has been studied individually, the pathogenesis of gastric cancer is likely to be multifactorial. Epidemiologic data strongly suggest the importance of environmental, particularly dietary, factors. For example, fresh fruit and vegetable consumption appears to be protective, possibly by providing β-carotene, vitamin E, ascorbic acid, and other naturally occurring antioxidants. High concentrations of nitrate and nitrites, present in preserved food, may increase risk. *H. pylori,* however, appears to be the key etiologic agent for the development of noncardia adenocarcinoma.

HELICOBACTER PYLORI—STRUCTURE AND BIOLOGY

Although spiral organisms were first identified in the mammalian stomach more than 100 yr ago, *H. pylori* was brought to international attention only in 1983 *(13)*. Named *Campylobacter pyloridis* when first isolated from mucosal biopsy specimens of patients with chronic active gastritis and peptic ulcer disease, it was reclassified to a new genus, *Helicobacter,* in 1989. The genome of *H. pylori* was entirely sequenced in 1997 *(14);* wide genomic diversity is thought to reside principally in a single hypervariable region *(15)*.

H. pylori is a relatively slow-growing, microaerophilic, Gram-negative, helical-shaped rod that lives beneath the mucus overlaying the gastric epithelium. The organism is between 2.5 and 5.0 µm long and has four to six unipolar flagellae that enable it to swim in a corkscrewlike fashion through the gastric mucus to take residence adjacent to the surface and pit epithelial cells. Beneath the mucus, many *H. pylori* remain freeliving, with approximately one fifth of organisms attaching to the cells *(16)*. Receptors for adherence of both the host and the bacterium are under investigation; potential host receptors include Lewis b (Leb) histo-blood group antigen *(17)* and phosphatidylethanolamine. Putative bacterial adhesins include a lipopolysaccharide, and the proteins BabA (which binds Leb) and AlpAB *(18–20)*. Adherence of *H. pylori* causes epithelial cell protein phosphorylation, resulting in actin polymerization and cytoskelton rearrangement (cup/pedestal formation) in the host cell *(21)*.

H. pylori is characterized by its abundant, constitutive production of urease, an enzyme that splits urea into ammonia and carbon dioxide. Urease constitutes up to 6% of the bacterial cell protein production *(22);* why so much of this enzyme is produced is not known. It is possible that the ammonia released by urease buffers the organism as it travels through the extremely low gastric pH of the stomach until reaching the more hospitable environment beneath the gastric mucus *(22,23)*. Urease may also serve nutritional functions for *H. pylori* and/or directly damage the gastric mucosa, allowing nutrients to be released into its environment *(24,25)*. Other important proteins produced by all *H. pylori* included catalase, oxidase, superoxide dismutase, and the heat shock proteins, HspA and HspB.

H. pylori causes chronic and acute inflammation of the gastric mucosa in all infected people. Infection is associated with epithelial cell release of interleukin (IL)-1, IL-6,

IL-8, tumor necrosis factor-α (TNF-α), and growth-regulated oncogene-α (Gro-α); these chemokines cause chemotaxis and activation of neutrophils *(26–29)*. *H. pylori*-associated proteins also directly cause activation of macrophages and lymphocytes, inducing a Th-1 type immune response and production of mucosal IgA and serum IgG to *H. pylori* antigens. Some of these antibodies may crossreact with gastric epithelial or other antigens, which implies that *H. pylori*-related inflammation may have an autoimmune component *(30,31)*.

The amount of inflammation produced by *H. pylori* infection correlates with specific characteristics of the infecting bacterium. Two basic phenotypes are widely recognized: one that produces a 90-kDa vacuolating cytotoxin (VacA) and one that does not, although all strains possess the *vacA* gene. VacA induces vacuole formation in tissue culture cells, and oral administration of purified cytotoxin to mice results in vacuolization, inflammation, and gastric ulceration *(32)*. In humans, those with VacA-expressing infections have higher degrees of inflammation than those without VacA expression. The *vacA* gene has several families of alleles, both of the signal sequence (s1a, s1b, s1c, s2) and of the middle region (m1, m2a, m2b). The geographic distribution of these alleles is currently being explored; for example, isolates from Northern Europe are mostly subtype s1a, from Central and South America subtype s1b, and from East Asia subtype s1c *(34)*. Cytotoxin production appears to correlate principally with the s1m1 strains *(34,35)*.

vacA s1m1 genotype also correlates with the presence of a 40-kb segment of DNA containing 31 open reading frames termed the *pathogenicity island (14)*. The functions of many genes in this pathogenicity island are unknown, although six genes appear to code for a type 4 searcher system *(36)*. One gene, found primarily in strains of the *vacA* s1 signal type, encodes a highly antigenic protein, the cytotoxin-associated gene A (CagA). Anti-CagA antibodies are easy to detect and can be used to indicate infection with these more inflammatory or virulent strains of *H. pylori (37)*. Two genes closely linked to *cagA, picA* and *picB*, are thought to be responsible for the proinflammatory activity associated with cagA-positive strains *(38)*; the virulence potential of another linked gene, *iceA*, is currently under investigation *(39)*.

EPIDEMIOLOGY OF INFECTION

H. pylori occurs worldwide and infects 50% of the world's population *(40)*. Its prevalence varies, depending on age and country. In developing countries, most children are infected by the age of 10 yr and infection is virtually universal by mid-life. By contrast, in developed countries, infection in children is uncommon, and is present in only 40–50% of adults. In addition, there is a clear age-related increase in prevalence. The fact that older people are more likely to be infected probably represents a cohort phenomenon in that acquisition of *H. pylori* infection was more common in children in the past than it is today *(41,42)*.

At the present date, *H. pylori* incidence in the United States is quite low across all age groups, estimated as approx 0.4% per year for adults *(43)*. In developing countries, this rate may be much higher, from 2% to 10% *(43,44)*. The reinfection rate is unlikely to be greater than the estimated primary incidence rate in adults and could be lower, suggesting a degree of immunity. Recurrence of infection after antibiotic therapy is more likely to be recrudescence than true reinfection *(45)*.

How *H. pylori* is transmitted remains controversial. Circumstantial evidence suggests that *H. pylori* transmission most probably occurs through direct person-to-person contact *(46,47),* possibly via human feces or regurgitated gastric material. *H. pylori* has been cultured recently from saliva, vomitus, air samples collected during bouts of vomiting, and diarrheal stools *(48–50).* Although a variety of environmental sources has been examined, including water, animals and insects, *H. pylori* has not been cultured from any sources other than primates. Furthermore, *H. pylori* has few regulatory genes, suggesting that the organism would have difficulty adapting to environments outside its natural human host *(14).*

Studies have indicated that lower socioeconomic status, particularly during childhood, is associated with a higher risk of *H. pylori* acquisition *(51,52).* This is most probably due to the association of low socioeconomic status with increased household crowding and lower levels of household sanitation and hygiene. Thus, racial and ethnic groups with lower socioeconomic status would be expected to have higher infection prevalence. Even when analyses are controlled for socioeconomic status, however, some populations have higher infection prevalence than others *(41,53,54).* For example, in the United States, blacks and Hispanics exhibit two- or threefold more *H. pylori* than do non-Hispanic whites. The reasons for these ethnic and racial differences are not known. Also for unknown reasons, men in some populations have up to 30% higher rates of infection than do women *(33).*

EPIDEMIOLOGIC EVIDENCE FOR A LINK BETWEEN *H. PYLORI* AND GASTRIC CANCER

Because *H. pylori* causes the vast majority of chronic gastritis and because gastritis is known to precede noncardia gastric cancer, there has been much interest in *H. pylori* as a cause of cancer. A number of ecologic studies have compared rates of *H. pylori* infection in different populations with rates of gastric cancer in those same populations. In most areas, cancer rates have correlated well with *H. pylori* prevalence *(55,56).* Temporal studies have also indicated a correlation between trends in *H. pylori* prevalence and trends in cancer incidence. Similar to the gastric cancer rate, *H. pylori* incidence has been declining over time *(41,42).*

Many retrospective epidemiologic studies have evaluated whether *H. pylori* is more common in cancer patients than in persons without cancer. A number of these studies have been subject to bias, including poor control selection or lack of adjustment for known confounders or tumor site; this would tend to mask any association between infection and cancer. In addition, cancerous stomachs may lose the ability to harbor *H. pylori* *(57–59),* leading to a reduced antibody response in cases. Despite these biases, however, *H. pylori* has been significantly linked to cancer in a large proportion of studies. Two meta-analyses of all case-control studies suggest that infection increases the risk of cancer approximately twofold for both diffuse- and intestinal-type tumors *(60,61).*

The strongest epidemiologic evidence for an association between *H. pylori* and cancer comes from a series of prospective case-control studies that used stored serum from well-characterized populations that were being followed over time *(62–69).* In these studies, serum titers were not biased by the coexistence of cancer in the cases; in addition, infection was known to precede malignancy. *H. pylori* was linked to both diffuse and intestinal histologic types of noncardia cancer. Additional analyses showed that in subjects followed for more than 10 yr, *H. pylori* increased the risk of cancer eightfold *(70)*. Furthermore, persons with CagA-positive *H. pylori* had a two- to threefold higher risk of cancer than those without CagA antibodies, and a 10-fold higher risk of cancer compared to those without *H. pylori* infection *(71,72)*.

H. pylori fulfills a number of the criteria used to determine whether an agent is a cause of disease. The epidemiologic associations between *H. pylori* and gastric cancer are strong and have shown remarkable consistency across studies. *H. pylori* strains that produce more inflammation appear to be more malignant, suggesting a biologic gradient or dose response. Chronic inflammation has been linked to cancer in other organs; *H. pylori* is thus a plausible cause of cancer by being a cause of chronic inflammation. Experimental evidence from laboratory and clinical studies suggests that *H. pylori* could lead to mutagenic damage. With the weight of this evidence, in 1994 *H. pylori* was declared a Group I carcinogen, a definite cause of cancer in humans *(73)*.

ANIMAL MODELS FOR *H. PYLORI* AND GASTRIC CANCER

Evidence to link *H. pylori* with gastric cancer has been provided by animal models. In mice, *H. hepaticus* causes low-grade infection of intrahepatic bile canaliculi; it produces hepatic carcinoma in males of the A/JCr strain *(74,75)*. Liver cells in these animals exhibit both increased cell turnover and increased oxidative damage; they also demonstrate a range of mutations *(75–77)*. This model, however, although useful for the understanding of carcinogenesis, has limited applicability to human gastric cancer.

H. mustelae, a pathogen of ferrets, has many parallels to *H. pylori (78)*. It attaches to the gastric mucosa in a manner similar to *H. pylori,* and causes chronic inflammation, hypochlorhydria and elevations in serum gastrin levels. Ferrets with *H. mustelae* frequently develop gastric atrophy *(79);* gastric adenocarcinoma occurs consistently when infected animals are exposed to the mutagen N-methyl-N-nitro-N'-nitrosoguanidine (MNNG) *(80)*.

Rhesus monkeys can be infected experimentally with *H. pylori*. As in humans, the infection can be transient or persistent, and may cause both gastritis and an elevated antibody response *(81,82)*. Interplay between characteristics of both the monkey host and the infecting *H. pylori* strain probably determine the type of gastric response that occurs, as individual monkeys differ in their susceptibility to the infection and the bacterial strains differ in their ability to sustain their presence *(83)*. Because monkeys in colonies tend to become naturally infected, monkey populations provide a useful place for the testing of potential anti-*H. pylori* therapies and vaccines *(84,85)*.

The most recent model to be identified has been that of the Mongolian gerbil *(86)*. Readily infected with *H. pylori*, Mongolian gerbils develop gastritis, gastric ulceration, intestinal metaplasia, and gastric adenocarcinoma *(87–89)*. Of note, *H. pylori* alone appears to be sufficient to cause cancer in this model. While much remains to be discovered, particularly with respect to epithelial alterations, this system should provide a particularly good model for the understanding of the progression from infection to malignancy.

MECHANISMS FOR CANCER DEVELOPMENT

H. pylori infection produces inflammation within the gastric mucosa. Inflammation generates reactive oxygen and nitrogen oxide species (ROS and RNOS); these mole-

Table 1
Possible Mechanisms by Which *H. pylori* Causes Mutations

DNA damage	Increased ROS production[a,b]
	Increased RNOS production[a,b]
	Decreased DNA repair enzyme activity
	Decreased antioxidant levels[b]
Cell proliferation[c]	Increased gastrin production[b]
	Increased apoptosis
	Increased COX2 activity

ROS, reactive oxygen species; RNOS, reactive nitrogen oxide species; COX2, cyclooxygenase-2.

[a] Associated with inflammation.

[b] Associated with hypochlorhydria.

[c] Associated with *H. pylori* phenotype (CagA).

cules can be both directly and indirectly mutagenic. Infection is also associated with changes in gastric physiology, including loss of gastric acidity (hypochlorhydria), increases in gastric hormone levels, and decreases in antioxidant levels. *H. pylori* infection is also associated with both a proliferation of epithelial cells and alterations in apoptosis. In combination, these events may lead to the formation or selection of mutated cells and the development of gastric cancer (Table 1).

Inflammation and Reactive Oxygen/Nitrogen Species

Chronic and acute inflammation caused by *H. pylori* infection in the gastric mucosa are related to host and bacterial factors. IL-8, produced by epithelial cells in response to infection, may cause a neutrophil and macrophage influx into the gastric mucosa *(90)*. Both epithelial cells and phagocytic cells, in response to *H. pylori* antigens and secreted proteins, release ROS *(91)*. Release of IL-8 and ROS and the density of both neutrophils and macrophages directly correlate with the density of organisms present on mucosal surfaces *(92,93)*.

ROS can either directly cause mutation or can react with other chemical species to form highly mutagenic compounds. One marker of oxidative damage by ROS is 8-hydroxy-2′-deoxyguanosine (8HdG), an adduct that, if unrepaired, leads to G→T transversions *(94)*. Mucosal levels of this adduct are higher in *H. pylori*-infected than in uninfected persons *(95–97)*, and they return to baseline after antibiotic therapy *(95)*. Deficiencies in DNA repair could also cause oxidative adducts to accumulate in the gastric mucosa, paralleling what occurs in other inflammatory conditions *(98,99)*.

Nitric oxide production is associated with *H. pylori* infection *(100,101)*. A relatively reactive species, it can induce mutagenic damage directly or by combining with other chemicals to form highly mutagenic species, causing the deamination of cytosine and C → T transitions. Macrophages and neutrophils exposed to *H. pylori* have increased expression of inducible nitric oxide synthase (iNOS) *(101–103);* urease may be involved in this process *(104)*. iNOS expression has been found to be high in subjects with *H. pylori* infection and atrophic gastritis *(105)*. Nitrotyrosine, a marker for damage induced by RNOS, has also been identified in the mucosa of infected patients. Eradication of infection or dietary supplementation with antioxidants or antinitrosating agents (such as β-carotene and ascorbic acid) produces a decrease in both iNOS and nitrotyrosine. Finally, nitric oxide has been found to inhibit a DNA repair enzyme, formamidopyrimidine–DNA glycosylase, which repairs 8HdG in bacteria *(106).*

Changes in Gastric Physiology

Gastric acid is produced by parietal cells in the body of the stomach in response to a variety of stimuli including the gastric hormome, gastrin *(107).* Gastrin, produced in the antrum of the stomach, is released in response to intraluminal protein, to neural and hormonal stimuli, and to intraluminal gastric acidity. Gastrin also stimulates epithelial cells to proliferate particularly within the gastric antrum *(108).*

Under normal conditions, *H. pylori* confines itself to the gastric antrum of the stomach where it lives beneath the mucus gel, shielded from intraluminal acid. Paradoxically, however, antral *H. pylori* stimulates gastrin release and increases acid secretion, at least postprandially *(109).* This type of response may precipitate duodenal ulcer disease, particularly in people with other predisposing factors for ulcers (e.g., family history, cigarette smoking or use of nonsteroidal antiinflammatory agents). In a substantial subset of people, however, *H. pylori* infection causes destruction of the gastric glands (chronic atrophic gastritis) either in the antrum and body of the stomach or almost exclusively in the body *(110).* Body involvement may be a function of duration of infection, host genetic factors, or other cofactors, such as diet and nutrition *(107,111,112).* Extension of *H. pylori* into the body coincides with glandular destruction, loss of acid-secreting ability (hypochlorhydria), and an increased likelihood of developing cancer *(113).*

Hypochlorhydria can contribute to carcinogenesis in several ways. Hypoacidity is associated with high levels of mutagenic *N*-nitrosamines *(114),* which have been epidemiologically linked to gastric cancer. It also decreases intraluminal concentrations of vitamin C *(115,116);* one form, ascorbic acid, is an antioxidant and a strong inhibitor of *N*-nitrosation. Hypochlorhydria causes feedback secretion of gastrin *(117),* which, in turn, causes proliferation of epithelial cells *(108).* Hypergastrinemia is a strong risk factor for subsequent development of gastric adenocarcinoma, independent of the presence of *H. pylori* infection *(118,119).* Hypochlorhydria appears to allow *H. pylori* to grow more extensively into the gastric body *(120–122).* Finally, hypoacidity may allow overgrowth of nitrate-fixing bacteria that can convert nitrates into nitrites and foster formation of *N*-nitrosamines *(123,124).*

Thus, the physiologic effects of *H. pylori* on the stomach would appear to predispose infected people to cancer. Alone, however, these effects are probably not sufficient to induce malignancy, as there is no evidence in humans or in animals that drug-induced acid suppression leads to an increased risk of gastric cancer *(125,126).*

Epithelial Cell Proliferation and Apoptosis

Cell proliferation increases the risk of cancer by increasing the number of cells that are dividing and are therefore susceptible to DNA damage. Hyperproliferation of gastric mucosal cells in *H. pylori*-infected people has been well documented *(127–129).* This proliferative effect is particularly prominent in patients infected with the CagA-positive phenotype of *H. pylori (130)* and in those with advanced preneoplastic lesions (atrophic gastritis, incomplete intestinal metaplasia and dysplasia) *(131–133).* When *H.*

pylori infection is cured with antibiotics, cell proliferation declines dramatically *(127,128)*.

H. pylori infection also causes cell loss, both through necrosis and apoptosis. *H. pylori* toxin damages cells, directly causing necrotic cell death *(134–136)*. Apoptosis is also increased with infection, however *(137,138)*, possibly through a Bak-dependent pathway *(139)* or by the Fas or CD95 antigen pathways *(140,141)*. Thus, hyperproliferation may be a necessary response to compensate for both necrotic and apopotic death. Interestingly, although patients with the CagA-positive phenotype of *H. pylori* have increased cell proliferation, apoptosis does not increase *(130,142)*. This suggests that CagA$^+$–VacA$^+$ *H. pylori* may induce higher rates of necrotic cell death than other forms of infection or that the gastric mucosa may be unable to compensate for DNA damage. In support of this, recent studies demonstrate that *H. pylori* infection may induce cyclooxygenase-2 (COX-2), a critical enzyme for prostaglandin synthesis. COX-2, which can inhibit *H. pylori*-induced apoptosis *(143)*, is overexpressed in gastric cancer and preneoplastic conditions.

FACTORS CONTRIBUTING TO MALIGNANCY

Only 1% of people infected with *H. pylori* developing gastric adenocarcinoma, and the vast majority of infected persons have no clinical symptoms. Any model that attempts to describe *H. pylori* as a risk factor for gastric cancer must explain why this disease develops in some people but not in others *(144)*. Factors that could explain this variability include: differences in *H. pylori* genotype, host genotype, age at infection, and exposures to environmental cofactors (Fig. 3).

H. pylori Genotype

The genetic diversity between strains of *H. pylori* is wide. Identical *H. pylori* strains are rarely, if ever, seen in unrelated individuals *(145)* and within families, strains frequently differ *(146)*. Even within an individual, variability of the infecting strain may exist *(147)*. Little is known about the clinical significance of these strain differences. The prognostic value of combinations of alleles for different virulence factors is being explored *(37–39)*. Strains containing the *H. pylori* pathogenicity island increase an individual's risk of intestinal-type gastric cancer when compared with strains that do not *(71,72)*. Similarly, *H. pylori*-infected people with CagA antibodies are two times more likely to progress from nonatrophic gastritis to atrophic gastritis than are *H. pylori*-infected people without these antibodies *(148)*.

Although the prevalence of strains with the pathogenicity island varies across populations *(149,150)*, it is not clear that this variation translates into differences in disease incidence. Moreover, variation in *H. pylori* strain type cannot explain the differences between population rates of peptic ulcer disease and gastric cancer, as CagA-positive strains appear to increase risk for both of these conditions *(151)*.

Human Genotype

A variety of human genetic factors have been associated with *H. pylori* carcinogenesis; any could predispose infected hosts to one disease outcome and prevent another. Glutathione-*S*-transferase-μ (GSTM1) conjugates and detoxifies carcinogenic compounds; specific genotypes may be associated with cancer risk *(152–154)* and, in combi-

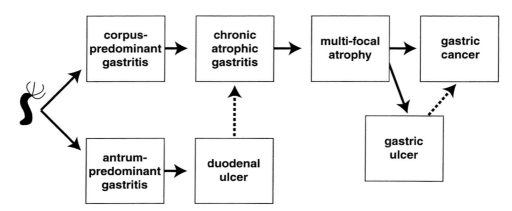

Fig. 3. Model of progression of *H. pylori*-associated clinical conditions. *H. pylori* causes gastritis, either confined to the antrum or corpus-wide; this distribution is probably associated with age at infection and/or host susceptibility. Antrum-based infection causes increased acid production and increased risk of duodenal ulcer (DU). Corpus infection leads to decreased acid levels via loss of parietal cells through atrophy. In a subset of persons with chronic atrophic gastritis, this low acid environment predisposes to the development of gastric ulcer and/or cancer. Of note, DU patients on long-term anti-acid regimens could potentially develop chronic atrophic gastritis. Each step in this model could be affected by environmental factors (e.g., diet or smoking), *H. pylori* genotype (e.g., *cagA*), or host genotype.

nation with *H. pylori,* may amplify this risk. The acid response to *H. pylori* may have a genetic basis, as may the rate of proliferation of the gastric mucosa *(155,156)*. Human leukocyte antigen (HLA) types show associations with atrophic gastritis, duodenal ulcer, and gastric cancer although associations with *H. pylori* remain unexamined *(157–159)*. Additional human genetic factors that are being explored in relation to infection include ABO blood group type, Lewis blood group type, and mucin genotype *(160–164)*.

Age at Infection

Similar to other cancers associated with an inflammatory process *(165–167)*, the risk of gastric cancer may correlate with the length of time that a person has been infected with *H. pylori*. People infected with *H. pylori* as children have more time to acquire necessary mutations over their lifetime compared to those infected as adults. In developed countries, it appears that the average age of acquiring infection is increasing over time *(41,42)*, possibly explaining in part the decline in cancer rates and the increase in age at which cancer occurs. It is difficult, however, to prove that the age of infection influences disease outcome. In mice, infection is more likely to persist if infection occurs at a young age, producing multifocal gastritis *(168)*, suggesting a different susceptibility of the young stomach. The stomach of a human child may be physiologically different that that of an adult. Children have less acute inflammation and more prominent lymphoid follicles than do adults *(169)*; they may also be more likely to have *H. pylori* in the corpus of the stomach *(170)*. This would increase their likelihood of hypochlorhydria, explaining why, even with antral gastritis, duodenal ulceration is a rare response to childhood *H. pylori* infection *(169)*.

It is possible that factors that cause hypochlorhydria in childhood, such as malnutrition and infectious diseases, are necessary for cancer formation. Under hypochlorhydric conditions, *H. pylori* could extend into the gastric corpus, initiating the chain of events that leads to malignancy. In the absence of malnutrition or infection, *H. pylori* would remain confined to the antrum and intraluminal acid levels would remain normal or high.

Environmental Cofactors for Infection

The effects of other known risk factors for gastric cancer could be modified by the concurrent presence of *H. pylori*. For example, it appears that diets high in salt and nitrates increase cancer risk while diets rich in fresh fruits and vegetables protect against gastric cancer *(123)*. Because *H. pylori* both induces nitric oxide formation (potentially fostering the formation of *N*-nitroso compounds from intraluminal nitrites) and destroys mucosal ascorbate, the interaction of infection with diet may have an effect far greater than each alone in causing cancer. In the same way, cigarette smoking potentially alters the outcome of *H. pylori* infection *(171,172)*, again via the nitric oxide pathway *(173)*. Also of interest, some gastric adenocarcinomas have clonal integration of Epstein–Barr virus *(174,175)*, although a relationship with *H. pylori* remains unclear.

PREVENTION OF *H. PYLORI*-RELATED GASTRIC CANCER

Within an individual, the development of cancer results from a combination of factors, including circumstances of infection, the individual's genetic makeup, *H. pylori* strain type, and other cofactors. Only some of these risk factors are amenable to intervention within a population. *H. pylori*-related gastric cancer could be prevented by preventing *H. pylori* infection (through either the interruption of *H. pylori* transmission or the immunization of susceptible people); by curing *H. pylori* infection (with the treatment of infected people via antibiotic therapy or therapeutic vaccination); or by removing other factors necessary for gastric cancer development.

Prevention of Infection

H. pylori is decreasing in prevalence with time. Estimates of the decline over the century range from 26% to 52% per decade *(41,42,176,177)*. It is not known why the organism is disappearing, but improvements in nutrition, household sanitation, and household crowding are likely factors. Thus as countries improve their socioeconomic conditions, infection rates should continue to decline around the world. At the current rate, *H. pylori* could disappear from some populations entirely within the next few generations (M. Rupnow, *personal communication*).

Meanwhile, prophylactic vaccines could prevent infection with *H. pylori* in uninfected at-risk persons, primarily children and young adults. Although several oral and intranasal vaccines have been shown to provide protective mucosal immunity against *H. pylori* in both mice and monkeys *(178–183)*, many years will be required until a vaccine shown to be successful in animal models is proven safe and efficacious in humans *(184,185)*. Because some of the damage caused by *H. pylori* may result from an autoimmune response, vaccination actually might induce a chronic inflammatory response *(181)*.

Treatment of H. pylori infection

H. pylori infection can be eradicated by antibiotic therapy. To date, screening for and treatment of *H. pylori* are recommended only for persons in specific high-risk groups *(186,187)*. A key reason for this selection is that it is not known whether eradication of infection prevents gastric cancer. If antibiotic therapies could prevent a small percentage of cancers (e.g., 20–30%), screening and treatment of *H. pylori* would be a cost-effective strategy to preventing cancer *(188,189)*. Current trials in Europe and China *(190)* are examining the preventive ability of *H. pylori* eradication and have randomized thousands of infected people to *H. pylori* therapy or placebo with follow-up for gastric cancer incidence over 10–20 yr. If treatment is shown to be effective in reducing cancer rates, these studies will prove that *H. pylori* causes malignancy and that screening and treatment are warranted. Unfortunately, studies of this type are extremely expensive in both logistics and follow-up time; they also run the risk of insufficient statistical power due to decreasing cancer rates and *H. pylori* prevalence.

An alternative and cheaper study design examines intermediate biomarkers instead of cancer. Subjects with gastric preneoplastic conditions are randomized to receive either *H. pylori* therapy or placebo and monitored for the progression or regression of these conditions. These studies, also ongoing, will not be able to prove that treatment of *H. pylori* will prevent cancer, as even if preneoplastic conditions regress, cancer could still occur. To date, small case series that have looked at regression of preneoplastic conditions have yielded mixed results *(191–195)*, although one has suggested that *H. pylori* eradication not only can prevent cancer, but it can also do so at a very late stage in tumor development *(195)*.

It is important to recognize that *H. pylori* infection might actually have a beneficial effect. For example, recent studies suggest that *H. pylori* infection protects against the development of reflux esophagitis, and adenocarcinoma of the gastric cardia and gastroesophageal junction *(196,197)*. Thus, trials of *H. pylori* eradication should assess all-cause mortality, not just mortality from noncardia gastric cancer.

Cofactors for Cancer

Alternative targets for gastric cancer prevention involve environmental cofactors. As mentioned previously, dietary supplementation with antioxidants, or diets rich in fresh fruit have been associated with a decreased gastric cancer risk and are beneficial for many reasons *(198,199)*. Cigarette smoking has also been linked to gastric tumors, among many other conditions *(171)*.

SUMMARY

Both epidemiologic and pathophysiologic evidence exist to support *H. pylori* as a cause of noncardia gastric cancer. Further study is needed, however, to understand how *H. pylori* infection causes tumor development. Data are accumulating to suggest that *H. pylori* eradication may be a useful strategy to prevent gastric cancer, particularly in certain populations. Studies that evaluate the cost-effectiveness and role of therapies such as antibiotic treatment or vaccination will clarify this issue.

REFERENCES

1. Parkin DM, Pisani P, Ferlay J. Estimates of the worldwide incidence of 25 major cancers in 1990. Int J Cancer 1999; 80:827–841.
2. Murray CJL, Lopez AD. Mortality by cuase for eight regions of the world: Global Burden of Disease study. Lancet 1997; 349:1269–1276.
3. Coleman MP, Esteve J, Damiecki P, Arslan A. Renard H. Tends in cancer incidence and mortality. Lyon: International Agency for Research on Cancer, 1993; pp. 192–224.
4. Ries LAG, Kosary CL, Hankey BF, Miller BA, Edwards BK (eds). SEER Cancer Statistics Review, 1973–1996, National Cancer Institute. Bethesda, MD, 1999.
5. Rios-Castellanos E, Sitas F, Shepard NA, Jewell DP. Changing pattern of gastric cancer in Oxfordshire. Gut 1992; 33:1312–1317.
6. Wang HH, Antonioli DA, Goldman H. Comparative features of esophageal and gastric adenocarcinomas: recent changes in type and frequency. Hum Pathol 1986; 17:482–487.
7. Salvon-Harman JC, Cady B, Nikulasson S, Khettry U, Stone MD, Lavin P. Shifting proportions of gastric adenocarcinomas. Arch Surg 1994; 129:381–388; discussion 388–9.
8. Lauren P. The two histological main types of gastric cancer: diffuse and so-called intestinal type carcinoma. Acta Pathol Microbiol Scand 1965; 64:31–49.
9. Correa P, Cuello C, Duque E, et al. Gastric cancer in Colombia. III. Natural history of precursor lesions. J Natl Cancer Inst 1976; 57:1027–1035.
10. Munoz N, Connelly R. Time trends of intestinal and diffuse types of gastric cancer in the United States. Int J Cancer 1971; 8:158–164.
11. Fukao A, Tsubono Y, Tsuji I, Hisamichi S, Sugahara N, Takano A. The evaluation of screening for gastric cancer in Miyagi Prefecture, Japan: a population-based case-control study. Int J Cancer 1995; 60:45–48.
12. Faive J, Forman D, Esteve J, Gatta G. Survival of patients with oesophageal and gastric cancers in Europe. Eur J Cancer 1998; 34:2167–2175.
13. Marshall BJ. History of the discovery of *C. pylori*. In: Blaser MJ (ed). *Campylobacter pylori* in gastritis and peptic ulcer disease. New York: Igaku-Shoin, 1989, pp. 7–23.
14. Tomb JF, White O, Kerlavage AR, et al. The complete genome sequence of the gastric pathogen *Helicobacter pylori*. Nature 1997; 388:539–547.
15. Alm RA, Ling LS, Moir DT, Brown ED, et al. Genomic-sequence comparison of two unrelated isolates of the human gastric pathogen *Helicobacter pylori*. Nature 1999; 14:176–180.
16. Lee A, Fox J, Hazell S. Pathogenicity of *Helicobacter pylori:* a perspective. Infect Immun 1993; 61:1601–1610.
17. Boren T, Normark S, Falk P. *Helicobacter pylori:* molecular basis for host recognition and bacterial adherence. Trends Microbiol 1994; 2:221–228.
18. Osaki T, Yamaguchi H, Taguchi H, et al. Establishment and characterisation of a monoclonal antibody to inhibit adhesion of *Helicobacter pylori* to gastric epithelial cells. J Med Microbiol 1998; 47:505–512.
19. Ilver D, Arnqvist A, Ogren J, et al. *Helicobacter pylori* adhesin binding fucosylated histo-blood group antigens revealed by retagging. Science 1998; 279:373–377.
20. Odenbreit S, Till M, Hofreuter F, Faller G, Haas R. Genetic and functional characterization of the alpAB gene locus essential for the adhesion of *Helicobacter pylori* to human gastric tissue. Mol Microiol 1999; 31:1537–1548.
21. Segal ED, Falkow S, Tompkins LS. *Helicobacter pylori* attachment to gastric cells induces cytoskeletal rearrangements and tyrosine phosphorylation of host cell proteins. Proc Natl Acad Sci USA 1996; 93:1259–1264.
22. Hu LT, Mobley HL. Purification and N-terminal analysis of urease from *Helicobacter pylori*. Infect Immun 1990; 58:992–998.

23. Eaton KA, Brooks CL, Morgan DR, Krakowka S. Essential role of urease in pathogenesis of gastritis induced by *Helicobacter pylori* in gnotobiotic piglets. Infect Immun 1991; 59:2470–2475.

24. Hazell SL, Mendz GL. The metabolism and enzymes of *Helicobacter pylori:* function and potential virulence effects. In: Goodwin CS, Worsley BW (eds). *Helicobacter pylori:* Biology and Clinical Practice. Boca Raton, FL: CRC Press, 1993, pp. 115–142.

25. Emond JP, Mahe D, Cattan D, Launay JM, Courillon-Mallet A. *H. pylori* uses urea nitrogen for the synthesis of histamine and N alpha methylhistamine. Gastroenterology 1999; 116:G0604 (Abstr).

26. Ernst PB, Crowe SE, Reyes VE. How does *Helicobacter pylori* cause mucosal damage? The inflammatory response. Gastroenterology. 1997; 13:S35–42; discussion S50.

27. Crabtree JE. Role of cytokines in the pathogenesis of *Helicobacter pylori*-induced mucosal damage. Dig Dis Sci 1998; 43(Suppl):46S–55S.

28. Lindhilm C, Quinding-Jarbrink M, Lonroth H, Hamlet A, Svennerholm AM. Local cytokine response in *Helicobacter pylori*-infected subjects. Infect Immun 1998; 66:5964–5971.

29. Suzuki H, Mori M, Sakaguch A, Suzuki M, Miura S, Ishii H. Enhanced levels of C-X-C chemokine, human GRO alpha, in *Helicobacter pylori*-associated gastric disease. J Gastroenterol Hepatol 1998; 13:516–520.

30. Faller G, Seininger H, Appelmelk B, Kirchner T. Evidence of novel pathogenic pathways for the formation of antigastric autoantibodies in *Helicobacter pylori* gastritis. J Clin Pathol 1998; 51:244–245.

31. Fastame L, Tocci A, Mura D, et al. Is *Helicobacter pylori* infection responsible for abnormal humoral immune reactions and cryo globulins? Gastroenterology 1999; 116:G3098 (Abstr).

32. Telford JL, Ghiara P, Dell'Orco M, et al. Gene structure of the *Helicobacter pylori* cytotoxin and evidence of its key role in gastric disease. J Exp Med 1994; 179:1653–1658.

33. Van Doorn LJ, Figueiredo C, Megraud F, et al. Geographic distribution of vacA allelic types of *Helicobacter pylori*. Gastroenterology 1999; 116:823–830.

34. Gunn MC, Stephens JC, Stewart JA, Rathbone BJ, West KP. The significance of cagA and vacA subtypes of *Helicobacter pylori* in the pathogenesis of inflammation and peptic ulceration. J Clin Pathol 1998; 10:761–764.

35. Yamaoka Y, Kodama T, Kita M, Imanishi J, Kashima K, Graham DY. Relationship of vacA genotypes of *Helicobacter pylori* to cagA status, cytotoxin production, and clinical outcome. Helicobacter 1998; 3241–3253.

36. Covacci A, Telford JC, Giudice GD, Parsonnet J, Rappouli R. *Helicobacter pylori* virulence and genetic geography. Science 1999; 284:1328–1333.

37. Cover TL, Glupczynski Y, Lage AP, et al. Serologic detection of infection with cagA+ *Helicobacter pylori* strains. J Clin Microbiol 1995; 33:1496–1500.

38. Blaser MJ. Role of vacA and the cagA locus of *Helicobacter pylori* in human disease. Aliment Pharmacol Ther 1996; 10 (Suppl 1):73–77

39. Peek RM, Thompson SA, Donahue JP, et al. Adherence to gastric epithelial cells induces expression of a *Helicobacter pylori* gene, iceA, that is associated with clinical outcome. Proc Assoc Am Physicians 1998; 110:531–544.

40. Smith KL, Parsonnet J. *Helicobacter pylori*. In: Evans A, Brachman P (eds). Bacterial Infections of Humans. New York: Plenum Publishing, 1998, pp. 337–353.

41. Parsonnet J, Blaser MJ, Perez-Perez GI, Hargrett-Bean N, Tauxe RV. Symptoms and risk factors of *Helicobacter pylori* infection in a cohort of epidemiologists. Gastroenterlogy 1992; 102:41–46.

42. Banatvala N, Mayo K, Megraud F, Jennings R, Deeks JJ, Feldman RA. The cohort effect and *Helicobacter pylori*. J Infect Dis. 1993; 168:219–221.

43. Parsonnet J. The incidence of *Helicobacter pylori* infection. Aliment Pharmacol Ther 1995; 9(Suppl 2):45–52.

44. Becker SI, Smalligan RD, Frame JD, et al. Risk of *Helicobacter pylori* infection among long-term residents in developing countries. Am J Trop Med Hyg 1999; 60:267–270.

45. Gisbert JP, Pajares JM, Garcia-Vilriberas R, et al. Recurrence of *Helicobacter pylori* infection after eradication: incidence and variables influencing it. Scand J Gastroenterol 1998; 33:1144–1145.

46. Rothenbacher D, Bode G, Berg G, et al. *Helicobacter pylori* among preschool children and their parents: evidence of parent–child transmission. J Infect Dis 1999; 179:398–402.

47. Wang JT, Sheu JC, Lin JT, Wang TH, Wu MS. Direct DNA amplification and restriction pattern analysis of *Helicobacter pylori* in patients with duodenal ulcer and their families. J Infect Dis 1993; 168:1544–1548.

48. Shmuely H, Haggerty T, Villacorta R, Yang S, Parsonnet J. H. pylori in vomitus, saliva and air after experimentally-induced emesis (Abstr). Program and Abstracts, IDSA '98; 1998 Nov 12–15; Denver. Alexandria: Infectious Diseases Society of America, 1998, p. 77.

49. Haggerty T, Shmuely H, Parsonnet J. Uniformity of *Helicobacter* fingerprints in isolates from stool vomitus, air, and saliva of individual subjects. (Abstr) Program and Abstracts, IDSA '98; 1998 Nov 12–15; Denver. Alexandria: Infectious Diseases Society of America, 1998, p. 102.

50. Shmuely H, Haggerty T, Villacorta R, Yang S, Parsonnet J. *H. pylori* in stools of infected people with and without experimentally-induced diarrhea. (Abstr) Program and Abstracts, IDSA '98; 1998 Nov 12–15; Denver. Alexandria: Infectious Diseases Society of America, 1998, p. 102.

51. Malaty HM, Graham DY. Importance of childhood socioeconomic status on the current prevalence of *Helicobacter pylori* infection. Gut 1994; 35:742–745.

52. Malaty HM, Graham DY, Isaksson I, Engstrand L, Pedersen NL. Co-twin study of the effect of environment and dietary elements on acquisition of *Helicobacter pylori* infection. Am J Epidemiol 1998; 149:793–797.

53. Replogle ML, Glaser SL, Hiatt RA, Parsonnet J. Biological sex as a risk factor for *Helicobacter pylori* infection in healthy young adults. Am J Epidemiol 1995; 142:856–863.

54. Eurogast Study Group. Epidemiology of, and risk factors for, *Helicobacter pylori* infection among 3194 asymptomatic subjects in 17 populations. Gut 1993; 34:1672–1676.

55. Forman D, Sitas F, Newell DG, et al. Geographic association of *Helicobacter pylori* antibody prevalence and gastric cancer mortality in rural China. Int J Cancer 1990; 46:608–611.

56. Eurogast Study Group. An international association between *Helicobacter pylori* infection and gastric cancer. Lancet 1993; 341:1359–1362.

57. Masci E, Viale E, Freschi M, Porcellati M, Tittobello A. Precancerous gastric lesions and *Helicobacter pylori*. Hepatogastroenterology 1996; 43:854–858.

58. Osawa H, Inoue F, Yoshida Y. Inverse relation of serum *Helicobacter pylori* antibody titres and extent of intestinal metaplasia. J Clin Pathol 1996; 49:112–115.

59. Genta RM, Graham DY. Intestinal metaplasia, not atrophy or achlorhydria, creates a hostile environment for *Helicobacter pylori*. Scand J Gastroenterol 1993; 28:924–928.

60. Huang J, Sridhar S, Chen Y, Hunt RH. Meta-analysis of the relationship between *Helicobacter pylori* seropositivity and gastric cancer. Gastroenterology 1998; 114:1169–1179.

61. Eslick GD, Talley NJ. *Helicobacter pylori* infection and gastric carcinoma: a meta-analysis. Gastroenterology 1998; 114:2871 (Abstr).

62. Parsonnet J, Friedman GD, Vandersteen DP, et al. *Helicobacter pylori* infection and the risk of gastric carcinoma. N Engl J Med 1991; 325:1127–1131.

63. Forman D, Newell DG, Fullerton F, et al. Association between infection with *Helicobacter pylori* and risk of gastric cancer: evidence from a prospective investigation. Br Med J 1991; 302:1302–1305.

64. Nomura AMY, Stemmerman GN, Chyou P, Kato I, Perez-Perez GI, Blaser MJ. *Helicobacter pylori* infection and gastric carcinoma in a population of Japanese-Americans in Hawaii. N Engl J Med 1991; 325:1132–1136.

65. Siman JH, Forsgren A, Berglund G, Floren CH. Association between *Helicobacter pylori* and gastric carcinoma in the city of Malmo, Sweden. A prospective study. Scand J [???]Gastroenterol[???] 1997; 32:1215–1221.

66. Watanable Y, Kurata JH, Mizuno S, et al. *Helicobacter pylori* infection and gastric cancer. A nested case-control study in a rural area of Japan. Dig Dis Sci 1997; 42:1383–1387.

67. Aromaa A, Kosunen TU, Knekt P, et al. Circulating anti-*Helicobacter pylori* immunoglobulin A antibodies and low serum pepsinogen I level are associated with increased risk of gastric cancer. Am J Epidemiol 1996; 144:142–149.

68. Webb PM, Yu MC, Forman D, et al. An apparent lack of association, between *Helicobacter pylori* infection and risk of gastric cancer in China. Int J Cancer 1996; 67:603–607.

69. Lin JT, Wang LY, Wang JT, Wang TH, Yang CS, Chen CJ. A nested case-control study on the association between *Helicobacter pylori* infection and gastric cancer risk in a cohort of 9775 men in Taiwan. Anticancer Res 1995; 15:603–606.

70. Forman D, Webb P, Parsonnet J. *H. pylori* and gastric cancer. Lancet 1994; 343:243–244.

71. Blaser MJ, Perez-Perez GI, Kleanthous H, et al. Infection with *Helicobacter pylori* strains possessing cagA is associated with an increased risk of developing adenocarcinoma of the stomach. Cancer Res 1995; 55:2111–2115.

72. Parsonnet J, Friedman G, Orentreich N, Vogelman J. Risk for gastric cancer in persons with CagA positive and CagA negative *Helicobacter pylori* infection. Gut 1997; 40:297–301.

73. IARC Working Group on the Evaluation of Carcinogenic Risks to Humans. *Helicobacter pylori.* In: Schistosomes, Liver Flukes and *Helicobacter pylori:* Views and Expert Opinions of an IARC Working Group on the Evaluation of Carcinogenic Risks to Humans. Lyon: IARC, 1994, pp. 177–240.

74. Ward JM, Fox JG, Anver MR, et al. Chronic active hepatitis and associated liver tumors in mice caused by a persistent bacterial infection with a novel *Helicobacter* species. J Natl Cancer Inst 1994; 86:1222–1227.

75. Fox JG, Li X, Yan L, et al. Chronic proliferative hepatitis in A/JCr mice associated with persistent *Helicobacter hepaticus* infection: a model of *Helicobacter*-induced carcinogenesis. Infect Immun 1996; 64:1548–1558.

76. Sipowicz MA, Chomarat P, Diwan BA, et al. Increased oxidative DNA damage and hepatocyte overexpression of specific cytochrome P450 isoforms in hepatitis of mice infected with *Helicobacter hepaticus*. Am J Pathol 1997; 151:933–941.

77. Sipowicz MA, Weghorst CM, Shiao YH, et al. Lack of p53 and ras mutations in *Helicobacter hepaticus*-induced liver tumors in A/JCr mice. Carcinogenesis 1997; 18:233–236.

78. Fox JG, Otto G, Murphy JC, Taylor NS, Lee A. Gastric colonization of the ferret with *Helicobacter* species: natural and experimental infections. Rev Infect Dis 1991; 13 (Suppl 8):S671–680.

79. Fox JG, Dangler CA, Sager W, Borkowski R, Gliatto JM. *Helicobacter mustelae*-associated gastric adenocarcinoma in ferrets *(Mustela putorius furo)*. Vet Pathol 1997; 34:225–229.

80. Fox JG, Wishnok JS, Murphy JC, Tannenbaum SR, Correa P. MNNG-induced gastric carcinoma in ferrets infected with *Helicobacter mustelae*. Carcinogenesis 1993; 14:1957–1961.

81. Dubois A, Fiala N, Heman-Ackah LM, et al. Natural gastric infection with *Helicobacter pylori* in monkeys: a model for spiral bacteria infection in humans. Gastroenterology 1994; 106:1405–1417.

82. Dubois A, Berg DE, Incecik ET, et al. Transient and persistent experimental infection of nonhuman primates with *Helicobacter pylori:* implications for human disease. Infect Immun 1996; 64:2885–2891.

83. Dubois A, Berg D, Incecik ET, et al. Host specificity of *Helicobacter pylori* strains and host reponses in experimentally challenged nonhuman primates. Gastroenterology 1999; 116:90–96.

84. Dubois A, Berg DE, Fiala N, Hmen-Ackah LM, Perez-Perez GI, Blaser MJ. Cure of *Helicobacter pylori* infection by omeprazole-clarithromycin-based therapy in non-human primates. J Gastroenterol 1998; 33:18–22.

85. Dubois A, Lee CK, Fiala N, Keanthous H, Mehlman PT, Monath T. Immunization against natural *Helicobacter pylori* infection in nonhuman primates. Infect Immun 1998; 66:4340–4346.

86. Hirayama F, Takagi S, Yokoyama Y, Iwao E, Ikeda Y. Establishment of gastric *Helicobacter pylori* infection in Mongolian gerbils. J Gastroenterol 1996; 31(Suppl):24–28.

87. Honda S, Fujioka T, Tokieda M, Gotoh T, Nishizono A, Nasu M. Gastric ulcer, atrophic gastritis, and intestinal metaplasia caused by *Helicobacter pylori* infection in Mongolian gerbils. Scand J Gastroenterol 1998; 33:45–60.

88. Watanabe T, Tada M, Nagai H, Sasaki S, Nakao M. *Helicobacter pylori* infection induces gastric cancer in Mongolian gerbils. Gastroenterology 1998; 115:642–648.

89. Ikeno T, Ota H, Sugiyama A, et al. *Helicobacter pylori*-induced chronic active gastritis, intestinal metaplasia, and gastric ulcer in Mongolian gerbils. Am J Pathol 1999; 154:951–960.

90. Zhang QB, Dawodu JB, Husain A, Etolhi G, Gemmell CG, Russell RI. Association of antral mucosal levels of interleukin 8 and reactive oxygen radicals in patients infected with *Helicobacter pylori*. Clin Sci (Colch) 1997; 92:69–73.

91. Bagchi D, Bhattacharya G, Stohs SJ. Production of reactive oxygen species by gastric cells in association with *Helicobacter pylori*. Free Radical Res 1996; 24:439–450.

92. Zhang Q, Dawodu JB, Etolhi G, Husain A, Gemmell CG, Russell RI. Relationship between the mucosal production of reactive oxygen radicals and density of *Helicobacter pylori* in patients with duodenal ulcer. Eur J Gastroenterol Hepatol 1997; 9:261–265.

93. Davies GR, Banatvala N, Collins CE, et al. Relationship between infective load of *Helicobacter pylori* and reactive oxygen metabolite production in antral mucosa. Scand J Gastroenterol 1994; 29:419–24.

94. Cheng KC, Cahill DS, Kasai H, Nishimura S, Loeb LA. 8-Hydroxyguanine, an abundant form of oxidative DNA damage, causes G–T and A–C substitutions. J Biol Chem 1992; 267:166–172.

95. Hahm KB, Lee KJ, Choi SY, et al. Possibility of chemoprevention by the eradiation of *Helicobacter pylori:* oxidative DNA damage and apoptosis in *H. pylori* infection. Gastroenterology 1997; 92:1853–1857.

96. Baik SC, Youn HS, Chung MH, et al. Increased oxidative DNA damage in *Helicobacter pylori*-infected human gastric mucosa. Cancer Res 1996; 56:1279–1282.

97. Farinati F, Cardin R, Degan P, et al. Oxidative DNA damage accumulation in gastric carcinogenesis. Gut 1998; 42:351–356.

98. Harris G, Asbery L, Lawley PD, Denman AM, Hylton W. Defective repair of $O(6)$-methylguanine in autoimmune diseases. Lancet 1982; 2:952–956.

99. Badawi AF, Cooper DP, Mostafa MH, et al. O^6-alkylguanine-DNA alkyltransferase activity in schistosomiasis-associated human bladder cancer. Eur J Cancer 1994; 30A:1314–1319.

100. Rachmilewitz D, Karmeli F, Eliakim R, et al. Enhanced gastric nitric oxide synthase activity in duodenal ulcer patients. Gut 1994; 35:1394–1397.

101. Wilson KT, Ramanujam KS, Mobley HL, Musselman RF, James SP, Meltzer SJ. *Helicobacter pylori* stimulates inducible nitric oxide synthase expression and activity in a murine macrophage cell line. Gastroenterology 1996; 11:1524–1533.

102. Shapiro KB, Hotchkiss JH. Induction of nitric oxide synthesis in murine macrophages by *Helicobacter pylori*. Cancer Lett 1996; 102:49–56.

103. Tsuji S, Kawano S, Tsujii M, et al. *Helicobacter pylori* extract stimulates inflammatory nitric oxide production. Cancer Lett 1996; 108:195–200.

104. Konturek SJ, Konturek PC, Brzozowski T, Stachura J, Zembala M. Gastric mucosal damage and adaptive protection by ammonia and ammonium ion in rats. Digestion 1996; 57:433–445.

105. Mannick EE, Bravo LE, Zarama G, et al. Inducible nitric oxide synthase, nitrotyrosine, and apoptosis in *Helicobacter pylori* gastritis: effect of antibiotics and antioxidants. Cancer Res 1996; 56:3238–3243.

106. Wink DA, Laval J. The Fpg protein, a DNA repair enzyme, is inhibited by the biomediator nitric oxide in vitro and in vivo. Carcinogenesis 1994; 15:2125–2129.

107. Parsonnet J. *Helicobacter pylori* in the stomach—a paradox unmasked. N Engl J Med 1996; 335:278–280.

108. Walsh JH. Role of gastrin as a trophic hormone. Digestion 1990; 47 (Suppl 1):11–6; discussion 49–52.

109. Mulholland G, Ardill JE, Fillmore D, Chittajallu RS, Fullarton GM, McColl KE. *Helicobacter pylori* related hypergastrinaemia is the result of a selective increase in gastrin 17. Gut 1993; 34:757–761.

110. Ruiz B, Correa P, Fontham ET, Ramakrishnan T. Antral atrophy, *Helicobacter pylori* colonization, and gastric pH. Am J Clin Pathol 1996; 105:96–101.

111. Sonnenberg A. Temporal trends and geographical variations of peptic ulcer disease. Aliment Pharmacol Ther. 1995; 9 (Suppl 2):3–12.

112. Graham DY. *Helicobacter pylori* infection in the pathogenesis of duodenal ulcer and gastric cancer: a model. Gastroenterology 1997; 113:1983–1991.

113. el-Omar EM, Oien K, El-Nujumi A, et al. *Helicobacter pylori* infection and chronic gastric acid hyposecretion. Gastroenterology 1997; 113:15–24.

114. Pignatelli B, Malaveille C, Rogatko A, et al. Mutagens, *N*-nitroso compounds and their precursors in gastric juice from patients with and without precancerous lesions of the stomach. Eur J Cancer 1993; 29A:2031–2039.

115. Zhang ZW, Patchett SE, Perrett D, Katelaris PH, Domizio P, Farthing MJ. The relation between gastric vitamin C concentrations, mucosal histology, and CagA seropositivity in the human stomach. Gut 1998; 43:322–326.

116. Sobala GM, Schorah CJ, Sanderson M, et al. Ascorbic acid in the human stomach. Gastroenterology 1989; 97:357–363.

117. Feldman M. Gastric secretion in health and disease. In: Sleisenger MH, Fordtran JS (eds). Gastrointestinal Disease, 4th edit. Philadelphia: WB Saunders, 1989, pp. 713–734.

118. Parsonnet J, Kim P, Yang S, Orentreich N, Vogelman JH, Friedman GD. Gastrin and gastric adenoacarcinoma: a prospective evaluation. Gastroenterology 1996; 110:A574 (Abstr).

119. Wang TC, Dangler CA, Chen D, et al. Hypergastrinemia leads to atrophy and invasive gastric cancer in transgenic mice. Gastroenterology 1999; 116:G2314 (Abstr).

120. Sakaki N, Arakawa T, Katou H, et al. Relationship between progression of gastric mucosal atrophy and *Helicobacter pylori* infection: retrospective long-term endoscopic follow-up study. J Gastroenterol 1997; 32:19–23.

121. Logan RPH, Walker MM, Misiewicz JJ, Gummett PA, Karim QN, Baron JH. Changes in the intragastric distribution of *Helicobacter pylori* during treatment with omeprazole. Gut 1995; 36:12–16.

122. Kuipers EJ, Lundell L, Klinkenberg-Knol EC, et al. Atrophic gastritis and *Helicobacter pylori* infection in patients with reflux esophagitis treated with omeprazole or fundoplication. N Engl J Med 1996; 334:1018–1022.

123. Howson C, Hiyama T, Wynder E. The decline in gastric cancer: epidemiology of an unplanned triumph. Epidemiol Rev 1986; 8:1–27.

124. Correa P, Haenszel W, Cuello C, Tannenbaum S, Archer M. A model for gastric cancer epidemiology. Lancet 1975; 2:58–60.

125. Moller H, Nissen A, Mosbech J. Use of cimetidine and other peptic ulcer drugs in Denmark 1977–1990 with analysis of the risk of gastric cancer among cimetidine users. Gut 1992; 33:1166–1169.

126. Colin-Jones DG, Langman MJ, Lawson DH, Logan RF, Paterson KR, Vessey MP. Postmarketing surveillance of the safety of cimetidine: 10 year mortality report. Gut 1992; 33:1280–1284.

127. Lynch DAF, Mapstone NP, Clarke AMT, et al. Cell proliferation in *Helicobacter pylori* associated gastritis and the effect of eradication therapy. Gut 1995; 36:345–350.

128. Murakami K, Fujioka T, Kodama R, Kubota T, Tokieda M, Nasu M. *Helicobacter pylori* infection accelerates human gastric mucosal cell proliferation. J Gastroenterol 1997; 32:184–188.

129. Fan XG, Kelleher D, Fan XJ, Xia HX, Keeling PW. *Helicobacter pylori* increases proliferation of gastric epithelial cells. Gut 1996; 38:19–22.

130. Peek RM, Moss SF, Tham KT, et al. *Helicobacter pylori* cag A$^+$ strains and dissociation of gastric epithelial cell proliferation from apoptosis. J Natl Cancer Inst 1997; 89:863–868.

131. Yabuki N, Sasano H, Tobita M, et al. Analysis of cell damage and proliferation in *Helicobacter pylori*-infected human gastric mucosa from patients with gastric adenocarcinoma. Am J Pathol 1997; 151:821–829.

132. Abdel-Wahab M, Attallah AM, Elshal MF, et al. Cellular proliferation and ploidy of the gastric mucosa: the role of *Helicobacter pylori*. Hepatogastroenterology 1997; 44:880–885.

133. Fraser AG, Sim R, Sankey EA, Dhillon AP, Pounder RE. Effect of eradication of *Helicobacter pylori* on gastric epithelial cell proliferation. Aliment Pharmacol Ther 1994; 8:167–173.

134. Fiocca R, Luinetti O, Villani L, Chiaravalli AM, Capella C, Solcia E. Epithelial cytotoxicity, immune responses, and inflammatory components of *Helicobacter pylori* gastritis. Scand J Gastroenterol (Suppl) 1994; 205:11–21.

135. Dekigai H, Murakami M, Kita T. Mechanism of *Helicobacter pylori*-associated gastric mucosal injury. Dig Dis Sci 1995; 40:1332–1339.

136. Smoot DT. How does *Helicobacter pylori* cause mucosal damage? Direct mechanisms. Gastroenterology 1997; 113:S31–4.

137. Moss SF, Calam J, Agarwal B, Wang S, Holt PR. Induction of gastric epithelial apoptosis by *Helicobacter pylori*. Gut 1996; 38:498–501.

138. Jones NL, Shannon PT, Cutz E, Yeger H, Sherman PM. Increase in proliferation and apoptosis of gastric epithelial cells early in the natural history of *Helicobacter pylori* infection. Am J Pathol 1997; 151:1695–1703.

139. Chen G, Sordillo EM, Ramey WG, et al. Apoptosis in gastric epithelial cells in induced by Helicobacter pylori and accompanied by increased expression of BAK. Biochem Biophys Res Commun 1997; 239:626–632.

140. Houghton J, Korah RM, Condon MR, Kim KH. Apoptosis in *Helicobacter pylori*-associated gastric and duodenal ulcer disease is mediated via the Fas antigen pathway. Dig Dis Sci 1999; 44:465–478.

141. Rudi J, Kuck D, Strand S, et al. Involvement of the CD95 (APO-1/Fas) receptor and ligand system in *Helicobacter pylori*-induced gastric epithelial apoptosis. J Clin Invest 1998; 102:1506–1514.

142. Rokkas T, Ladas S, Liatsos C, et al. Relationship of *Helicobacter pylori* CagA status to gastric cell proliferation and apoptosis. Dig Dis Sci 1999; 44:487–493.

143. Wilson KT, Ramanujam KW, Shirin H, Delohery T, Moss SF. Prostaglandin E2 inhibits *Helicobacter pylori*-induced apoptosis. Gastroenterology 1999; 116:G2327 (Abstr).

144. Hannson L, Nyren O, Hsing AW, et al. Risk of stomach cancer in patients with gastric or duodenal ulcer disease. N Engl J Med 1996; 335:242–249.

145. Akopyanz N, Bukanov NO, Westblom TU, Berg DE. PCR-based RFLP analysis of DNA sequence diversity in the gastric pathogen *Helicobacter pylori*. Nucleic Acids Res 1992; 20:6221–6225.

146. Wang JT, Sheu JC, Lin JT, Wang TH, Wu MS. Direct DNA amplification and restriction pattern analysis of *Helicobacter pylori* in patients with duodenal ulcer and their families. J Infect Dis 1993; 168:1544–1548.

147. Enroth H, Nyren O, Engstrand L. One stomach—one strain: does *Helicobacter pylori* strain variation influence disease outcome? Dig Dis Sci 1999; 44:102–107.

148. Kuipers EJ, Perez-Perez GI, Meuwissen SG, Blaser MJ. *Helicobacter pylori* and atrophic gastritis: importance of the cagA status. J Natl Cancer Inst 1995; 87:1777–1780.

149. Perez-Perez GI, Bhat N, Gaensbauer J, et al. Country-specific constancy by age in cagA+ proportion of *Helicobacter pylori* infections. Int J Cancer 1997; 72:453–456.

150. Parsonnet J, Replogle M, Yang S, Hiatt R. Seroprevalence of CagA-positive strains among *Helicobacter pylori*-infected, healthy young adults. J Infect Dis 1997; 175:1240–1242.

151. Webb PM, Crabtree JE, Forman D. Gastric cancer, cytotoxin-associated gene A-positive *Helicobacter pylori,* and serum pepsinogens: an international study. The Eurogst Study Group. Gastroenterology 1999; 116:269–276.

152. Katoh T, Nagata N, Kuroda Y, et al. Glutathione *S*-transferase M1 (GSTM1) and T1 (GSTT1) genetic polymorphism and susceptibility to gastric and colorectal adenocarcinoma. Carcinogenesis 1996; 17:1855–1859.

153. Deakin M, Elder J, Hendrickse C, et al. Glutathione *S*-transferase GSTT1 genotypes and susceptibility to cancer: studies of interactions with GSTM1 in lung, oral, gastric and colorectal cancers. Carcinogenesis 1996; 17:881–884.

154. Ng EK, Sung JJ, Ling TK, et al. *Helicobacter pylori* and the null genotype of glutathione-*S*-transferase-mu in patients with gastric adenocarcinoma. Cancer 1998; 82:268–273.

155. el-Omar E, Oien K, E1-Nujumi A, et al. Prevalence of atrophy and hypochlorhydria is high in gastric cancer relatives and related to *H. pylori* status. Gastroenterology 1998; 114:3318 (Abstr)

156. Meining A, Hackelsberger A, Daenecke C, Stolte M, Bayerdorffer E, Ochsenkuhn T. Increased cell proliferation of the gastric mucosa in first-degree relatives of gastric carcinoma patients. Cancer 1998; 83:876–881.

157. Larrea M, Barrios Y, Jimenez A, Salifo E, Quintero E. Interaction between host HLA-DQB1 and *Helicobacter pylori* genotype predicts the development of peptic ulcer disease. Gastroenterology 1999; 116:G1009 (Abstr).

158. Spanish Group for *Helicobacter* Research. Host DBQ1 alleles and *Helicobacter pylori* genotype interact to predict the development of gastric cancer in the Spanish population. Gastroenterology 1999; 116:G2236 (Abstr).

159. Azuma T, Ito S, Sato F, et al. The role of the HLA-DQA1 gene in resistance to atrophic gastritis and gastric adenocarcinoma induced by *Helicobacter pylori* infection. Cancer 1998; 82:1013–1018.

160. Hallstone AE, Perez EA. Blood type and the risk of gastric disease. Science 1994; 264:1386–1388.

161. Boren T, Falk P, Roth KA, Larson G, Normark S. Attachment of *Helicobacter pylori* to human gastric epithelium mediated by blood group antigens. Science 1993; 262:1892–1895.

162. Sipponen P, Aarynen M, Kaariainen I, Kettunen P, Helske T, Seppala K. Chronic antral gastritis, Lewis(a+) phenotype, and male sex as factors in predicting coexisting duodenal ulcer. Scand J Gastroenterol 1989; 24:581–588.

163. Mentis A, Blackwell CC, Weir DM, Spiliadis C, Dailianas A, Skandalis N. ABO blood group, secretor status and detection of *Helicobacter pylori* among patients with gastric or duodenal ulcers. Epidemiol Infect 1991; 106:221–229.

164. Yamashita Y, Chung YS, Sawada T, et al. F1 alpha: a novel mucin antigen associated with gastric carcinogenesis. Oncology 1998; 55:70–76.

165. Payne RJ, Nowak MA, Blumberg BS. Analysis of a cellular model to account for the natural history of infection by the hepatitis B virus and its role in the development of primary hepatocellular carcinoma. J Theor Biol 1992; 159:215–240.

166. Stewenius J, Adnerhill I, Anderson H, et al. Incidence of colorectal cancer and all cause mortality in non-selected patients with ulcerative colitis and indeterminate colitis in Malmo, Sweden. Int J Colorectal Dis 1995; 10:117–122.

167. Wening JV, Stein M, Langendorff U, Delling G. Chronic osteomyelitis and cancer of the fistula. Langenbecks Arch Chir 1989; 374:55–59.

168. Fox JG, Taylor NS, Dangler CA. Colonization and persistence of *H. pylori* in ICR mice is dependent of age of infection. Gastroenterology 1999; 116:G3117 (Abstr).

169. Mitchell HM, Bohane TD, Tobias V, et al. *Helicobacter pylori* infection in children: potential clues to pathogenesis. J Pediatr Gastroenterol Nutr 1993; 16:120–125.

170. Queiroz DM, Rocha GA, Mendes EN, et al. Differences in distribution and severity of *Helicobacter pylori* gastritis in children and adults with duodenal ulcer disease. J Pediatr Gastroenterol Nutr 1991; 12:178–181.

171. Tredaniel J, Boffetta P, Buiatti E, Saracci R, Hirsch A. Tobacco smoking and gastric cancer: review and meta-analysis. Int J Cancer 1997; 72:565–573.

172. Kurata JH, Nogawa AN. Meta-analysis of risk factors for peptic ulcer. J Clin Gastroenterol 1997; 24:2–17.

173. Wang HY, Ma L, Li Y, Cho CH. Cigarette smoking increases apoptosis in gastric mucosa through reactive oxygen species-mediated and p53-independent pathwya. Gastroenterology 1999; 116:G1526 (Abstr).

174. Moritani S, Kushima R, Sugihara H, Hattori T. Phenotypic characteristics of Epstein–Barr-virus-associated gastric carcinomas. J Cancer Res Clin Oncol 1996; 122:750–756.

175. Osato T, Imai S. Epstein–Barr virus and gastric carcinoma. Semin Cancer Biol 1996; 7:175–182.

176. Roosendall R, Kuipers EJ, Buitenwerf J, et al. *Helicobacter pylori* and the birth cohort effect: evidence of a continuous decrease of infection rates in childhood Am J Gastroenterol 1997; 92:1480–1482.

177. Replogle ML, Kasumi W, Ishikawa KB, et al. Increased risk of *Helicobacter pylori* associated with birth in wartime Japan. Int J Epidemiol 1996; 25:210–214.

178. Gomez-Duarte OG, Lucas B, Yan ZX, Panthel K, Haas R, Meyer TF. Protection of mice against gastric colonization by *Helicobacter pylori* by single oral dose immunization with attenuated *Salmonella typhimurium* producing urease subunits A and B. Vaccine 1998; 16:460–471.

179. Corthesy-Theulaz IE, Hopkins S, Bachmann D, et al. Mice are protected from *Helicobacter pylori* infection by nasal immunization with attenuated *Salmonella typhimurium* phoPc expressing urease A and B subunits. Infect Immun 1998; 66:581–586.

180. Radcliff FJ, Hazell SL, Kolesnikow T, Doidge C, Lee A. Catalase, a novel antigen for *Helicobacter pylori* vaccination. Infect Immun 1997; 65:4668–4674.

181. Czinn SJ. What is the role for vaccination in *Helicobacter pylori?* Gastroenterology 1997; 113:S149–153.

182. Lee CK, Soike K, Hill J, et al. Immunization with recombinant *Helicobacter pylori* urease decreases colonization levels following experimental infection of rhesus monkeys. Vaccine 1999; 17:1493–1505.

183. Saldinger PF, Porta N, Launois P, et al. Immunization of BALB/c mice with Helicobacter urease B induces a T helper 2 response absent in Helicobacter infection. Gastroenterology 1998; 115:891–897.

184. Rijpkema SG. Prospects for therapeutic Helicobacter vaccines (editorial). J Med Microbiol 1999; 48:1–3.

185. Michetti P, Kreiss C, Kotloff KL, et al. Oral immunization with urease and Escherichia coli heat-labile enterotoxin is safe and immunogenic in Helicobacter pylori-infected adults. Gastroenterology 1999; 116:804–812.

186. NIH Consensus Conference. *Helicobacter pylori* in peptic ulcer disease. NIH Consensus Development Panel on Helicobacter pylori in Peptic Ulcer Disease. JAMA 1994 Jul 6; 272:65–69.

187. Malfertheiner P, Megraud F, O'Morain C, et al. Current European concepts in the management of *Helicobacter pylori* infection—the Maastricht Consensus Report. The European Helicobacter Pylori Study Group (EHPSG). Eur J Gastroenterol Hepatol 1997; 9:1–2.

188. Parsonnet J, Harris R, Hack HM, Owens DK. Modelling cost effectiveness of *Helicobacter pylori* screening to prevent gastric cancer: a mandate for clinical trials. Lancet 1996; 348:150–154.

189. Fendrick AM, Chernew ME, Hirth RA, Bloom BS, Bandekar RR, Scheiman JM. Clinical and economic effects of population-based *Helicobacter pylori* screening to prevent gastric cancer. Arch Intern Med 1999; 159:142–148.

190. Forman D. Ongoing studies of *H. pylori* treatment to prevent gastric cancer. Aliment Pharmacol Ther 1998; 12 (Suppl 1):3–7.

191. Ciok J, Dzieniszewski J, Lucer C. *Helicobacter pylori* eradication and antral intestinal metaplasia—two years follow-up study. J Physiol Pharmacol 1997; 48 (Suppl 4):115–122.

192. Maconi G, Lazzaroni M, Sangaletti O, Bargiggia S, Vago L, Porro GB. Effect of *Helicobacter pylori* eradication on gastric histology, serum gastrin and pepsinogen I levels, and gastric emptying in patients with gastric ulcer. Am J Gastroenterol 1997; 92:1844–1848.

193. Forbes GM, Warren JR, Glaser ME, Cullen DJ, Marshall BJ, Collins BJ. Long-term follow-up of gastric histology after *Helicobacter pylori* eradication. J Gastroenterol Hepatol 1996; 11:670–673.

194. van der Hulst RW, van der Ende A, Dekker FW, et al. Effect of *Helicobacter pylori* eradication on gastritis in relation to cagA: a prospective 1-year follow-up study. Gastroenterology 1997; 113:25–30.

195. Uemura N, Mukai T, Okamoto S, et al. Effect of *Helicobacter pylori* eradication on sub194. sequent development of cancer after endoscopic resection of early gastric cancer. Cancer Epidemiol Biomarkers Prev 1997; 6:639–642.

196. Chow W, Blaser MJ, Blot WJ, et al. An inverse relation between *cagA*+ strains of *Helicobacter pylori* infection and risk of esophageal and gastric cardia adenocarcinoma. Cancer Res 1998; 58:588–590.

197. el-Serag HB, Sonnenberg A. Opposing time trends of peptic ulcer and reflux disease. Gut 1998; 43:327–333.

198. Blot WJ, Li JY, Taylor PR, et al. Nutrition intervention trials in Linxian, China: supplementation with specific vitamin/mineral combinations, cancer incidence, and disease-specific mortality in the general poulation. J Natl Cancer Inst 1993; 85:1483–1492.

199. Garay J, Bravo JC, Ruiz BA, et al. Change in gastric atrophy after long-term intervention with antioxidants and antimicrobials. Gastroenterology 1999; 116:G0729 (Abstr).

22

Gastric Mucosa-Associated Lymphoid Tissue Lymphoma

Andrew C. Wotherspoon

INTRODUCTION

Although lymphomas are normally associated with a presentation primarily within lymph nodes, up to 40% of lymphomas arise at sites outside those considered to be the major lymphoid organs *(1–3)*. The majority of these extranodal lymphomas arise within the gastrointestinal tract *(3)*, which contains a very high quantity of lymphoid tissue in the normal individual but is not considered to be a primary lymphoid organ. Of lymphomas that arise in the gastrointestinal tract, the most common site for these tumors to develop is within the stomach.

The definition of a primary extranodal lymphoma and its distinction from secondary involvement of an extranodal site by a primary node-based lymphoma is problematic. Originally the definition restricted extranodal lymphomas to those that were confined to a single extranodal site and contiguous lymph node groups without dissemination to more distant areas (including bone marrow) *(4)*. This definition is obviously very restrictive and by definition ensured that all primary extranodal lymphomas were of low stage and therefore associated with a favorable prognosis. With better knowledge of the biology of extranodal lymphomas and modern staging procedures, the rigidity of this definition of these tumours has been relaxed and most investigators would now consider a lymphoma to by extranodal if the main bulk of the tumour is found at an extranodal site.

The relaxation of the definition of these tumors has been associated with an appreciation that lymphomas with characteristic clinicopathologic features are frequently found as extranodal lymphomas and are less frequently encountered within lymph nodes. In 1983 Isaacson and Wright described a group of lymphomas that arose at extranodal sites and that had clinical and pathologic features that were distinct from those commonly encountered in lymph nodes *(5)*. The similarity of the organization and phenotype of these lymphomas to the lymphoid tissue that is encountered at extranodal sites, predominantly within the mucosa of the intestinal tract and particularly in the Peyer's patches of the terminal ileum, termed mucosa-associated lymphoid tissue (MALT), has led to these tumors being designated MALT lymphomas *(5,6)*. Subsequently lymphomas of this type have been described at many extranodal sites.

From: *Infectious Causes of Cancer: Targets for Intervention*
Edited by: J. J. Goedert © Humana Press Inc., Totowa, NJ

As with extranodal lymphomas in general, MALT lymphomas are most commonly encountered in the stomach. For this reason and due to the possibility of close exami- nation of the organ *in situ* by endoscopy, gastric MALT lymphomas have been widely studied. These lymphomas thus form the prototype for the group of MALT lymphomas as a whole.

MUCOSA-ASSOCIATED LYMPHOID TISSUE

In the normal individual MALT is found constitutively to be almost entirely con- fined to the intestinal tract, with the highest concentration within the terminal ileum in the form of Peyer's patches. These are areas of organized lymphoid tissue that differ from lymph nodes in that they are unencapsulated and do not possess afferent lymphat- ics. Peyer's patches consist of a central lymphoid follicle that is similar to that seen in lymph nodes. The follicle is egg shaped and contains a reactive germinal center with the light zone at the apex nearest the luminal surface. A mantle zone composed of small lymphoid cells surrounds the germinal center. The mantle zone is thin at the base and thickest at the point nearest the luminal epithelium. Outside the mantle zone is a further zone of B cells in which the cells are slightly larger and with more abundant pale cytoplasm than mantle zone B cells. This is the marginal zone, which is not nor- mally encountered in lymph nodes (with the exception of mesenteric nodes) but is a normal constituent of the splenic white pulp. The broadest aspect of the marginal zone is found in the area of greatest potential antigenic challenge—the lumen; and cells from this zone extend into the overlying dome epithelium to form a lymphoepithelium. The majority of the cells that constitute the marginal zone B-cell population are mem- ory B cells. Within the dome epithelium there are specialized epithelial cells—the M cells—which are thought to facilitate the transport and presentation of luminal derived antigen to the underlying lymphoid tissue *(7)*. Antigens are transported across the epithelium by the M cells and are presented to the Peyer's patches, where antigen-spe- cific B cells are stimulated to undergo switching from immunoglobulin M (IgM) to IgG production. Following stimulation these B cells leave the mucosa, and pass through the mesenteric nodes and into the thoracic duct. These cells home back to the mucosa, where they are present as plasma cells in the lamina propria around the lymphoid folli- cles and in the subepithelial region *(8–10)*. The T-cell compartment present around the sides and the base of the lymphoid follicle and the intraepithelial T-cell compartment make up the other constituents of MALT.

The vast majority of the histologically low grade (small cell) lymphomas found at extranodal sites are of MALT type. The great paradox that surrounds the development of lymphomas of MALT is that these lymphomas invariably arise in extranodal sites that are normally devoid of organized lymphoid tissue. Indeed the site at which MALT is found constitutively in normal humans—the terminal ileum—is an uncommon site for the development of MALT lymphomas. Rather, this site is more often associated with lymphomas of nodal type (mantle cell lymphoma, follicle center cell lymphoma), diffuse large B cell lymphoma, or Burkitt's lymphoma. The first step toward the devel- opment of a primary extranodal lymphoma requires the acquisition of the organized lymphoid tissue from within which the lymphoma can develop. Unsurprisingly the lymphoma that develops has a significant association with the condition responsible for the acquisition of the lymphoid tissue, such as close association of thyroid MALT lymphoma with Hashimoto's thyroiditis *(11)* and of salivary gland lymphoma with myoepithelial sialadenitis (MESA) and Sjögren's disease *(12)*. In the stomach, acquisition of MALT is associated with a few clinical situations, of which the most frequent is colonization of the gastric mucosa by *Helicobacter pylori (13–17)*. The relatively high frequency of gastric MALT lymphoma and the ability to make the diagnosis before definitive surgery has allowed the collection of fresh tissue for in vitro studies of the functional properties of the lymphoma cells. This has led to advances in our understanding of gastric MALT lymphoma (and MALT lymphomas in general) leading to changes in the clinical management of these tumours.

ACQUISITION OF GASTRIC MALT

The lamina propria of the gastric mucosa in the normal individual contains scattered B cells, plasma cells, and a small number of T cells. Intraepithelial T cells are also present but are less numerous than is seen in the small intestine. There is no organized lymphoid tissue in the form of MALT within the normal gastric mucosa. Immunohistochemical studies suggest that the normal gastric microenvironment is quiescent as there is no expression of antigens associated with inflammation such as epithelial HLA class II or CD25 (interleukin-2 receptor) on lamina propria macrophages or T lymphocytes *(18)*.

As the normal stomach is a hostile environment for infective organisms, and the lamina propria is protected from luminal derived antigens by a thick layer of viscous mucus and an intact epithelium that is generally nonabsorptive and lacks M cells, there is little stimulation to lymphoid tissue. However, there are circumstances in which these barriers can be overcome, resulting in the stimulation of lymphoid tissue and the acquisition of MALT. This is most commonly seen in association with colonization of the stomach by *H. pylori,* an organism that is ideally adapted to living within the gastric environment associated with its motility, ability to penetrate the mucus layer and adhere to the gastric epithelium, and to secrete enzymes (in particular urease) that are active at low pH and that increase the local pH within the organism's microenvironment.

H. pylori infection is associated with a spectrum of abnormalities in the stomach. All patients infected by *H. pylori* have an abnormal gastric mucosa. Active chronic gastritis with neutrophil penetration predominantly of the superficial epithelium is maximal around the surface and neck regions, where the organism shows the highest concentration. In many instances, the neutrophils and *H. pylori* organisms are spatially related. Infiltration of the epithelium by acute inflammatory cells is likely to cause damage to the integrity of the epithelial barrier and to result in the potential leak of antigen into the lamina propria and stimulation of lymphoid tissue. This has been confirmed by studying gastric permeability to sucrose, which is higher in patients with *H. pylori* infection *(19)* and which normalizes after eradication of the organism *(20)*. Increased permeability of the epithelium together with the presence of *H. pylori*-derived antigens may be responsible for the subsequent acquisition of MALT within the gastric mucosa.

Several studies have shown that infection with *H. pylori* is associated with the accumulation of MALT within the stomach. Although lymphoid follicles are not found in endoscopic biopsies from normal individuals *(13,14,16)*, they can be found in 27–100% of patients infected with *H. pylori* (13–16). In the most comprehensive study, Genta et al. *(16)* demonstrated that lymphoid follicles can be detected in all patients with *H. pylori* infection if the biopsies are sufficiently large and numerous. Wotherspoon et al. *(15)* showed that the lymphoid tissue that accumulates in *H. pylori* infection has features of MALT, with the formation of a lymphoepithelium by the marginal zone B cells around the follicles that infiltrated the foveolar epithelium of the gastric glands.

Although *H. pylori* is probably the most common association with acquired gastric MALT, it is not the only stimulus to accumulation of lymphoid tissue in the gastric mucosa. The related organism *Helicobacter heilmannii* is also associated with acquired gastric MALT *(21)*, and MALT-type lymphoid tissue has been described in the stomachs of patients with celiac disease.

MUCOSA-ASSOCIATED LYMPHOID TISSUE LYMPHOMA

Clinical features

Gastric MALT lymphomas affect males and females equally. The age range at which these lymphomas occur is wide, but the majority of patients are over the age of 50 yr. The majority of patients present with rather nonspecific symptoms including dyspepsia, nausea, and vomiting, while weight loss or the presence of an epigastric mass is rare. The symptoms may have been present for many years, and in some patients multiple endoscopies may have been performed before the diagnosis of lymphoma is reached. In these cases retrospective review of the gastric biopsy material may reveal changes consistent with low-grade MALT lymphoma from the start. The endoscopic picture is variable. In some patients the gastric mucosa may appear normal or show very minor changes such as hyperaemia, while others may show enlarged gastric folds, gastritis, superficial erosions, or ulceration. Mass lesions are relatively rare. Although any region of the stomach may be involved, the majority of gastric MALT lymphomas occur in the distal stomach within the antrum or distal body regions. Gastric MALT lymphoma, in common with MALT lymphomas arising at other sites, is an indolent tumor that disseminates in a minority of cases. Bone marrow involvement can be detected in up to 10% of cases, but spread to peripheral lymph nodes away from the immediate vicinity of the tumor is rare. When spread to other sites does occur, it frequently is to other extranodal organs.

Histology, Immunophenotype, and Genotype

The organization, cellular morphology and immunophenotype of MALT lymphomas mimic that of Peyer's patches and are constant irrespective of the location at which the lymphomas arise *(22)*. Neoplastic cells infiltrate around preexisting lymphoid follicles initially with a marginal zone arrangement (outside a preserved mantle zone) but eventually spreading to become a more diffuse infiltrate within the lamina propria. The morphology of the neoplastic cells can be quite variable not only among cases of MALT lymphoma but also within an individual case. The classical appearance of the MALT lymphoma cell is of a small to intermediate sized cell with a pale cytoplasm and irregular nucleus. The resemblance of these to the small centrocyte cell of the follicle center led this cell to be called the "centrocyte-like (CCL) cell" and is considered the characteristic cell of these lymphomas. However, the cellular morphology may vary, ranging from a cell more reminiscent of a mature small lymphocyte with a rounder nucleus and scantier cytoplasm to a monocytoid B cell with abundant pale/clear cytoplasm, round nucleus, and well-demarcated cytoplasmic borders. There is invariably some plasma cell differentiation that in some cases may be very striking, and Dutcher bodies may be seen in a proportion of cases. Transformed or blast cells, which are larger with vesicular nuclei and prominent nucleoli, are seen scattered within the infiltrate. The neoplastic CCL cells have a specific interaction with the epithelium in a mimic of the interaction between marginal zone B cells and the dome epithelium above a Peyer's patch. In the lymphoma, however, the infiltration of the CCL cells into the glandular epithelium results in damage to the epithelial calls and eventual destruction of the gland. The structures resulting from this interaction are called lymphoepithelial lesions (LELs) and are an invariable finding in all MALT lymphomas, although LELs are not absolutely specific to this lymphoma type. High-grade transformation of a low-grade MALT lymphoma can occur. Such a transformation can be confidently confirmed only by the identification of a preexisting low-grade MALT lymphoma or of a concurrent low-grade component in a high-grade lesion.

Lymphoid follicles are important structures in low-grade MALT lymphomas *(23)*. Reactive follicles are identified frequently, but on occasion the presence of lymphoid follicles can be inferred only by the identification of residual disrupted follicular dendritic cell networks in an otherwise diffuse appearing infiltrate of CCL cells. The lymphoid follicles play an essential role in the development and growth of MALT lymphoma. In all cases there is some interaction between the lymphoma and the lymphoid follicles. In many cases this takes the form of the CCL cells overrunning the follicles giving a vaguely nodular appearance to the infiltrate, but in some cases specific colonization of the lymphoid germinal center by the neoplastic CCL cells can be identified. In these cases the follicle centers are populated by cells that show light chain restriction of the same type as seen in the diffuse infiltrate, although they are separated from the surrounding infiltrate by an intact mantle zone. The intrafollicular component may appear more activated with large cell size, larger nuclei, and higher proliferation. They also may loose their bcl-2 antigen expression. Plasma cell differentiation may be seen in the intrafollicular component.

Immunophenotypically the CCL cells express pan-B cell markers but do not express CD5, CD10, or CD23. They are usually bcl-2 protein positive and many cases express CD43. They express surface and to a lesser extent cytoplasmic immunoglobulin (usually IgM or IgA, rarely IgG) and show immunoglobulin light chain restriction.

Genotypically all cases show clonal rearrangement of the immunoglobulin genes *(24)*. There is some controversy over the characteristic genetic abnormality of this lymphoma. The t(11;18) may be seen as a sole abnormality in some cases of low-grade MALT lymphoma but appears rare in high-grade tumors *(25,26)*. Trisomy 3 has been seen in up to 60% of cases in series reported by some authors using both conventional metaphase and interphase cytogenetic techniques *(27,28)*. The translocation t(1;14) also has been described in a small proportion of cases *(29)* associated with an increased cell survival in in vitro culture systems. The breakpoint in t(1;14) recently has been cloned revealing a novel gene, *bcl-10,* on chromosome 1 that may substantially affect the behavior of these lymphomas *(30)*.

The cell of origin of MALT lymphoma is thought to be the marginal zone B cell within the acquired MALT tissue. This is supported by the organization of the lymphoma—initially occupying the marginal zone—the cellular morphology, and the close immunophenotypic relationship between marginal zone B cells and the CCL cells of MALT lymphoma.

GASTRIC MALT LYMPHOMA AND *H. PYLORI*

The recognition that infection with *H. pylori* is invariably associated with acquisition of MALT-type lymphoid tissue in the stomach and the knowledge that this lymphoid tissue is most frequently acquired as a result of *H. pylori* infection suggests that there should be a close association between the organism and the lymphoma that develops within that acquired lymphoid tissue. Studies of low-grade MALT lymphoma support this. Initial studies suggested that *H. pylori* could be identified in 92–98% of cases of low-grade MALT lymphoma *(15,31)*, but some subsequent studies have suggested an association in the region of 70–77% *(32,33)*. In Japan the association is of similar proportion (72%) to that seen Western cases *(34)*, although in small series in the United Kingdom and Hong Kong only 62% of cases were associated with *H. pylori* infection *(35,36)*. The presence of *H. pylori* appears to be less with high-grade lymphomas. In high-grade cases that also have a low grade component, *H. pylori* is seen in 52–71% *(32,33)*. In contrast, the organism is detected in only 25–38% of cases with a pure high-grade lesion, some of which may be unrelated to MALT *(32,35)*. Gisbertz et al. *(32)* have studied non-*H. pylori* organisms in MALT lymphoma and have discovered that these organisms can be seen in up to 35% of low-grade MALT lymphomas in association with *H. pylori* and in a further 17% of cases without concomitant *H. pylori* infection. They reported only a single case in which low-grade lymphoma was seen in the absence of an infective organism. The presence of non-*H. pylori* organisms was found more frequently in high-grade lesions. When *H. pylori* infection has been correlated with the stage of the lymphoma it has been shown that the organism is present in 90% of cases limited to the mucosa and superficial submucosa, falling to 76% when the deep submucosa is involved and to only 48% when the lymphoma extends beyond the submucosa *(34)*.

Parsonnet et al. *(37)* have performed an elegant retrospective serum-based study, confirming that infection with *H. pylori* predated the development of the lymphoma and was associated with a odds ratio for the development of lymphoma of 6.3. Furthermore Nakamura et al. *(38)*, in a retrospective analysis of two subject groups, demonstrated that B-cell monoclonality was present in the gastric biopsies of 79% of patients who subsequently went on to develop overt lymphoma compared to 24% of patients in whom lymphoma did not develop in the follow-up period. Zucca et al. *(39)* have had the opportunity to study two patients in whom a series of biopsies prior to the diagnosis of low-grade MALT lymphoma showed only chronic *H. pylori*-associated gastritis. In these patients small clonal populations could be detected in the apparently reactive lymphoid infiltrates using a polymerase chain reaction (PCR) technique to look for immunoglobulin gene rearrangements with patient specific primers.

The accumulated evidence would therefore suggest that the majority of low-grade MALT lymphomas are associated with *H. pylori* infection and that a neoplastic clone may develop within the acquired lymphoid tissue associated with the infection. This abnormal population of B cells may expand gradually over a number of years before overt lymphoma develops. The close association between lymphoma and organism diminishes with increasing stage and grade of the lymphoma.

There is controversy surrounding the role of the organism's own genetic features and the development of lymphoma. *H. pylori* shows considerable genetic diversity but all stains appear to be equally associated with the acquisition of MALT tissue. There are conflicting results in studies of *H. pylori cagA* genotypes with MALT lymphoma. Some groups have not detected an association between *cagA*-positive strains and development of low grade lymphoma *(40,41)*, while others have found *cagA*-positive strains in up to 95% of cases *(42)*. Peng et al. *(41)* have found that although *cagA*-positive strains are not associated with low-grade lymphomas they are more frequently associated with high-grade tumors.

CELLULAR BASIS FOR THE ASSOCIATION BETWEEN LOW-GRADE GASTRIC MALT LYMPHOMA AND *H. PYLORI*

There are several features that suggest that there is a residual immunologic drive to low-grade MALT lymphomas. This includes the presence of plasma cell differentiation, particularly in the subepithelial zone and the presence of scattered blastic cells within the infiltrate. Migration into the follicle center is a characteristic feature of normal marginal zone B cells under immunologic/antigen stimulus *(43,44)*, and the follicular colonization seen in low-grade MALT lymphomas appears to be a mimic of this. As MALT lymphoma is a lymphoma derived from marginal zone B cells, this morphologic feature strongly suggests an antigenic stimulus associated with these lymphomas. At the molecular level this is supported by the demonstration of ongoing somatic mutations that occur over a period of time after neoplastic transformation has occurred, suggesting that the clonal expansion of the lymphoma has been driven by an antigen *(45–47)*. Further evidence comes from a study of the third complementary determining region of the immunoglobulin heavy chain gene in these lymphomas, which showed a pattern of change associated with the generation of antibody diversity and increased antigen-binding affinity *(48)*.

When unseparated cells isolated from low-grade MALT lymphomas were incubated in vitro with heat-treated whole cell preparations of *H. pylori,* the tumor cells proliferated whereas those cultured without *H. pylori* or with an unrelated mitogenic stimulus rapidly died *(49)*. The proliferative response to the *H. pylori* was strain specific, with each case responding to a single, distinct *H. pylori* strain *(49)*. When T cells were removed from this culture system no proliferative response to coculturing with *H. pylori* was not seen, demonstrating a clear T-cell dependence to this proliferative response. The proliferative response could not be replicated if supernatants from other cultures containing unseparated cell populations were added, implying that the tumor cells require contact dependant T-cell help for their proliferative drive *(50)*.

The specificity of the T cells from the low-grade MALT lymphoma and from the spleen of a single patient has also been studied. In this case the T cells derived from the tumor bulk proliferated in response to exposure to *H. pylori* while the splenic T cells did not *(50)*. This T-cell response was to the same strain to which the unseparated tumor cell suspensions proliferated. Tumor cells cultured in the absence of the tumor infiltrating T cells using a CD40 system failed to respond to the *H. pylori (50)*. This suggests that the proliferative drive is associated with contact-dependent help specifically from tumor infiltrating T cells that are themselves responding to the presence of *H. pylori*.

Studies of immunoglobulin expression by the lymphoma cells have shown that they recognized auto-antigens (51,52). Although some crossreactivity between auto-antigens and *H. pylori*-associated antigens have been described (53), there is no evidence for crossreactivity between those recognized by the lymphoma-derived immunoglobulin and *H. pylori*.

REGRESSION OF GASTRIC MUCOSA ASSOCIATED LYMPHOID TISSUE LYMPHOMA FOLLOWING ERADICATION OF *H. PYLORI*

Given the close relationship between *H. pylori* and gastric MALT lymphoma and the *in vitro* evidence that the lymphoma cells proliferate in response to the presence of the organism, Wotherspoon and co-workers (54) enrolled six patients with low-grade gastric MALT lymphoma into a trial in which the patients received a standard anti-*H. pylori* therapy. In five of these six patients, the lymphoma regressed to undetectable levels. Subsequent larger studies confirmed these findings, with a complete regression rate of 67–84% (55,56). In the study of Thiede et al. (55) the patients who showed no change in their tumors underwent surgical resection, and these patients were shown to have high-grade lymphoma. In general, high-grade lymphomas do not respond to simple *H. pylori* eradication, although low-grade areas may regress in cases that have both high- and low-grade components (57). The time taken to achieve remission may be highly variable. Some patients respond very quickly with regression of the tumor to undetectable levels within 4–6 wk. In other patients remission may only be achieved after 12–18 mo. In general the more superficial the tumor the higher the chances of inducing remission by *H. pylori* eradication alone. Ninety percent or more of lymphomas confined to the mucosa and submusosa respond, whereas the response rate falls with involvement of the deeper submucosa, muscularis propria, and serosa.

The stability of the regressions induced by the eradication of *H. pylori* is still under investigation. Of the six patients originally reported by Wotherspoon et al., three patients have remained in complete remission for 6 yr; one patient who took 1 yr to obtain complete remission has maintained this for 5 yr (54). Two patients relapsed histologically during the follow-up period but returned to undetectable tumor without further therapy and continue in this state 6 yr after initial diagnosis (A.C. Wotherspoon and P.G. Isaacson, *unpublished data*). In a separate study Neubauer et al. found four local relapses in 40 patients achieving complete remission during a mean follow-up period of 24 mo (58).

SUMMARY

The normal stomach is devoid of organized lymphoid tissue. Organized gastric lymphoid tissue with morphologic features characteristic of organised extranodal lymphoid tissue—termed mucosa associated lymphoid tissue (MALT)—is acquired most commonly but not exclusively in association with infection by *H. pylori*. It is from within this lymphoid tissue that the vast majority of primary gastric lymphomas develop. These lymphomas, termed gastric MALT lymphomas, have very characteristic clinicopathologic features that are distinct from those of the more common node based B-cell lymphomas. Given the close association between acquired gastric MALT and *H. pylori*, it is unsurprising to find that most low-grade gastric MALT lymphomas are associated with infection by this organism. In vitro studies of *H. pylori*-associated cases of low-grade gastric MALT lymphomas have demonstrated that the lymphoma cells proliferate in response to the presence of the organism in an immunocompetent mechanism associated with contact-dependent help from tumor infiltrating T cells. It would be assumed that a similar mechanism would be seen for those lymphomas associated with other gastric infections. Clinical trials have shown that simple eradication of the organism results in complete regression of the lymphoma in the majority of cases although the chance of inducing regression becomes less with increasing depth of invasion of the tumor. Although long-term studies are still needed to assess the stability of these regressions, early indication are that these may be stable for many years. At present, eradication of *H. pylori* should form part of any treatment plan for patients with gastric lymphoma. In low-grade cases, *H. pylori* eradication can be used as a single treatment modality at least in the first instance, particularly if the tumor is superficial. In view of the lack of information about long-term disease-free survival, these patients need continued and regular follow-up to monitor the remission.

REFERENCES

1. Freeman C, Berg JW, Cutler SJ. Occurrence and prognosis of extranodal lymphomas. Cancer 1972; 29:252–260.
2. Otter R, Beiger R, Kluin PM, Hermans J, Willemze R. Primary gastrointestinal non-Hodgkin's lymphoma in a population-based registry. Br J Cancer 1989; 60:745–750.
3. Siebert JD, Mulvaney DA, Potter KL, Fishkin PAS, Geoffroy FJ. Relative frequencies and sites of presentation of lymphoid neoplasms in a community hospital according to the revised European-American classification. Am J Clin Pathol 1999; 111:379–386.
4. Dawson IMP, Cornes JS, Morson BC. Primary malignant lymphoid tumours of the intestinal tract. Report of 37 cases with a study of factors influencing prognosis. Br J Surg 1961; 49:80–89.
5. Isaacson P, Wright DH. Malignant lymphoma of mucosa-associated lymphoid tissue. A distinctive type of B-cell lymphoma. Cancer 1983; 52:1410–1416.
6. Isaacson PG, Wright DH. Extranodal lymphomas arising from mucosa-associated lymphoid tissue. Cancer 1984; 53:2515–2525.
7. Owen RL, Jones AL. Epithelial cell specialization within human Peyer's patches: an ultrastructural study of intestinal lymphoid follicles. Gastroenterology 1974; 66:189–203.
8. Gowens JL, Knight EJ. The route of recirculation of lymphocytes in the rat. Proc R Soc Lond B Biol Sci 1964; 159:257–282.
9. Hall JG, Smith ME. Homing of lymph-borne immunoblasts to the gut. Nature 1970; 226:262–263.
10. Husband AJ. Kinetics of extravasation and redistribution of IgA specific antibody containing cells in the intestine. J Immunol 1982; 128:1355–1359.
11. Hyjek E, Isaacson PG. Primary B cell lymphoma of the thyroid and its relationship to Hashimoto's thyroiditis. Hum Pathol 1988; 19:1315–1326.
12. Hyjek E, Smith WJ, Isaacson PG. Primary B-cell lymphoma of salivary glands and its relationship to myoepithelial sialadenitis. Hum Pathol 1988; 19:766–776.
13. Wyatt JI, Rathbone BJ. Immune response of the gastric mucosa to *Campylobacter pylori*. Scand J Gastroenterol 1988; 23(Suppl 142):44–49.
14. Stolte M, Eidt S. Lymphoid follicles in antral mucosa: immune response to *Campylobacter pylori?* J Clin Pathol 1989; 42:1269–1271.
15. Wotherspoon AC, Ortiz-Hidalgo C, Falzon MR, Isaacson PG. *Helicobacter pylori*-associated gastritis and primary B-cell gastric lymphoma. Lancet 1991; 338:1175–1176.
16. Genta RM, Hamner W, Graham DY. Gastric lymphoid follicles in *Helicobacter pylori* infection: frequency, distribution and response to triple therapy. Hum Pathol 1993; 24:577–583.

17. Zaitoun AM. The prevalence of lymphoid follicles in *Helicobacter pylori* associated gastritis in patients with ulcers and non-ulcer dyspepsia. J Clin Pathol 1995; 48:325–329.

18. Valnes K, Huitfeldt HS, Brandtzaeg P. Relation between T cell number and epithelial HLA class II expression quantified by image analysis in normal and inflamed human gastric mucosa. Gut 1990; 31:647–652.

19. Rabassa A, Goodgame R, Sutton F, Ou C, Rognerud C, Graham D. Effects of aspirin and H. pylori in the gastroduodenal mucosa permeability to sucrose. Gut 1996; 39:159–163.

20. Goodgame RW, Malaty HM, El-Zimaity HMT, Graham DY. Decrease in gastric permeability to sucrose following cure of *Helicobacter pylori* infection. Helicobacter 1997; 2:44–47.

21. Stolte M, Kroher G, Morgner A, Bayerdorffer E, Bethke B. A Comparison of *Helicobacter pylori* and *H. heilmannii* gastritis. A matched control study involving 404 patients. Scand J Gastroenterol 1997; 32:28–33.

22. Isaacson PG, Spencer J. Malignant lymphoma of mucosa associated lymphoid tissue. Histopathology 1987; 11:44–49.

23. Isaacson PG, Wotherspoon AC, Diss TC, Pan L. Follicular colonization in B-cell lymphoma of mucosa associated lymphoid tissue. Am J Surg Pathol 1991; 15:819–828.

24. Wotherspoon AC, Pan LX, Diss TC, Isaacson PG. A genotypic study of low grade B-cell lymphomas including lymphomas of mucosa associated lymphoid tissue (MALT). J Pathol 1990; 162:135–140.

25. Auer IA, Gascoyne RD, Connors JM, Cotter FE, Greiner TC, Sanger WG, et al. t(11;18)(q21;q21) is the most common translocation in MALT lymphomas. Ann Oncol 1997; 8:979–985.

26. Ott G, Katzenberger T, Greiner A, Kalla J, Rosenwald A, Heinrich U, Orr M, Muller-Hermelink HK. The t(11;18)(q21;q21) chromosome translocation is a frequent and specific aberration in low-grade hut not high-grade malignant non-Hodgkin's lymphomas of the mucosa-associated lymphoid tissue (MALT-) type. Cancer Res 1997; 57:3944–3948.

27. Wotherspoon AC, Pan L, Diss TC, Isaacson PG. Cytogenetic study of B-cell lymphoma of mucosa-associated lymphoid tissue. Cancer Genet Cytogenet 1992; 58:35–38.

28. Wotherspoon AC, Finn TM, Isaacson PG. Trisomy 3 in low-grade B-cell lymphomas of mucosa-associated lymphoid tissue. Blood 1995; 85:2000–2004.

29. Wotherspoon AC, Soosay GN, Diss TC, Isaacson PG. Low-grade primary B-cell lymphoma of the lung. An immunohistochemical, molecular and cytogenetic study of a single case. Am J Clin Pathol 1990; 94:655–660.

30. Willis AG, Jadayel DM, Du M-Q Peng H, Perry AR, Abdul-Rauf M, et al. Bcl10 is involved in t(1;14)(p22;q32) of MALT B cell lymphoma and mutated in multiple tumor types. Cell 1999; 96:35–45.

31. Eidt S, Stolte M, Fischer R. Helicobacter pylori gastritis and primary gastric non-Hodgkin's lymphomas. J Clin Pathol 1994; 47:436–439.

32. Gisbertz IAM, Jonkers DMAE, Arends JW, Bot FJ, Stockbrugger RW, Vrints LW, et al. Specific detection of *Helicobacter pylori* and non-*Helicobacter pylori* flora in small- and large-cell primary gastric B-cell non-Hodgkin's lymphoma. Ann Oncol 1997; 8(Suppl 2); S33–S36.

33. Bouzourene H, Haefliger T, Delacretaz F, Saraga E. The role of *Helicobacter pylori* in primary gastric MALT lymphoma. Histopathology 1999; 34:118–123.

34. Nakamura S, Yao T, Aoyagi K, Iida M, Fujishima M, Tsuneyoshi M. *Helicobacter pylori* and primary gastric lymphoma. A histological and immunohistochemical analysis of 237 patients. Cancer 1997; 79:3–11.

35. Karat D, O'Hanlon DM, Hayes N, Scott D, Raimes SA, Griffin SM. Prospective study of *Helicobacter pylori* infection in primary gastric lymphoma. Br J Surg 1995; 82:1369–1370.

36. Xu WS, Ho FCS, Chan ACL, Srivastave G. Pathogenesis of gastric lymphoma: the enigma in Hong Kong. Ann Oncol 1997; 8(Suppl 2): S41–S44.

37. Parsonnet J, Hansen S, Rodriguez L, Gelb AB, Warnke RA, Jellum E, et al. *Helicobacter pylori* infection and gastric lymphoma. N Engl J Med 1994; 330:1267–1271.

38. Nakamura S, Aoyagi K, Furuse M, Suekane H, Matsumoto T, Yao T, et al. B-cell monoclonality precedes the development of gastric MALT lymphoma in *Helicobacter pylori*-associated chronic gastritis. Am J Pathol 1998; 152:1271–1279.

39. Zucca E, Bertoni F, Roggero E, Bosshard G, Cazzaniga G, Pedrinis E, et al. Molecular analysis of the progression from *Helicobacter pylori*-associated chronic gastritis to mucosa-associated lymphoid tissue lymphoma of the stomach. N Eng J Med 1998; 338:804–810.

40. De Jong D, van der Hulst RWM, Pals G, van Dijk WC, van der Ende A, Tytgat GNJ, et al. Gastric non-Hodgkin lymphomas of mucosa-associated lymphoid tissue are not associated with more aggressive *Helicobacter pylori* strains as identified by CagA. Am J Clin Pathol 1996; 106:670–675.

41. Peng H, Ranaldi R, Diss TC, Isaacson PG, Bearzi I, Pan L. High frequency of CagA+ *Helicobacter pylori* infection in high-grade gastric MALT B-cell lymphomas. J Pathol 1998; 185:409–412.

42. Eck M, Schauber B, Hass R, Greiner A, Czub S, Muller-Hermelink HK. MALT-type lymphoma of the stomach is associated with *Helicobacter pylori* strains expressing the CagA protein. Gastroterology 1997; 112:1482–1486.

43. Gray D, Kammaratne DS, Lortan J, Khan M, MacLennan IC. Relation of intra-splenic migration of marginal zone B cells to antigen localization on follicular dendritic cells. Immunology 1984; 52:659–669.

44. MacLennan IC, Liu YJ, Oldfield S, Zhang J, Lane PJ. The evolution of B cell clones. Curr Top Microbiol Immunol 1990; 159:37–63.

45. Qin Y, Greiner A, Trunk MJF, Schmausser B, Ott MM, Muller-Hermelink HK. Somatic mutation in low-grade mucosa-associated lymphoid tissue-type B-cell lymphoma. Blood 1995; 86:3528–3534.

46. Du M, Diss TC, Xu C, Peng H, Isaacson PG, Pan L. Ongoing mutation in MALT lymphoma immunoglobulin gene suggests that antigen stimulation plays a role in the clonal expansion. Leukaemia 1996; 10:1190–1197.

47. Chapman CJ, Dunn-Walters DK, Stevenson FK, Hussell T, Isaacson PG, Spencer J. Sequence analysis of immunoglobulin genes that encode autoantibodies expressed by lymphomas of mucosa associated lymphoid tissue. J Clin Mol Biol 1996; 49:M29–M32.

48. Bertoni F, Cazzaniga G, Bosshard G, Roggero E, Barbazza R, de Boni M, et al. Immunoglobulin heavy chain diversity genes rearrangement pattern indicates that MALT-type gastric lymphoma B cells have undergone an antigen selection process. Br J Haematol 1997; 97:830–836.

49. Hussell T, Isaacson PG, Crabtree JE, Spencer J. The response of cells from low-grade B-cell gastric lymphomas of mucosa associated lymphoid tissue to *Helicobacter pylori*. Lancet 1993; 342:571–574.

50. Hussell T, Isaacson PG, Crabtree JE, Spence J. *Helicobacter pylori* specific tumour infiltrating T cells provide contact dependent help for the growth of malignant B cells in low grade gastric lymphoma of mucosa associated lymphoid tissue. J Pathol 1996; 178:122–127.

51. Hussell T, Isaacson PG, Crabtree JE, Dogan A, Spencer J. Immunoglobulin specificity of low grade B cell gastric lymphoma of mucosa associated lymphoid tissue. Am J Pathol 1993; 142:285–292.

52. Greiner A, Marx A, Heesman J, Leebman J, Schmausser B, Muller-Hermelink HK. Idiotype identity in a MALT-type lymphoma and B cells in *Helicobacter pylori* associated chronic gastritis. Lab Invest 1994; 70:572–578.

53. Negrini R, Lisato L, Zanelli I, Cavazzini L, Gullini S, Villanacci V, et al. *Helicobacter pylori* infection induces antibodies cross reacting with gastric mucosa. Gastroenterology 1991; 101:437–445.

54. Wotherspoon AC, Doglioni C, Diss TC, Pan L, Moschini A, de Boni M, et al. Regression of primary low grade B cell gastric lymphomas of mucosa-associated lymphoid tissue (MALT) following eradication of *Helicobacter pylori*. Lancet 1993; 342:575–577.

55. Thiede C, Morgner A, Alpen B, Wundisch T, Herrmann J, Ritter M, et al. What role does *Helicobacter pylori* eradication play in gastric MALT and gastric MALT lymphoma? Gastroenterology 1997; 113:S61–S64.
56. Pinotti G, Zucca E, Roggero E, Pascarella A, Bertoni F, Savio A, et al. Clinical features, treatment and outcome of 93 patients with low-grade gastric MALT lymphoma Leukaemia Lymphoma 1997; 26:527–537.
57. Boot H, de Jong D, van Heerde P, Taal B. Role of *Helicobacter pylori* eradication in high-grade MALT lymphoma. Lancet 1995; 346:448–449.
58. Neubauer A, Thiede C, Morgner A, Alpen B, Ritter M, Neubauer B, et al. Cure of *Helicobacter pylori* infection and duration of remission of low-grade gastric mucosa-associated lymphoid tissue lymphoma. J Natl Cancer Inst 1997; 89:1350–1355.

23

Salmonella typhi/paratyphi and Gallbladder Cancer

Christine P. J. Caygill and Michael J. Hill

INTRODUCTION

Malignant neoplasms of the gallbladder and biliary tract are rare in most populations, and this is not a disease with which the average physician is familiar. It usually arises in the fundus (55%) or mid-section (30%), with the remainder arising in the neck of the gallbladder. Histologically, they are usually adenocarcinomas (83–95%), with squamous cell carcinomas accounting for the rest. They usually appear as infiltrative or scirrhous lesions, whereas those that are papillary often are confused with dysplastic adenomas.

Although there are no specific presenting symptoms, patients typically experience upper quadrant or epigastric pain (75%), as well as anorexia and nausea (50%) leading to vomiting and progressive weight loss. Tumors often arise in patients with preexisting gall stones, among whom a change from sporadic to continuous pain, of steadily increasing severity, should arouse suspicion of malignancy. Jaundice is seen in 48–87% of patients, and this is deep, progressive, and unremitting. The most consistent laboratory finding is raised serum alkaline phosphatase (45–75% of cases). In 50–75% of cases, there is a right upper quadrant mass that can be seen definitively by computed tomography or ultrasonography. However, fewer than 5% of cases are diagnosed before laparotomy or necropsy. The clinical aspects of the disease are reviewed by Moertal and by Sherman and Finlayson *(1,2)*.

EPIDEMIOLOGY OF GALLBLADDER CANCER

Descriptive Epidemiology

The epidemiology of cancer of the gallbladder and biliary tract has been reviewed by Mack and Menck *(3)*, by Hill *(4)*, and by Zatonski et al. *(5)*. It is a relatively uncommon cancer in Europe but with a very poor prognosis. Table 1 shows data *(6)* in which the mortality from gallbladder cancer can be compared with that of cancer of the stomach and of the large bowel. In men there is no country for which it is higher than the 12th commonest cancer site, although for women it reaches as high as 6th to 8th commonest site in central European countries. It is one of the few cancers for which the mortality in women exceeds that in men. During the 20 yr from 1965–69 to 1985–89

From: *Infectious Causes of Cancer: Targets for Intervention*
Edited by: J. J. Goedert © Humana Press Inc., Totowa, NJ

Table 1
**Mortality from Cancer of the Gallbladder and Biliary Tree in European Countries
Compared with Mortalities for Gastric and Colorectal Cancer**

| | Mortality per annum per 10^5 age adjusted | | | | | |
| | Stomach | | Gallbladder | | Colorectum | |
Country	M	F	M^b	F	M	F
Hungary	31.6	14.0	3.5 (15)	8.1 (6)	24.3	18.1
Czechoslovakia	25.7	12.1	3.3 (12)	5.5 (7)	27.3	17.1
Austria	25.5	12.3	3.2 (14)	5.0 (8)	23.8	16.0
Germany	21.2	11.0	2.6 (12)	4.6 (8)	18.0	14.4
Sweden	12.8	6.7	2.4 (16)	4.4 (8)	16.5	12.6
Denmark	12.2	6.2	1.6 (17)	2.5 (11)	24.3	18.5
Finland	20.2	10.5	2.1 (17)	3.5 (9)	12.1	9.6
England/Wales	16.8	7.4	1.0 (18)	1.1 (17)	21.1	15.7
Netherlands	17.5	7.4	2.3 (13)	3.5 (9)	20.0	15.9
France	12.5	5.4	1.2 (18)	1.7 (11)	22.9	14.3
Italy	22.7	10.7	1.4 (19)	2.1 (11)	18.2	13.3
Spain	19.8	9.8	0.9 (19)	1.6 (11)	11.8	9.5
Yugoslavia	21.1	10.2	1.2 (18)	2.5 (1)	11.8	8.7

Data from ref. *6.*

[a] Mortality rates are per 100,000 per annum, age adjusted.

[b] Ranking of site for cancer mortality within the country.

the mortality increased by 30% in Hungary and Czechoslovakia and by similar amounts in Sweden and Denmark *(5).* However not all high-risk countries showed such an increase and the mortality decreased in Austria and Germany *(5).*

Mortality rates in North America, much of Asia and South America, and Oceania tend to be similar to those in Europe. The mortality rates in African countries tend to be relatively low, whereas those in the Andean countries of South and Central America tend to be relatively high, because the rates are very high indeed in all American Indian populations *(7).*

In addition to these variations among populations, there are also within-population variations. The mortality increases sharply with age and is inversely related to socioeconomic status. Within the United States the disease is much more common in Catholic than in Protestant or Jewish communities *(3).* It is also much more common in Spanish Californians than in the Black, White, Japanese, or Chinese Californians. However, all of these within-population differences are seen only in women and are not detectable in men, suggesting that risk factors are different in the two sexes.

High-Risk Disease States

The high-risk disease states for gallbladder cancer are gallstones and previous Polya partial gastrectomy for peptic ulcer, in which the vagal nerves are severed resulting in impaired bile stimulation. The latter is associated with a 10-fold excess risk of gallbladder cancer *(8)* with a latency period of 20 yr. Other gastric surgery is associated with a much smaller increased risk. Ulcerative colitis and choledochal cysts also are high-risk states for cancer of the bile ducts, as discussed elsewhere in depth *(4)*. The common feature of all the predisposing diseases is their association with biliary stasis or infection.

In 1982 Devor *(9)* reviewed 69 reports of series of gallbladder cancer cases, making a total of 6478 cases. In only 59 reports (with 4184 cases) were there details of gall-stone status. Among those 4184 cases 77% were associated with gallstone carriage. The association was much stronger in white than in black patients. The nature of the association is unclear but it is known that gallstones are associated with bacterial infection of the gallbladder *(10)*.

Other Risk Factors

The risk factors that are most consistently reported are overweight *(11)* and smoking *(5)*. Overweight is one of the main risk factors for gallstones, and so it is difficult to determine which of these is the primary association and which is secondary. The bile is the main route of excretion of the carcinogens from tobacco smoke.

TYPHOID AND PARATYPHOID INFECTION

Typhoid and Paratyphoid Fever

Typhoid and paratyphoid fevers have been described in detail by Benenson *(12)*. Typhoid fever is a systemic disease characterized by onset of sustained fever, headache, malaise, anorexia, etc. It is caused by the bacterium *Salmonella typhi,* which can be isolated from the blood, feces, and urine of patients. The usual fatality rate of 10% can be reduced to $\leq 1\%$ with prompt antibiotic treatment. Paratyphoid fever presents a similar clinical picture but tends to be milder and the case fatality rate is much lower. The infectious agents are *Salmonella paratyphi* A, B, and C. *Paratyphi* B is the most common whereas C is extremely rate. All are transmitted by food and water contaminated by the feces and urine of patients and carriers.

With the development of sanitary facilities, typhoid and paratyphoid fever have been virtually eliminated from Europe and the Western world, but they are still endemic in many parts of the world such as Asia, the Middle East, and Latin America. In 1950 2484 cases of typhoid fever were reported in the United States, but for several years it has been fairly constant, with fewer than 500 cases *(12)*. In England and Wales the number of cases have been relatively constant since 1982 (Table 2), and the cases of typhoid fever (as compared with paratyphoid fever) have been mainly contracted abroad. However, outbreaks such as the one in Aberdeen in 1964 do occur. In May 1964, 507 people were infected by *S. typhi,* phage type 34 *(13),* a phage type strain common in South America and Spain, but almost unknown in the United Kingdom. This was traced to contaminated sliced corned beef originating in South America. This outbreak left a legacy of six chronic carriers, in spite of antibiotic treatment *(14)*.

Typhoid Carriers

A chronic faecal typhoid carrier is defined as one whose feces contain typhoid bacilli, but who does not give a history of typhoid fever within the preceding year *(15)*.

Table 2
Statutory Notifications of Typhoid and Paratyphoid Fever in England and Wales
1982–1987 Communicable Disease Surveillance Centre, Public Health Laboratory,
Colindale, London, UK[a]

Year	Typhoid fever contracted				Paratyphoid fever contracted			
	Abroad	UK	Unknown	Total	Abroad	UK	Unknown	Total
1982	125	27	13	165	53	8	8	69
1983	145	16	21	182	56	16	5	77
1984	104	32	16	152	54	4	12	70
1985	139	20	18	177	62	5	8	75
1986	120	21	15	156	64	10	9	83
1987	95	20	25	140	46	7	10	63
1988	117	22	35	174	52	115	13	180
1989	114	15	35	164	60	7	21	88
1990	123	22	33	178	64	18	16	93
1991	134	16	32	182	79	8	12	99
1992	134	32	35	201	56	8	17	81
1993	122	21	32	175	63	12	18	93
1994	149	21	61	231	104	9	26	139
1995	164	28	54	246	83	13	28	124
1996	117	20	38	175	77	2	22	101
1997	99	16	25	140	74	7	80	101
Total	2001	349	488	2838	1047	244	245	1536

[a] Personal communication.

The most famous carrier, "Typhoid Mary," a cook in New York, is thought to have caused more than 1300 cases of typhoid between 1901 and 1914 *(16)*. In another unusual case in Scotland, a 65-yr-old housewife developed typhoid fever, having been infected by her husband, who had had typhoid fever in Poland 31 yr previously *(17)*.

Foci of *S. typhi* (or less commonly *S. paratyphi*) infection may persist in the gall-bladder, liver, biliary tract, kidney, or renal tract (although the latter two give chronic urinary excretion, not faecal excretion). Some 2–4% of patients infected with *S. typhi* become chronic carriers *(18–24)*. Various factors determine the likelihood of a person becoming a carrier; among these are increasing age (0.3% of those under 20 yr becoming carriers compared with 10.2% of those over 50 yr) and gender (women are twice as likely as men to become carriers) *(20)*. Patients with preexisting cholecystitis or pyelitis are particularly vulnerable, and may excrete for many years *(18–20)*. The same risk factors influence carriage of *S. paratyphi* B, but there is a lower overall chronic carriage rate of 2.1% *(19)*. Chronic carriage can be eradicated in a proportion of cases by antibiotic therapy *(20)*. The success of cholecystectomy has varied from zero of 8 patients *(20)* to as high as 53 of 64 patients *(21)*.

BILE, BACTERIA, AND GALLBLADDER CANCER

Biliary stasis and/or infection is a common feature of all the predisposing diseases. Gallstones and choledochal cysts impair the free flow of bile. As noted earlier, Polya surgery impairs bile stimulation due to severing of the vagal nerves. Ulcerative colitis is associated with biliary infection by a number of colonic organisms *(25)*. Colonization of the gallbladder and bile ducts is a feature of typhoid carriage; the colonisation by *S. typhi/paratyphi,* and the resultant mucosal irritation, would normally facilitate a subsequent mixed bacterial infection.

Bile is a rich source of detoxified carcinogens or promoters of carcinogenesis. Polycyclic aromatic hydrocarbons (PAHs) are potent carcinogens that are present in tobacco smoke, cooking fumes, and motor exhaust fumes. After inhalation they are absorbed and are then detoxified in the liver by hydroxylation and glucuronidation. The (harmless) glucuronide is excreted in bile. However, many bacteria produce a β-glucuronidase that releases the hydroxy-PAH. Although the hydroxy-PAHs are not carcinogenic, a high-energy intermediate is released during β-glucuronidase action that binds to DNA and so is potentially carcinogenic *(26)*. The organisms present in infected bile are generally good sources of β-glucuronidase *(4)*, and the best producers of the enzyme would be the enterobacteria that include *S. typhi/paratyphi.*

The bile also is rich in bile salts—the bile acids conjugated with either taurine or glycine. These bile salts are nontoxic to human mucosal cells, but after deconjugation deoxycholic and lithocholic acids are released, both of which are potent tumour promoters *(4)*. More importantly, free lithocholic acid causes bile duct hyperplasia *(27)*, which would be an important step in promotion of biliary tract cancer. The organisms in infected bile are rich in the bile salt hydrolase enzyme *(4)*.

Finally, bile is a rich source of nitrosatable nitrogen compounds and of nitrate. It has been demonstrated that bacteria (perhaps but not definitively shown to include *S. typhi*) can catalyse the formation of locally acting *N*-nitroso compounds (NNCs) *(4)*. High levels of such locally acting NNCs are associated with an increased risk of gastric cancer in patients with gastric bacterial overgrowth *(8)*, and of bladder cancer in patients with chronic bladder infections *(4)*.

Thus, there are good reasons for suspecting that bacteria in infected bile can produce carcinogens or cancer promoters that could cause local gallbladder cancers. Furthermore, all of the disease states associated with increased risk of gallbladder cancer are also associated with gallbladder colonization. The bile is most certainly colonized, however, in typhoid carriers.

BILIARY TRACT CANCER IN TYPHOID CARRIERS

There is a growing body of evidence that typhoid carriers are at increased risk of biliary tract cancer. There have been numerous single case reports of biliary tract cancer in typhoid carriers, but the earliest study of a large number of cases was by Vogelsang *(28)*, who in 1950 reported a cohort of 71 typhoid carriers of whom 47 had died. Of those, three (6.49%) died of biliary tract cancers. A cohort of 210 Californian carriers was reported in 1962 *(29)*, of whom 13 died of hepatobiliary cancers (6.1%).

A case-control study in 1979 of 471 carriers registered by the New York City Health Department and 942 age- and sex-matched controls is the largest study reported to date. It showed that chronic carriers were six times as liable to die of hepatobiliary cancer as controls *(30)*, and this finding was confirmed by Mellemgaard et al. (1988) *(31)*.

Thus, there is an established high risk of hepatobiliary carcinoma in typhoid carriers. By looking at the proportion of gallbladder cancers that are former or current carri-

Table 3
Cohorts of Patients with Chronic Carriage of or Acute Infection with
S. typhi **or** *S. paratyphi*

	Scotland Register of chronic *S. typhi* and *S. paratyphi* carriers	Aberdeen outbreak of acute *S. typhi* and *S. paratyphi*
Total number	102	507
Suitable for analysis	83	386
Deaths	58	81
Sex		
M	21	148
F	62	238
Ratio F/M	3.0	1.6
Mean age at infection (years)		
M	44	29
F	54	33
Year of infection	Various	1964
Infecting organism		
S. typhi	21	359
S. paratyphi	61	6
Type A	9	0
Type B	36	0
Type C	1	0
Unspecified	15	6
S. typhi and *S. paratyphi*	1	21

ers the contribution that this makes to the total gallbladder cancer risk can be determined. In a study in Egypt *(32)* 9 out of 23 (39.1%) patients with bile duct carcinoma tested positive for *S. typhi* and *S. paratyphi* A in stool cultures, compared with 1 in 50 (2%) of healthy individuals. In a similar study in India *(33),* 13 out of 28 patients (46.4%) with carcinoma of the gallbladder tested positive for these organisms, compared with 2 out of 17 (11.8%) in the control group.

In our studies *(34,35)* we investigated the long-term cancer risk in two cohorts, starting with data maintained by the Communicable Diseases Unit (Glasgow, Scotland) of all isolates of *S. typhi* and *S. paratyphi* A, B, and C reported by microbiology laboratories since 1967. One was a cohort of 507 people in the 1964 Aberdeen acute outbreak described earlier. Excluding the six cases who became chronic carriers, 386 of the people in the acute cohort were traced through the General Register Office for Scotland (GROS); death certificates were obtained for 81 and 305 were still alive (Table 3). The chronic cohort included 102 typhoid/paratyphoid carriers from the Scottish Carrier Register (Table 3). Study subjects were regarded as chronic carriers if they were excreting 2 yr after infection. Unlike the acute cases, the chronic carriers were not from a single outbreak and, therefore, included a mixture of different

Table 4
Deaths from Cancer and from All Causes in a Cohort of Acute Typhoid Cases from the 1964 Aberdeen Outbreak

Cause of death	ICD no.	O	E		O/E		95% CI	
Biliary tract	156	0	0.23	(0.23)	0	(0)	0–16.0	(0–16.0)
Pancreas	157	0	1.47	(1.46)	0	(0)	0–2.51	(0–2.53)
Colorectum	152–4	3	4.40	(4.09)	0.68	(0.73)	0.14–1.99	(0.15–2.14)
Stomach	151	2	2.18	(1.86)	0.92	(1.08)	0.11–3.31	(0.13–3.88)
Lung	162	6	8.55	(6.84)	0.70	(0.88)	0.26–1.53	(0.32–1.91)
All neoplasms	140–208	23	32.55	(29.00)	0.71*	(0.79)	0.45–1.06	(0.50–1.19)
Death from all causes		81	141.68	(126.93)	0.55**	(0.64)	0.45–0.71	(0.51–0.79)

O, observed; E, expected.

* $p < 0.05$; ** $p < 0.001$.

Expected mortality using Grampian Area statistics are in parentheses.

typhoid and paratyphoid phage types. Of the 102, 83 were flagged with GROS; 58 had died and death certificates were obtained; 25 were still alive (Table 3). The data obtained from GROS was supplemented by information from the Information and Statistics Division (ISD) of the Common Services Agency in Edinburgh on linkage between our cohorts and (1) cholecystectomy subsequent to infection and (2) cause of death. The expected deaths from a number of various cancers and for "all causes" were calculated for the two cohorts, as were years of potential life lost by those from the carrier cohort who developed cancer. The odds ratio of cholecystecomy in carriers was compared with cases.

The two cohorts basically followed the expected pattern, with greater numbers of women in both, and the carrier cohort having a greater female/male ratio. The mean age at infection of the carriers, again as expected, was also greater.

There was no excess cancer mortality in the cohort of acute Aberdeen typhoid cases using either local (Grampian) area statistics or all Scotland statistics, and the drop in mortality from all neoplasms was not significant when local statistics were used (Table 4). There was a significant deficit in death from all causes.

In contrast, among the chronic typhoid/paratyphoid carriers from the Glasgow Register, there was a 167-fold excess of death from cancer of the gallbladder, an 8-fold excess of death from cancer of the pancreas, and a 2.6-fold excess of death from cancer overall (Table 5). There was also a significant excess of mortality from all causes. Among these chronic carriers, the estimated lifetime risk of death from cancer of the gallbladder was 8.6%.

The characteristics of those carriers who died of cancer (Table 6) show that although age at death was not particularly low, the mean number of years of potential life lost was 7.2 yr for those with cancer of the gallbladder and 9.7 yr for cancer of the pancreas. If the cancers were a result of bacterial colonisation, by analogy with other situations, we would expect a latency of 15–20 yr. There are too few cases to calculate this, but it is of interest that the interval between diagnosis of carrier status and death from cancer was more than 10 yr in 12 out of 20 cases.

Table 5
Deaths from Cancer and from all Causes in the Cohort of Typhoid/Paratyphoid Chronic Carriers

Cause of Death	ICD no.	Male				Female				Total			
		O	E	O/E	95% CI	O	E	O/E	95% CI	O	E	O/E	95% CI
Gallbladder	1560	0	<0.005	0		5	0.03	167	(54–389)	5	0.03	167***	(54–391)
Pancreas	157	3	0.13	23.1***	(4.8–67.4)	0	0.24	0	(0–15.4)	3	0.37	8.1***	(1.7–23.7)
Colorectum	152–4	0	0.32	0	(0–11.5)	3	0.68	4.4*	(0.9–12.9)	3	1.00	3.8	(0.6–8.8)
Lung	162	0	1.10	0	(0–3.35)	5	0.88	5.7**	(1.8–13.3)	5	1.98	2.5	(0.8–5.9)
All neoplasms	140–208	6	2.94	2.0	(0.7–4.4)	14	4.86	2.9***	(1.6–4.8)	20	7.80	2.6***	(1.6–4.0)
All causes		13	13.64	1.0	(0.5–1.6)	45	24.60	1.8***	(1.3–2.5)	58	38.24	1.5**	(1.2–2.0)

O, observed; E, expected.

*$p < 0.05$; **$p < 0.01$; ***$p < 0.001$.

Based on ref. 34.

Table 6
Characteristics of Carrier Cohort Who Died of Cancer

Patient no.	Sex	Age at death	Year of infection[a]	Year of death	Cancer site	ICD no.	Minimum interval between infection and death (yr)	Years of potential life lost
1	F	79	1936	1972	Gallbladder	1560	36	7.0
2	F	77	1923	1977	Gallbladder	1560	54	8.4
3	F	84	1974	1977	Gallbladder	1560	3	5.4
4	F	77	1923	1976	Gallbladder	1560	53	8.8
5	F	82	1979	1981	Gallbladder	1560	2	6.4
6	M	67	1975	1977	Pancreas	1570	2	10.8
7	M	62	1953	1974	Pancreas	1570	21	13.4
8	M	83	1965	1986	Pancreas	1571	21	5.1
9	F	82	1965	1972	Lung	1621	7	6.0
10	F	63	1975	1976	Lung	1621	1	17.2
11	F	76	1975	1984	Lung	1621	9	9.5
12	F	88	1956	1992	Lung	1629	32	—
13	F	67	1982	1990	Lung	1629	8	15.3
14	M	75	1976	1987	Esophagus	1509	11	7.8
15	M	70	1959	1973	Larynx	1619	14	9.0
16	M	80	1972	1988	Kidney	1890	16	5.9
17	F	84	1974	1990	Colon	1531	16	6.1
18	F	89	1965	1986	Colon	1534	21	—
19	F	75	1940	1978	Rectum	1541	38	9.5
20	M	99	1962	1969	Myeloma	203	7	—

[a] This is earliest recorded year, but in many cases infection will have occurred earlier. Years of potential life lost were not calculated for persons who died aged 85 yr or over, because of a lack of data.

Table 7
Characteristics of Patients Who Underwent Cholecystectomy (CC)

Cohort/patients no.	Sex	Age at infection	Age at CC	Reason for CC	Cause of death/alive
Carriers					
1	F	31	32	N/K	Alive
2	F	46	57	Gallstones	Duodenal ulcer
3	F	40	41	N/K	Alive
4	F	41	42	Gallstones	Alive
5	F	67	68	Cholecystitis	Ca lung
6	F	27	25	Gallstones	Alive
7	F	35	62	N/K	Diabetes mellitus
8	F	43	51	N/K	Alive
9	F	63	29	N/K	Cerebrovascular accident
10	F	39	39	Gallstones	Alive
11	F	60	60	N/K	Atheroselerosis
12	M	62	70	Gallstones	Ca body of pancreas
13	F	43	43	N/K	Alive
14	F	80	81	N/K	Senile dementia
15	F	78	78	Gallstones	Ca gallbladder
16	M	17	28	Cholecystitis	Alive
Aberdeen cases					
17	M	51	73	Cholecystitis	Alive
18	F	34	59	Gallstones	Alive
19	F	56	83	Epigastric pain	Alive
20	M	44	64	Gallstones	Alive
21	M	47	68	Cholecystitis	Alive
22	F	70	74	Gallstones	Acute leukaemia
23	F	62	66	Gallstones	Heart disease (ischemic)
24	F	28	40	Gallstones	Alive

Through the ISD linkage system we identified those members of our cohorts who had had cholecystectomy between infection and death (Table 7), and therefore could not develop subsequent gallbladder cancer. Of the 83 carriers, 16 (19%) had undergone cholecystecomy. In comparison, only 8 of the 386 noncarrier cases (2%) had had cholecystecomy. Thus, the prevalence of cholecystecomy in carriers was 6.1 times higher than in cases. Thus, the risk of gallbladder cancer in typhoid carriers with an intact gallbladder is likely to be more than 200-fold.

Earlier studies (e.g., *31*) have concluded that the vast majority, if not all, of typhoid carriers have gallstones. However, as the excess risk of gallbladder cancer with gall-stones is only 2–15-fold *(36)* this explains only a small proportion of the more than 200-fold excess risk of gallbladder cancer seen in our study.

CONCLUSIONS

1. It is clear that chronic bacterial colonisation of the gallbladder, as in chronic carriage of typhoid and paratyphoid, confers an excess risk of gallbladder cancer. Typhoid infection *per se* (without biliary colonisation) confers no excess risk.
2. The magnitude of the excess gallbladder cancer risk (> 200-fold) in typhoid/paratyphoid carriers makes the gallbladder the most common cancer site (equal to the lung) when normally it would be insignificant.
3. Gallstones have been identified as the major risk factor for gallbladder cancer in the general population. Although typhoid carriers have a very high prevalence of gallstones, these cannot be responsible for even 10% of the total excess risk. We need an alternative explanation, therefore, for the bulk of the excess risk.
4. The bile is a rich source of detoxified carcinogens and tumor promoters that can be reactivated by bacterial action. Thus, there are good reasons why we might expect bacterial colonisation of the bile to increase the risk of local cancers and this is what we see.
5. From a public health point of view the lifetime risk of gallbladder cancer of at least 8.6% and the possible excess risk of other gastrointestinal cancers strengthen the arguments for trying to eradicate carriage using antibiotics or surgery. Accordingly, we recommend that known carriers be reviewed to assess the potential for eradication of their carrier state. To be able to do this, however, it is essential to keep registers of known carriers. In addition to screening for carrier status, consideration should be given to surveillance of known carriers for gallbladder, pancreas, or colorectal cancer by whatever methods are available.

REFERENCES

1. Moertal CG. The gallbladder. In: (Holland JF, Frei F, eds). Cancer Medicine. Philadelphia: Lea & Febriger, 1982, pp. 1782–1785.
2. Shearman DJ, Finlayson ND. Diseases of the Gastrointestinal Tract and Liver. Edinburgh: Churchill Livingstone, 1989, pp. 1043–1044.
3. Mack TM, Menck HR (1982). Epidemiology of cancer of the gallbladder and biliary passages. In: Correa P, Haenszel W (eds). Epidemiology of Cancer of the Digestive Tract. The Hague: Martinus Nijhoff, 1982, pp. 227–242.
4. Hill MJ (ed). Microbes and Human Cancer. London: Edward Arnold, 1986.
5. Zatonski W, La Vecchia C, Levi F, Negri E, Lucchini F. Descriptive epidemiology of gallbladder cancer in Europe. Cancer Res Clin Oncol 1993; 119:165–713.
6. Levi F, Maisonneuve P, Filiberti R, La Vecchia C, Boyle P. Cancer incidence and mortality in Europe. Soc Prev Med 1989; 34(Suppl 2):S1–S84.
7. Creagan ET, Fraumeni JF. Cancer mortality among American Indians, 1950–67. J Natl Cancer Inst 1972; 49:959–967.
8. Caygill C, Hill M, Kirkham J, Northfield TC. Increased risk of biliary tract cancer following gastric surgery. Br J Cancer 1988; 57:434–436.
9. Devor EJ. Ethnogeographic patterns in gallbladder cancer. In: Correa P, Haenszel W (eds). Epidemiology of Cancer of the Digestive Tract. The Hague: Martinus Nijhof, 1982, pp. 197–225.
10. England DM, Rosenblatt JE. Anaerobes in human biliary tracts. J Clin Microbiol 1977; 6:494–500.
11. Hill MJ. Overweight and cancer. Eur J Cancer Prev 1996; 5:151–152.
12. Benenson AS. Control of Communicable Disease in Man, 15th edit. An official report of the American Public Health Association, 1990, pp. 469–470.
13. Walker W. The Aberdeen typhoid outbreak of 1964. Scottish Med J 1965; 10:466–479.

14. Brodie J, McQueen IA, Livingstone D. Effect of trimethoprim-sulphamethoxazole on typhoid and salmonella carriers. Br Med J 1970; ii:318.

15. Ames WR, Robins M. Age and sex as factors in the development of the typhoid carrier state and a method for estimating carrier prevalence. Am J Pub Health 1943; 33:221–230.

16. Parry WH (ed). Communicable Diseases, 3rd edit. London: Hodder and Stongton, 1979, p. 106.

17. Sharp JCM. Typhoid fever—thirty years after. Health Bull 1967; XXV:1–5.

18. Ledingham JCG. The carrier problem in enteric fever. In: Ledingham JCG, Arkwright JA (eds). The Carrier Problem in Infectious Diseases. London: Arnold, 1912, pp. 5–135.

19. Vogelsang TM, Boe J. Temporary and chronic carriers of *Salmonella typhi* and *Salmonella paratyphi* B. J Hyg (Lond) 1948; 46:252–261.

20. Tynes BS, Utz JP. Factors influencing the cure of salmonella carriers. Ann Intern Med 1962; 57:871–882.

21. Vogelsang TM. The campaign against typhoid and paratyphoid B in western Norway. Results of cholecystectomy. J Hyg Camb 1964; 62:443–449.

22. Sharp JCM, Brown PP, Sangster G. Outbreak of paratyphoid in the Edinburgh area. Br Med J 1964; 1:1282–1285.

23. McFadzean AJS, Ong GB. Intrahepatic typhoid carriers. Br Med J 1966; 1:1567–571.

24. El-Shabrawy Ali M, Al-Sekait MA, Al-Nasser AAN. Typhoid carriers in Riyadh City, Saudi Arabia. JRSH 1988; 3:97–101.

25. Brooke BN, Slaney G. Portal bacteraemia in ulcerative colitis. Lancet 1958; i:1206–7.

26. Kinoshita N, Gelboin HV. Beta glucuronidase catalysed hydrolysis of benzo[a]pyrene-3-glucuronide and binding to DNA. Science 1978; 199:307–310.

27. Palmer RH, Hruban Z. Production of bile duct hyperplasia and gallstones by lithocholic acid. J Clin Invest 1966; 45:1255.

28. Vogelsang TM. Typhoid and paratyphoid carriers and their treatment. Universitetet I Bergen Arbok 1950, Medisinskrekke Nr. 1, AS John Griegs Boktrykkeri, Bergen, Norway, November 1950.

29. Beck MD, Hollister AC. Typhoid fever cases and carriers—an analysis of records of the California State Department of Public Health, Berkley, California, 1962.

30. Welton JC, Marr JS, Friedman SM. Association between hepatobiliary cancer and typhoid carrier state. Lancet 1979; i:791–794.

31. Mellemgaard A, Gaarslev K. Risk of hepatobiliary cancer in carriers of *Salmonella typhi*. J Natl Cancer Inst 1988; 80:288.

32. El-Zayadi A, Ghoneim M, Kabil SM, et al. Bile duct carcinoma in Egypt; possible etiological factors. Hepato-Gastroenterology 1991; 38:337–340.

33. Nath G, Singh H, Shukla VK. Chronic typhoid carriage and carcinoma of the gallbladder. Eur J Cancer Prev 1997; 6:557–559.

34. Caygill CPJ, Hill MJ, Braddick M, Sharp JCM. Cancer mortality in chronic typhoid and paratyphoid carriers. Lancet 1994; i:83–84.

35. Caygill CPJ, Braddick M, Hill MJ, Knowles RL, Sharp JCM. The association between typhoid carriage, typhoid infection and subsequent cancer at a number of sites. Eur J Cancer Prev 1995; 4:187–193.

36. Diehl AK. Epidemiology of gallbladder cancer: a synthesis of recent data. J Natl Cancer Inst 1980; 65:1209–1214.

24

Schistosoma hematobium and Bladder Cancer

Monalisa Sur and Kum Cooper

INTRODUCTION

It has been estimated that more than 250 million people in the tropical and subtropical regions of the world suffer from schistosomiasis, also known as bilharziasis. The parasitic disease may cause morbidity that is protean in character, and it has a mortality rate that is difficult, if not impossible, to calculate, especially in Third World countries. Of the major species of human schistosomes, *Schistosoma japonicum,* is restricted to the Far East while *S. hematobium* is almost confined to the African continent and parts of Asia Minor and the Arabian peninsula. *S. mansoni* is found in Africa and tropical parts of the Western hemisphere.

Apart from the granulomatous reaction to the eggs, with its unique complications that may be seen in almost any organ, a causal relationship between parasitic infection and malignancy has long been suggested. This association is more clearly defined in *S. hematobium* infection (the causative agent of urinary or bladder schistosomiasis) than in *S. mansoni* or *S. japonicum,* which generally inhabit the portal venous circulation and involve the intestines and lungs.

HISTORICAL BACKGROUND

Theodor Bilharz first found adult worms of the trematode, now known as *S. hematobium,* in the portal veins of a cadaver in Cairo in 1851 *(1)*. As early as 1905, Goebel *(2)* noted the geographic association between endemic *S. hematobium* infections and incidence of bladder carcinoma, later to be supported by Hashem *(3)*, Gillman and Prates *(4)*, Prates and Torres *(5)*, and Brand *(6)*, among others. In 1911, Ferguson postulated a causal relationship between the parasite and bladder carcinoma *(7)*. Proof of this association has remained somewhat elusive, with proponents both for and against the debate, the latter perhaps being in the minority, especially in recent years when possible interactions between the parasite and urinary carcinogens have emerged.

SCHISTOSOMAL EPIDEMIOLOGY AND INCIDENCE OF BLADDER CANCER

In nonendemic urinary schistosomiasis areas, for example, in the West, the peak incidence of bladder carcinomas occurs in the sixth decade of life, with only 12% of

From: *Infectious Causes of Cancer: Targets for Intervention*
Edited by: J. J. Goedert © Humana Press Inc., Totowa, NJ

cases occurring in people under the age of 50 yr *(8)*. In contrast, in lower Egypt, a hyperendemic region for *S. hematobium,* the mean age of patients with carcinoma of the bladder is 46 yr *(14)*, with 73% of patients below the age of 50 yr *(9)*.

Carcinoma of the bladder is the most common malignancy seen in Egypt with prevalence rates varying between 11% and 40% *(9–11)*, with a male-to-female ratio of 5:1 being recorded *(12,13)*.

The mean age at presentation of carcinoma of the bladder in endemic areas of Malawi is also lower (44.9 yr) than and in nonendemic areas *(15)*; similar patterns are seen in Zambia *(16)*, where most of the people are younger than 50 yr. In Iraq, bladder carcinoma is the second most common malignancy recorded, with areas bordering Kuwait showing bladder carcinoma to be the third most common malignancy reported in men *(17)*. An interesting observation with respect to the differences in epidemiology is that cryptogenic or aromatic amine-induced cancers seen in Western countries occur in the most dependent trigonal region of the bladder whereas the schistosome-associated group rarely affects that trigone *(18–20)*.

SCHISTOSOMAL EGGS AND CANCER

A definite association exists between the presence of eggs and carcinoma of the bladder, especially in squamous carcinoma. In Egypt, 82.5% of bladder tumors are associated with schistosomiasis *(21)*, while in Malawi 67.1% of bladder tumors contain schistosome eggs *(15)*. Ninety-four percent of bladder tumors in Zambia contain *S. hematobium* eggs, of which 72% are squamous carcinomas, 18% transitional carcinomas, and 10% adenocarcinomas or undifferentiated carcinomas *(16)*. In Southern Iraq, schistosome eggs are present in 70% of squamous carcinomas, in 17.1% of transitional carcinomas, and in 12.8% of adenocarcinomas and anaplastic carcinomas of the bladder *(22)*. A study from King Edward VIII hospital in Durban, South Africa reported a 61% association between chronic urinary schistosomiasis and bladder carcinomas in black patients *(23)*.

A published series from Egypt showed squamous carcinomas to be the most common, with ratios of 70:25:5 between squamous carcinomas, transitional cell carcinomas, and adenocarcinomas *(18)*. This contrasts sharply with squamous carcinoma, transitional carcinoma, and adenocarcinoma ratios of 5:94:1, respectively, reported in Western countries *(24,25)*. It thus becomes evident that the ratio between transitional cell carcinoma and squamous carcinoma clearly differs when comparing tumor incidence in endemic and nonendemic areas with urinary bladder schistosomiasis. However, not all bladder malignancies in endemic schistosomiasis areas are associated with the parasite: 17.6% of bladder cancers in Egypt do not harbor eggs of *S. hematobium (21)*. These cases represent either patients with schistosomiasis from nonbilharzial areas, patients with mild schistosomal disease or those in whom the disease had burnt itself out, or those patients who have been successfully treated and cured *(21)*. In the treated group, tumors present at a later age, comparable with those in industrialized countries, as opposed to the younger age (46 yr) reported from endemic schistosomal areas *(14)*.

Although the incidence of bladder malignancies, notably squamous carcinoma, is much higher in areas endemic for schistosomiasis, subtle differences occur within these endemic areas. Fripp and Keen *(26)* have reported a higher prevalence in the

Shangaan tribes of Mozambique and Eastern Transvaal, South Africa, especially in women, when compared to different ethnic groups of the Northern Transvaal. Egg load, naturally occurring carcinogens, dietary factors, and cultural or behavioral patterns may possibly explain these differences, although the nature of dietary factors remains elusive. One dietary factor that has been shown to be associated with raised incidence of bladder cancer in Ugandans is 3-hydroxyanthranilic acid. The source of this tryptophan derivative is the Matoke plantain, a staple food of some of the inhabitants. It should, however, be noted that this particular dietary factor is of importance in nonendemic *S. hematobium* areas *(27)*.

URINARY TRACT INFECTIONS AND SCHISTOSOME-INFECTED BLADDERS

A report from Egypt demonstrated that males between the ages of 10 and 25 infected with *S. hematobium* consistently had a load of 10^3–10^5 bacterial organisms per milliliter of urine *(28)*. Bacteriuria in endemic regions is 10 times greater than in nonendemic regions. In Western populations, most bladder infections comprise monocultures of *Escherichia coli* (88%) or *Proteus mirabalis* (10%), the remainder divided over a range of organisms *(29)*. In Egypt, *Escherichia coli* is the most common cause of bacterial infections in bladders affected by schistosomiasis, although mixed cultures, with anaerobes and *Escherichia coli,* can occur *(29–31)*. Bacterial infections in schistosomal bladders seldom, if ever, disappear totally, and it has been postulated that this constant presence of predominantly mixed infections may act synergistically on naturally occurring carcinogens in the urine *(29)*. Stasis of urine as a result of the many obstructive complications of bladder schistosomiasis, and if eggs are present, whether alive, dead, or calcified, they may act as foreign bodies, thereby promoting bacterial infections, have been also considered to be significant.

CARCINOGENS, METABOLITES, CHRONIC BACTERIAL INFECTIONS, AND SCHISTOSOMIASIS

Hicks et al. *(28,32)* have shown that the *N*-nitroso compound, *N*-butyl-*N*-(4-hydroxybutyl) nitrosamine (BBN), when fed to baboons infected with *S. hematobium,* induced bladder tumor formation. Uninfected control baboons fed on BBN did not develop tumors more than 2 yr after exposure, whereas baboons infected with *S. hematobium* and not receiving BBN only developed the usual schistosomal polyps and hyperplastic lesions. It therefore seems likely that bladder schistosomiasis acts as a proliferative stimulus in the already altered epithelium of carcinogen-exposed bladders.

Small amounts of nitrosamines are formed endogenously by nitrosation of ingested or metabolically derived secondary and tertiary amines. There is therefore a significant and constant, albeit low, concentration of carcinogens present in human urine. Furthermore, urinary bacteria can produce large quantities of nitroso compounds over a wide urinary pH range as many bacterial species are able to reduce diet-derived nitrates to nitrites, followed by the formation of *N*-nitrosamines through nitrosation of amine precursors *(33)*. This augments the action of the already existing small quantities of naturally occurring free nitrosamines in the urine.

E. coli and *Proteus* are examples of bacteria able to nitrosate amine precursors, and high levels of urinary *N*-nitrosamines can be present in urinary infections caused by these species. As many bacteria, especially *E. coli,* contain the enzyme nitrate reductase, it is not surprising that higher nitrite levels are present in severe bacterial infections *(30).* Data from the Qalyub area in Egypt, which is endemic for *S. hematobium,* showed that relatively healthy young men, who would be at risk for developing bladder carcinoma 20–30 yr later, had elevated concentrations of *N*-nitroso substances in their urine. The level of *N*-nitroso compounds therefore seems to reflect the presence and metabolic activity of nitrate-reducing organisms that commonly contribute to chronic bladder infections, which are known to occur with greater frequency in the presence of *S. hematobium (27).* In addition, various *N*-nitroso compounds are known to be bladder carcinogens in rodents and dogs. These include *N*-nitrosomethylurea (MNU), BBN, and *N*-nitrosomethyl-dodecyclamine (NMDCA) *(34–36).*

A study from Egypt demonstrated that in individuals with schistosome-associated bladder carcinoma, 66.2% tested positive for nitrites and 5.7% had dysplastic changes in the bladder epithelium *(37),* demonstrating the increased susceptibility of schistosome-infected bladders with raised nitrite levels to the development of bladder cancers.

β-Glucuronidase, which splits glucuronide conjugates formed in the liver, plays an important role in activating naturally occurring or dietary carcinogens in the bladder. It is present in blood leukocytes, occurs free in plasma, and is filtered through the glomerulus. It is also present in the epithelial cells of the ureters and bladder *(38).* It has therefore been suggested that urothelial cells damaged by the passage of schistosome eggs released into the lumen may significantly contribute to the high levels of the enzyme. Bacteria, notably *E. coli,* are another source of the enzyme, and higher levels of β-glucuronidase activity have been detected in schistosomal bladders infected by this organism *(30).* The pH of the urine may, however, reduce the activity of the bacterial enzyme *(38).*

Levels of the carcinogen 3-hydroxyanthranilic acid (3-OHAA), present in low quantities in normal urine, were found elevated in urine specimens of people living in certain rural areas of Transvaal, South Africa, with a high incidence of bladder cancers *(39).* β-glucuronidase has been found responsible for the hydrolysis of the conjugate in this population *(39).* The raised levels of the enzyme in response to the higher concentration of precarcinogenic substrate may well explain the differences in bladder cancer incidence as seen in different areas of the Transvaal where schistosomiasis of the bladder is endemic.

Whether vitamin deficiencies or the abnormal metabolism of certain vitamins play a role in carcinogenesis of the bladder is still to a great extent unclear. Reports from Egypt have shown that patients with schistosomiasis of the bladder, as well as those with squamous carcinoma of the bladder associated with schistosomiasis, had reduced levels of vitamin A compared with normal controls *(40).* As vitamin A is synthesized in the liver, and as the liver is often the target in schistosomiasis, even in mixed infections, the connection seems to be obvious that vitamin A deficiency may have some role in bladder carcinogenesis in association with schistosomiasis.

Abnormal tryptophan metabolism has long been suspected of playing a partial role in bladder carcinogenesis. Abnormal tryptophan metabolism has also been observed in patients with schistosome-associated bladder cancer with a significant increase in the secretion of kynurenic acid, acetyl kynurenine, kyunurenine, and 3-hydroxykynurenine. Tryptophan metabolites, however, require a local abnormality such as a foreign body, for example, urinary schistosomiasis, in the bladder to function as a promoter *(41,42)*.

High levels of urinary kynurenine are often found in Vitamin B_6 deficiency *(43)*. Bladder cancer patients also have high urinary levels of kynurenine *(43)*. Some kynurenine metabolites are carcinogenic, and it is possible that a vitamin B_6 deficiency with consequent high secretory levels of kynurenine derivatives in the urine may augment the action of other carcinogenic factors already present in the bladder, but only if the latter are unconjugated.

Proline has a regulating effect on fibroblast proliferation and occurs in high levels in schistosome eggs, which are known to elicit a strong fibroblastic reaction *(44)*. It has been postulated that a change in the stromal environment of tumors is necessary before tumor infiltration can take place. Because proline diffuses across the egg shell into the environment surrounding the eggs, changes in stromal integrity or altered interaction between stroma and epithelium could possibly promote tumor formation or infiltration *(45)*.

MOLECULAR EVENTS: CHROMOSOMAL ALTERATIONS ASSOCIATED WITH *SCHISTOSOMA*-RELATED BLADDER CANCERS

Although the association of carcinoma with bilharziasis has long been evident in epidemiologic studies, the exact mechanism by which chronic bilharzial infestation leads to carcinoma is not entirely clear. Among the mechanisms that have been postulated, are specific chromosomal aberrations of tumor suppressor genes known to play a role in the pathogenesis of other carcinomas. These genetic abnormalities result in the production of mutant proteins that distort control of the cell cycle, thereby affecting proliferative potential *(46–50)*.

Ghaleb et al. *(57)* examined 27 paraffin-embedded bladder specimens from 18 Egyptian patients with schistosome-associated carcinoma. Fluorescence *in situ* hybridization results, in the carcinoma and from benign mucosa of patients with schistosomiasis, were compared with flow cytometric DNA ploidy and cell cycle assays. Numerical aberrations of chromosomes 9 and 17 were identified in schistosome-associated bladder carcinoma, similar to that demonstrated in nonendemic carcinomas of the bladder.

Thus it appears that numerical aberrations of chromosomes 9 and 17 may occur in chronically inflamed and metaplastic but still histologically benign mucosa of at least some patients with schistosomal cystitis, and in other areas of carcinoma *in situ* *(57)*. Aberrations of chromosome 9 and 17 have also been implicated in the development and progression of transitional cell carcinoma of the urinary tract *(58)*. It is therefore possible that schistosome-associated bladder cancer in Egypt and sporadic cases of bladder cancer in the United States may develop through the same genetic mechanisms.

MOLECULAR EVENTS UNDERLYING *SCHISTOSOMA*-RELATED BLADDER CANCER

Molecular events underlying urothelial neoplastic progression have identified alterations associated with specific genes along this pathway. Results collected from patient populations in North America, where transitional cell carcinomas predominate and multiple etiologic agents are implicated in progression, shows interesting findings: H-*ras* activation *(59–61)*, *p53 (62)* and retinoblastoma gene *(Rb) (63)* inactivation and overexpression of the epidermal growth factor receptor (EGFR) *(64)* and C-*erbB-2 (65)*. The prospective analysis of bladder tumors involving each of the genetic loci implicate *p53* inactivation as a late event associated with the transition of tumor from a low-grade to a high-grade lesion *(66)*. Loss of expression of the *Rb* gene product (pRB) and overexpression of the EGFR are correlated with the invasive phenotype and along with *p53* have been proposed as independent prognostic indicators of progression in bladder cancer. In contrast, H-*ras* activation has been consistently found to be represented in all grades of bladder tumors.

Ramchurren et al. *(67)* examined the molecular alterations reported in transitional cell carcinomas from Western countries in schistosomiasis-related squamous cell carcinomas of the bladder and whether genetic changes identified were indicative of the action of a specific etiologic agent. Preferential activation of the H-*ras* gene in approx 14% of the schistosomiasis-related squamous cell carcinoma lesions was demonstrated. No mutational events associated with codon hot spots in N- or K-*ras* genes were found using single strand conformation polymorphism (SSCP) analysis *(67)*. In addition, the most common mutational event reported in transitional cell carcinoma, involving a G-T transversion at codon 12 resulting in a glycine-to-valine change *(59,60,68)*, was not found in this group of schistosomiasis-related bladder cancers. Of the three *ras* activation events identified, two displayed codon-13 mutations, an occurrence recorded only rarely in transitional cell carcinoma.

Inactivation events associated with the *p53* tumor suppressor gene are the most common molecular changes recorded in transitional cell carcinomas *(62,69)*. Genetic changes associated with this locus are generally considered late events, possibly linked to transition from a low-grade to a high-grade transitional cell carcinoma *(66)*. The frequency of detection of *p53* alterations in bladder tumors has been reported in a range between 29% and 61% where such events have been shown to be indicative of a significantly lower progression-free interval *(70)*. In the study by Ramchurren et al. *(67)*, *p53* inactivation was found in 57% tumors involving 23 point mutations and one deletion/insertion event. In addition, the preponderance of G-A transitions in the schistosomiasis cases harboring multiple mutations is also characteristic of the molecular changes elicited by the action of alkylating *N*-nitroso compounds. The *p53* mutations found in schistosomiasis-bladder lesions are limited mainly to exons 7 and 8, with multiple mutations being a common occurrence. Therefore, *p53* mutational events would be unlikely to occur as late events in schistosome-associated bladder squamous cell carcinomas and probably occur early on in bladder carcinogenesis. A study by Habuchi et al. *(71)* from Egypt showed *p53* missense mutations involving exons 5, 6, 8, and 10. This may indicate the involvement of alternative carcinogenic cofactors in different schistosomiasis-infested regions.

pRB is altered in bladder carcinoma cell lines and is an important prognostic variable in patients presenting with invasive bladder cancer *(72,73)*. Altered patterns of pRB expression detected with immunocytochemistry are represented by undetectable or heterogeneous nuclear staining throughout tumor tissue and is considered indicative of more aggressive biologic behavior *(72,73).* Unlike the transitional cell carcinoma, which is characterized by *Rb* inactivation, pRB is expressed in a majority of invasive schistosomiasis-related squamous cell carcinoma of the bladder.

High-level expression of EGFR is a common property of squamous cell carcinomas and occurs during the progression of normal epidermal cells to the malignant state *(74).* Many studies have described an association between increased expression of EGFR and high stage of bladder tumors *(75).* Ramchurren et al. *(67)* found strong immunoreaction for the EGFR in 67% of the schistosoma-associated bladder tumors. This finding is similar to the overexpression recorded in transitional cell carcinomas of the bladder reported in the Western population.

C-*erbB-2,* a member of the tyrosine-kinase-receptor family, that encodes a transmembrane protein, is also amplified and/or overexpressed in bladder cancer *(65).* The findings are similar in schistosomiasis-associated bladder tumors, with strong immunostaining and frequent amplification and higher gene-copy number in high grade tumors *(67).*

In summary, the molecular changes occurring in schistosomal bladder carcinoma differ in several ways from those recorded in transitional cell carcinomas in the Western population.

MOLECULAR EVENTS UNDERLYING SQUAMOUS CELL CARCINOMA OF THE BLADDER

Ramchurren et al. conducted a study which examined whether the mutational changes recorded in schistosomal bladder squamous cell carcinoma are a result of *S. hematobium* infection or a function of squamous rather than transitional cell carcinoma. They examined the H-*ras* and *p53* genes in squamous cell carcinoma of the bladder not associated with schistosoma infections in South Africa *(76).* None of the squamous cell carcinomas harbored an H-*ras* mutation, suggesting that the H-*ras* gene may not be involved in the tumorogenesis of squamous cell carcinoma of the bladder in the absence of schistosomiasis infection. *p53* mutations were present in 80% of the bladder squamous cell carcinomas. The prevalence of mutations at this locus in squamous cell carcinoma appeared to be higher than that reported for transitional cell carcinoma (29–61%), suggesting that the *p53* gene has a greater involvement in the development of squamous rather than transitional cell carcinoma of the bladder. Genetic changes associated with this locus are generally considered late events, possibly linked to transition from a low-grade to a high-grade lesion *(66).* Squamous cell carcinomas at the time of diagnosis are generally more advanced with deep muscle invasion and typically more aggressive than transitional cell carcinoma. It is therefore not unexpected that the *p53* gene sustains a high incidence of mutations in squamous cell carcinoma compared to transitional cell carcinoma.

Ramchurren et al. *(76)* detected five silent mutations in *p53* occurring at codon 264 involving leucine, with the remainder being scattered throughout exons 4–9. Mutations at codons 146 and 192 were also identified, with the change at codon 192 being glutamine to a stop codon (CAG-TAG). Another observation regarding the *p53* locus in bladder squamous cell carcinoma in the South African population is that whereas tumors *without* schistosomiasis infection possess mutations in exons 4, 5, 6, 7, 8, and 9,

96% of the mutations in schistosome-associated squamous cell carcinoma are confined to exons 7 and 8. This would suggest that the involvement of the parasite in tumorogenesis of bladder squamous cell carcinoma results in the targeting of *p53* mutations to a very restricted region of the gene. Further, in the study by Ramchurren et al. *(76)*, 72% of the mutations were transitions of which 65% were C-T/T-C substitutions. In contrast, the schistosomal bladder squamous cell carcinomas showed a 79% prevalence of transitional changes with 65% being G-A/A-G base substitutions *(67)*. It therefore appears that molecular changes occurring in H-*ras* and *p53* genes in squamous cell carcinomas of the bladder associated with schistosomiasis are different from those *not* associated with the parasite.

HPV AND SCHISTOSOMIASIS-ASSOCIATED BLADDER CANCER

Cooper et al. *(77)* examined the human papillomavirus (HPV) DNA status in schistosomal associated squamous cell carcinoma of urinary bladder in South Africa by using nonisotopic *in situ* hybridization (NISH) and polymerase chain reaction (PCR) against 6, 11, 16, 18, 31, and 33 genotypes. None of the cases was shown to harbor HPV DNA. This study abrogates the role of HPV in schistosoma-associated bladder cancer in South Africa. Other factors including nitrosamine exposure, *p53* mutations, and additional unknown chromosomal events may play a major role in the development of this parasite-associated neoplasm.

SCREENING FOR *S. HEMATOBIUM*

Ideally, screening for S. *hematobium* should be done in endemic and hyperendemic areas. Microscopic detection of schistosome eggs in feces or urine is the most reliable and cost-effective means of diagnosis *(78)*. The preferred diagnostic method for *S. hematobium* infection is microscopic examination of filtered urine. *S. hematobium* eggs are counted at ×100 magnification. Egg counts of fewer than 50 eggs/10 mL urine indicate light infection; all other are designated as heavy infection. After chemotherapy, most or all eggs may appear dark, that is, nonviable, even before egg excretion ceases. However, morbidity can persist in inactive infections and in such patients, rectal or bladder biopsy or serodiagnosis should be performed.

In large-scale campaigns, for control of endemic *S. hematobium,* simple dipstick urine tests have proven accurate and advantageous. Commercially available reagent strips capable of detecting 5–15 red cells per microliter of urine and 10–25 mg of protein/100 mL of urine are up to 89% specific in spotting *S. hematobium* infection among endemic children *(79)*. Although the dipstick greatly facilitates field studies, it should not replace parasitologic diagnosis.

Most diagnostic laboratories in endemic countries today perform enzyme-linked immunosorbent assays (ELISAs) or radioimmunoassay (RIA) tests using a variety of crude or fractionated worm or egg antigens including purified *S. mansoni* egg antigen *(80)*.

In the United States, the Centers for Disease Control and Prevention offers a two-step procedure based on adult worm microsomal antigen fractions in which sera are first screened by FAST-ELISA, followed by immunoblotting with schistosome species-specific fractions. Field adoptable versions of these have recently been developed *(81)*.

TREATMENT OF *S. HEMATOBIUM*

It has been observed that a close relationship exists between vesical schistosomiasis and vesical carcinoma, particularly in areas where the infection is highly endemic. Early treatment of *S. hematobium* is likely to reduce the risk of bladder cancer. However, because all drugs currently used for treatment of schistosomiasis have potentially serious side effects, the relative risks of treatment must be weighted, particularly in lightly infected patients. Only patients with active infection should be treated. Embryonated eggs can be found in the excreta of nearly all actively infected cases. Drugs commonly used for treatment are Niridazole, trivalent antimonials, and Hycanthone. The results of treatment are best followed by quantitation of eggs in the feces or urine, as chemotherapy may greatly reduce the number of parasites without eradicating them. Therefore, the effectiveness of a drug and benefit to the patient should be judged in large part by reduction in the intensity of infection.

CONCLUSION

Schistosomal carcinogenesis may therefore be summarized as follows (Fig. 1):

1. The presence of *S. haematobium* eggs in the mucosal layers of the bladder results in metaplasia as well as reparative hyperplasia of the epithelium, leading to an increased cell turnover that may escape growth control mechanisms. It may also enhance already existing minute foci of intra-epithelial neoplasia.
2. As bacterial infection, notably mixed, forms part of the pathology of schistosomal bladders, the effect of naturally occurring carcinogens may be enhanced by accelerated nitrosation of precursor substrates through nitrate reductase activity.
3. Hydrolytic enzymes such as β-glucuronidase, originating from many sources, split nontoxic glucuronide conjugates into active carcinogenic moities.
4. Altered metabolism of vitamins, and/or deficiencies may enhance carcinogenesis especially through the action of kynurenine metabolites, in themselves carcinogenic. The protective role of certain vitamins such as A and B_6 will be absent, either through diet deficiencies or liver and intestinal disease.
5. Differences in diet with a resultant different intake of a variety of naturally occurring carcinogens (although still illusive) may explain focal differences of tumor incidence in endemic schistosomiasis areas.
6. Changes in the stroma underlying and surrounding mucosal lesions may well promote the development of infiltrative lesions; alternatively, interactions between stroma and epithelium may be impaired. Stromal proliferation caused by excess of proline in the vicinity of viable schistosome eggs may possibly have a counterpart in epithelial proliferation.
7. Aberrations of chromosome 9 and 17 have been implicated in the development and progression of transitional cell carcinoma of the urinary bladder. Similar aberrations may occur in chronically inflamed and metaplastic mucosa with bilharzial cystitis and in carcinoma *in situ*. Bilharzial-associated bladder cancer in Egypt and sporadic cases of bladder cancer in the United States may develop through the same genetic mechanisms.
8. The molecular changes involving H-*ras* and *p53* occurring in schistosomiasis related squamous cell carcinoma are different from those recorded in transitional cell carcinoma in the Western countries. Multiple mutations found at the *p53* locus in schistosomiasis related bladder tumors is consistent with the involvement of a specific etiologic agent, possibly nitrosamine(s), responsible for the neoplastic progression in bilharzial bladder cancer.

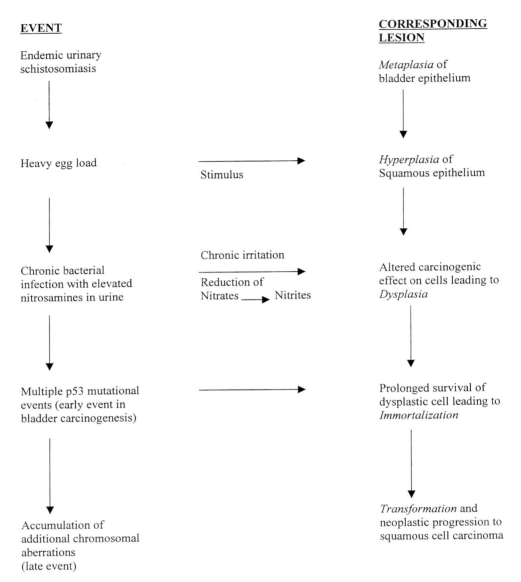

EVENT

Endemic urinary
schistosomiasis

Heavy egg load

Chronic bacterial
infection with elevated
nitrosamines in urine

Multiple p53 mutational
events (early event in
bladder carcinogenesis)

Accumulation of
additional chromosomal
aberrations
(late event)

Stimulus

Chronic irritation

Reduction of
Nitrates ⟶ Nitrites

**CORRESPONDING
LESION**

Metaplasia of
bladder epithelium

Hyperplasia of
Squamous epithelium

Altered carcinogenic
effect on cells leading to
Dysplasia

Prolonged survival of
dysplastic cell leading to
Immortalization

Transformation and
neoplastic progression to
squamous cell carcinoma

Fig. 1. Proposed pathogenetic pathway of neoplastic progression for squamous cell carcinogenesis associated with schistosomiasis.

9. Molecular changes occurring in the H-*ras* and *p53* genes in squamous cell carcinomas
of the bladder associated with schistosomiasis are different from those not infected
with the parasite. The H-*ras* gene is unaltered in the absence of bilharzial infection and
may therefore not be directly involved in the tumorogenesis of squamous cell carcinoma of the bladder. Multiple mutations and transitional base changes are a common
occurrence in squamous cell carcinoma of the bladder, particularly in the South African
population. However, the interaction of the carcinogenic agents in the presence of the
parasite produces mutations in the *p53* tumor suppressor gene that are different in profile from those seen in the absence of schistosomiasis infection.

REFERENCES

1. Bilharz T. Further observations concerning *Distomum hematobium* in the portal vein of man and its relationships to certain pathological formations. Zeitschrift Fur Wissenschaftliche Zoologie 1852; 4:72–76.

2. Goebel C. On bilharzia disease occurring with bladder tumors with special reference to carcinoma. Zeitschrift Fur Krebsforschung 1905; 3:369–513.

3. Hashem M. The etiology and pathogenesis of the bilharzial bladder cancer. J Egypt Med Assoc 1961; 44:857–966.

4. Gillman J, Prates MD. Histological types and histogenesis of bladder cancer in the Portuguese East African with special reference to bilharzial cystitis. Acta Unio Internationalis Contra Cancrum 1962; 18:560–574.

5. Prates MD, Torres FO. A cancer survey in Lourenco Marques, Portuguese East Africa. J Natl Cancer Inst 1965; 35:729–756.

6. Brand KG. Schistosomiasis-cancer: etiological considerations. A review. Acta Trop 1979; 36:203–214.

7. Ferguson AR. Associated bilharziasis and primary malignant disease of the urinary bladder, with observations in the series of forty cases. J Path Bacteriol 1911; 16:76–94.

8. Payne P. Sex, age, history, tumor type and survival. In: Wallace DM, ed. Tumours of the Bladder. Edinburgh and London: E&S Livingstone, 1959, pp. 258–306.

9. Fawzi RM. Carcinoma of the bladder in Egypt. Proceedings of the 7th International Cancer Congress. London: Urine International Control Concern, 1958; 57.

10. Aboul Nasr AL, Gazayerli ME, Fawzi RM, El-Sebai I. Epidemiology and pathology of cancer of the bladder in Egypt. Acta Unio Internationalis Contra Cancrum 1962; 18:528–537.

11. Pfister E. Uber den endemischen Blasenkrebs bei Bilharziasis. Zeitschrift fur Urologie 1921; 15:51–57.

12. Ishak KG, Le Golvan PC, El-Sebai I. Malignant bladder tumors associated with bilharziasis. A gross and microscopic study. In: Mostofi F (eds). Bilharziasis. New York: Springer-Verlag, 1967, pp. 58–83.

13. El-Sebai I. Parasites in the etiology of cancer-bilharziasis and bladder cancer. CA 1977; 27:100–106.

14. El Bolkainy MN; Ghoneim MA, Mansour MA. Carcinoma of the bilharzial bladder in Egypt: clinical and pathological features. Br J Urol 1983; 55:275–278.

15. Lucas. SB Bladder tumors in Malawi. Br J Urol 1982; 54:275–279.

16. Elem B, Purohit R. Carcinoma of the urinary bladder in Zambia. A quantitative estimation of *Schistosoma haematobium* infection. Br J Urol 1983; 55:275–278.

17. Al-Fouadi A. Parkin DM. Cancer in Iraq: seven year's data from the Baghdad Tumor registry. Int J Cancer 1984; 34:207–213.

18. Khafagy MM, El-Bolkainy MN, Mansour MA. Carcinoma of the bilharzial urinary bladder; a study of the associated mucosal lesions in 86 cases. Cancer 1972; 30:150–159.

19. Makar NA. Some observations in pseudoglandular proliferations in the bilharzial bladder. Acta Unio Internationalis Contra Cancrum 1962; 18:599–607.

20. Prates MD, Gillman J. Carcinoma of the urinary bladder in Portuguese east African with special reference to bilharzial cystitis and pre neoplastic reactions. S Afr J Med Sci 1959; 24:13–40.

21. El-Bolkainy MN, Mokhtar NM, Ghoneim MD, Hussein MH. The impact of schistosomiasis on the pathology of bladder carcinoma. Cancer 1981; 48:2643–2648.

22. Al Adnani MS, Saleh KM. Schistosomiasis and bladder carcinoma in Southern Iraq. J Trop Med Hyg 1983; 86:93–97.

23. Cooppan RM, Bhoola KDN, Mayet FGH. Schistosomiasis and bladder cancer in Natal. S Afr Med J 1984; 66:841–843.

24. Mostofi FK. A study of 2678 patients with initial carcinoma of the bladder: survival rates. J Urol 1956; 75:480–491.

25. Mostofi FK, Leestma JE. The genitourinary tract. In: Brunson JG, Gall EA (eds). Concepts of Disease. New York: Macmillan, 1971, p. 835.

26. Fripp PJ, Keen P. Bladder cancer in endemic schistosomiasis area: geographical and sex distribution. South Afr J Sci 1980; 76:228–230.

27. Manek PV, Fripp PJ. The free amino acids of the green banana `Matoke' (*Musa* sp.) Biochem J 1963; 89:75.

28. Hicks RM. The canopic worm: role of bilharziasis in the aeitiology of human bladder cancer. J R Soc Med 1983; 76:16–22.

29. Hill MJ. Bacterial metabolism and human carcinogenesis. Br Med Bull 1980; 36:89–94.

30. El-Aaser AA, El-Merzabani MM, Higgy NA, El-Habet AE. A study on the etiological factors of bilharzial bladder cancer in Egypt.6. The possible role of urinary bacteria. Tumori 1982; 68:23–28.

31. Hicks RM, Walters CL, El-Sebai I, El-Aaser AA, El-Merzabani MM, Gough TA. Demonstration of nitrosamines in human urine: preliminary observations on a possible etiology for bladder cancer in association with chronic urinary infections. Proc R Soc Med 1977; 70:413–417.

32. Hicks RM, James C, Webbe G. Effect of schistosoma haematobium and *N*-butyl-*N* (4-hydroxy-butyl) nitrosamine on the development of urothelial neoplasia in the baboon. Br J Cancer 1980; 42:730–755.

33. Hill MJ, Hawksworth G. Bacterial production of Nitrosamines in vitro and in vivo. In: Bogovski P, Preusmann R, Walker EA (eds). N-Nitroso compounds: Analysis and Formation (IARC Publications No. 3). Lyons: International Agency for Research on Cancer, 1972, pp. 111–121.

34. Druckrey H, Preussman R, Ivankovic S, Schmidt CH, Mennel HD, Stahl KW. Selektive erzeugung von blasenkrebs an ratten durch Dibutyl und *N*-butyl-*N*-Butamol (4) Nitrosamin. Zeitschrift fur Krebsforschung 1964; 66:280–290.

35. Hicks R, Wakefield J. Rapid induction of bladder cancer in rats with *N*-methyl-*N*-nitrosurea. Chem Biol Interact 1972; 5:139–152.

36. Lijinsky W, Taylor HW. Induction of urinary bladder tumors in rats by administration of nitrosomethyldodecylamine. Cancer Res 1975; 35:958–961.

37. El-Aaser AA, El-Merzabani MM, El-Bolkainy MN, Ibrahim AS, Zakhary NI, El-Morsi B. A study on the etiological factors of bilharzial bladder cancer in Egypt: 5 urinary nitrite in rural population. Tumori 1980; 66:409–414.

38. Fripp PJ. The origin of urinary B-glucuronidase. Br J Cancer 1965; 19:330–335.

39. Fripp PJ, Keen P. Bladder cancer in an endemic *Schistosoma hematobium* area. The excretion patterns of 3-hydroxyanthranilic acid and kynurenine. S Afr J Sci 1980; 76:212–215.

40. El-Aaser AA, El-Merzabani MM, Abdel-Reheem KA, Hamza BM. A study on the etiological factors of bilharzial bladder cancer in Egypt: Part 4. β-Carotene and vitamin A level in serum. Tumori 1982; 68:19–22.

41. Oyasu R, Hopp ML. Collective review: the etiology of cancer of the bladder. Surg Gynecol Obstet 1974; 138:97–108.

42. Bryan GT. Neoplastic response of various tissues to systemic administration of the 8-methyl ether of xanturenic acid. Cancer Res 1968; 28:183–185.

43. Abdel-Tawab GA, Ibrahim EK, El Masri A, Al-Ghorab M, Makhyoun N. Studies on tryptophan metabolism in bilharzial bladder cancer patients. Invest Urol 1968; 5:591–601.

44. Rojkind M, De Leon LD. Collagen biosynthesis in cirrhotic rat liver slices; a regulatory mechanism. Biochem Biophys Acta 1970; 217:512–522.

45. Van den Hooff A. The part played by the stroma in carcinogenesis. Perspect Biol Med 1984; 27:498–509.

46. Dolcetti R, Doglioni C, Maestro R, et al. p53 overexpression is an early event in the development of human squamous cell carcinoma of the larynx: genetic and prognostic implications. Int J Cancer 1992; 52:178–182.

47. Maesawa C, Tamura G, Suzuki Y, et al. Aberrations of tumor-suppressor genes (*p53, apc, mcc* and *Rb*) in esophageal squamous cell carcinoma. Int J Cancer 1994; 57:21–25.

48. Friedell GH. Current concepts of the etiology, pathogenesis and pathology of bladder cancer. Urol Res 1978; 6:179–182.

49. Mercer WE, Shields MT, Lin D, Appella E, Ullrich SJ. Growth suppression induced by wild-type p53 protein is accompanied by selective down-regulation of proliferation cell nuclear antigen expression. Proc Natl Acad Sci USA 1991; 88:1958–1962.

50. Jerry DL, Ozbun MA, Kittrell FS, et al. Mutations in p53 are frequent in the preneoplastic state in the mouse mammary tumor development. Cancer Res 1993; 53:3374–3381.

51. Rosin M, Anwar W. Chromosomal damage in urothelial cells from Egyptians with chronic *Schistosoma haematobium* infections. Int J Cancer 1992; 50:539–543.

52. Rubin CM. Technical advances in the cytogenetic analysis of malignant tissues. Cancer 1992; 69:1567–1571.

53. Poddighe PJ, Ramaekers FCS, Smeets AWGB, Vooijs GP, Hopman AHN. Structural chromosome 1 aberrations in transitional cell carcinoma of the bladder: Interphase cytogenetics combining a centromeric, telomeric and library DNA probe. Cancer Res 1992; 52:4929–4934.

54. Meloni AM, Peier AM, Haddad FS, et al. A new approach in the diagnosis and follow up of bladder cancer. FISH analysis of urine, bladder washings and tumors. Cancer Genet Cytogenet 1993; 71:105–118.

55. Hamilton SR. Molecular genetics alterations as potential prognostic indicators in colorectal carcinoma. Cancer 1992; 69:1589–1591.

56. Hopman AHN, Poddighe PJ, Smeets AWGB, et al. Detection of numerical chromosome aberrations in bladder cancer by in situ hybridization. Am J Pathol 1989; 135:1105–1117.

57. Ghaleb AH, Pizzolo JG, Myron RM. Aberrations of chromosomes 9 and 17 in Bilharzial bladder cancer as detected by fluorescence in-situ hybridization. Am J Clin Pathol 1996; 106:234–241.

58. Tsai YC, Nichols P, Hiti AL, et al. Allelic losses of chromosome 9, 11 and 17 in human bladder cancer. Cancer Res 1990; 50:44–47.

59. Czernaik B, Deitch D, Simmons H, Etkind P, Herz F, Koss LG. Ha-*ras*-gene codon-12 mutation and DNA ploidy in urinary bladder carcinoma. Br J Cancer 1990; 62:762–763.

60. Levesque P, Ramchurren M, Saini K, Joyce A, Libertino J, Summerhayes IC. Screening of human bladder tumors and urine sediments for the presence of H-*ras* mutations. Int J Cancer 1993; 55:785–790.

61. Knowles MA, Williamson M. Mutation of H-*ras* is infrequent in bladder cancer: confirmation by single strand conformation-polymorphism analysis, designed restriction-fragment length polymorphisms, and direct sequencing. Cancer Res 1993; 53:133–139.

62. Sidransky D, Von Eschiebach A, Tsai YC, et al. Identification of *p53* gene mutations in bladder cancers and urine samples. Science 1991; 252:706–709.

63. Ishikawa J, XU H-J, Hu S-X, Yandell DW, Maeda S, Kamidono S, Benedict WF, Takahashi R. Inactivation of the retinoblastoma gene in human bladder and renal cell carcinomas. Cancer Res 1991; 51:5736–5743.

64. Neal DW, Marsh C, Bennet MK, Abel PD, Hall RR, Sainsbury JRC, Harris AL. Epidermal growth factor receptors in human bladder cancer. Comparison of invasive and superficial tumors. Lancet 1985; I:366.

65. Coombs LM, Pigott DA, Sweeney E, Proctor AJ, Eydmann ME, Parkinson C, Knowles MA. Amplification and overexpression of c-*erb B-2* in transitional cell carcinoma of the urinary bladder. Br J Cancer 1991; 63:601–608.

66. Olumi AF, Tsai YC, Nichols PW, et al. Allelic loss of chromosome 17p distinguishes high grade from low grade transitional cell carcinomas of the bladder. Cancer Res 1990; 50:7081–7083.

67. Ramchurren N, Cooper K, Summerhayes IC. Molecular events underlying schistosomiasis related bladder cancer. Int J Cancer 1995; 62:237–244.

68. Burchill SA, Neal DE, Lunec J. Frequency of H-*ras* mutations in human bladder cancer detected by direct sequencing. Br J Urol 1994; 73:516–521.

69. Fujimoto K, Yamada Y, Okajima E, Kakizoe T, Sasaki H, Sugimura T, Terada M. Frequent association of *p53* gene mutations in invasive bladder cancer. Cancer Res 1992; 52:1393–1398.

70. Sarkis AS, Dalbagni G, Cordon-Cardo C, et al. Nuclear over-expression of p53 protein in transitional cell bladder carcinoma: a marker for disease progression. J Nat Cancer Inst 1993; 85:53–59.

71. Habuchi T, Takahashi R, Yamada H, et al. Influence of cigarette smoke and schistosomiasis on p53 gene mutation in urothelial cancer. Cancer Res 1993; 53:3795–3799.

72. Cordon-Cardo C, Wartinger D, Petrylak D, et al. Altered expression of the retinoblastoma gene product: prognostic indicator in bladder cancer. J Natl Cancer Inst 1992; 84:1251–1256.

73. Logothetis CJ, Xu H-J, Ro JY, et al. Altered expression of retinoblastoma protein and known prognostic variables in locally advanced bladder cancer. J Nat Cancer Inst 1992; 84:1256–61

74. Cowley G, Smith J, Gusterson B, Hendler F, Ozanne B. The amount of EGF receptor is elevated in squamous cell carcinomas. Cancer Cells 1984; 1:5–10.

75. Neal D, Sharples L, Smith K, Fennelly J, Hall R, Harris A. The epidermal growth factor receptor and the prognosis of bladder cancer. Cancer 1990; 65:1619–1625.

76. Ramchurren N, Cooper K, Summerhayes IC. Molecular events underlying squamous cell carcinoma of the bladder submitted for publication.

77. Cooper K, Haffazee Z, Taylor L. Human papilloma virus and schistosomiasis associated bladder cancer. J Clin Pathol 1997; 50:145–148.

78. World Health Organization. Basic Laboratory Methods in Medical Parasitology. Geneva: WHO, 1991, pp. 25–36.

79. Stephenson LS, Latham MC, Kinoti SN, Oduori ML. Sensitivity and specificity of reagent strips in screening Kenyan children for *Schistosoma hematobium* infection. Am J Trop Med Hyg 1984; 33:862–871.

80. Maddison SE. The present status of serodiagnosis of sero-epidimiology of schistosomiasis. Diagn Microbiol Infect Dis 1987; 7:93–105.

81. Mahmoud AAR. Trematodes (schistosomiasis) and other Flukes. In: Mandell GL, Douglas Jr RG, Bennett JE (eds) Principles and Practice of Infectious Diseases, 3rd edit. New York: Churchill Livingstone, 1990, pp. 2145–2151.

VII
Other Infections and Human Neoplasms

25

Does Childhood Acute Lymphoblastic Leukemia Have an Infectious Etiology?

Mel F. Greaves

"We incline on our evidence to the belief that the solution to the problem of leukaemia lies rather in some peculiar reaction to infection than in the existence of some specific infective agent."

F.J. Poynton, H. Thursfield, and D. Paterson
Hospital for Sick Children, Great Ormond Street, London. 1922 (1)

INTRODUCTION

The idea that infection may play a causal role in the etiology of leukemia has an antiquity equivalent to the recognition of leukemia as a disease; indeed some early descriptions regarded leukemia as a pathological response to infection rather than a malignancy. It was recognized that the general age-associated incidence of pediatric leukemia appeared to mirror that of common infections such as diphtheria and measles. Reports of infections preceding or copresenting with a diagnosis of leukemia (2,3) were considered to reflect causal linkage although other interpretations of this association were obviously possible. Stewart in particular argued that infections occurring in children prior to diagnosis were likely to have arisen as a consequence of the immunosuppressive effects of leukemia (4). Attempts to implicate infectious spread of leukemia via contact with patients drew negative conclusions (5). These early and incomplete studies therefore left any etiologic association of leukemia and microorganisms unsubstantiated and generally disbelieved.

Unrelated to these clinical observations was a separate, although relevant, history of animal leukemias, both "spontaneous" and experimentally induced, that convincingly demonstrated that viruses could be leukemogenic (6,7). It would have been surprising if humans were an exception in this respect and HTLV-I (in adult T-cell leukemia) (8) and Epstein–Barr virus (EBV; in endemic/tropical Burkitt's lymphoma) (9) fulfilled expectations in providing two clear examples of human lymphoid malignancies in which viruses are causally involved. As yet, however, there has been no equivalent, direct evidence linking common types of childhood or adult leukemia with viruses or other infectious agents.

From: *Infectious Causes of Cancer: Targets for Intervention*
Edited by: J. J. Goedert © Humana Press Inc., Totowa, NJ

Many epidemiologic case/control studies over the past few decades have attempted to identify associations that might point to major causal links for childhood leukemia. On the whole, these have provided either weak or contentious associations, for example, with environmental exposure to ionizing radiation, pesticides, or electromagnetic fields (reviewed in *[10–12]*). A small proportion (<5%) of cases of pediatric leukemia involve inherited genetic predisposition *(13)* and in the past there was a small but significantly increased risk (approx 1.4-fold) associated with X-ray pelvimetry during pregnancy *(14,15)*. This unsatisfactory impasse arises in part because of the difficulty in design and executing case/control epidemiologic studies on an adequate scale for a relatively rare disease. The overall rate of childhood leukemia in the United States (whites) and Europeans is around $35/10^6$/yr, giving a cumulative risk of about 1 in 2000 between birth and age 15 yr *(16)*. This problem is then compounded by the biologic heterogeneity of childhood leukemia. Clearly this is not one cancer but a family of related malignancies derived from different stem cells in the hemopoietic hierarchy and/or driven by distinctive molecular mechanisms *(17,18)*. *A priori* it is unlikely that these all have a single causal explanation or that even a well-defined hematologic subtype has an exclusive etiology.

Over the past few years very large-scale case/control studies have been set up, in the United Kingdom and United States in particular, to try and address this issue, taking on board the biology of the disease. A few component studies have so far been reported, for example, on electromagnetic fields *(19),* and others will shortly follow. The United States (CCG) study was not designed to assess any possible role of infection *(20)* but that in the United Kingdom was (along with other possible mechanisms). This distinction arises in part because the hypothesis that infection might be involved in childhood leukemia has been resurrected and given some priority in the United Kingdom. I summarize here the rationale for this and what data appear to support it.

EVIDENCE FOR THE PROSECUTION

If childhood leukemia were indeed linked to infection, then one might expect this to be reflected in demographic features of communities, that is, with instances of clustering or linked to population density or movement and mixing and perhaps with socioeconomic status. This does not necessarily follow of course if leukemia were to be, say, a very rare outcome of a common infection. Moreover, nonrandom clusters could have other, noninfectious causes. Still, there is now rather convincing evidence along these lines. The first and almost classic case of childhood leukemia clustering was reported in 1963 *(21)*.

Between autumn 1957 and summer 1960, eight cases of acute lymphoblastic or "stem cell" leukemia (ALL) occurred in children (aged 3–13 yr) living in a single parish of the town of Niles, a Chicago suburb. In the 1950s Niles underwent a sixfold population expansion, mostly in the parish in which the leukemias occurred. A striking, though possibly incidental, feature of the cluster was the simultaneous occurrence of a miniepidemic of rheumatic-like illness at the school. Acute arthropathy and (false) rheumatic fever are established, if uncommon, sequelae of common bacterial and viral infections. The features of the cluster in Niles were interpreted as indicating the involvement of an agent of high infectivity but low pathogenicity.

Population increases are well recognized to alter the dynamics of infection endemnicity for domestic animals and humans *(22);* and indeed over the centuries have probably had a major impact on disease prevalence, preferential survival, and genetic selection in human populations as both Charles Darwin and the geneticist J. B. S. Haldane prescribed. One interpretation of the Niles time/space cluster of cases was that the admixture of people brought a few infectious carriers of microbe species "X" into contact with a large cohort of previously unexposed and therefore nonimmune individuals; this then facilitated infectious spread and in a few cases, leukemia resulted. In the United Kingdom, epidemiologist Leo Kinlen has vigorously pursued this possibility *(23).* Niles provided the precedent but the real prompt was actually the cluster of childhood leukemia cases around the nuclear reprocessing plant in the village of Seascale in northeast England. This was popularly attributed to environmental contamination or somewhat more evocatively with exposed fathers working at the plant passing on mutant genes to their offspring *(24).* The evidence for these two possibilities was at best very weak and has not been substantiated *(25).*

Kinlen initiated studies to test the idea that population mixing and infection might best explain this cluster based upon the premise that the village of Seascale was an unusual example of a community artificially "assembled" for employment purposes with individuals drawn from all over the United Kingdom, although mostly from professional, middle to high income families. His subsequent series of eight independent studies *(23)* all involve special examples of population movement and mixing in the United Kingdom and have consistently shown an increased relative risk of childhood acute leukemia (averaging around twofold for acute myeloid leukemia [AML] and ALL combined) shortly after the mixing occurred. A similar finding has since been recorded outside of the United Kingdom—in new towns in the New Territories region of Hong Kong *(26).* Here, the increased risk was selective for the common (B-cell precursor) subset of acute lymphoblastic leukemia (cALL). Other demographic studies, particularly by Alexander and colleagues, have provided evidence commensurate with an infectious etiology, particularly for ALL (*see* Table 1).

Other studies have suggested an increased risk of ALL with higher socioeconomic status or affluence *(27,28)* and in our international collaborative studies, we showed that cALL in particular appears to be considerably more common, perhaps by an order of magnitude, in more economically advanced countries or ethnic groups within countries *(29).* Costa Rica appeared to be an exception to this, but this in itself helped prompt a novel explanation for these associations *(29).* It is perhaps paradoxical that improving living standards may increase risk of a disease linked with infection in the young.

These studies certainly raise the spectre of an infectious mechanism but fall considerably short of direct evidence. But then what kind of evidence might one seek and expect to find? Kinlen, drawing on the analogy with the biology and epidemiology of cat leukemia, suggested that a transforming retrovirus might be involved. No evidence to support this view has been forthcoming, but it is unclear if it has been adequately tested. In collaboration with R. Jarrett and colleagues, we have used polymerase chain reaction (PCR) degenerate primers to screen for other candidate viruses, including Herpes family and BK virus *(30)* in leukemic samples. To date, these have produced no positive results *(31)* (and R. Jarrett and M. Greaves, *unpublished data*). If transforming

Table 1
Epidemiologic Evidence for an Infectious Etiology of Childhood ALL[a]

	Parameter	Reference
1. Geographic variation:	"Developed" societies ($\uparrow$ 10×)	*(29,46)*
2. Time trends:	"Emergence" of age (2–5 yr) peak in developed countries[b]	*(47)*
3. Sociodemography:	Socioeconomic status[c]	*(27,28,48,49)*
	Isolated areas	*(48)[d]*
	Time/space clusters	*(21,50–52)*
	Population mixing	*(23,26)*

[a] Evidence reviewed in refs. *(35,47)*.

[b] 1920–1945 in the United Kingdom and the United States (whites); later in Japan. See ref. *(47)* for further discussion.

[c] Status of *community* appears to be more important than that of patient's immediate family.

[d] Association with distance from metropolitan centres and with relatively low population density. Another study, from Sweden, has reported a *higher* incidence rate of ALL in built-up areas with higher population densities *(53)*.

viruses were involved, then one might expect to see an elevated incidence of leukemia in immunodeficient or immunosuppressed children. It is recognized that such individuals do have an increased frequency of EBV-associated lymphomas and of leukemia/lymphoma overall but only very few cases are of cALL (or AML) *(32,33)*. Taking this observation into account along with the apparent risk of ALL with improving living circumstances suggested an alternative idea that has gone under various titles but in essence is a "delayed infection" hypothesis in which the immune response is not the missing protector but rather the instigator of the problem. This idea is very much along the lines hinted at by clinicians treating leukemia in London in 1922; see the quote heading this chapter *(1)*.

The hypothesis (Fig. 1) *(34,35)* emphasizes the critical importance of the pattern and timing of infections in early life in relation to the developmental programming of the immune system. The idea is that the biologic "norm" is for many common or endemic infections to be encountered around birth through the mother, or during infancy through breast milk or other siblings or contacts. Moreover, these early infectious exposures should occur in the context of the immune protection or dose limitation that derives from the mother's transplacental immunoglobulins in the first month after birth and from breast milk thereafter. The naïve neonatal immune system has a distinct cellular composition and response pattern to microbial challenge. Early exposures are educational for the immune system, much as early environmental exposures are critical for the brain and will modulate or prime the infant's immunologic repertoire in a stable fashion as a contingency for potential exposures in the future. These changes include both expansion and elimination or suppression of certain T-cell subsets or clones. In mice, and presumably in humans also, the immunologic response of the neonate is strongly influenced by inherited alleles of the major histocompatibility complex (MHC) class II locus. Recent lifestyle changes in developed countries, including childrearing and breastfeeding practices, inadvertently compromise this evolutionary

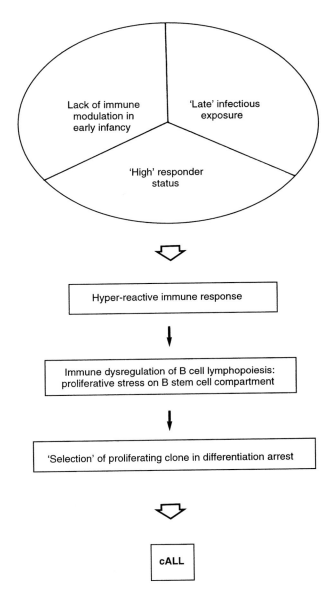

Fig. 1. "Delayed" infection hypothesis for cALL. (From ref. *[35]* with permission.)

adaptation of the immune system. First, pregnant mothers may not themselves have been exposed and therefore are not competent to provide immune protection or modulation. Second, exposure of children themselves to infection has been much reduced through improvements in hygiene and altered patterns of social contacts. These changes have occurred concomitantly with a withdrawal, for social reasons, of prolonged breastfeeding. Breastfeeding has multiple nutritional and immunologic effects on offspring, including the oral transmission of bacteria and viruses, which may constitute early first exposure.

Lack of early exposure may therefore leave the immune system unmodulated or uneducated, and subsequent infection, via social "mixing", with some common microbes then occurs in a biologically abnormal time frame for which the immune system is inappropriately programmed. In some individuals, perhaps rendered susceptible or predisposed by genotype, this could lead to an abnormal immunologic response that increases the risk of leukemia. A simple parallel would be with the high rate of cytomegalovirus and *Haemophilus* infections occurring when previously nonexposed young children attend playgroups *(36)*. The pathologic precedent or model is paralytic poliomyelitis, long considered to be a consequence of delayed infection in "modernized" societies. Delayed first exposure is thought to contribute to the pathogenesis of several diseases associated with affluence and in which infection is implicated. It applies to Epstein–Barr virus infection and infectious mononucleosis in young adults, and a similar idea has been proposed for Hodgkin's disease in young adults *(see* Chapter 7) *(37)*, although the time frame of relevant exposures for these disorders differs from that proposed for childhood leukemia. A similar explanation may hold true for some autoimmune diseases, especially multiple sclerosis *(35)*, for which epidemiologic evidence implicates a delayed but common infection of low pathogenicity in genetically susceptible individuals.

NATURAL HISTORY OF ALL

If a nonspecific or indirect response to infection was to be causally involved in ALL, then one would need to place this in the context of the natural history of the disease. Would infection be expected to *initiate* leukemia or promote it (or both)? Some insight has been gained recently into the natural history of childhood ALL by the use of acquired gene fusions that are associated with pathogenesis and provide stable and unique clonal markers *(18)*. Studies on identical twins *(38)* and retrospective PCR analysis of neonatal blood spots (Guthrie cards) *(39)* have provided convincing evidence that the *MLL–AF4* fusion gene characteristic of infant ALL is generated *in utero* during fetal hemopoiesis, probably as an initiating event. This is perhaps as to be expected in patients less than 2 yr of age. But the same now appears to apply to most children with ALL. Twin pairs and Guthrie spot data again provide evidence for a prenatal, fetal *initiation,* in this instance via *TEL–AML1* gene fusion *(40–42)*.

The twin studies provide another clue also. The concordance rates for leukemia in identical twins will reflect the requirements for additional events after the initiation of leukemogenesis in the fetus *(18)*. For infant ALL with *MLL* fusion genes, the concordance rate is very high. Accurate figures are not available but rates are around 25–50% and may approach 100% for those with a single placenta. Latency is also remarkably brief. An implication of the very high concordance rate plus very brief latency or time frame of clonal evolution to clinical disease is that the *MLL* gene fusion may be *sufficient* for leukemogenesis. Alternatively, the fusion gene would have to very efficiently provoke whatever other secondary changes are necessary *(18)*. But for cALL in children, the story is different. The precise concordance rate for identical twins is again not known but is around 5% with an average postnatal latency of 3 yr *(18)*. This then implies that fetal initiation, by *TEL–AML1,* is *insufficient* for overt leukemia development; from this follow two important predictions. First, many more children are born

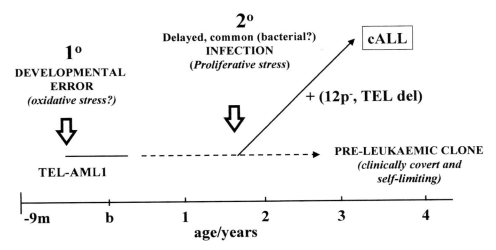

Fig. 2. A two-step model for the natural history of cALL. (From ref. *[18]* with permission.)

with a *TEL–AML1*-driven preleukemic clone than ever become diagnosed with leukemia. This is currently being assessed by molecular screening of unselected cord blood samples. Second, something else is required after birth for cALL to develop. As with other medical studies on twins (e.g., autoimmune disease), the suspicion then falls on environmental exposures that, in this case, might provoke or promote evolution of the fetal "preleukemic" clones.

Although we obviously cannot rule out that the infectious event, if it is relevant at all, occurs *in utero,* the most plausible model becomes one in which delayed infection provides the necessary noncarcinogenic *promoting* event (Fig. 2). The recent suggestion of a seasonal onset of clinical symptoms for cALL *(43)* is in accord with this possibility. There are a number of ways by which infection might provoke the critical second event including via transient marrow hypoplasia induced by T-cell derived γ-interferon followed by florid regeneration.

There are both animal *(44)* and clinical *(45)* precedents for lymphoid malignancies originating via indirect immunologic or infectious mechanisms. The nature of the infections involved remains entirely conjectural at present although there is no appealing logic in considering only viruses; bacteria, and particularly common bacteria with super-antigens, are plausible candidates. Can this idea be stringently tested? Obviously it is difficult to substantiate an indirect infectious mechanism, particularly if common infections are involved, and if no single species of microorganism is responsible. But there are epidemiologic predictions that follow on from the hypothesis (Table 2). These are being assessed in the UK National Case/Control Study of Childhood Cancer and in fact already have some support from prior studies (Table 2).

Clearly this model mechanism is speculative but it is plausible and there is a reasonable expectation that it will be refuted or endorsed by ongoing epidemiologic studies. If it is correct, then the implication is that it might be possible to prevent a substantial fraction of childhood leukemias by some kind of prophylactic vaccination in infancy. Alternatively, or in addition, changes in lifestyle factors influencing social 'exposures' of infants could have a beneficial impact.

Table 2
Predictions of the Delayed Infection Hypothesis for Childhood ALL

Parameter	Relative risk	Provisional supporting evidence
1. *Decreased* infections in first year of life	↑	*(54–56)*
2. *Decreased* social contacts in infants	↑	*(57)*
3. *Decreased* length of breastfeeding	↑	*(58)*
4. Others: HLA associations	↑ or ↓	*(59)*

REFERENCES

1. Poynton FJ, Thursfield H, Paterson D. The severe blood diseases of childhood: a series of observations from the Hospital for Sick Children, Great Ormond Street. Br J Child Dis 1922; XIX:128–144.
2. Cooke JV. The incidence of acute leukemia in children. JAMA 1942; 119:547–550.
3. Pierce M. Childhood leukemia. J Pediatr 1936; 8:66–95.
4. Kneale GW, Stewart AM. Pre-cancers and liability to other diseases. Br J Cancer 1978; 37:448–457.
5. Ward G. The infective theory of acute leukaemia. Br J Child Dis 1917; 14:10–20.
6. Gross L. Viral etiology of cancer and leukemia: a look into the past, present and future. Cancer Res 1978; 38:485–493.
7. Goldman JM, Jarrett O (eds). Mechanisms of viral leukaemogenesis. Edinburgh: Churchill Livingstone, 1984.
8. Gallo RC, Essex ME, Gross L (eds). Human T-cell leukemia/lymphoma virus. The family of human T-lymphotropic retroviruses: their role in malignancies and association with AIDS. Cold Spring Harbor, NY: Cold Spring Harbor Laboratory Press, 1984.
9. Lenoir GM, O'Conor GT, Olweny CLM (eds). Burkitt's lymphoma: a human cancer model. Lyon: World Health Organization International Agency for Research on Cancer, 1985.
10. Linet MS, Devesa SS. Descriptive epidemiology of childhood leukaemia. Br J Cancer 1991; 63:424–429.
11. Neglia JP, Robison L. Epidemiology of the childhood acute leukemias. Pediatr Clin North Am 1988; 35:675–692.
12. Ross JA, Davies SM, Potter JD, Robison LL. Epidemiology of childhood leukemia, with a focus on infants. Epidemiol Rev 1994; 16:243–272.
13. Taylor GM, Birch JM. The hereditary basis of human leukemia. In: Henderson ES, Lister TA, Greaves MF (eds). Leukemia, 6th edit. Philadelphia: WB Saunders, 1996, pp. 210–245.
14. Boice JDJ, Inskip PD. Radiation-induced leukemia. In: Henderson ES, Lister TA, Greaves MF (eds). Leukemia, 6th edit. Philadelphia: WB Saunders, 1996, pp. 195–209.
15. Doll R, Wakeford R. Risk of childhood cancer from fetal irradiation. Br J Radiol 1997; 70:130–139.
16. Parkin DM, Stiller CA, Draper GJ, Bieber CA. The international incidence of childhood cancer. Int J Cancer 1988; 42:511–520.
17. Greaves M. The new biology of leukemia. In: Henderson ES, Lister TA, Greaves MF (eds). Leukemia, 6th edit. Philadelphia: WB Saunders, 1996, pp. 34–45.
18. Greaves M. Molecular genetics, natural history and the demise of childhood leukaemia. Eur J Cancer 1999; 35:173–185.
19. Linet MS, Hatch EE, Kleinerman RA, et al. Residential exposure to magnetic fields and acute lymphoblastic leukemia in children. N Engl J Med 1997; 337:1–7.

20. Robison LL, Buckley JD, Bunin G. Assessment of environmental and genetic factors in the etiology of childhood cancers: the children's cancer group epidemiology program. Environ Health Perspect 1995; 103:111–116.
21. Heath CW Jr, Hasterlik RJ. Leukemia among children in a suburban community. Am J Med 1963; 34:796–812.
22. Anderson RM, May RM. Immunisation and herd immunity. Lancet 1990; 335:641–645.
23. Kinlen LJ. Infective cause of childhood leukaemia. Lancet 1989; i:378–379.
24. Gardner MJ, Hall AJ, Downes S, Terrell JD. Follow-up study of children born to mothers resident in Seascale, West Cumbria (birth cohort). Br Med J 1987; 295:822–827.
25. Bridges BA. Committee on Medical Aspects of Radiation in the Environment (COMARE) Fourth Report. UK Department of Public Health, 1996.
26. Alexander FE, Chan LC, Lam TH, et al. Clustering of childhood leukaemia in Hong Kong: association with the childhood peak and common acute lymphoblastic leukaemia and with population mixing. Br J Cancer 1997; 75:457–463.
27. Rodrigues L, Hills M, McGale P, Elliott P. Socio-economic factors in relation to childhood leukaemia and non-Hodgkin lymphomas: an analysis based on small area statistics for census tracts. In: Draper G (ed). The Geographical Epidemiology of Childhood Leukaemia and Non-Hodgkin's Lymphoma in Great Britain 1966–83. London: OPCS, 1991, pp. 47–56.
28. Draper GJ, Vincent TJ, O'Conor CM, Stiller CA. Socio-economic factors and variation in incidence rates between county districts. In: Draper G (ed). The Geographical Epidemiology of Childhood Leukaemia and Non-Hodgkin's Lymphoma in Great Britain 1966–83. London: OPCS, 1991, pp. 37–46.
29. Greaves MF, Colman SM, Beard MEJ, et al. Geographical distribution of acute lymphoblastic leukaemia subtypes: second report of the collaborative group study. Leukemia 1993; 7:27–34.
30. Smith M. Consideration on a possible viral etiology for B-precursor acute lymphoblastic leukemia of childhood. J Immunother 1997; 20:89–100.
31. MacKenzie J, Perry J, Ford AM, Jarrett RF, Greaves M. JC and BK virus sequences are not detectable in leukaemic samples from children with common acute lymphoblastic leukaemia. Br J Cancer 1999; 81:898–899.
32. Filipovich AH, Zerbe D, Spector BD, Kersey JH. Lymphomas in persons with naturally occurring immunodeficiency disorders. In: Magrath IT, O'Conor GT, Ramot B (eds). Pathogenesis of Leukemias and Lymphomas: Environmental Influences. New York: Raven Press, 1984, pp. 225–234.
33. Filipovich AH, Mathur A, Kamat D, Kersey JH, Shapiro RS. Lymphoproliferative disorders and other tumors complicating immunodeficiencies. Immunodeficiency 1994; 5:91–112.
34. Greaves MF. Speculations on the cause of childhood acute lymphoblastic leukemia. Leukemia 1988; 2:120–125.
35. Greaves MF. Aetiology of acute leukaemia. Lancet 1997; 349:344–349.
36. Ferson MJ. Infections in day care. Curr Opin Pediatr 1993; 5:35–40.
37. Gutensohn N, Cole P. Childhood social environment and Hodgkin's disease. N Engl J Med 1981; 304:135–140.
38. Ford AM, Ridge SA, Cabrera ME, et al. *In utero* rearrangements in the trithorax-related oncogene in infant leukaemias. Nature 1993; 363:358–360.
39. Gale KB, Ford AM, Repp R, et al. Backtracking leukemia to birth: identification of clonotypic gene fusion sequences in neonatal blood spots. Proc Natl Acad Sci USA 1997; 94:13950–13954.
40. Ford AM, Bennett CA, Price CM, Bruin MCA, Van Wering ER, Greaves M. Fetal origins of the *TEL–AML1* fusion gene in identical twins with leukemia. Proc Natl Acad Sci USA 1998; 95:4584–4588.
41. Wiemels JL, Ford AM, Van Wering ER, Postma A, Greaves M. Protracted and variable latency of acute lymphoblastic leukaemia after *TEL–AML1* gene fusion in utero. Blood 1999; 94:1057–1062.

42. Wiemels JL, Cazzaniga G, Daniotti M, et al. Pre-natal origin of acute lymphoblastic leukaemia in children. Lancet 1999; 354:1499–1503.

43. Westerbeek RMC, Blair V, Eden OB, et al. Seasonal variations in the onset of childhood leukaemia and lymphoma. Br J Cancer 1998; 78:119–124.

44. Tsiagbe VK, Yoshimoto T, Asakawa J, Cho SY, Meruelo D, Thorbecke GJ. Linkage of superanti-gen-like stimulation of syngeneic T cells in a mouse model of follicular center B cell lymphoma to transcription of endogenous mammary tumor virus. EMBO J 1993; 12:2313–2320.

45. Wotherspoon AC, Doglioni C, Diss TC, et al. Regression of primary low-grade B-cell gastric lymphoma of mucosa-associated lymphoid tissue type after eradication of *Helicobacter pylori.* Lancet 1993; 342:575–577.

46. Ramot B, Magrath I. Hypothesis: the environment is a major determinant of the immunological sub-type of lymphoma and acute lymphoblastic leukaemia in children. Br J Haematol 1982; 52:183–189.

47. Greaves MF, Alexander FE. An infectious etiology for common acute lymphoblastic leukemia in childhood? Leukemia 1993; 7:349–360.

48. Alexander FE, Ricketts TJ, McKinney PA, Cartwright RA. Community lifestyle characteristics and risk of acute lymphoblastic leukaemia in children. Lancet 1990; 336:1461–1465.

49. Petridou E, Trichopoulos D, Kalapothaki V, et al. The risk profile of childhood leukaemia in Greece: a nationwide case-control study. Br J Cancer 1997; 76:1241–1247.

50. Alexander FE. Space-time clustering of childhood acute lymphoblastic leukaemia: indirect evidence for a transmissible agents. Br J Cancer 1992; 65:589–592.

51. Alexander FE, Wray N, Boyle P, et al. Clustering of childhood leukaemia: a European study in progress. J Epidemiol Biostat 1996; 1:13–24.

52. Petridou E, Revinthi K, Alexander FE, et al. Space-time clustering of childhood leukaemia in Greece: evidence supporting a viral aetiology. Br J Cancer 1996; 73:1278–1283.

53. Hjalmars U, Gustafsson G. Higher risk for acute childhood lymphoblastic leukaemia in Swedish population centres 1973–1994. Br J Cancer 1999; 79:30–33.

54. van Steensel-Moll HA, Valkenburg HA, van Zanen GE. Childhood leukemia and infectious diseases in the first year of life: a register-based case/control study. Am J Epidemiol 1986; 124:590–594.

55. Robison LL, Neglia J. Personal communication to author. August 1998.

56. McKinney PA, Juszczak E, Findlay E, Smith K, Thomson CS. Pre- and perinatal risk factors for childhood leukaemia and other malignancies: a Scottish case control study. Br J Cancer, 1999; 80:1844–1851.

57. Petridou E, Kassimos D, Kalmanti M, et al. Age of exposure to infections and risk of childhood leukaemia. Br Med J 1993; 307:774.

58. Shu XO, Linet MS, Steinbuch M, et al. Breast feeding and risk of childhood acute leukemia. J Natl Cancer Inst 1999; 91:1765–1772.

59. Taylor GM, Robinson MD, Binchy A, et al. Preliminary evidence of an association between HLA-DPB1*0201 and childhood common acute lymphoblastic leukaemia supports an infectious aetiology. Leukemia 1995; 9:440–443.

26

Polyoma Viruses (JC Virus, BK Virus, and Simian Virus 40) and Human Cancer

Keerti V. Shah

Polyomaviruses are widely distributed in nature and are known to infect humans, monkeys, cattle, rabbits, mice, hamsters, rats, and parakeets. Of the 12 polyomaviruses described to date *(1)*, the two human polyomaviruses, BK virus (BKV) and JC virus (JCV), and a polyomavirus of monkeys designated simian virus 40 (SV40) have been investigated for their potential role in human cancers. BKV and JCV are common infections of childhood, and they persist indefinitely in the infected individuals. Human exposure to SV40 occurred in the late 1950s and early 1960s mainly as a result of immunization with poliovirus vaccines inadvertently prepared in SV40-contaminated monkey kidney cultures.

INFECTIOUS AGENT

Polyomaviruses and papillomaviruses constitute the two subfamilies of the family *Papovaviridae.* Papovaviruses are small, nonenveloped viruses with icosahedral capsids and circular, covalently closed, double-stranded DNA genome. They multiply in the nucleus. Viruses of the two subfamilies are not related genetically or immunologically and differ in the following respects. Polyomaviruses have a smaller genome (5 kb), and about one half of the genetic information is carried on each DNA strand. Papillomaviruses have a larger genome (8 kb), and all of the genetic information is carried on a single strand. After initial infection, polyomaviruses reach their target organs by viremia, whereas papillomaviruses do not have a viremic phase; they multiply and produce pathology at the site of infection. The role of polyomaviruses in human cancer is equivocal but that of human papillomaviruses in genital cancer is firmly established (*see* Chapters 14 and 15).

The polyomavirus DNA is condensed into a tight superhelical minichromosome by four cellular histones. The viral genome consists of (1) a noncoding regulatory region of about 400 basepairs that is involved in the regulation of viral transcription and replication; (2) an early region that codes for the nonstructural large and small T antigens and that is expressed prior to viral DNA replication; and (3) a late region that codes for the viral capsid proteins VP1, VP2, and VP3 and that is expressed following viral DNA replication.

From: *Infectious Causes of Cancer: Targets for Intervention*
Edited by: J. J. Goedert © Humana Press Inc., Totowa, NJ

The large T antigen is a multifunctional protein that interacts with specific DNA sequences and with a wide variety of host cell proteins *(2)*. It is essential for virus multiplication, mediates cell transformation, and is responsible for the oncogenic properties of polyomaviruses in laboratory animals. During the lytic cycle, the T antigen, through its interaction with cellular proteins, stimulates cells to enter the cell cycle and to replicate their DNA. It initiates viral DNA replication through its ability to assist in the assembly of preinitiation complexes at the origin of viral DNA replication. It regulates the shift from early- to late-region viral transcription during lytic infection.

BKV, JCV, and SV40 display a high degree of nucleotide sequence homology. Overall, JCV genome shares 75% of BKV's sequences and 69% of SV40's sequences *(3)*.

TRANSFORMATION AND ONCOGENICITY

In permissive cells (derived generally from the natural hosts of the viruses), polyomavirus infection is productive and results in the synthesis of large numbers of virions and death of the infected cells. In cells of heterologous species, the polyomavirus infection is nonpermissive and may lead to transformation. The ability of the polyomaviruses to transform established cell lines and primary cultures and to produce tumors in laboratory animals has been studied extensively. The presence of T antigen is required for the initiation as well as for the maintenance of transformation. In transformed cells, as a rule, the viral genome is integrated into the cellular DNA. The capacity of T antigen to transform cells is mediated, in part, by its ability to complex with and to inactivate tumor suppressor proteins pRb and p53.

BKV, JCV, and SV40 are tumorigenic for laboratory animals, especially Syrian hamsters. The animal species, the age of the animal, the route of inoculation, and the amount of virus in the inoculum are important determinants of oncogenicity. Table 1 lists the species in which the viruses produce tumors and the histologic types of the main tumors. Brain tumors are induced by all three viruses. BKV most often produces tumors of the ventricular surfaces, such as ependymomas and choroid plexus papilloma *(4,5)*, whereas JCV produces predominantly tumors of neural origin, such as medulloblastoma, glioblastoma, and astrocytoma *(6,7)*. JCV is unique among viruses in its ability to produce experimental brain tumors in primates, specifically astrocytomas in owl and squirrel monkeys *(8)*. SV40 produces a large variety of tumors in laboratory rodents, including mesotheliomas in hamsters.

The site and phenotypes of experimentally produced tumors have provided leads for the study of whether polyomaviruses contribute to the etiology of human cancers. This is quite appropriate. However, it should be recognized that in experimental infections, very large amounts of virus are introduced directly into a susceptible tissue (e.g., in the brain of a newborn animal by intracerebral inoculation) and that such exposures are never encountered in natural situations. Also, experimental tumors are produced in species in which the viruses do not multiply to produce lytic infections.

BIOLOGY, EPIDEMIOLOGY, AND CLINICAL FEATURES

Polyomaviruses have a narrow host range. BKV and JCV infect only humans. SV40 naturally infects a number of species of the genus *Macaca* *(9)*. In animal colonies, SV40 infection may be naturally transmitted to other old-world species of the same family *(Cercopithidae)* as the macaques, but not to new-world simian species, which

Table 1
Oncogenicity of BKV, JCV, and SV40 for Laboratory Animals

Virus	Species	Tumor types
JCV	Hamster	Medulloblastoma, glioblastoma, astrocytoma, pineocytoma, retinoblastoma, neuroblastoma
	Owl and squirrel monkeys	Astrocytoma
BKV	Hamster, mouse, rat (in one or more of the above species)	Ependymoma, choroid plexus papilloma, glioma, pineal gland tumors, neuroblastoma, insulinoma, nephroblastoma, osteosarcoma, fibrosarcoma, lymphoma
SV40	Hamster	Ependymoma, lymphoma, osteogenic sarcoma, fibrosarcoma, mesothelioma

belong to other families. BKV and JCV infect cells by binding to sialic acid based receptors. SV40 does not interact with sialic acid, but binds to major histocompatibility (MHC) class I proteins for entry into cells *(10)*.

BKV infections occur early and JCV infections late in childhood. Serologic data indicate that, in the United States, 50% of the children are infected with BKV by the age of 3 and nearly everyone is infected by 10–11 yr of age. The route of transmission is not known but is suspected to be through the respiratory tract. Antibodies to JCV are acquired at later ages, with a 50% prevalence by 10–14 yr of age and a 75% prevalence among adults. Tonsil tissue may be the primary site of JCV infection. After entry into the body, the viruses reach their target organs, the kidneys, by viremia. They persist indefinitely in the kidneys and in the B lymphocytes of the infected hosts. BKV and JCV are reactivated and excreted in urine in times of immunosuppression (such as with AIDS or organ transplant) and also during pregnancy and old age. JCV is shed frequently in the urine of nonimmunosuppressed adults.

Natural SV40 infection of rhesus macaques is comparable to BKV and JCV infections of humans. In the wild, antibodies to SV40 are detected in almost all adult rhesus and in a proportion of juvenile animals *(9)*. In captivity, the infection spreads rapidly to susceptible animals. The virus remains latent in rhesus kidneys after primary infection. Experimentally, the rhesus is readily infected after oral (or intragastric), subcutaneous, and intravenous inoculation of SV40.

Primary infections with these polyomaviruses are almost always completely asymptomatic and unrecognized. Nearly all serious illnesses associated with polyomavirus infection occur as complications of diseases in which cell-mediated immunity is compromised *(1)*. JCV is the etiologic agent of progressive multifocal leukoencephalopathy (PML), a subacute, fatal, demyelinating disease of the central nervous system that occurs in patients with AIDS or other chronic conditions such as cancer or organ transplants. Prior to 1982, PML was a rare disease affecting individuals in the fifth and sixth decades of life. With the advent of AIDS, PML now occurs in younger individuals and the number of cases has increased manifold. It is recognized in 1–2% of human immunodeficiency virus(HIV)-related deaths.

The broad outline of the pathogenesis of PML is well understood. It results from the productive infection of oligodendrocytes in the brain by JCV, most often by the virus reactivated in the immunocompromised host. The oligodendrocytes produce large amounts of JCV virions and are destroyed by the infection. Oligodendrocytes produce and maintain myelin; their destruction is the hallmark of the disease. In addition to the oligodendrocytes with enlarged nuclei, the PML lesions also contain large, bizarre, often multinucleated astrocytes that resemble malignant cells *(11)*.

BKV infection is associated with hemorrhagic cystitis in bone marrow transplant recipients, with occasional cases of cystitis and renal disease in immunosuppressed individuals, and rarely with encephalitis *(1,12)*. In rhesus monkeys immunocompromised by simian immunodeficiency virus (SIV), SV40 produces a PML-like illness *(13)*. SV40 also is associated with occasional cases of renal and lung disease in rhesus macaques *(14)*. Almost all recognized illnesses associated with JCV, BKV and SV40 result from productive infections and destruction of specific cell types. However, the report of an SV40-positive malignant astrocytoma in an SIV-infected pigtail macaque suggests the possibility that polyomaviral infection may lead to tumors in the immunosuppressed host *(15)*.

ROLE OF JCV, BKV, AND SV40 IN HUMAN CANCERS

This has been studied by examination of tumors or tumor-derived cells for polyomavirus virions, viral T antigen, and viral sequences. Sera of cancer patients have been tested for antibodies to virus-coded proteins. A large number of tumor types has been studied. Special attention has been given to human tumors that occur at the sites of polyomavirus multiplication and to tumors that resemble experimentally induced cancers, particularly brain tumors, bone tumors, and mesotheliomas. In the first publication on this subject, in 1976 Fiori and DiMayorca *(16)* reported that BKV sequences were detected by Southern hybridization of DNAs from a variety of tumors. Since that time a large number of studies have been published. Comprehensive recent reviews of these studies *(17–20)* as well as the published proceedings of an international conference in January, 1997 on "SV40: a possible human polyomavirus" *(21)* are available. Most of the data relate to detection of viral sequences in cancers using polymerase chain reaction (PCR) technology. For virtually all tumors examined, both positive and negative data have been reported. JCV has been associated with brain tumors and recently with colon cancer. BKV sequences have been detected in a large variety of tumors, including, most recently, childhood neuroblastoma. SV40 sequences have been reported from pediatric brain tumors, common brain tumors, pituitary adenomas, osteosarcomas and other bone tumors, mesotheliomas, and thyroid carcinomas. The role of the three viruses in human tumors, especially tumors of the nervous system, osteosarcomas, and mesotheliomas are reviewed in the following sections, focusing mostly on studies conducted in the 1990s.

JC Virus

Brain Tumors Coexistent with PML

Several cases of brain tumors coexisting in brains with PML have been reported *(22–25)*. Some of these tumors were topographically close to PML lesions and may have arisen in areas of the brain affected by PML *(22,23,25)*. The PML lesions in these

Table 2
JCV, BKV, and SV40 Sequences in Selected Nervous System Tumors: A Summary of Recent Studies

| Tumor type | Reference | Virus (no. positive/no. tested) | | |
		JCV	BKV	SV40
Choroid plexus papilloma	*(41)*			10/20
	(31)	1/16	0/16	6/16
	(36,37)			5/6
Ependymoma	*(41)*			10/11
	(31)	0/16	0/16	9/16
	(42)			0/10
	(36,37)			8/11
	(66)			4/13
Medulloblastoma	*(30)*	10/11		
	(31)	0/17	1/17	9/17
Xanthoastrocytoma	*(27)*	1/1		
Other gliomas	*(28)*	0/75	0/75	
	(26)	1/1		
	(29)	0/52		
	(31)	3/150	5/150	51/150
	(36,37)			10/30
	(66)			3/20
Neuroblastoma	*(38)*		18/18	
	(41)			0/12

cases contained large amounts of JCV *(22,23)*. The astrocytes in PML lesions have JCV DNA, and they morphologically resemble "transformed" cells. Therefore, it is plausible that the tumors arise from multiplication of JCV-transformed astrocytes in the immunocompromised host. On the other hand, immunocompromising conditions that favor the development of PML may also independently favor the emergence of brain tumors unrelated to JCV infection. A complete characterization of the JCV–tumor cell association may be helpful in assessing if the virus is etiologically linked to these tumors.

JCV Sequences in Brain Tumors

JCV sequences have been reported recently in some brain tumors (Table 2). Rencic et al. *(26)* described a single case of oligoastrocytoma in a 61-yr-old, HIV-negative immunocompetent male. The tumor was an oligodendroglioma with distinct areas of fibrillary astrocytoma. There were large areas of hypomyelinated white matter in areas of tumor infiltration. JCV DNA, RNA, and T antigen were detected in the tumor tissue. JCV T antigen was identified in the nuclei of tumor cells in the oligodendroglioma component, but not in tumor cells in the astrocytoma component of the tumor. Boldorini et al. *(27)* identified JCV DNA in a pleomorphic xanthoastrocytoma of a 9-yr-old immunocompetent child. They examined the tumor for JCV because the histopathologic features of pleomorphic xanthoastrocytoma resemble those of lytic

JCV infection. Other studies of gliomas have been negative. Arthur et al. *(28)* did not detect JCV (or BKV) sequences in 75 glial tumors or tumor-derived cell lines, and Herbarth et al. *(29)* also failed to detect JCV DNA in 52 gliomas or tumor-derived cell lines.

Khalili et al. *(30)* have reported JCV DNA in all but one of 11 childhood medulloblastomas. JCV T antigen was detected in a majority of the cases. In contrast, Huang et al. *(31)* did not detect JCV genome in any of 17 medulloblastomas, but they recovered SV40 genome from five of these tissues.

In a recent report, JCV DNA sequences were recovered from a large majority of colorectal cancers as well as of normal mucosal tissues adjacent to the cancers *(32)*. Cancer tissues contained greater quantities of JCV DNA than did normal tissues. Treatment of the specimens with topoisomerase 1 (which would relax the supercoiled viral DNA) improved the efficiency of JCV detection.

JCV and Genetic Instability

Neel and co-workers *(33)* have proposed a hypothesis that JCV infection (and perhaps BKV infection) may result in chromosomal damage in cells at the site of virus multiplication and that some of the altered cells may progress to cancer.

JCV and Acute Lymphocytic Leukemia (ALL)

An infectious etiology for ALL has been suspected for a long time (*see* Chapter 25), and JCV was noted to have several likely characteristics of an infectious agent able to cause ALL in children *(34)*. However, JCV, BKV, or SV40 sequences were not identified in leukemia cells of 2- to 5-yr-old children *(35)*.

BK Virus

BKV sequences have been identified in a large variety of human cancers, including lung and liver carcinomas; kidney, prostate, bladder, and urethral carcinomas; almost all histologic types of common brain tumors; osteosarcomas; carcinomas of the uterine cervix and vulva; carcinomas of the lip and tongue; Kaposi's sarcoma; and retinoblastomas. A comprehensive review by Barbanti-Brodano and his colleagues *(17)*, who have made the major contributions to this topic, should be consulted for details. The most recent studies are reviewed here.

BKV and Tumors of the Nervous System

BKV sequences frequently have been amplified from brain tumors (Table 2). It is curious that the specimens from which BKV sequences were recovered most frequently were also found to be SV40-positive in subsequent studies *(36,37)*.

In a recent article, Flaegstad et al. *(38)* raised the possibility that BK virus may contribute to the development of neuroblastoma in young children. Neuroblastomas are tumors of the autonomic nervous system located in the adrenal glands. BKV sequences were recovered by PCR from all 18 neuroblastomas studied, and in 17 cases BKV DNA was localized to tumor cells by *in situ* hybridization. BKV T antigen was detected in 16 specimens. Five normal adrenal glad specimens were virus negative.

BKV and Kaposi's Sarcoma

In one report, BKV sequences were found in 100% of Kaposi's skin lesions and 75% of Kaposi's sarcoma cell lines (*see also* Chapter 10) *(39)*.

SV40

SV40 has no reservoir in the United States or Europe. As described in detail in previous reviews *(9,40),* the major documented human exposure to SV40 was between 1955 and 1963 as a result of immunization with SV40-contaminated poliovirus vaccines. Although about 100 million people in the United States were immunized with inactivated Salk poliovirus vaccines in that time period, only a small minority probably received live SV40 with the vaccines *(9).*

SV40 and Brain Tumors

In 1992, Bergsagel and colleagues first reported detection of SV40 sequences in two types of rare pediatric brain tumors, ependymomas and choroid plexus papillomas *(41)* (Table 2). As they had been born long after SV40's contamination of poliovirus vaccines, it was suggested that these young children may have become infected by transplacental transmission of SV40 from infected mothers. Krainer et al. *(42)* could not confirm the presence of SV40 in ependymomas. Subsequent studies reported SV40 sequences not only from pediatric brain tumors but also from many histologic types of adult gliomas *(31).* In this regard, the results from an earlier study (not listed in Table 2) are pertinent. Greenlee et al. *(43)* cultured tumor cells from 80 brain tumors and stained them for SV40 T antigen. Cells from all of the tumors were clearly negative for SV40 T antigen. In contrast, tumor cells cultured from SV40 tumors experimentally produced in hamsters stained uniformly positive for SV40 T antigen.

SV40 and Osteosarcoma

In several recent studies, a significant proportion of osteosarcomas was positive for SV40 sequences by PCR *(44–46).* Using Southern hybridization, Mendoza et al. examined 10 unamplified tissue DNAs (that previously were SV40-positive by PCR) and found patterns of hybridization suggestive of viral integration in five tissues *(45).* In one instance, the pattern of viral integration was seen in DNA of normal tissue of a tumor-bearing patient. Many of the tissues that were PCR-positive for SV40 also contained the BKV genome.

SV40 and Mesothelioma

SV40 sequences were recovered from mesotheliomas in several studies in the United States, United Kingdom, and Europe (Table 3). However, two laboratories, one in Europe *(47)* and the other in the United States *(48),* failed to detect SV40 sequences in mesothelioma tissues. In addition, Griffiths et al. *(49)* expressed some doubt about the positive data from their own laboratory. They remarked on the possibility of obtaining false-positive PCR by contamination with the many laboratory reagents, such as mammalian expression vectors, that contain SV40 sequences.

SV40 and Other Cancers

SV40 sequences have also been reported in thyroid carcinoma *(50).*

ARE POLYOMAVIRUSES ETIOLOGICALLY LINKED TO HUMAN CANCER?

There are three polyomaviruses and each is associated with several types of cancers. Therefore, there are 15–20 virus-cancer associations. However, we discuss them as a group where possible, and point out specific details when necessary.

Table 3
SV40 Sequences in Mesothelioma Tissues by PCR Technology

Study (reference)	Country	Proportion with SV40	Comment
Carbone et al., 1994 *(53)*	USA	29/48	
Cristaudo et al., 1995 *(54)*	Italy	8/11	
Pepper et al., 1996 *(55)*	UK	4/9	
Strickler et al., 1996 *(48)*	USA	0/48	
DeLuca et al., 1997 *(56)*	Italy	30/35	
Galateau-Salle et al., 1998 *(57)*	France	10/21	Also found SV40 in 18 of 63 bronchopulmonary carcinomas
Griffiths et al., 1998 *(49)*	UK	?/26	Questioned the positive data of their own laboratory
Testa et al., 1998 *(58)*	USA	9/12	In each of four participating laboratories
Mulatero et al., 1999 *(47)*	UK	0/12	

In 1965, A. Bradford Hill proposed that an association between an environmental exposure and disease could be examined from many different viewpoints to assess if the exposure caused the disease *(51)*. We will examine the polyomavirus-cancer associations in the light of these criteria.

(1) *Strength of association: Is the effect of the exposures large?*

None of the polyomavirus-cancer studies have been performed in a case-control setting or as cohort studies. Therefore it is not possible to estimate the strength of the association. In viral infections that have been etiologically linked to human cancers, the relative risks of exposure are estimated to be high, about 20 for hepatitis B virus (HBV) and hepatocellular carcinoma and about 62 for human papilloma viruses (HPVs) and squamous cell carcinoma of the cervix *(52)*.

(2) *Consistency of association: Is the effect seen consistently in different studies?*

None of the associations are completely consistent. The observation that ependymomas have SV40 sequences *(41)* was contradicted in another study *(42)*. Medulloblastomas were reported to have JCV sequences in one study *(30)*, and SV40 sequences (but no JCV sequences) in another study *(31)*. The high prevalence of SV40 in gliomas in one study *(31)* was not reproduced in other studies *(28,29)*. Several studies, in different parts of the world, reported the association of SV40 with mesothelioma *(53–58)*. However, two laboratories *(47,48)* reported negative data, and a third *(49)* expressed reservations about their own positive findings. There also are wide variations in the proportion of normal tissues found to be virus positive. For example, SV40 was reported to be positive in 45% of semen fluids in one study *(37)* and in 0% in another study *(49)*.

Most of the studies for the three viruses have been conducted with sensitive but error-prone PCR methods. Positive PCR results have been difficult to confirm with more robust, if less sensitive assays such as Southern hybridization of unamplified tumor DNAs. The repeated finding of polyomavirus sequences in human cancers by such a large number of laboratories, and the identification of viral transcripts and virus-coded proteins in some of the studies, is intriguing but the significance of these observations remains unclear at present. Methodologic artifacts and presence of latent genomes may account for some of the positive findings.

(3) *Specificity: Is the exposure related to a specific type of disease at a specific site?*

Taken together, the three polyomaviruses are recovered from a bewildering variety of cancers and from many different sites. As for individual viruses, JCV has some specificity for brain tumors. BKV genomes have been reported from a large number of unrelated sites. SV40 has been recovered from carcinomas and sarcoma, from very young children and from adults, and from tumors at disparate sites such as the brain, the bone, and the mesothelium. None of the polyomavirus-tumor associations have the specificity comparable to that of HBV for hepatocytes and of HPVs for squamous epithelia.

(4) *Temporality: Does exposure precede the disease?*

Prospective studies that might answer this question have not been carried out for any of the polyomaviruses. BKV infections are universal and occur so early in childhood that it would be difficult to set up a study of BKV-negative and BKV-positive cohorts.

However, human SV40 exposure occurred over a limited time period (1955–1963) so it was possible to inquire if the incidence of specific cancers was influenced by SV40 exposure. Such analyses have not revealed that SV40 exposure is associated with excess risk for all brain tumors, for ependymomas, for osteosarcomas or for medulloblastomas *(59–61)*. The SV40-exposed cohort has not yet reached the age of peak incidence for mesothelioma *(59)*. The increase in incidence of mesothelioma after 1950 is well explained by exposure to asbestos around the Second World War. It would be possible to examine prospectively if SV40 increases the risk of asbestos-associated mesothelioma. The SV40 status of the large number of asbestos-exposed individuals who are now healthy but at a high risk of developing mesothelioma could be determined, and the incidence of mesothelioma in SV40-infected and uninfected individuals could be estimated.

(5) *Biological gradient: Is there a dose–response relationship between exposure and disease?*

This criterion is appropriate for exposures such as smoking, radiation, and asbestos, but not for an infectious disease.

(6) *Plausibility: Is the association plausible?*

The T antigens of polyomaviruses are capable of transforming cells, so the viruses have a biologic mechanism for initiating cancer. However, there are questions related to virus–tumor cell relationship in these cancers. In a large proportion of the polyomavirus studies, the viral genomes are found in very small amounts, less than one copy per tumor cell. In most instances, the virus has not been localized to the tumor cell and the viral transcripts have not been characterized. This pattern is very different from the one seen in experimentally induced polyomavirus tumors or in naturally occurring HPV-related cancers in which the viral genome is present in every tumor cell and viral transcripts and virus-coded proteins are located in the tumor cells.

There is a major difficulty with respect to the plausibility of SV40-positive studies. In the United States, there has been no documented human exposure to SV40 since 1963. A large number of the cancer patients in whom SV40 sequences were identified were born long after 1963, implying that SV40 now readily circulates in the communities by person-to-person transmission.

There is no unequivocal evidence that this is true. Polyomaviruses have evolved with their natural hosts and are highly species specific. Humans exposed to SV40 by aerosol or oral administration of contaminated poliovaccines had transient asymptomatic infections with little viral shedding *(9)*. To determine if SV40 circulates at present in human communities, we examined urines of 166 homosexual men, half of them HIV-seropositive, for polyomavirus genomic sequences *(62)*. JCV and BKV sequences were detected in 34% and 14% of the urines, respectively, but SV40 sequences were detected in none. Bofill et al. *(63)* tested 28 samples of urban sewage collected in Spain, France, Sweden, and South Africa to determine if SV40 was an environmental contaminant. Seventy percent of the samples were positive for both BKV and JCV, but none were positive for SV40. While these studies are not comprehensive, they do point to the need for firm evidence that the virus is circulating in humans by person-to-person transmission.

Investigators who have identified SV40 sequences from human cancers have concluded that the sequences are of SV40 itself and not of any related polyomavirus. Comparisons of human-derived and rhesus-derived SV40 sequences show that there are no "human-specific" or "tumor-specific" sequences in the human isolates *(64)*. These observations led to two alternative interpretations: (1) SV40 has a broad host range, which includes both simians and humans; or (2) SV40, a simian virus, has become a human pathogen, without any adaptive changes in its genome. It is difficult to accept either of these two possibilities without additional evidence.

(7) Coherence: Is the association consistent with the known facts of the natural history of disease?

JCV: Astrocytomas arising in PML lesions in the brain constitute the most coherent of the polyomavirus–human cancer associations. There are abundant amounts of JCV at the site, and the astrocytes in PML lesions look "malignant" and have JCV DNA but no JCV virions. The multiplication of these astrocytes in an immunocompromised host could lead to JCV-caused astrocytomas. The case report of an oligoastrocytoma in which JCV DNA, RNA, and protein were detected *(26)* had areas of "hypomyelination," which suggests the possibility of JCV infection of the brain. The relationship of JCV to medulloblastomas requires confirmation. The identification of JCV in colonic mucosa and colon cancer *(32)* proposes a site of JCV multiplication that was not previously recognized. This observation also needs to be confirmed.

BKV: Although BKV genomic sequences have been reported from tumors at a large number of sites, there are no data indicating that the biology of these tumors is affected in any way by the purported presence of BKV.

SV40: In the absence of any knowledge about the biology and epidemiology of human infection with SV40, it is not possible to evaluate if the SV40–human cancer association is coherent.

(8) Experiment: Does reduction of exposure reduce or prevent disease?

This criterion is applicable for cancer-associated infections that can be prevented by immunization, for example, HBV and hematocellular carcinoma (*see* Chapter 17). At present it is not applicable to the polyomavirus–human cancer associations.

(9) Analogy: Do other agents, similar to the one in question, produce the effect?

Mouse polyomavirus has been shown to produce tumors in thymectomized mice after natural infection *(65)*. The reported case of an SV40-positive malignant astrocytoma in an SIV-infected macaque *(15)* and of cases of brain tumors in PML patients may represent analogous situations.

CONCLUSIONS

The data, available to date, have not firmly established an etiologic link between any human cancer and infections with polyomaviruses JCV, BKV, or SV40. The plausibility of such an association is strongest for the rare cases of astrocytoma that originate in JCV-caused PML lesions and weakest for the tumors linked to SV40 infection.

REFERENCES

1. Shah KV. Polyomaviruses. In: Fields BN, Knipe DM, Howley PM, et al. (eds). Virology, 3rd edit. Philadelphia: Lippincott-Raven, 1996, pp. 2027–2043.
2. Cole CN. Polyomavirinae: The viruses and their replication. In: Fields BN, Knipe DM, Howley PM, et al. (eds). Virology. Philadelphia: Lippincott-Raven, 1996, pp. 1997–2025.
3. Walker DL, Frisque RJ. The biology and molecular biology of JC virus. In: Salzman NP (eds). The Papovaviridae, vol. 1: The Polyomaviruses. New York: Plenum Press, 1985, pp. 327–377.
4. Corallini A, Altavilla G, Cecchetti MG, et al. Ependymomas, malignant tumors of pancreatic islets, and osteosarcomas induced in hamsters by BK virus, a human papovavirus. J Natl Cancer Inst 1978; 61:875–880.
5. Costa J, Yee C, Tralka TS, et al. Hamster ependymomas produced by intracerebral inoculation of a human papovavirus (MMV). J Natl Cancer Inst 1976; 56:863–864.
6. Varakis J, ZuRhein GM, Padgett BL, Walker DL. Induction of peripheral neuroblastomas in Syrian hamsters after injection as neonates with JC virus, a human polyoma virus. Cancer Res 1978; 38:1722.
7. Walker DL, Padgett BL, ZuRhein GM, Albert AE, Marsh RF. Human papovavirus (JC): induction of brain tumors in hamsters. Science 1973; 181:674–676.
8. Houff SA, London W, ZuRhein GM, Padgett BL, Walker DL, Sever J. New world primates as a model of virus-induced astrocytomas. In: Sever JL, Madden DL[???],[???] (eds). Polyomaviruses and human neurological diseases. New York: Alan R. Liss, 1983, pp. 223–226.
9. Shah KV, Nathanson N. Human exposure to SV40: review and comment. Am J Epidemiol 1976; 103:1–12.
10. Atwood WJ, Norkin LC. Class I major histocompatibility proteins as cell surface receptors for simian virus 40. J Virol 1989; 63:4474–4477.
11. Aksamit AJ, Sever JL, Major EO. Progressive multifocal leukoencephalopathy: JC virus detection by in situ hybridization compared with immunohistochemistry. Neurology 1986; 36:499–504.
12. Voltz, R., Jager G, Seelos K, Fuhry L, Hohlfeld R. BK virus encephalitis in an immunocompetent patient. Arch Neurol 1996; 53:101–103.
13. Holmberg C, Gribble D, Takemoto K, Howley P, Espana C, Osborn B. Isolation of simian virus 40 from rhesus monkeys *(Macaca mulatta)* with spontaneous progressive multifocal leukoencephalopathy. J Infect Dis 1977; 136:593–596. ·
14. Sheffield W, Strandberg J, Braun L, Shah K, Kalter S. Simian virus 40 associated fatal interstitial pneumonia and renal tubular necrosis in a rhesus monkey. J Infect Dis 1980; 142:618–622.
15. Hurley JP, Ilyinskii PO, Horvath CJ, Simon MA. A malignant astrocytoma containing simian virus 40 DNA in a macaque infected with simian immunodeficiency virus. J Med Primatol 1977; 26:172–180. ·

16. Fiori M, DiMajorca G. Occurrence of BK virus DNA in DNA obtained from certain human tumors. Proc Natl Acad Sci USA 1976; 73:4662–4666.

17. Barbanti-Brodano G, Martini F, De Mattei M, Lazzarin L, Corallini A, Tognon M. BK and JC human polyomaviruses and simian virus 40: natural history of infection in humans, experimental oncogenicity, and association with human tumors. Adv Virus Res 1998; 50:69–99.

18. Butel JS, Lednicky JA. Cell and molecular biology of simian virus 40: implications for human infection and disease (review). J Natl Cancer Inst 1999; 91:119–134.

19. Dorries K. New aspects in the pathogenesis of polyomavirus-induced disease. Adv Virus Res 1997; 48:205–261.

20. Shah KV. Does SV40 infection contribute to the development of human cancers? Rev Med Virol 1999, in press.

21. Brown F, Lewis AJ. Simian virus 40 (SV40): a possible human polyomavirus. Basel: Karger, 1998.

22. Gullotta F, Masini T, Scarlato G, Kuchelmeister K. Progressive multifocal leukoencephalopathy and gliomas in a HIV-negative patient. Pathol Res Pract 1992; 188:964–972.

23. Sima AAF, Finkelstein SD, McLachlan DR. Multiple malignant astrocytomas in a patient with spontaneous progressive multifocal leukoencephalopathy. Ann Neurol 1983; 14:183–188.

24. Richardson E. Progressive multifocal leukoencephalopathy. N Engl J Med 1961; 265:315–316.

25. Castaigne P, Rondot P, Escourolle R, et al. Leucoencephalopathie multifocale progressive et gliomes multiples. Rev Neurol 1974; 130:379–392.

26. Rencic A, Gordon J, Otte J, Curtis M, Kovatich A, Zoltick P, et al. Detection of JC virus DNA sequence and expression of the viral oncoprotein, tumor antigen, in brain of immunocompetent patient with oligoastrocytoma. Proc Natl Acad Sci USA 1996; 93:7352–7357.

27. Boldorini R, Caldarelli-Stefano R, Monga G, Zocchi M, Mediati M, Tosoni A, et al. PCR detection of JC virus DNA in the brain tissue of a 9-year-old child with pleomorphic zanthoastrocytoma. J Neurovirol 1998; 4:242–245.

28. Arthur RR, Grossman SA, Ronnett BM, Bigner SH, Vogelstein B, Shah KV. Lack of association of human polyomaviruses with human brain tumors. J Neurooncol 1994; 20:55–58.

29. Herbarth B, Meissner H, Westphal M, Wegner M. Absence of polyomavirus JC in glial brain tumors and glioma-derived cell lines. Glia 1998; 22:415–420.

30. Khalili K, Krynska B, Del Valle L, Katsetos CD, Croul S. Medulloblastomas and the human neurotropic polyomavirus JC virus [letter]. Lancet 1999; 353:1152–1153.

31. Huang H, Reis R, Yonekawa Y, Lopes JM, Kleihues P, Ohgaki H. Identification in human brain tumors of DNA sequences specific for SV40 large T antigen. Brain Pathol 1999; 9:33–44.

32. Laghi L, Randolph AE, Chauhan DP, Marra G, Major EO, Neel JV, et al. JC virus DNA is present in the mucosa of the human colon and in colorectal cancers. Proc Natl Acad Sci USA 1999; 96:7484–7489.

33. Neel JV, Major EO, Awa AA, Glover T, Burgess A, Traub R, et al. Hypothesis: rogue cell-type chromosomal damage in lymphocytes is associated with infection with the JC human polyoma virus and has implications for oncogenesis. Proc Natl Acad Sci USA 1996; 93:2690–2695.

34. Smith M. Considerations on a possible viral etiology for B-precursor acute lymphoblastic leukemia of childhood. J Immunother 1997; 20:89–100.

35. Smith MA, Strickler HD, Granovsky M, Reaman G, Linet M, Daniel R, et al. Investigation of leukemia cells from children with common acute lymphoblastic leukemia for genomic sequences of the primate polyomaviruses JC virus, BK virus, and simian virus 40. Med Pediatr Oncol 1999, in press.

36. DeMattei M, Martini F, Corallini A, Gerosa M, Scotlandi K, Barbanti-Brodano G, et al. High incidence of BK virus large-T-antigen-coding sequences in normal human tissues and tumors of different histotypes. Int J Cancer 1995; 61:756–760.

37. Martini F, Iaccheri L, Lazzarin L, Carinci P, Corallini A, Gerosa M, et al. SV40 early region and large T antigen in human brain tumors, peripheral blood cells, and sperm fluids from healthy individuals. Cancer Res 1996; 56:4820–4825.

38. Flaegstad T, Andresen PA, Johnsen JI, Asomani SK, Jorgensen GE, Vignarajan S, et al. A possible contributory role of BK virus infection in neuroblastoma development. Cancer Res 1999; 59:1160–1163.

39. Monini P, Rotola A, DeLellis L, Corallini A, Secchiero P, Albini A, et al. Latent BK virus infection and Kaposi's sarcoma pathogenesis. Int J Cancer 1996; 66:717–722.

40. Strickler HD, Goedert JJ. Exposure to SV40-contaminated poliovirus vaccine and the risk of cancer—a review of the epidemiological evidence. In: Brown F, Lewis AJ (eds). Simian Virus 40 (SV40): A Possible Human Polyomavirus. Basel: Karger, 1998, pp. 235–244.

41. Bergsagel DJ, Finegold MJ, Butel JS, Kupsky WJ, Garcea RL. DNA sequences similar to those of simian virus 40 in ependymomas and choroid plexus tumors of childhood. N Engl J Med 1992; 326:988–993.

42. Krainer M, Schenk T, Zielinski CC, Muller C. Failure to confirm presence of SV40 sequences in human tumours. Eur J Cancer 1995; 31A:1893.

43. Greenlee JE, Becker LE, Narayan O, Johnson RT. Failure to demonstrate papovavirus tumor antigen in human cerebral neoplasms. Ann Neurol 1978; 3:479–481.

44. Lednicky JA, Stewart AR, Jenkins JJI, Finegold MJ, Butel JS. SV40 DNA in human osteosarcomas shows sequence variation among T-antigen genes. Int J Cancer 1997; 72:791–800.

45. Mendoza SM, Konishi T, Miller CW. Integration of SV40 in human osteosarcoma DNA. Oncogene 1998; 17:2457–2462.

46. Carbone M, Rizzo P, Procopio A, Giuliano M, Pass HI, Gebhardt MC, et al. SV40-like sequences in human bone tumors. Oncogene 1996; 13:527–535.

47. Mulatero C, Surentheran T, Breuer J, Rudd RM. Simian virus 40 and human pleural mesothelioma. Thorax 1999; 54:60–61.

48. Strickler HD, Goedert JJ, Fleming M, Travis WD, Williams AE, Rabkin CS, et al. Simian virus 40 and pleural mesothelioma in humans. Cancer Epidemiol Biomarkers Prev 1996; 5:473–475.

49. Griffiths DJ, Nicholson AG, Weiss RA. Detection of SV40 sequences in human mesothelioma. Dev Biol Stand 1998; 94:127–136.

50. Pacini F, Vivaldi A, Santoro M, Fedele M, Fusco A, Romei C, et al. Simian virus 40-like DNA sequences in human papillary thyroid carcinomas. Oncogene 1998; 16:665–669.

51. Hill AB. The environment and disease: association or causation? Proc R Soc Med 1965; 58:295–300.

52. Parkin DM, Pisani P, Munoz N, Ferlay J. The global health burden of infection associated cancers. In: Newton R, Beral V, Weiss WA (eds). Infections and Human Cancer. Cold Spring Harbor, NY: Cold Spring Harbor Laboratory Press, 1999, pp. 5–33.

53. Carbone M, Pass HI, Rizzo P, Marinetti M, Di Muzio M, Mew DJY, et al. Simian virus 40-like sequences in human pleural mesothelioma. Oncogene 1994; 9:1781–1790.

54. Cristaudo A, Vivaldi A, Sansales G, Guglielmi G, Ciancia E, Elisei R, et al. Molecular biology studies onmesothelioma tumor samples: preliminary data on H-*Ras, P21,* and SV40. J Environ Pathol Toxicol Oncol 1995; 14:29–34.

55. Pepper C, Jasani B, Navabi H, Wynford-Thomas D, Gibbs AR. Simian virus 40 large T antigen (SV40LTAg) primer specific DNA amplification in human pleural mesothelioma tissue. Thorax 1996; 51:1074–1076.

56. De Luca A, Baldi A, Esposito V, Howard CM, Bagella L, Rizzo P, et al. The retinoblastoma gene family *pRb/p105, p107, pRb2/p130* and simian virus-40 large T-antigen in human mesotheliomas. Nat Med 1997; 3:913–916.

57. Galateau-Salle F, Iwatsubo Y, Gennetay E, Renier A, Letourneux M, Pairon JC et al. SV40-like DNA sequences in pleural mesothelioma, bronchopulmonary carcinoma, and non-malignant pulmonary diseases. J Pathol 1998; 184:252–257.
58. Testa JR, Carbone M, Hirvonen A, Khalili K, Krynska B, Linnainmaa K, et al. A multi-institutional study confirms the presence and expression of simian virus 40 in human malignant mesotheliomas. Cancer Res 1998; 58:4505–4509.
59. Strickler HD, Rosenberg PS, Devesa SS, Hertel J, Fraumeni JF, Goedert JJ. Contamination of poliovirus vaccines with simian virus 40 (1955–1963) and subsequent cancer rates. JAMA 1998; 279:292–295.
60. Strickler HD, Rosenberg PS, Devesa SS, Fraumeni JF, Jr, Goedert JJ. Contamination of poliovirus vaccine with SV40 and the incidence of medulloblastoma. Med Pediatr Oncol 1999; 32:77–78.
61. Olin P, Giesecke J. Potential exposure to SV40 in polio vaccines used in Sweden during 1957: No impact on cancer incidence rates 1960 to 1993. In: Brown F, Lewis AM (eds). Simian Virus 40 (SV40): A Possible Human Polyomavirus. Basel: Karger, 1998, pp. 227–233.
62. Shah KV, Daniel RW, Strickler HD, Goedert JJ. Investigation of human urine for genomic sequences of the primate polyomaviruses simian virus 40, BK virus, and JC virus. J Infect Dis 1997; 176:1618–1621.
63. Bofill S, Pina S, Girones R. Detection of polyomaviruses BK and JC but not SV40 in urban sewage from widely divergent geographical areas. Abstract presented at the 1998 molecular biology of small DNA tumor viruses meeting, July 14–19, 1998, University of Wisconsin, Madison, 104.
64. Stewart AR, Lednicky JA, Butel JS. Sequence analyses of human tumor-associated SV40 DNAs and SV40 viral isolates from monkeys and humans. J Neurovirol 1998; 4:182–193.
65. Law LW. Neoplasms in thymectomized mice following room infection with polyoma virus. Nature 1965; 205:672.
66. Suzuki SO, Mizoguchi M, Iwaki T. Detection of SV40 T antigen genome in human gliomas. Brain Tumor Pathol 1997; 14:125–129.

27

In Pursuit of a Human Breast Cancer Virus, from Mouse to Human

Marjorie Robert-Guroff and Gertrude Case Buehring

MOUSE MAMMARY TUMOR VIRUS MODEL

For decades researchers have been fascinated with the idea that human breast cancer might be caused by a virus. This idea derives primarily from the mouse model, the only naturally occurring mammary cancer in an animal for which the cause is known. We briefly review the hallmarks of mouse mammary cancer and its causative virus to set the stage for discussion of possible links with human breast cancer. There are numerous comprehensive reviews of the mouse mammary tumor literature, a few of which have been resources for this chapter *(1–5)*.

Mammary cancer in wild mice was first described by Crisp in 1854 and Livingood in 1896 (reviewed in *[1]*). In the early 1900s C.C. Little and his colleagues utilized brother–sister mating of wild mice to develop genetically homogeneous strains of laboratory mice differing widely in their frequency of mammary carcinoma (reviewed in *[2]*). This increased the availability of mammary neoplasias and allowed detailed morphologic studies. Although several pathologists in the early 1900s attempted classification of mouse mammary tumors, it was the painstaking work of Apolant, published in 1906, that made the most lasting impact and is the scheme still used today (reviewed in *[1]*). Apolant established five important characteristics of mouse mammary tumors: (1) tumors had many diverse forms but all seemed to originate from a common cell type, the mammary epithelial cell; (2) there were both benign adenomas and malignant adenocarcinomas, and the adenocarcinomas developed from the adenomas rather than directly from unaltered tissue; (3) tumors, when present, were usually present at multiple foci; (4) tumors appeared histologically the same in inbred as in wild mice; (5) metastases occurred, usually to the lungs. The work of later investigators (reviewed in *[2]*) enlarged on these early conclusions of Apolant. Most notably, DeOme and colleagues *(6)* definitively established the precancerous nature of the benign adenomas, which came to be known as hyperplastic alveolar nodules (HAN).

The first inkling that mammary tumors were hormone responsive came, of course, from the fact that they were observed only in female mice. A more definitive connection with hormones was forged by the discovery that pregnancy increased the likeli-

From: *Infectious Causes of Cancer: Targets for Intervention*
Edited by: J. J. Goedert © Humana Press Inc., Totowa, NJ

hood of mammary tumors *(7)* whereas ovariectomy decreased it *(8)*. Lacassagne in 1933 was able to induce mammary cancer in male mice by estrogen treatment (reviewed in *[2]*).

It was Borrel in 1903 who first formulated the hypothesis that mouse mammary tumors might be caused by a virus. He was vigorously supported by Haaland. The hypothesis was based on their observations of inclusions in some mammary cancer cells that were similar to inclusions seen in certain viral diseases. Borrel believed that a nematode commonly infesting mice carried the causative virus (reviewed in *[1]*). Most investigators in the early 1900s, however, believed that the cause of the mammary carcinomas was genetic, as some laboratory strains had a high incidence and others a low incidence. When crosses were done to determine what Mendelian pattern was involved, it was surprisingly found that the inheritance was non-Mendelian. A now classic paper authored by the staff of the Jackson Laboratory, Bar Harbor, Maine *(9)* reported that when low- and high-incidence strains were crossed, the inheritance of mammary tumor susceptibility was maternal. This suggested that an extrachromosomal gene or agent was responsible. It remained for John Bittner to prove in another milestone study, that what was passed from mother to offspring was not a gene, but rather an infectious agent in milk. When pups born of high-incidence strain mothers were foster nursed on low-incidence strain mothers, their incidence of mammary tumors was low *(10)*. Likewise, offspring of low-incidence mothers foster nursed on high-incidence mothers developed mammary cancer at a higher frequency *(11)*.

With the advent of the electron microscope in the 1940s, the infectious milk agent was identified as a virus. Although the first electron microscope studies utilized pelleted extracellular virus material, the most definitive study utilized cultured cells so that virus morphology was more clearly defined and the life cycle could be delineated *(12)*. The authors described two forms of the virus, an intracytoplasmic form consisting of the nucleopcapsid only, and an enveloped particle consisting of the nucleocapsid plus envelope acquired by budding from the cell surface. These forms were later named A particles and B particles, respectively, by Bernhard *(13)*. Subsequent studies by many investigators pieced together the biochemical and biophysical properties of the virus (reviewed in *[3]*), placing it in the large family of *Retroviridae,* subfamily *oncovirinae*. The virions of the mouse mammary tumor virus (MMTV), as it is now known, contain two copies of single-stranded RNA, surrounded by a nucleocapsid consisting primarily of p27 (capsid protein). In mature particles the nucleocapsid is surrounded by an envelope permeated with the envelope glycoprotein (gp52) and the transmembrane protein (gp36). A reverse transcriptase (RT) enzyme (polymerase) enables the virus to make a DNA copy of its genome that then integrates into the cellular genome as a provirus. As in other retroviruses, the major areas of the MMTV genome (in the provirus form) are the 5′ and 3′ long-terminal repeat (LTR) promoter regions, the *gag* region coding for the capsid protein, the *pol* region coding for the polymerase, and the *env* region coding for the envelope glycoprotein.

The humoral and cell-mediated immune responses of the host mouse to MMTV are primarily to the envelope glycoprotein gp52. Both an antibody-dependent complement-mediated cytotoxicity and a cell-mediated cytotoxicity response develop as a result of exposure to MMTV, but they are not always sufficient to prevent the appearance of mammary tumors. The immune responses of neonatally infected mice are detectable with sensitive methods but are considerably weaker than the responses of animals first infected as adults. The strength of both the humoral and the cell-mediated cytotoxicity response increases with increasing number of pregnancies *(4)*.

Heston et al. *(14)* discovered that some mammary tumors developed in mice free of the milkborne virus, that is, in high-incidence strains (C3Hf) that were foster nursed on virus-free mothers. This, coupled with the observation of MMTV-like particles in the mammary cells of the C3Hf mice *(15)*, led to the hypothesis that in the germ line there might be endogenous MMTV sequences whose inheritance would be Mendelian *(16)*. This was borne out with the advent of molecular techniques and the work of many investigators that ultimately allowed the detection and characterization of more than 25 loci of endogenous MMTV sequences *(17)*.

Molecular analysis of the genomes of mammary tumor cells indicated certain pre-ferred sites of integration of exogenous MMTV proviral DNA *(18)*. Eventually through the efforts of many scientists, the picture emerged that conserved integration sites were adjacent to cellular protooncogenes and that MMTV insertion at these sites perturbed the normal growth regulating functions of the protooncogenes leading eventually to malignant transformation (reviewed in *[3]*). This form of viral tumorigenesis is called insertional mutagenesis (*see also* Chapter 13).

An early clue that MMTV might be directly stimulated by hormones was the observa-tion that mammary tumors from late-pregnant and lactating MMTV-infected mice con-tained more particles than tumors from nonlactating infected mice *(19)*. Another clue was the work of Smoller et al. *(20)*, who observed by electron microscopy increased numbers of cytoplasmic virus aggregations in tissue sections of mammary tumors from cortisol-treated mice. With the advent of efficient cell culture systems for mouse mam-mary epithelium, corticosteroid-induced virus replication was detected more definitively by fluorescent antibodies *(21)*, DNA–RNA hybridization *(22,23)*, and immunoassay of MMTV proteins *(22)*. Attempts to unravel the mechanism of this hormone stimulation culminated in the discovery of the glucocorticoid response element (GRE), a short DNA sequence to which glucocorticoid receptor binds and enhances transcription *(24,25)*. MMTV was found to have multiple GREs in its LTR promoter regions.

The most profound work on MMTV in recent years has to do with the transportation of MMTV from the gut to the mammary gland. The work of Tsubura et al. *(26)* revealed that MMTV ingested by the newborn in milk may first infect B lymphocytes of intestinal Peyer's patches, and then get transferred to T lymphocytes, which circu-late to the mammary gland and transfer the virus to mammary epithelial cells. One of the most intriguing findings that greatly advanced our understanding of MMTV biol-ogy was the discovery of the MMTV superantigen encoded by a 3′ LTR sequence, for many years a mysterious open reading frame (ORF) with an unknown function (reviewed in *[3]*). Evidence now suggests that the superantigen orchestrates the multi-plication of T cells and MMTV-infected B cells, thus increasing the number of key lymphocytes and ultimately enhancing the probability of successful delivery of MMTV to the epithelial cells of the mammary gland (reviewed in *[5,27]*).

EARLY SEARCHES FOR A HUMAN BREAST CANCER VIRUS

Based on the extensive studies of MMTV, the hypothesis that a retrovirus might also cause human breast cancer was compelling, and rigorously pursued in the 1970s. The methodology at the time included not only electron microscopy, but much more sensitive biochemical techniques for detecting the signature enzyme of retroviruses, RT, as a footprint of a retroviral agent, and a simultaneous detection technique for detecting RT activity in association with the viral 60–70S RNA genome. Using such methodology, evidence accumulated in support of a retroviral agent–human breast cancer link. The findings included detection of type B and D retroviral-like particles in milk of women from familial breast cancer families and certain ethnic groups with high breast cancer incidence (28–30), detection of RT activity in particulate fractions of human milk (31), detection of RNA homologous to MMTV in human breast tumors (32), detection of retrovirus-like particles associated with RT activity in the breast carcinoma cell line MCF-7 (33), and simultaneous detection of RT and viral RNA in human milk and breast tumors (34).

With more extensive investigations, however, such retroviral markers were not correlated with breast cancer risk, casting doubt on the overall hypothesis, and suggesting that a retrovirus-like agent might have a wide distribution. Thus, if it participated in the development of breast cancer, or was even necessary, it could not be sufficient for disease induction. For example, in an extensive study of milk specimens from women with or without a family history of breast cancer, although virus-like particles were correlated with the presence of RT activity and 70S viral RNA in the samples, no association with a family history of disease was obtained (35). A further rigorous investigation failed to correlate the milk RT activity itself with a family history of breast cancer (36). Also, epidemiologic studies failed to show that breast-fed babies had a higher incidence of breast cancer than bottle-fed babies (37). Other studies argued that virus-like particles observed by electron microscopy were merely cytoplasmic debris or milk microsomes (38,39). In view of these conflicting results and the fact that no human breast cancer agent was ever isolated, interest in the hypothesis of an exogenous retroviral etiology of human breast cancer waned.

DO ENDOGENOUS ELEMENTS CONTRIBUTE TO HUMAN BREAST CANCER?

MMTV causes breast cancer in mice not only as an exogenous agent, but also as an endogenous one as discussed above (40). In the 1980s it became apparent that human DNA contained endogenous retroviral sequences, some highly related to MMTV (41,42) with the typical retroviral genomic organization including gag, pol, and env genes (43). The discoveries that retrovirus-like particles immunologically related to MMTV were produced by a human breast cancer cell line, T47D (44), and that expression of the MMTV-related human endogenous provirus in these cells was stimulated by female steroid hormones (45), stimulated interest into whether endogenous proviral elements might contribute to breast cancer development. Such elements could potentially play a role in the disease process by insertional mutagenesis or by alteration of normal cellular transcriptional processes resulting from enhancer/promoter elements in the endogenous LTR regions. A review of human endogenous elements is beyond the scope of this chapter; Wilkinson et al. provide a recent thorough review (46). Here we summarize studies on two types of endogenous element in which links to human breast cancer have been pursued: so-called LINE elements as well as the human endogenous retrovirus type K (HERV-K).

LINEs (long interspersed elements) are retroelements that transpose via an RNA intermediate and lack the LTRs characteristic of retroviruses and noninfectious retrotransposons. They possess a 3' terminal poly (A) tract, similar to messenger RNAs, and an internal RNA polymerase II promoter. L1, the most extensively studied human LINE, contains two ORFs, with the longer 3' ORF encoding a protein with RT activity *(47)*. Although most L1 copies within the human genome are defective, new integrations of L1 have been observed including an insertion into c-*myc* in a human breast carcinoma *(48)*, an insertion into an APC tumor-suppressor gene in a colorectal cancer *(49)*, and two integrations into factor VIII genes leading to hemophilia A *(50)*. These few examples suggest not only that some functional L1 elements exist, but as with the latter case, the possibility of disease induction is real. Using an antibody to the L1 p40 protein encoded by the first ORF, L1 was found to be frequently expressed in human cells and tissues, including teratocarcinomas and choriocarcinomas *(51)* and adult and pediatric germ cell cancers *(52)*. Ten percent of adult testicular germ cell cancers were found to express L1 *(53)*, although a causative relationship could not be established.

The L1 c-*myc* insertion in a breast adenocarcinoma *(48)*, suggested the possibility of a more general association with human breast cancer. In support of this hypothesis, expression of the L1 p40 protein was observed in seven of eight breast cancer cell lines and in nine of twelve primary infiltrating ductal carcinomas *(54)*. In contrast, normal breast cell lines, malignant B- and T-cell lines, normal breast tissue, or breast tumors of other types were found to be negative for p40 expression. Later, however, using more sensitive methodology, all breast tissues examined were shown to express the p40 protein, although breast cancer cells expressed significantly higher levels than normal cells *(55)*. Perhaps if L1 is routinely expressed in breast tissue, high expression levels might lead to a greater chance of retrotransposition and consequent insertional mutagenesis. This possibility and the underlying hypothesis of an L1–breast cancer association remain to be proven.

HERV-K, so called because it has a lysine tRNA primer binding site, is present in the human genome at about 30–50 copies, and has also been studied with regard to breast cancer development. HERV-K is a class II endogenous retrovirus related to type B and D retroviruses. In fact, it shares significant homology with MMTV. Of six human MMTV-like (HML) families of viruses *(56)*, HERV-K is identical to HML-2 *(57)*. Unlike most HERVs, nearly complete copies of HERV-K exist with open reading frames for *gag, pol,* and *env* genes *(58)* which are transcribed and translated in some cells. Full-length, singly, and multiply spliced transcripts have been observed in teratocarcinoma cells *(59)*. One of the doubly spliced transcripts encodes a putative regulatory protein similar to the rev protein of human immmnuodeficiency virus (HIV) *(60)*. HERV-K particles, for which HERV-K gag protein is required, were first described in teratocarcinoma cell lines *(61)*. Significant expression of HERV-K gag protein is further inferred by the detection of anti-gag antibodies in patients with seminomas *(62)*. Antibodies to HERV-K envelope protein have also been described *(63)* and other HERV-K encoded proteins are not only expressed, but possess functional activity, including the protease *(64)* and RT *(65)*. Recently, a recombinant HERV-K under the control of a CMV promoter was shown to retrotranspose at a low level in vitro in dog osteosarcoma cells *(66)*, supporting the notion that active retrotransposition of some HERV-K elements might be able to occur in vivo. The report of a subset of HERV-K elements with human-specific integrations indicates that some HERVs may have amplified much later in humans than previously thought *(67),* and fuels speculation that some elements may still be able to actively transpose. However, infectious HERV-K particles have not been observed, perhaps due to an inefficient c-ORF-related signal peptide, low levels of env expression, or lack of appropriate processing of the envelope precursor protein *(68).*

The relatedness of HERV-K to MMTV, its possession of a glucocorticoid response element in the LTR region *(58),* and its steroid hormone-dependent expression in the human breast carcinoma cell line, T47-D *(45),* stimulated the hypothesis that it might contribute to breast cancer development in humans. However, evidence for such a role has not been forthcoming. Although the T47-D cell line releases viral particles that exhibit RT activity *(69),* like HERV-K particles produced by teratocarcinoma cell lines, they are noninfectious. Recently, the cell line was reported to release particles in which retroviral transcripts of both type B and type C origin are packaged *(70).* Some particles, termed HERV-K-T47D, were shown to package nearly full length, but highly defective sequences with 40–60% homology to HERV-K10. Thus, while high levels of transcription were seen in human placenta and T47D cells in response to steroid hormone, the *env* gene was not transcribed *(71).*

A further extensive investigation of transcription of five of the six HML families in placenta and breast tissue revealed that expression in general was greater in placenta than in breast tissue, and that it varied among individuals *(72).* Overall, expression of the endogenous sequences was comparable in both malignant and nonmalignant tissues. Of interest, however, was very high expression of HML-6 sequences in breast cancer tissue of a young woman with bilateral breast cancer, ductal carcinoma *in situ,* and concomitant ovarian carcinoma, raising the possibility that HML expression might be augmented in some cases leading to a certain subset of breast cancer types. No evidence for this has been presented however.

In addition to studies of HERV transcription, serologic studies probing possible endogenous virus–breast cancer links at the protein level have also been carried out. In one study, a low percentage (~4%) of normal, healthy blood donors exhibited antibody reactivity to HERV-K antigens *(73),* while increased percentages of reactive sera were seen in patients with germ cell tumors (62%), and in pregnant women (~8%). No reactivity was seen in four sera from breast cancer patients. In a second study, 12.6% of healthy blood donor sera and 11.7% of breast cancer sera, unspecified with regard to pre- or post-therapy, were reactive with recombinant HERV-K envelope protein *(63).* Thus by serologic criteria, HERV-K would appear unassociated with breast cancer development. It is possible, however, that sera obtained at the time of breast cancer diagnosis might reveal greater reactivity than that seen following treatment, as was shown in individuals with germ cell tumors compared to those whose tumors had been surgically removed *(73).* In addition, certain subsets of breast cancer or certain ethnic groups, for example, Tunisian women with particularly aggressive breast cancers cross-reactive to MMTV *(74),* might reveal an endogenous virus–breast cancer link.

Transcription of HERV-K is limited to specific cell types. The cellular transcription factor YY1 enhances HERV-K expression *(75),* and it is likely that a spectrum of regulatory factors contribute to transcriptional control. In addition, expression of both HERV-K gag and L1 sequences appear to be regulated by methylation *(76–78).* In fact, transcriptional silencing by DNA methylation has been proposed as the main defense of the host against transposable genetic elements *(79,80)*. In view of the complex regulatory controls and the vast number of endogenous elements in the human genome, individual instances of an endogenous element contributing to disease might occur. The challenge, however, would be in establishing an etiologic relationship.

OTHER CANDIDATE BREAST CANCER AGENTS

Because many of the attempts to find an MMTV-related exogenous human agent have led to endogenous elements with no conspicuous relationship to breast cancer, Pogo and her colleagues have searched for evidence of an agent closely resembling MMTV but with no homology to HERVs. They used the polymerase chain reaction (PCR) to probe normal and malignant breast tissue DNAs for a 660-bp sequence with 98% homology to the MMTV *env* gene and minimal homology to HERVs. They recently reported that 40% of breast cancer patients possessed this sequence compared to only 2% of normal donors *(81)*. In a follow-up study they observed that 66% of the samples positive for the MMTV *env* DNA sequence also transcribed the sequence *(82)*. Their results have not yet been independently confirmed by any other investigator.

The involvement of several other viruses with human breast cancer has also been suggested, but again, the findings have not been confirmed and causal relationships have not been established. The group headed by Beverly Griffin in England detected Epstein–Barr virus (EBV) by PCR more frequently in malignant breast tissues (primarily invasive ductal carcinomas) than in nonmalignant tissues *(83)*. *In situ* hybridization on the same specimens indicated that the positive signal was in epithelial cells rather than in lymphocytes infiltrating the tissues. In Japan, Horiuchi et al. *(84)* also found by PCR that two out of three breast carcinomas were positive for EBV, but upon *in situ* hybridization, the EBV was localized to infiltrating lymphocytes, not breast epithelium. Three other groups in the United States, Belgium, and Taiwan failed to find evidence of EBV by PCR in medullary breast carcinomas *(85,86)* or invasive ductal carcinomas *(86–88)*. The discrepancies among these studies have not yet been untangled, but may be due to technical differences or geographic variation in the presence of EBV in breast cancers.

Rakowicz-Szulczynska and her colleagues found evidence of human immunodeficiency virus (HIV)-like sequences and proteins in breast cancer tissues significantly more frequently than in nonmalignant breast tissues. They propose that not HIV, but perhaps a virus crossreacting with HIV, could be what they are detecting and may be an etiologic agent of human breast cancer *(89)*. No studies supporting this work have as yet appeared.

Finally, some believe that breast cancer may be caused by an as yet unidentified virus, and that more general methods are needed to detect it *(90)*. In this vein, Al-Sumidaie et al. *(91)* returned to earlier approaches and reported RT activity in monocytes of 97% of breast cancer patients compared to 11% of age- and gender-matched normal controls. In contrast, other investigators using essentially the same radioactive methodology did not find significant RT activity in any culture of human monocytes *(92,93)*. Recently, a group using a highly sensitive enzyme-linked immunosorbent assay for RT did find RT activity in cultures of monocytes from five out of ten breast cancer patients but not in any of the 20 cultures from normal controls *(94)*. It will take further studies to clarify these discrepancies.

CONCLUDING REMARKS

Clearly the mouse mammary tumor model has provided an inspiration so strong that, despite many failures to implicate a virus as the cause of human breast cancer, there are still researchers willing to persevere in the quest. The major difficulty in applying the model to humans, is the fact that mice are inbred, which no doubt facilitated elucidation of MMTV oncogenesis. The situation in humans is much more complex. Nevertheless, the similarities of mouse mammary cancer to human breast cancer makes it a useful model. The pathology of human breast cancer resembles that of mouse mammary cancer in originating primarily from the secretory mammary epithelial cell and progressing from precancerous to malignant to metastatic. Like the mouse system, human breast cancers are usually responsive to estrogens and progestins, and approximately 30% are multicentric. The fact that some MMTV genomes are endogenous and vertically transmitted, while others are exogenous and horizontally transmitted, is now paralleled, in a way, in human breast cancer where approx 5% of cases appear to be due to vertically transmitted genes, for example, *BRCA1* and *BRCA2,* and the other 95% to exogenous environmental factors *(95)* such as hormones, radiation, diet, etc. The recent report that a HERV possesses a superantigen that is etiologically linked to insulin-dependent diabetes myelitis *(96),* although controversial *(97–99),* suggests another way in which a human endogenous element may parallel MMTV.

Have the complexities of the human system simply masked our ability to detect virally induced oncogenesis? Human breast cancer may arise from amplification of oncogenes (*erbB-2, myc, cyclin D*) or mutation or loss of suppressor genes (*p53, Rb-1, cyclin E*) (reviewed in *[100]*). Other oncogene and suppressor gene candidates may also play a role in breast neoplasia. To determine if a possibly ubiquitous virus or viral element triggers one or more of these events is a formidable task.

What else can we glean from the mouse studies to guide us in further pursuit of a human breast cancer virus? Having extensively pursued retroviruses, should we now consider other types of viruses? Should we look for a virus that is hormone responsive and therefore more adaptable to the reproductive cycles of the human female? Should we consider lymphocytes as well as mammary epithelial cells as pertinent target cells for a causative virus? Should we look for a connection between superantigens and breast cancer? The mouse model has been a continuing source of powerful insights. Hopefully one of its revelations will provide the critical clue allowing resolution of the question of whether viruses are linked to human breast cancer.

REFERENCES

1. Dunn TB. Morphogenesis and histogenesis of mammary tumors. In: Mammary Tumors in Mice. Washington, DC: American Association for the Advancement of Science, Publ No 22, 1945, pp. 13–38.
2. Nandi S, McGrath CM. Mammary neoplasia in mice. Adv Cancer Res 1973; 17:353–414.
3. Dickson C. Molecular aspects of mouse mammary tumor virus biology. Int Rev Cytol 1987; 108:119–147.
4. Blair PB. Immune responses to mammary tumor virus-induced mammary tumors. In: Blasecki JW (eds). Mechanisms of Immunity to Virus-Induced Tumors. New York: Marcel Dekker, 1981, pp. 181–257.
5. Matsuzawa A. Biology of mouse mammary tumor virus (MMTV). Cancer Lett 1995; 90:3–11.

6. DeOme KB, Faulkin LJ, Bern HA, Blair PB. Development of mammary tumors from hypersplastic alveolar nodules transplanted into gland-free mammary fat pads of female C3H mice. Cancer Res 1959; 19:515–520.

7. Lathrop AEC, Loeb L. The influence of pregnancies on the incidence of cancer in mice. Proc Soc Exp Biol 1913; 11:38–40.

8. Lathrop AEC, Loeb L. Further investigations on the origin of tumors in mice. III. On the part played by internal secretion in the spontaneous development of tumors. J Cancer Res 1916; 1:1–20.

9. Staff of the Roscoe B. Jackson Memorial Laboratory. The existence of nonchromosomal influence in the incidence of mammary tumors in mice. Science 1933; 78:465.

10. Bittner JJ. Some possible effects of nursing on the mammary tumor incidence in mice. Science 1936; 84:162–169.

11. DeOme, KB. The incidence of mammary tumors among low-tumor strain C57BLK mice when foster-nursed by high-tumor strain A females. Am J Cancer 1940; 40:231–234.

12. Porter KR, Thompson HP. A particulate body associated with epithelial cells cultured from mammary carcinomas of mice of a milk-factor strain. J Exp Med 1948; 88:15–23.

13. Bernhard W. Electron microscopy of tumor cells and tumor viruses. Cancer Res 1958; 18:491–509.

14. Heston WE, Deringer MK, Dunn TB, Levillain WD. Factors in the development of spontaneous mammary gland tumors in agent-free strain C3Hb mice. J Natl Cancer Inst 1950; 10:1139–1155.

15. Pitelka DR, Nandi S, De Ome KB. On the significance of virus-like particles in mammary tissues of C3Hf mice. J Natl Cancer Inst 1964; 33:867–885.

16. Bentvelzen P. Endogenous mammary tumor viruses in mice. Cold Spring Harbor Symp Quant Biol 1975; 39 Pt 2:1145–1150.

17. Kozak C, Peters G, Pauley R, Morris V, Michalides R, Dudley J, et al. A standard nomenclature for endogenous mammary tumor virus. J Virol 1987; 61:1631–1654.

18. Nusse R, Varmus HE. Many tumors induced by the mouse mammary tumor virus contain provirus integrated in the same region of the host genome. Cell 1982; 31:99–109.

19. Hairstone MA, Sheffield JB, Moore DH. Study of B particles in the mammary tumors of different mouse strains. J Natl Cancer Inst 1964; 33:825–836.

20. Smoller CG, Pitelka DR, Bern HA. Cytoplasmic inclusion bodies in cortisol-treated mammary tumors of C3H/Crgl mice. J Biophys Biochem Cytol 1961; 9:915–920.

21. McGrath CM. Replication of mammary tumor virus in tumor cell cultures: dependence on hormone-induced cellular organization. J Natl Cancer Inst 1971; 47:455–467.

22. Parks WP, Scolnik EM, Kozikowski EH. Dexamethasone stimulation of murine mammary tumor virus expression: a tissue culture source of virus. Science 1974; 184:158–160.

23. Ringold GM, Yamamoto KR, Tompkins GM, Bishop JM, Varmus HE. Dexamethasone-mediated induction of mouse mammary tumor virus RNA: a system for studying glucocorticoid action. Cell 1975; 6:299–305.

24. Chandler VL, Maier BA, Yamamoto, KR. DNA sequences bound specifically by glucocorticoid receptor in vitro render a heterologous promoter hormone responsive in vivo. Cell 1983; 33:489–499.

25. Payvar F, De Franco D, Firestone GL, Edgar B, Wrange Ö, Okret S, et al. Sequence-specific binding of the glucocorticoid receptor to MTV-DNA at sites within and upstream of the transcribed region. Cell 1983; 35:381–392.

26. Tsubura A, Inaba M, Imai S, Murakami A, Oyaizu N, Yasumizu R, et al. Intervention of T-cells in transportation of mouse mammary tumor virus (milk factor) to mammary gland cells in vivo. Cancer Res 1988; 48:6555–6559.

27. Ross SR. Mouse mammary tumor virus and its interaction with the immune system. Immuno-logic Res 1998; 2:209–216.

28. Moore DM, Sarkar NH, Kelly CE, Pillsbury N, Charney J. Type B particles in human milk. Texas Rep Biol Med 1969; 27:1027–1039.

29. Chopra H, Ebert P, Woodside N, Kvedar J, Albert S, Brennan M. Electron microscopic detection of simian-type virus particles in human milk. Nature New Biol 1973; 243:159–160.

30. Moore DH, Charney J, Kramarsky B, Lasfargues EY, Sarkar NH, Brennan MJ, et al. Search for a human breast cancer virus. Nature 1971; 229:611–614.

31. Schlom J, Spiegelman S, Moore D. RNA-dependent DNA polymerase activity in virus-like particles isolated from human milk. Nature 1971; 231:97–102.

32. Axel R, Schlom J, Spiegelman S. Presence in human breast cancer of RNA homologous to mouse mammary tumour virus RNA. Nature 1972; 235:32–36.

33. McGrath CM, Grant PM, Soule HD, Glancy T, Rich MA. Replication of oncornavirus-like particles in human breast carcinoma cell line, MCF-7. Nature 1974; 252:247–250.

34. Schlom J, Spiegelman S, Moore DH. Reverse transcriptase and high molecular weight RNA in particles from mouse and human milk. J Natl Cancer Inst 1972; 48:1197–1203.

35. Sarkar NH, Moore DH. On the possibility of a human breast cancer virus. Nature 1972; 236:103–106.

36. Gerwin BI, Ebert PS, Chopra HC, Smith SG, Kvedar JP, Albert S, et al. DNA polymerase activities of human milk. Science 1973; 180:198–201.

37. Henderson BE. Type B virus and human breast cancer. Cancer 1974; 34(Suppl):1386–1389.

38. Wooding RBP. Milk microsomes, viruses, and the milk fat globule membrane. Experientia 1972; 28:1077–1079.

39. Calafat J, Hageman PC. Remarks on virus-like particles in human breast cancer. Nature 1973; 242:260–262.

40. Bentvelzen P, Daams, JH, Hageman P, Calafat J. Genetic transmission of viruses that incite mammary tumor in mice. Proc Natl Acad Sci USA 1970; 67:377–384.

41. Callahan R, Drohan W, Tronick S, Schlom J. Detection and cloning of human DNA sequences related to the mouse mammary tumor virus genome. Proc Natl Acad Sci USA 1982; 79:5503–5507.

42. May FEB, Westley BR, Rochefort H. Mouse mammary tumour virus related sequences are present in human DNA. Nucleic Acids Res 1983; 11:4127–4139.

43. Callahan R, Chiu I-M, Wong JFH, Tronick SR, Roe BA, Aaronson SA, et al. A new class of endogenous human retroviral genomes. Science 1985; 228:1208–1211.

44. Keydar I, Ohno T, Nayak R, Sweet R, Simoni F, Weiss F, et al. Properties of retrovirus-like particles produced by a human breast carcinoma cell line: immunological relationship with mouse mammary tumor virus proteins. Proc Natl Acad Sci USA 1984; 81:4188–4192.

45. Ono M, Kawakami M, Ushikubo H. Stimulation of expression of the human endogenous retrovirus genome by female steroid hormones in human breast cancer cell line T47D. J Virol 1987; 61:2059–2062.

46. Wilkinson DA, Mager DL, Leong JC. Endogenous human retroviruses. In: Levy JA, (eds). The Retroviridae, vol. 3. New York: Plenum Press, 1994, pp. 465–535.

47. Mathias S, Scott A, Kazazian H, Jr, Boeke J, Gabriel A. Reverse transcriptase encoded by a human transposable element. Science 1991; 254:1808–1810.

48. Morse B, Rotherg PG, South VJ, Spandorfer JM, Astrin SM. Insertional mutagenesis of the *myc* locus by a LINE-1 sequence in a human breast carcinoma. Nature 1988; 333:87–90.

49. Miki Y, Nishisho I, Horii A, Miyoshi Y, Utsunomiya J, Kinzler KW, et al. Disruption of the APC gene by a retrotransposal insertion of L1 sequence in a colon cancer. Cancer Res 1992; 52:643–645.

50. Kazazian HH, Wong C, Youssoufian H, Scott AF, Phillips DG, Antonarakis S. Haemophilia A resulting from de novo insertion of L1 sequences represents a novel mechanism for mutation in man. Nature 1988; 332:164–166.

51. Leibold DM, Swergold GD, Singer MF, Thayer RE, Dombroski BA, Fanning TG. Translation of LINE-1 DNA elements in vitro and in human cells. Proc Natl Acad Sci USA 1990; 87:690–694.

52. Bratthauer GL, Fanning TG. LINE-1 retrotransposon expression in pediatric germ cell tumors. Cancer 1993; 71:2383–2386.

53. Bratthauer GL, Fanning TG. Active LINE-1 retrotransposons in human testicular cancer. Oncogene 1992; 7:507–510.

54. Bratthauer GL, Cardiff RD, Fanning TG. Expression of LINE-1 retrotransposons in human breast cancer. Cancer 1994; 73:2333–2336.

55. Asch HL, Eliacin E, Fanning TG, Connolly JL, Bratthauer G, Asch BB. Comparative expression of the LINE-1 p40 protein in human breast carcinomas and normal breast tissues. Oncol Res 1996; 8:239–247.

56. Medstrand P, Blomberg J. Characterization of novel reverse transcriptase encoding human endogenous retroviral sequences similar to type A and type B retroviruses: differential transcription in normal human tissues. J Virol 1993; 67:6778–6787.

57. Tonjes RR, Lower R, Boller K, Denner J, Hasenmaier B, Kirsch H, et al. HERV-K: the biologically most active human endogenous retrovirus family. J Acq Imm Def Syndr Hum Retrovirology 1996; 13(Suppl 1):S261–S267.

58. Ono M, Yasunaga T, Miyata T, Ushikubo H. Nucleotide sequence of human endogenous retrovirus genome related to mouse mammary tumor virus genome. J Virol 1986; 60:589–598.

59. Lower R, Boller K, Hasenmaier B, Korbmacher C, Mueller-Lantzsch N, Lower J, et al. Identification of human endogenous retroviruses with complex mRNA expression and particle formation. Proc Natl Acad Sci USA 1993; 90:4480–4484.

60. Lower R, Tonjes RR, Korbmacher C, Kurth R, Lower J. Identification of a rev related protein by analysis of spliced transcripts of the human endogenous retroviruses HTDV/HERV-K. J Virol 1995; 69:141–149.

61. Boller K, Konig H, Sauter M, Mueller-Lantzsch N, Lower R, Lower J, et al. Evidence that HERV-K is the endogenous retrovirus sequence that codes for the human teratocarcinoma-derived retrovirus HTDV. Virology 1993; 196:349–353.

62. Sauter M, Schommer S, Kremmer E, Remberger K, Dolken G, Lemm I, et al. Human endogenous retrovirus K10: expression of gag protein and detection of antibodies in patients with seminomas. J Virol 1995; 69:414–421.

63. Vogetseder W, Dumfahrt A, Mayersbach P, Schonitzer D, Dierich MP. Antibodies in human sera recognizing a recombinant outer membrane protein encoded by the envelope gene of the human endogenous retrovirus K. AIDS Res Hum Retroviruses 1993; 9:687–694.

64. Schommer S, Sauter M, Krausslich H-G, Best B, Mueller-Lantzsch N. Characterization of the human endogenous retrovirus K proteinase. J Gen Virol 1996; 77:375–379.

65. Berkhout B, Jebbink M, Zsiros J. Identification of an active reverse transcriptase enzyme encoded by a human endogenous HERV-K retrovirus. J Virol 1999; 73:2365–2375.

66. Nan X-L, Tonjes RR, Kurth R. Retrotransposition of recombinant endogenous and exogenous retrovirus in cultured mammalian cells. Presented at the Meeting on Retroviruses, Cold Spring Harbor Laboratory, May 26–31, 1998.

67. Medstrand P, Mager DL. 1998. Human-specific integrations of the HERV-K endogenous retrovirus family. J Virol 1998; 72:9782–9787.

68. Tonjes RR, Limbach C, Lower R, Kurth R. Expression of human endogenous retrovirus type K envelope glycoprotein in insect and mammalian cells. J Virol 1997; 71:2747–2756.

69. Patience C, Simpson GR, Colletta AA, Welch HM, Weiss RA, Boyd, MT. Human endogenous retrovirus expression and reverse transcriptase activity in the T47D mammary carcinoma cell line. J Virol 1996; 70:2654–2657.

70. Seifarth W, Skladny H, Krieg-Schneider F, Reichert A, Hehlmann R, Leib-Mosch C. Retrovirus-like particles released from the human breast cancer cell line T47-D display type B- and C-related endogenous retroviral sequences. J Virol 1995; 69:6408–6416.

71. Seifarth W, Baust C, Murr A, Skladny H, Krieg-Schneider F, Blusch J, et al. Proviral structure, chromosomal location, and expression of HERV-K-T47D, a novel human endogenous retrovirus derived from T47D particles. J Virol 1998; 72:8384–8391.

72. Yin H, Medstrand P, Andersson M-L, Borg A, Olsson H, Blomberg J. Transcription of human endogenous retroviral sequences related to mouse mammary tumor virus in human breast and placenta: similar pattern in most malignant and nonmalignant breast tissues. AIDS Res Hum Retroviruses 1997; 13:507–516.

73. Boller K, Janssen O, Schuldes H, Tonjes RR, Kurth R. Characterization of the antibody response specific for the human endogenous retrovirus HTDV/HERV-K. J Virol 1997; 71:4581–4588.

74. Levine PH, Mesa-Tejada R, Keydar I, Tabbane F, Spiegelman S, Mourali N. Increased incidence of mouse mammary tumor virus-related antigen in Tunisian patients with breast cancer. Int J Cancer 1984; 33:305–308.

75. Knossl M, Lower R, Lower J. Expression of the human endogenous retrovirus HTDV/HERV-K is enhanced by cellular transcription factor YY1. J Virol 1999; 73:1254–1261.

76. Thayer RE, Singer MF, Fanning TG. Undermethylation of specific LINE-1 sequences in human cells producing a LINE-1-encoded protein. Gene 1993; 133:273–277.

77. Alves G, Tatro A, Fanning T. Differential methylation of human LINE-1 retrotransposons in malignant cells. Gene 1996; 176:39–44.

78. Gotzinger N, Sauter M, Roemer K, Mueller-Lantzsch N. Regulation of human endogenous retrovirus-K gag expression in teratocarcinoma cell lines and human tumours. J Gen Virol 1996; 77:2983–2990.

79. Yoder JA, Walsh CP, Bestor TH. Cytosine methylation and the ecology of intragenomic parasites. Trends Genet 1997; 13:335–340.

80. Henikoff S, Matzke MA. Exploring and explaining epigenetic effects. Trends Genet 1997; 13:293–295.

81. Wang Y, Holland JF, Bleiweiss IJ, Melana S, Liu X, Pelisson I, et al. Detection of mammary tumor virus *env* gene-like sequences in human breast cancer. Cancer Res 1995; 55:5173–5179.

82. Wang Y, Go V, Holland JF, Melana SM, Pogo BG. Expression of mouse mammary tumor virus-like *env* gene sequences in human breast cancer. Clin Cancer Res 1998; 4:2565–2568.

83. Labrecque LG, Barnes DM, Fentiman IS, Griffin BE. Epstein–Barr virus in epithelial cell tumors: a breast cancer study. Cancer Res 1995; 55:39–45.

84. Horiuchi K, Mishima K, Ohasawa M, Aozasa K. Carcinoma of stomach and breast with lymphoid stroma: localisation of Epstein–Barr virus. J Clin Pathol 1994; 47:538–540.

85. Gaffey MJ, Frierson HF Jr, Mills SE, Boyd JC, Zarbo RJ, Simpson JF, et al. Medullary carcinoma of the breast: identification of lymphocytes subpopulations and their significance. Mod Pathol 1993; 6:721–728.

86. Lespagnard L, Cochaux P, Larsimont D, Degeyter M, Velu T, Heimann R. Absence of Epstein–Barr virus in medullary carcinoma of the breast as demonstrated by immunophenotyping, in situ hybridization and polymerase chain reacation. Am J Clin Pathol 1995; 103:449–452.

87. Chu J-S, Chen C-C, Chang, K-J. In situ detection of Epstein–Barr virus in breast cancer. Cancer Letters 1998; 124:53–57.

88. Glaser SL, Ambinder RF, DiGiuseppe JA, Horn-Ross PL, Hsu JL. Absence of Epstein–Barr virus EBER-1 transcripts in an epidemiologically diverse group of breast cancers. Int J Cancer 1998; 75:555–558.

89. Rakowicz-Szulczynska E, Jackson B, Szulczynska A, Smith M. Human immunodeficiency virus type 1-like DNA sequences and immunoreactive viral particles with unique association with breast cancer. Clin Diag Lab Immunol 1998; 5:645–653.

90. Labat ML. Possible retroviral etiology of human breast cancer. Biomed Pharmacother 1998; 52:6–12.

91. Al-Sumidaie AM, Leinster SJ, Hart CA, Green CD, McCarthy K. Particles with properties of retroviruses in monocytes from patients with breast cancer. Lancet 1988; 5–9.

92. Kahl LP, Carroll AR, Rhodes P, Wood J, Reid NG. An evaluation of the putative human mouse mammary tumour retrovirus associated with peripheral blood monocytes. Br J Cancer 1991; 63:534–540.

93. Hallam N, McAlpine L, Puszcynska E, Bayliss G. Absence of reverse transcriptase activity in monocyte cultures from patients with breast cancer. Lancet 1990; 336:1079.

94. Hughes G, McKerr G, Allen J, Barnett Y. Are retroviruses involved in the aetiology of human breast cancer? Cancer Lett 1996; 103:219–225.

95. Henderson BE, Powell D, Rosario I, Keys C, Hanisch R, Young M, et al. An epidemiologic study of breast cancer. J Natl Cancer Inst 1974; 53:609–614.

96. Conrad B, Weissmahr RN, Boni J, Arcari R, Schupbach J, Mach B. A human endogenous retroviral superantigen as candidate autoimmune gene in type I diabetes. Cell 1997; 90:303–313.

97. Jaeckel E, Heringlake S, Berger D, Brabant G, Hunsmann G, Manns MP. No evidence for association between IDDMK(1,2)22, a novel isolated retrovirus and IDDM. Diabetes 1999; 48:209–214.

98. Badenhoop K, Donner H, Neumann J, Herwig J, Kurth R, Usadel KH, et al. IDDM patients neither show humoral reactivities against endogenous retroviral envelope protein nor do they differ in retroviral mRNA expression from healthy relatives or normal individuals. Diabetes 1999; 48:215–218.

99. Muir A, Ruan QG, Marron MP, She JX. The IDDMK(1,2)22 retrovirus is not detectable in either mRNA or genomic DNA from patients with type 1 diabetes. Diabetes 1999; 48:219–222.

100. Dickson RB, Lippman ME. Oncogenes and Suppressor Genes. In: Harris JR, Morrow M, Lippman ME, Hellman S (eds). Diseases of the Breast. Philadelphia: Lippincott-Raven, 1996, pp. 221–235.

Index